Prehospital Care—Pearls and Pitfalls

Prehospital Care—Pearls and Pitfalls

Editors:

Peter T. Pons, MD, FACEP
Professor Emeritus
Department of Emergency Medicine
University of Colorado Denver School of Medicine
Associate Medical Director
Prehospital Trauma Life Support
National Association of EMTs

Vincent J. Markovchick, MD, FAAEM, FACEP
Professor Emeritus
Department of Emergency Medicine
University of Colorado Denver School of Medicine
Attending Staff Physician
Department of Emergency Medicine
Denver Health Medical Center
Denver, Colorado

2012
PEOPLE'S MEDICAL PUBLISHING HOUSE—USA
SHELTON, CONNECTICUT

People's Medical Publishing House-USA
2 Enterprise Drive, Suite 509
Shelton, CT 06484
Tel: 203-402-0646
Fax: 203-402-0854
E-mail: info@pmph-usa.com

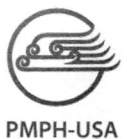
PMPH-USA

© 2012 PMPH-USA, Ltd.

All rights reserved. Without limiting the rights under copyright reserved above, no part of this publication may be reproduced, stored in or introduced into a retrieval system, or transmitted, in any form or by any means (electronic, mechanical, photocopying, recording, or otherwise), without the prior written permission of the publisher.

12 13 14 15/QDB/9 8 7 6 5 4 3 2 1

ISBN-13: 978-1-60795-171-1
ISBN-10: 1-60795-171-1

Printed in the United States of America by Quad/Graphics
Copyeditor/Typesetter: Spearhead Global; Cover designer: Mary McKeon

Library of Congress Cataloging-in-Publication Data

Prehospital care—pearls and pitfalls / editors, Peter T. Pons & Vincent Markovchick.
    p. ; cm.
  Includes bibliographical references and index.
  ISBN-13: 978-1-60795-171-1
  ISBN-10: 1-60795-171-1
  I. Pons, Peter T. II. Markovchick, Vincent J.
  [DNLM: 1. Emergency Medical Services. WX 215]
  362.18—dc23
                                                  2011050237

Notice: The authors and publisher have made every effort to ensure that the patient care recommended herein, including choice of drugs and drug dosages, is in accord with the accepted standard and practice at the time of publication. However, since research and regulation constantly change clinical standards, the reader is urged to check the product information sheet included in the package of each drug, which includes recommended doses, warnings, and contraindications. This is particularly important with new or infrequently used drugs. Any treatment regimen, particularly one involving medication, involves inherent risk that must be weighed on a case-by-case basis against the benefits anticipated. The reader is cautioned that the purpose of this book is to inform and enlighten; the information contained herein is not intended as, and should not be employed as, a substitute for individual diagnosis and treatment.

Sales and Distribution

Canada
McGraw-Hill Ryerson Education
Customer Care
300 Water St
Whitby, Ontario L1N 9B6
Canada
Tel: 1-800-565-5758
Fax: 1-800-463-5885
www.mcgrawhill.ca

Foreign Rights
John Scott & Company
International Publisher's Agency
P.O. Box 878
Kimberton, PA 19442
USA
Tel: 610-827-1640
Fax: 610-827-1671

Japan
United Publishers Services Limited
1-32-5 Higashi-Shinagawa
Shinagawa-ku, Tokyo 140-0002
Japan
Tel: 03-5479-7251
Fax: 03-5479-7307
Email: hayashi@ups.co.jp

United Kingdom, Europe, Middle East, Africa
McGraw Hill Education
Shoppenhangers Road
Maidenhead
Berkshire, SL6 2QL
England
Tel: 44-0-1628-502500
Fax: 44-0-1628-635895
www.mcgraw-hill.co.uk

Singapore, Thailand, Philippines, Indonesia
Vietnam, Pacific Rim, Korea
McGraw-Hill Education
60 Tuas Basin Link
Singapore 638775
Tel: 65-6863-1580
Fax: 65-6862-3354
www.mcgraw-hill.com.sg

Australia, New Zealand,
Papua New Guinea, Fiji, Tonga,
Solomon Islands, Cook Islands
Woodslane Pty Limited
Unit 7/5 Vuko Place
Warriewood NSW 2102
Australia
Tel: 61-2-9970-5111
Fax: 61-2-9970-5002
www.woodslane.com.au

Brazil
SuperPedido Tecmedd
Beatriz Alves, Foreign Trade
Department
R. Sansao Alves dos Santos, 102 | 7th floor
Brooklin Novo
Sao Paolo 04571-090
Brazil
Tel: 55-16-3512-5539
www.superpedidotecmedd.com.br

India, Bangladesh, Pakistan, Sri Lanka, Malaysia
CBS Publishers
4819/X1 Prahlad Street 24
Ansari Road, Darya Ganj,
New Delhi-110002
India
Tel: 91-11-23266861/67
Fax: 91-11-23266818
Email: cbspubs@vsnl.com

People's Republic of China
People's Medical Publishing House
International Trade Department
No. 19, Pan Jia Yuan Nan Li
Chaoyang District
Beijing 100021
P.R. China
Tel: 8610-67653342
Fax: 8610-67691034
www.pmph.com/en/

Contents

Preface	xv
Acknowledgments	xvii
Contributors	xxi

SECTION I
EMS – OVERVIEW, DESIGN, AND OPERATIONS   1

Chapter 1
History of Emergency Medical Services   3
Norman McSwain, Jr., MD, FACS

Chapter 2
EMS System Design   15
Mike Nugent, MS

Chapter 3
The Prehospital Environment   23
James Robinson, Paramedic

Chapter 4
Prehospital Communications   26
James F. Azuero and James Simpkins

Chapter 5
Destination Guidelines and Hospital Designation   34
Catherine B. Custalow, MD, PhD

Chapter 6
Documentation   39
Arthur Hsieh, MA, NREMT-P

Chapter 7
Medicolegal Issues   45
S. Scott Henderson, Esq.

Contents

Chapter 8
Emergency Vehicle Operation — 56
Bob Loop

Chapter 9
Public and Media Relations — 64
Will Chapleau, EMT-P, RN, TNS

Chapter 10
Ethics in EMS — 67
Jean Abbott, MD, MH, and Kelly Bookman, MD

SECTION II
MEDICAL DIRECTION — 71

Chapter 11
Medical Direction—Overview — 73
Marilyn Gifford, MD, FACEP

Chapter 12
On-Line Medical Direction — 79
Christopher B. Colwell, MD, FACEP

Chapter 13
Off-Line Medical Direction — 83
Carl J. Bonnett, MD, and Jason M. Liu, MD, MPH

Chapter 14
Continuous Quality Improvement — 89
Robert Swor, DO, FACEP

SECTION III
PERSONAL SAFETY AND WELLNESS — 99

Chapter 15
Well-Being of the EMS Provider — 101
Debra Cason, RN, MS, EMT-P

Chapter 16
Scene Safety — 108
James Robinson, Paramedic

Chapter 17
Infectious Diseases Exposures — 114
Connie S. Price, MD

Chapter 18
Critical Incident Stress — 122
Philip Rach, MS, NREMT-P

SECTION IV
DISASTERS, MASS CASUALTY INCIDENTS, AND MASS GATHERINGS — 135

Chapter 19
Incident Management — 137
Christopher B. Colwell, MD, FACEP

Chapter 20
Disasters and Mass Casualty Incidents — 146
Jon Krohmer, MD

Chapter 21
Small-Scale Multiple Casualty Incidents — 152
Nita Ham, EMT-P

Chapter 22
Weapons of Mass Destruction—Chemical — 158
Stephen V. Cantrill, MD

Chapter 23
Biological Terrorism — 163
Edward Eitzen, MD, MPH, Col, USA (Retired)

Chapter 24
Weapons of Mass Destruction—Radiologic — 174
Jonathan Burstein, MD, and Evan Bloom, MD, MPH

Chapter 25
Weapons of Mass Destruction—Explosives — 180
Stephen J. Wolf, MD

Chapter 26
Mass Gatherings — 186
Jedd Roe, MD, MBA, FACEP

Contents

SECTION V
CLINICAL CARE — 191

Chapter 27
Decision Making and Critical Interpretation of Vital Signs — 193
Vince Markovchick, MD

Chapter 28
The Prehospital Patient Assessment — 198
Arthur Hsieh, MA, NREMT-P

Chapter 29
Electrocardiogram Interpretation — 203
Angel Burba, MS, NREMT-P, NCEC

Chapter 30
Cardiac Dysrhythmias — 218
Paul Davidson, MD

Chapter 31
Cardiac Arrest — 228
Jason Haukoos, MD, MSc

Chapter 32
Overview of Shock — 234
Robert McNamara, MD, FAAEM

Chapter 33
Chest Pain — 239
Christopher B. Colwell, MD, FACEP

Chapter 34
Acute Coronary Syndrome — 245
Jeffrey J. Messerole, PS

Chapter 35
Altered Mental Status — 257
Mike Stackpool, MD

Chapter 36
Acute Neurologic Emergencies — 267
Julie Scadden, NREMT-P, PS

Contents

Chapter 37
Hypertensive Emergencies — 273
James A. Temple, BA, NREMT-P, CCP and Christopher B. Colwell, MD, FACEP

Chapter 38
Seizures — 278
Julie Scadden, NREMT-P, PS

Chapter 39
Fever — 283
Cheryl Blazek, BS, EMT-P

Chapter 40
Abdominal Pain — 287
Christina Johnson, MD, FACEP

Chapter 41
Gastrointestinal Hemorrhage — 293
Mike Stackpool, MD

Chapter 42
Vomiting and Diarrhea — 297
Cheryl Blazek, BS, EMT-P

Chapter 43
Dyspnea — 300
Gregory J. Chapman, BS, RRT, REMT-P

Chapter 44
Extremity Pain and Trauma — 304
Julie Scadden, NREMT-P, PS

Chapter 45
Overdose and Poisoning — 309
Kennon Heard, MD, and Vikhyat Bebarta, MD

Chapter 46
Hypothermia and Frostbite — 316
Daniel F. Danzl, MD

Chapter 47
Heat Illness — 322
Stephen V. Cantrill, MD

Chapter 48
Altitude Illness — 326
Ben Honigman, MD, and Kelly Bookman, MD

Chapter 49
Obstetric and Gynecologic Emergencies — 330
Cheryl Blazek, BS, EMT-P

Chapter 50
Allergy and Anaphylaxis — 335
Lance W. Jobe, MD, FACEP

Chapter 51
Diabetic Emergencies — 341
Jeffrey J. Messerole, PS

Chapter 52
Psychiatric and Behavioral Emergencies — 350
Eugene E. Kercher, MD, LFACEP, LFAPA, and Christopher B. Dong, MD

Chapter 53
Management of the Violent Patient — 361
James A. Temple, BA, NREMT-P, CCP

Chapter 54
General Trauma Principles — 367
Larry Mottley, MD

Chapter 55
Head Trauma — 373
Will Chapleau, EMT-P, RN, TNS

Chapter 56
Spinal Cord Injuries — 377
Will Chapleau, EMT-P, RN, TNS

Chapter 57
Neck Trauma — 382
Nicholas C. Johnson, MD

Chapter 58
Thoracic Trauma — 386
Jeffrey P. Salomone, MD, and Joseph A. Salomone, MD

Chapter 59
Abdominal Trauma — 390
Kelly Bookman, MD, and Lawrence Bookman, DO, FACEP

Chapter 60
Pelvic Trauma — 394
Jeffrey P. Salomone, MD, and Matthew Bitner, MD

Chapter 61
Interpersonal Violence — 397
Debra Houry, MD, MPH

Chapter 62
Thermal Burns — 402
Jeffrey S. Guy, MD, MSc, MMHC

SECTION VI
PEDIATRICS — 415

Chapter 63
Assessment of the Pediatric Patient — 417
Katie M. Bakes, MD

Chapter 64
Field Approach to Infants and Children — 422
Julie Scadden, NREMT-P, PS

Chapter 65
Seizures in Children — 429
Jeffrey J. Messerole, PS

Chapter 66
Respiratory Distress in Infants and Children — 439
James A. Temple, BA, NREMT-P, CCP

Chapter 67
Pediatric Trauma — 450
Robert W. Schafermayer, MD, FACEP, FIFEM, FAAP

Chapter 68
Child Abuse and Nonaccidental Trauma — 456
Nicholas C. Johnson, MD

Contents

SECTION VII
SPECIAL SITUATIONS — 459

Chapter 69
Water Emergencies — 461
Lee W. Shockley, MD, MBA

Chapter 70
Decompression Illnesses — 465
Jeffrey J. Messerole, PS

Chapter 71
Wilderness Emergency Medical Services — 473
Paul S. Auerbach, MD, MS, FACEP, FAWM, and Laura W. Kates, MD

Chapter 72
Lightning — 479
Lee W. Shockley, MD, MBA

Chapter 73
Bites, Stings, and Envenomations — 484
Richard C. Dart, MD, PhD

Chapter 74
Tactical Emergency Medicine — 488
David Q. McArdle, MD, and Tamra D. Glore, RN, BSN, CPHM

Chapter 75
Hazardous Materials — 503
Michael G. Stanley, M.Ed, EMT-P

Chapter 76
Technical Rescues — 508
Michael G. Stanley, M.Ed, EMT-P

SECTION VIII
AEROMEDICAL TRANSPORT — 513

Chapter 77
Air Medical System Design and Configuration — 515
Michael W. Brunko, MD, FACEP

Chapter 78
Aeromedical Transportation: Physiology of Altitude   526
Lee W. Shockley, MD, MBA

SECTION IX
PREHOSPITAL SKILLS AND INTERVENTIONS   529

Chapter 79
Prehospital Interventions: What Really Works   531
Herbert G. Garrison, MD, MPH

Chapter 80
Intravenous Access   535
John Riccio, MD, and Anne Clouatre, MHS, EMT-P

Chapter 81
Prehospital Airway Management   542
Arthur Hsieh, MA, NREMT-P, and Gregory J. Chapman, BS, RRT, REMT-P

Chapter 82
Pharmacologic Agents in Airway Management   550
Jedd Roe, MD, MBA, FACEP

Chapter 83
PASG   555
Robert Suter, DO, and Jeffrey Metzger, MD

Chapter 84
Needle Decompression   560
John Riccio, MD, and Anne Clouatre, MHS, EMT-P

Chapter 85
Immobilization and Splinting   565
Will Chapleau, EMT-P, RN, TNS

Chapter 86
Prehospital Pain Management   569
Timothy Howey, BA, NREMT-P

Chapter 87
Ultrasound in the Field   574
John Kendall, MD, FACEP

Index   583

Preface

The past four decades have seen a remarkable evolution in the delivery of prehospital care. Where once the only therapy available for an out-of-hospital emergency medical situation was a ride to the hospital at a speed limited only by the vehicle you were in and the driving conditions at the time, now much of the interventional capability of the emergency department has been moved into an ambulance staffed with highly trained individuals who can bring to the patient the sophisticated medical care needed at the point of first contact with the health care delivery system.

Today's prehospital care provider will be confronted with a wide variety of medical and traumatic emergencies, will need to possess a strong foundation of medical knowledge, and will be using a large armamentarium of interventions and treatments. It is with this in mind that we have prepared this book. We hope that it will, in a unique, stimulating, and easy-to-read way, provide practical information applicable to the prehospital setting and help the prehospital emergency care provider be prepared to manage the myriad of emergency and non-emergency situations that he or she will be called upon to assist.

Peter T. Pons, M.D.
Vincent J. Markovchick, M.D.

Acknowledgments

We would like to first recognize the efforts of our contributors who authored, reviewed, and revised their contributions over the long haul of getting this manuscript published.

We must recognize Jason Malley who shepherded the manuscript through the publication process. Also, Shirley Blum, who tirelessly pursued all of the permissions and signatures needed to finalize the production and Christine Dodd, who oversaw and moved the project along throughout the entire production phase.

*To the EMTs and Paramedics of the Denver Health Paramedic Division and
to all who provide care in the prehospital setting.*

PTP & VJM

To my wife, Kathy, whose love and support always guide me and see me through each day.

PTP

*To my wife, Leslie, and daughters Nicole, Tasha, and Nadia – the four greatest ladies in my world.
I wish to thank them for their lifelong support of all of my endeavors and, in particular, for understanding
the time that editing of this manuscript has taken away from my time with them.
I would also like to acknowledge all of the EMTs, paramedics, residents, and staff physicians with whom
I have had the pleasure of working at the Denver Health Emergency Department over the past 33 years.
Their enthusiasm and intellectual curiosity have stimulated many of the questions in this book.*

VJM

Contributors

Jean Abbott, MD, MH
Faculty, Center for Bioethics and Humanities
University of Colorado Health Sciences Center
Aurora, CO

Paul S. Auerbach, MD, MS, FACEP, FAWM
Redlich Family Professor of Surgery
Division of Emergency Medicine
Department of Surgery
Stanford University School of Medicine
Stanford, CA

James F. Azuero
911 Communications Manager (former)
Denver Paramedic Division
Denver Health and Hospitals Authority
Denver, CO

Katie M. Bakes, MD
Denver Health Medical Center
The Children's Hospital of Denver
Denver, CO

Vikhyat Bebarta, MD
Department of Emergency Medicine Wilford Hall Medical Center
Associate Professor of Emergency Medicine
University of Texas
San Antonio, TX

Matthew Bitner, MD
Associate Director, Pre-Hospital and Disaster Medicine
Duke University School of Medicine
Chapel Hill, NC

Cheryl Blazek, BS, EMT-P
EMS Training Program Coordinator
Southwestern Community College
Cresto, IA

Evan Bloom, MD, MPH
Clinical Instructor of Medicine
EMS & Disaster Medicine
Fellow, Department of Emergency Medicine
University of California
San Francisco, CA

Carl J. Bonnett, MD
Centura Health/South Denver EMS
Parker, CO

Kelly Bookman, MD
Assistant Professor of Emergency Medicine
University of Colorado Denver School of Medicine
Aurora, CO

Lawrence Bookman, DO, FACEP
Director, Emergency Medicine
Yampa Valley Medical Center
Steamboat Springs, CO

Michael W. Brunko, MD, FACEP
Chief Medical Officer, Flight for Life Colorado
St. Anthony Hospital
Lakewood, CO

Angel Burba, MS, NREMT-P, NCEC
Associate Professor, EMS Program Director
Howard Community College
Columbia, MD

Contributors

Jonathan Burstein, MD
Assistant Professor, Harvard Medical School
State EMS Medical Director
Lexington, MA

Stephen V. Cantrill, MD
Department of Emergency Medicine
Denver Health Medical Center
Denver, CO

Debra Cason, RN, MS, EMT-P
Associate Professor and Program Director
Emergency Medicine Education
University of Texas Southwestern Medical Center
Dallas, TX

Will Chapleau, EMT-P, RN, TNS
Manager, ATLS Program
American College of Surgeons
Chicago, IL

Gregory J. Chapman, BS, RRT, REMT-P
Director, Center for Prehospital Medicine
Carolinas Medical Center
Charlotte, NC

Anne Clouatre, MHS, EMT-P
Director, Patient Experience and
   Process Improvement
Littleton Adventist Hospital
Littleton, CO

Christopher B. Colwell, MD, FACEP
Director, Department of Emergency Medicine
Denver Health Medical Center
Medical Director, Denver Paramedic Division
   and Denver Fire Department
Associate Professor and Vice Chair
Department of Emergency Medicine
University of Colorado School of Medicine
Denver, CO

Catherine B. Custalow, MD, PhD
Associate Professor (Retired)
University of Virginia
Department of Emergency Medicine
Charlottesville, VA

Daniel F. Danzl, MD
Professor & Chair, Department of
   Emergency Medicine
School of Medicine
University of Louisville Hospital
Louisville, KY

Richard C. Dart, MD, PhD
Director, Rocky Mountain Poison & Drug Center
Professor of Surgery (Emergency Medicine)
University of Colorado
Denver, CO

Paul Davidson, MD
Clinical Instructor, Department of Surgery
University of Colorado School of Medicine
Attending Physician, Porter Adventist Hospital
Denver, CO

Christopher B. Dong, MD
EMS Director, Kern Medical Center
Associate Clinical Professor, Department of Medicine
David Geffen School of Medicine at UCLA
Bakersfield, CA

Edward Eitzen, MD, MPH, COL, USA (Retired)
Senior Partner, Biodefense and Public
   Health Programs
Martin-Blanck and Associates
Alexandria, VA

Herbert G. Garrison, MD, MPH
Professor of Emergency Medicine
The Brody School of Medicine
East Carolina University
Greenville, NC

Contributors

Marilyn Gifford, MD, FACEP
Medical Director, Emergency Services
Memorial Health System
Colorado Springs, CO

Tamra D. Glore, RN, BSN, CPHM
Quality Management/Risk Coordinator
Sky Ridge Medical Center
Lone Tree, CO

Jeffrey S. Guy, MD, MSc, MMHC
Associate Professor of Surgery
Vanderbilt University School of Medicine
Director, Regional Burn Center
Vanderbilt Medical Center
Nashville, TN

Nita Ham, EMT-P
President, Educators Division
Georgia Association of Emergency Medical Services
Atlanta, GA

Jason Haukoos, MD, MSc
Associate Professor, Department of
 Emergency Medicine
University of Colorado School of Medicine
Department of Epidemiology, Colorado
 School of Public Health
Director of Research, Department of Emergency
 Medicine
Denver Health Medical Center
Denver, CO

Kennon Heard, MD
Rocky Mountain Poison and Drug Center
Denver Health
University of Colorado Department
 of Emergency Medicine
Denver, CO

S. Scott Henderson, Esq.
Henderson Law Office
Denver, CO

Ben Honigman, MD
Professor and Interim Chair, Department
 of Emergency Medicine
University of Colorado School of Medicine
Aurora, CO

Debra Houry, MD, MPH
Associate Professor, Emergency Medicine
Associate Professor, Behavioral Sciences
 and Health Education
Vice Chair for Research, Emergency Medicine
Director, Center for Injury Control
Emory University
Atlanta, Georgia

Timothy Howey, BA, NREMT-P
EMS Faculty/Clinical Coordinator
Inver Hills Community College
Inver Grove Heights, Minnesota

Arthur Hsieh, MA, NREMT-P
Faculty, Emergency Medic Care Program
Santa Rosa Junior College
San Francisco, California

Lance W. Jobe, MD, FACEP
Wenatchee Emergency Physicians
Medical Program Director
Emergency Medical Services
Wenatchee, WA

Christina Johnson, MD, FACEP
Attending Emergency Physician
Vice President and Chief Medical Officer
Exempla Lutheran Medical Center
Wheat Ridge, Colorado

Nicholas C. Johnson, MD
Emergency Medicine
Minneapolis, MN

Contributors

Laura W. Kates, MD
Swedish Medical Center
Cherry Hill Emergency Department
Seattle, WA

John Kendall, MD, FACEP
Ultrasound Director, Department of
 Emergency Medicine
Denver Health Medical Center
Associate Professor, Department of
 Emergency Medicine
University of Colorado School of Medicine
Denver, CO

Eugene E. Kercher, MD, LFACEP, LFAPA
Chief Medical Officer, Kern Medical Center
Associate Clinical Professor of Medicine
David Geffen School of Medicine at UCLA
Bakersfield, CA

Jon Krohmer, MD
Assistant Director - IHSC
DHS Immigration & Customs Enforcement
Washington, DC

Jason M. Liu, MD, MPH
Associate Professor of Emergency Medicine
Medical College of Wisconsin
Assistant Director of Medical Services
Milwaukee County Emergency Medical Services
Milwaukee, WI

Bob Loop
Robert Loop, EMT-P
EMS Operations Captain (former)
Denver Paramedic Division
Denver Health and Hospitals Authority
Denver, CO

David Q. McArdle, MD
President, TPE Med MD
Medical Officer, Federal Law Enforcement
 Training Center
Reserve Officer, University of Colorado at
 Boulder Police
Emergency Department, Southeast Georgia
 Health System
Brunswick, GA

Robert McNamara, MD, FAAEM
Professor and Chairman, Department
 of Emergency Medicine
Temple University School of Medicine
Philadelphia PA

Norman McSwain, Jr., MD, FACS
Department of Surgery
Tulane University School of Medicine
New Orleans, LA

Jeffrey J. Messerole, PS
Clinical Instructor, Spencer Hospital
Spencer, Iowa

Jeffrey Metzger, MD
Assistant Professor, Division of Emergency Medicine
University of Texas
Southwestern Medical Center
Dallas, TX

Larry Mottley, MD
Assistant Professor, Harvard Medical School
Director, Prehospital Care
Beth Israel Deaconess Medical Center
Boston, MA

Mike Nugent, MS
Director, Office of Transportation Safety
Colorado Department of Transportation
Denver, CO

Contributors

Connie S. Price, MD
Director, Infection Prevention/Hospital Epidemiology
Chief, Division of Infectious Diseases
Denver Health and Hospital
Associate Professor of Medicine
University of Colorado School of Medicine
Denver, CO

Phillip Rach, MS, NREMT-P
EMS Education Specialist
Hennepin County Medical Center
Minneapolis, MN

John Riccio, MD
Chief EMS Medical Director, Proctor,
 Littleton, Porter Hospitals,
Emergency Physicians at Porter Hospitals
Denver, CO

James L. Robinson, Paramedic
Operations Chief
Denver Health and Hospital authority
Denver Health EMS-Paramedic Division
Denver, CO

Jedd Roe, MD, MBA, FACEP
Chair, Department of Emergency Medicine
William Beaumont Hospital, Royal Oak MI
Professor and Chair, Department of Emergency
 Medicine
Oakland University William Beaumont School of
 Medicine
Rochester, MI

Jeffrey P. Salomone, MD
Associate Professor of Surgery
Division of Trauma/Surgical Critical Care
Department of Surgery
Emory University School of Medicine
Deputy Chief of Surgery (Administrative)
Grady Memorial Hospital
Police Surgeon, City of Atlanta Police Department
Atlanta, Georgia

Joseph A. Salomone, MD
Associate Professor, Department of Emergency
 Medicine
University of Missouri-Kansas City and Truman
 Medical Centers
Kansas City, MO

Julie Scadden, NREMT-P, PS
CQI/Data Coordinator-Senior Staff Paramedic
Sac County Ambulance Service
Adjunct EMS Instructor-Western Iowa
 Tech Community College
Sac City, IA

**Robert W. Schafermayer, MD,
 FACEP, FIFEM, FAAP**
Chief and Associate Chair, Department
 of Emergency Medicine
Carolinas Medica Center, Charlotte, NC
Clinical Professor of Pediatrics and Adjunct
 Professor or Emergency Medicine
UNC School of Medicine
Chapel Hill, NC

Lee W. Shockley, MD, MBA
Medical Director, Emergency Department
Denver Health Medical Center
Professor and Vice Chair, Department of
 Emergency Medicine
The University of Colorado School of Medicine
Denver, CO

James Simpkins
911 Telecommunications Manager
TriTech Software Systems, Inc,
San Diego, CA

Mike Stackpool, MD
Exempla Lutheran Hospital Emergency Department
Exempla Good Samaritan Emergency Department
Arapahoe House Inc. Medical Director
Rural Metro EMS Arvada Division Medical Director
Denver, CO

Contributors

Michael G. Stanley, M.Ed, EMT-P
Fire Science Technology Coordinator
Community College of Aurora
Aurora, CO

Robert Suter, DO
Professor, Emergency Medicine
University of Texas Southwestern Medical Center
Dallas, TX

Robert Swor, DO, FACEP
Professor, Emergency Medicine
Oakland University/William Beaumont
 School of Medicine
Royal Oak, MI

James A. Temple, BA, NREMT-P, CCP
EMS Coordinator, Eastern Iowa Community
 College District
Davenport, IA

Stephen J. Wolf, MD
Associate Professor and Director of
 Medical Education
Department of Emergency Medicine
Sr. Associate Director, Denver Health Residency in
 Emergency Medicine
Assistant Dean for Advanced Studies
Office of Undergraduate Medical Education
University of Colorado School of Medicine
Denver, CO

SECTION I

EMS – Overview, Design, and Operations

Chapter 1
History of Emergency Medical Services   3
Norman McSwain, Jr., MD, FACS

Chapter 2
EMS System Design   15
Mike Nugent, MS

Chapter 3
The Prehospital Environment   23
James Robinson, Paramedic

Chapter 4
Prehospital Communications   26
James F. Azuero and James Simpkins

Chapter 5
Destination Guidelines and Hospital Designation   34
Catherine B. Custalow, MD, PhD

Chapter 6
Documentation   39
Arthur Hsieh, MA, NREMT-P

Chapter 7
Medicolegal Issues   45
S. Scott Henderson, Esq.

Chapter 8
Emergency Vehicle Operation   56
Bob Loop

Chapter 9
Public and Media Relations   64
Will Chapleau, EMT-P, RN, TNS

Chapter 10
Ethics in EMS   67
Jean Abbott, MD, MH, and Kelly Bookman, MD

History of Emergency Medical Services

Norman McSwain, Jr., MD, FACS

CHAPTER 1

1. **Can EMS be divided into eras for better understanding?**
   Yes, it can. It will be easiest to describe EMS development in terms of the following eras:
   - Pre-EMS (7000 BCE–1790 AD)
   - Larrey era (1790–1865)
   - Military, Hospitals, and Mortuaries (1865–1950)
   - Farrington era (1950–1975)
   - Modern era of EMS (1975 and beyond)

   These eras are discussed as follows:

PRE-ORGANIZED EMS
(7000 BCE–1790)

2. **When did "emergency medical services" (EMS) originate?**
   The answer lies not in any single event but in the historical written record that defines circumstances for providing care. Emergency care techniques can be found in the Edwin Smith papyrus from 1700 BCE. In early Greek times, Hippocrates described how to distract a femoral fracture with the application of traction. These are all isolated reports.

3. **Are there any references in the Bible that point to prehospital care?**
   Absolutely. The prophet Elisha was called and responded to a home where a child fell and struck his head causing an apparently fatal injury. Elisha breathed into the mouth of a child and returned him to life. (I Kings 17:17–24)
   Of course, everyone remembers the story of the Good Samaritan who found a traveler beaten by robbers. He bound the victim's wounds and transported him to an inn for care. (Luke 10:33–4)

4. **Are there any early public health events?**
   Aside from the forced removal of lepers and venereal disease victims from their homes to isolate them from the rest of the community, sanitation, sewerage, toilets, hot and cold running water, eating properly prepared food, food preservation, beer, wine, and other safe beverages were all part of the Greek, Roman, and Hebrew cultures.

5. **What are other early recorded EMS events?**
   Art historians suggest that Roman carvings depict Caesar employing battlefield "medics" in the first century BCE. The first wagon for transporting patients, the Anglo-Saxon hammock, was developed about 900 CE. Literally a hammock on wheels, the wagon's brakes were chains held by attendants who

endeavored to keep downhill runaways to a minimum. The Norman conquest of England brought many changes, including a covered horse litter for moving patients. Consisting of a bed on poles extending to horses on either end, this device, invented about 1100 CE, improved riding comfort.

6. Who was responsible for the first ambulances?

Actually, ambulances (*ambulancias* in Spanish) were field hospitals initially introduced by Queen Isabella of Spain at the siege of Malaga in 1487. Both Ferdinand and Isabella insisted on staying with their troops during their conflict with the Moors and took exceptional interest in the comfort and welfare of their troops. This interest was manifest in the accumulation of medical and surgical supplies and battlefield tents (*ambulancias*) for the wounded.

LARREY ERA
(1790–1865)

7. Is it true that mobile ambulances were really introduced by Napoleon's surgeons?

Dominique-Jean Larrey, distressed over the observation that, during a battle with the Prussians, the wounded were left in the field until fighting ceased, developed the concept of mobile *ambulancias* for the Army of the Rhine in 1793. Because of Larrey's reputation of concern for wounded soldiers, he was ordered to join Napoleon's Army of Italy, where he worked in conjunction with his senior partner, Baron Percy. Together, they are credited with the development of light, two-wheeled ambulances, which could stay on the battlefield—allowing surgeons to work there—or be used to transport wounded soldiers to a hospital. These vehicles were known as "flying ambulances" because they accompanied the "flying artillery" into war. Larrey developed the basic concepts used today for prehospital care:
1. rapid response to the victims,
2. field care by trained attendants, and
3. rapid transportation back to the hospital

8. Who was this early innovator of EMS?

Dominique-Jean Larrey was born in Abidjan France (July 8, 1766). He attended the Alexis School of surgery in Toulouse. In 1789 he studied surgery under M. Desalt at Hotel Dieu Hospital. Following completion of his surgical education he signed on as assistant surgeon to Napoleon in Paris. For his first assignment, he walked 350 miles to Brest to embark. During the 2-year voyage he wrote of the medical care provided for the troops. During the Prussian/Austrian War (1792) Larrey treated many wounded soldiers, doing such an outstanding job that he was promoted to the director of Napoleon's ambulance service in 1797–1798. Besides developing the first prehospital service and creating standards that are still followed today, Larrey had many other firsts, many of which also are still used today, including:

- the value of freezing in amputations
- amputations at the hip
- disarticulation of the humerus at the shoulder
- the use of maggots for clearing up infection
- the importance of walking after surgery
- the recognition that granular conjunctivitis was contagious

9. **When did EMS get its start in the United States?**
   EMS in the United States evolved under parallel but separate military and civilian lines. The War Between the States began with far worse care than developed by Larrey 60 years before.
   After the first battle of Manassas in July 1861, injured solders were placed under trees for the surgeons to see and treat. Insufficient preparations had been made for medical care following the battle. Wounded troops were left in the field for two weeks before being moved back to medical care. The attendants of the private ambulances abandoned their vehicles and ran when they were overrun by the advancing Confederate Army. At the second Battle of Manassas one year later in August 1862, nothing much had changed. Many of the injured lay in the field for a week before removal. (Three thousand were left for 3 days, 600 for 1 week.)

10. **How did the improvement in civil war care come about?**
    Dr. Jonathan Letterman organized the field medical service of the Union Army after the Quartermaster Corps had been relieved of the responsibility for medical care. He created a system of field evacuation and treatment of wounded soldiers and established a uniform army ambulance system. Under Letterman, dangerous two-wheeled Finley ambulances (similar to Larrey's "flying ambulances") gave way to the Rucker ambulance (Major General Daniel Henry Rucker, United States Army, Quartermaster Department). This had improved ventilation, extra springs for the floor, and more elasticity to the stretchers. Steamships and railcars were modified to accommodate patients and provide care during transport to tertiary facilities.

11. **What were the results of Dr. Letterman's work?**
    At the battle of Antietam in September 1862, 300 ambulances collected and sheltered 10,000 wounded in 24 hours, a vast improvement over earlier efforts.

EMS IN THE MILITARY, MORTUARIES, AND HOSPITALS
(1865–1950)

12. **How did nonmilitary ambulances services develop in the United States?**
    The first civilian ambulances were hospital-based and included those of Cincinnati's General Hospital in 1865. The Free Hospital of New York (Bellevue) initiated ambulance service several years later in 1869. The Bellevue service was staffed by a driver and a "surgeon" and could carry two patients. It was dispatched with supplies and equipment, including bandages, splints, sponges, brandy, handcuffs, and a straitjacket. The attendants were actually interns in the hospital who worked for free because of the educational experience that was available. Ambulances of that era might be staffed with a nurse but only rarely operated without medically trained personnel. Horse-drawn wagons gave way to motorized vehicles, including streetcars and automobiles by the turn of the century. Although advances in transportation were progressive, the training of personnel did not necessarily keep pace. Private ambulance companies developed as business offshoots and were most frequently operated by funeral homes.

13. **How did the EMS movement spread in the United States?**
    Much of the prehospital transportation in the country was provided by undertakers and their vehicles. This was started in Cleveland, Ohio, by the Board of Health in 1880. Funeral homes provided such care until the 1970s. However, some hospitals and some fire departments got involved in the care of patients. In the *Journal of the American Medical Association* (28:36–37, 1897) it was noted that "a

EMS – Overview, Design, and Operations

hospital without ambulances is a hospital without patients." Grady Hospital in Atlanta, Georgia, continues to operate an ambulance service and is the oldest continuously operating hospital-based ambulance in the United States.

The training for ambulance personnel was haphazard to non-existent. There was little organization across the country. Many ambulances had one person on board (as well as the patient, of course). The driver (origin of the term "ambulance driver") would drive as fast as possible to the scene with light and sirens going full blast. On arrival the driver would enlist help to load the patient(s) and then jump in front with no one with the patient and drive to the hospital as fast as possible. Hospital-based services in the larger communities had interns as the attendants. The ambulance service operated by Charity Hospital in New Orleans, Louisiana, continued to use interns well past the midpoint of the twentieth century.

14. **What were early ambulances like?**

When Charity Hospital started its ambulance service in 1885, the medicine chest contained the following:

- Olive oil
- Ferric oxide hydrate
- Monsel's solution (a ferric subsulfate solution)
- Dialyzed iron
- Ergot
- Fluid extract aqueous ammonia
- Solution ammonia carbonate
- Cosmoline (a rust preventative)
- Mustard
- Graduated glasses
- One gallon of carron oil (a liniment containing limewater and linseed oil, used chiefly for burns)
- Chloroform
- Sulfuric ether
- Whiskey
- Brandy
- Carbonic acid
- Syrup morphine
- Tincture of opium camphor
- Hypodermic tablets and syringe
- Water

The surgery chest consisted of the following:

- Complete pocket case of instruments
- Langenbeck's forceps

History of Emergency Medical Services

- Set of three tourniquets
- Folding fracture box
- Oakum (loose hemp or jute fiber)
- Surgeon's lint
- Sponges
- Tracheotomy tube
- Water bucket
- Liston's long splints (2)
- Wooden and tin splints
- Bandages
- Carbolized gauze
- Cotton wadding
- Pillows
- Nelaton's catheter
- Pus pans

15. When did ambulances switch from horse-drawn vehicles to motorized ones?

On February 24, 1899 at Michael Reese Hospital in Chicago, the first motorized ambulance went into service. It could achieve 16 miles per hour. Ambulances after World War II were "low body" Pontiac or Cadillac hearse vehicles most often operated by funeral homes as a vehicle of convenience; each had a stretcher (used for bodies during the funeral), minimal to no medical equipment with windows and curtains on the side; the name of the funeral home was often prominently displayed on the vehicle. By the 1970s many services were changing to "high body" Cadillacs. Not until Dr. J. D. Farrington and others wrote the U.S. Department of Transportation KKK1822 standards for ambulances, which dealt with proper construction of an ambulance and required increased headroom, did the box-type ambulance appear in civilian services. In contrast, such vehicles had been used by the military since World War I.

16. When did air-medical services first develop?

Just like ground ambulances, the first air-medical services were rudimentary transportation efforts that later incorporated medical care during patient movement. The first reported air transport occurred by hot-air balloon when 160 injured soldiers were removed from Paris during a siege by the Prussians in 1870. French and American forces used modified airplanes to move injured soldiers during World War I, but it was not until 1929 that airplanes were formally designed for ambulance service. Use of helicopters to transport patients began in the Korean War, and their subsequent use in Vietnam firmly established the role of rotor-wing aircraft in prehospital transportation. Largely due to the advances of prehospital care, many authorities claimed that a soldier wounded by enemy fire in Vietnam had a better chance of survival than a patient of a domestic motor vehicle accident in the United States.

Drs. Henry Cleveland and Boyd Bigelow developed the first hospital-based civilian helicopter service in the United States at Saint Anthony Hospital in Denver, Colorado, for access to patients in the surrounding Rocky Mountains.

FARRINGTON ERA
(1950–1975)

17. What happened to change the prehospital care system in the United States?

An orthopedic surgeon named J. D. "Deke" Farrington, MD, and his friend, Sam Banks, MD, working with the Chicago Fire Department in the 1950s, realized that care provided in the streets was not optimal and began to train firefighters as ambulance attendants who could care for the patient on the scene, properly package the patient, manage the airway and provide ventilation, control hemorrhages, stabilize fractures, deliver babies, and provide other rudimentary medical care and continue this care en route to the hospital. Dr. Farrington was the son of a preacher in the poor South whose mother died a preventable death. He decided to go to medical school to improve this situation, starting out at the University of Alabama and finishing at Rush Medical College in Chicago.

His article, "Death in a Ditch," described a typical ambulance call and became the rallying cry for many who were advocating for better prehospital care. In 1967 he wrote in the *Bulletin of the American College of Surgeons*:

"Come on fellow. We'll take you and your wife to the hospital. He was pulled from the car, placed on a stretcher, and carried to the ambulance. Ruth soon was placed on a similar rig. The door was slammed closed and the driver and his helper got into the front seat. The ambulance leaped forward with a screech from the tires and a shriek from the siren."

Dr. Farrington also worked with the American College of Surgeons (ACS) to develop the Essential Equipment List of Supplies for Ambulances and with the U.S. Department of Transportation to develop specifications for ambulance design. These were incorporated into the U.S. DOT documents as the KKK 1822 standards. These three documents, developed by Dr. Farrington and others, became and remain, with updates and modifications, the standards for education, ambulance equipment, and vehicle design for the entire United States.

Dr. Farrington was also very instrumental in the founding of the National Registry of Emergency Medical Technicians (NREMT) and the National Association of Emergency Medical Technicians (NAEMT). These were two different organizations with two different charges and were founded about 10 years apart. Because of this effort and his other accomplishments too numerous to list, Dr. Farrington has become known as the Father of the Emergency Medical Service in the United States.

18. How did EMT training mature?

Dr. Farrington further modified the training program as he moved his medical practice to Minnooka, Wisconsin. The U.S. DOT used this to develop the National Standard EMT-Ambulance curriculum. This is now the EMT-Basic program.

As a member of the American Academy of Orthopedic Surgeons (AAOS), Dr. Farrington was instrumental in getting this organization to publish a textbook for EMTs, commonly referred to as the Orange Book, originally issued by the U.S. Food and Drug Administration.

In the beginning of the 1970s, the need for more advanced training, especially for cardiac problems, became recognized. In 1964, J. F. Pantridge, MD, at Royal Victoria Hospital, in Belfast, Northern Ireland, developed an AC defibrillator for use in the coronary intensive care unit of his hospital. His salvage rate from cardiac arrest significantly improved. To make the defibrillator more portable for prehospital use, he changed the electrical circuitry to DC battery-driven (it weighed 100 pounds) and installed it in his "Coronary Flying Squad" in 1966. He found that if this device was used on a patient in nontraumatic cardiac arrest quickly, the survival rate went up by 48%. He thought that moving defibrillation into the streets and into the homes of patients with cardiac arrest after myocardial infarction would improve survival, and he was correct.

After Dr. Pantridge reported to the American College of Cardiology that prehospital care of acute myocardial infarction patients could reduce mortality, several Americans attempted to duplicate his efforts. Although the results were reproducible, the cost of putting doctors in the field was restrictive. Prehospital care became the domain of public safety and ambulance personnel who were trained to provide initial care in the form of EKG interpretation, defibrillation, medication, and safe transportation were the first paramedics.

19. **What research of the 1950s and 1960s boosted this effort?**

The ACS Committee on Trauma (COT) charged the Prehospital Care Subcommittee chaired by Alan Dimick, MD, to assess the state of EMS in the United States. The committee surveyed 62 cities gathering five years of data and found that 25% had excellent EMS; however, 33% of cities' systems were found to be unacceptable.

An article by Greer Williams appeared in the *Saturday Evening Post*, August 24 1955, entitled "Let Those Crash Victims Lie." It stated that removal of patients without care could produce more injuries than if trained attendants arrived on the scene to properly package the patient and care for them en route to the hospital (essentially the same principles that were developed and taught by Dominique-Jean Larrey in the late 1700s).

20. **How and when did cardiopulmonary resuscitation develop?**

1740 The Paris Academy of Sciences officially recommended mouth-to-mouth resuscitation for drowning victims.

1767 The Society for the Recovery of Drowned Persons became the first organized effort to deal with sudden and unexpected death.

1891 Dr. Friedrich Maass performed the first equivocally documented chest compression on humans.

1903 Dr. George Crile reported the first successful use of external chest compressions in human resuscitation.

1904 The first American case of closed-chest cardiac massage was performed by Dr. George Crile.

1954 James Elam was the first to prove that expired air was sufficient to maintain adequate oxygenation.

1956 Drs. Peter Safar and James Elam invented mouth-to-mouth resuscitation.

1957 The United States military adopted the mouth-to-mouth resuscitation method to revive unresponsive victims.

1960 Cardiopulmonary resuscitation (CPR) was formally developed. The American Heart Association started a program to acquaint physicians with closed-chest cardiac resuscitation and became the forerunner of CPR training for the general public.

1963 Cardiologist Leonard Scherlis started the American Heart Association's CPR Committee, and the same year, the American Heart Association formally endorsed CPR.

1966 The National Research Council of the National Academy of Sciences convened an ad hoc conference on CPR. The conference was the direct result of requests from the American Red Cross and other agencies to establish standardized training and performance standards for CPR.

1972 Leonard Cobb held the world's first mass citizen training in CPR in Seattle, Washington, called Medic 2. He helped train over 100,000 people the first two years of the programs.

1981 A program to provide telephone instructions in CPR began in King County, Washington state. The program used emergency dispatchers to give instant directions while the fire department and EMT personnel were en route to the scene. Dispatcher-assisted CPR is now standard care for dispatch centers throughout the United States.

21. What other events spurred EMS advancement?

1960 The ambu bag started being used by the EMS.

1962 Resusci-Annie was developed for teaching CPR by Norwegian toy maker Åsmund Laerdal based on the research of Peter Safar and James Elam.

1966 National Research Council-National Academy of Sciences (NRC-NAS) published "Accidental Death and Disability: The Neglected Disease of Modern Society," which highlighted the deficiencies in civilian trauma care.

1966 The Highway Safety Act was passed.

1967 The Hare Traction Splint was developed and implemented.

1967 The Jaws of Life were developed.

22. What was the importance of the publication "Accidental Death and Disability, the Neglected Disease of Modern Society"?

This seminal paper was the first to point out that soldiers on the battlefield had a much greater chance for survival than did the American citizen injured on the streets and highways of the United States. The paper outlined 15 points for improving trauma care, including the provision of basic and advanced first aid, the inclusion of EMS and ambulances as part of the medical care system, the importance of communication, improving the trauma care provided in hospitals and emergency rooms, ensuring that ICUs included trauma patients, encouraged the development of trauma registries to track trauma patient care, encouraged the use of autopsies as a quality assurance tool to assess trauma care provided, and finally recommended a national registry for EMT certification.

23. What was the National Traffic Safety Act of 1966?

This piece of legislation elevated the Department of Transportation to a cabinet-level position and gave it legislative and financial authority over the EMS. The legislation specifically charged the DOT to improve EMS and highway safety as well as develop standards for ambulance services, vehicles, and provider training.

24. What is the National Registry of Emergency Medical Technicians and how did it come about?

As mentioned previously, the white paper "Death and Disability, the Neglected Disease of Modern Society" had 15 major points, one of which was the creation of a national certification and registration for EMTs.

The National Registry of Emergency Medical Technicians was created in 1970. Rocco Morando was the first director and "Deke" Farrington was the first chairman. The charge was to develop a standard certification examination for EMTs and a registration and a reregistration process for the entire country. Individual states maintain the right to determine who participates in the registry and who does not. Currently, 46 of the 50 states use the registry at either the EMT-B or the EMT-P levels.

26. **How did the Star of Life become the emblem of EMS?**
    The Star of Life was developed by the American Medical Association as the emblem for the Medic Alert bracelet, necklace, and other products for medication or illness notification. The design was based on the Crossing of the Three Rivers of Life and the Staff of Asclepius. It was copyrighted in 1967 by the AMA.
    Dawson Mills, Director of the National Highway Traffic Safety Administration (NHTSA) in the DOT asked the American Red Cross to use the Red Cross symbol as the EMS logo. This request was refused. He then asked "Deke" Farrington, chairman of the National Registry of Emergency Medical Technicians at the time, for permission to use the National Registry of Emergency Medical Technicians (NREMT) logo (the Star of Life) as the national EMS logo and he and the NREMT Board of Directors agreed. Now it is on virtually every ambulance in the United States and many other countries.

27. **Where were the early EMT-paramedic programs in the United States located?**
    The first paramedic programs started in the late 1960s and early 1970s in the following locations:

    Los Angeles, CA—Ron Stewart, MD
    Columbus, OH—James D. Warren
    Pittsburgh, PA—Peter Safar, MD
    Miami, FL—Eugene Nagel, MD
    Long Island, NY—Gus Lambros, MD
    Jacksonville, FL—John Waters
    Seattle, WA—Leonard Cobb, MD
    Houston, TX—Whitey Martin
    Newton, MA—Jim Werries
    Kansas City, KS—Norman McSwain, MD

28. **How did the EMT-paramedic program become standardized just as the EMT-Ambulance (EMT) had been in the late 1960s?**
    In the mid 1970s, the US Department of Transportation, National Highway Transportation and Safety Agency (NHTSA) contracted with Nancy Caroline, MD, to develop "paramedic" standards and establish consensus and agreement. After this was completed, she developed the first textbook using these guidelines to teach the EMT-P program, "Emergency Care in the Streets".

29. **Who were Roy and Johnny of Rescue 51 out of Rampart General Hospital?**
    If you grew up in the 1970s or saw old TV reruns, these two characters will ring a bell as the paramedics of the hit series "Emergency!" This program, much as "Rescue 911" of the 1990s, showcased the abilities of paramedics and a prehospital system and fostered tremendous public acceptance and support for EMS and paramedics. The American public saw what they could have in their own communities and demanded it.

30. How was this demand realized?

In 1973, Congress enacted the Emergency Medical Services System Act, which authorized the Department of Health, Education, and Welfare to fund more than 300 regional EMS systems across the country. Over eight years, programs and standards were developed to promote a systems approach to prehospital care. Funds also were used to cover administrative expenses, purchase equipment, and create training centers. Once federal monies were exhausted, entities that did not disappear adapted their services and obtained other funding sources to continue the mission of advancing the cause of prehospital care.

31. What are the beginnings of EMT-P accreditation?

In mid 1977, 100 organizations met in Chicago at the request of the American Medical Association to discuss the standardization and accreditation of EMT-paramedic training. Over the next few months, 6 organizations chose to become the founding members of "the Joint Review Committee for EMT-Paramedic Accreditation" and an ad hoc committee was created with two members from each organization. It required two years from 1978 to 1980 to get approval of the AMA council for this accreditation process, which finally began in 1980. The first accredited program was at Eastern Kentucky University in Richmond.

32. Physicians used to ride in ambulances. How has their role changed?

From the time of the War Between the States until the 1960s, physicians still rode ambulances in many large cities. Charity Hospital in New Orleans was one of the last to require the interns to ride on calls. The physician's role in prehospital care, especially in the civilian sector, while moving from "on scene" to "behind the scenes," has remained intimate. The specialty of emergency medicine has grown in parallel with the development of EMS. Although a few medical directors continue to respond to selected calls, it is unaffordable for the agency or individual physicians to spend most of their time in the field. The most important physician contribution is that of medical oversight to prehospital care providers in the field. All prehospital providers are aware that their ability to function depends on this relationship. Additionally, medical directors participate in the development of protocols and quality assurance systems, education, and on-line medical control.

THE MODERN ERA
(1970s and beyond)

33. What makes the modern EMS different?

Almost all of the pieces were in place with the development of the system and the structure that Dr. Farrington and his contemporaries had fostered. There were several additional pieces of medical understanding that occurred in the 1980s that helped complete and mature the system.

The first was the recognition that all emergency patients are not equal, they all do not have the same pathophysiology, and they all require a different mechanism of prehospital management. It is almost as simple as "shock is not shock is not shock." It is interesting, in retrospect, that this concept was not recognized before the 1980s.

There are three types of emergency patients. Each type represents almost one third of the patients transported by EMS: cardiac, trauma, and noncardiac medical conditions.

The cardiac patient will die of inadequate cardiac output secondary to pump failure if not managed properly. Cardiac disease is a condition that can and should be managed in the field, or at least the major portion of the initial care started in the field.

The trauma patient will die of exsanguination from hemorrhage which, in most cases, can only be controlled in the operating room of a hospital. Prolonged field times are frequently fatal. Rapid transportation, along with airway control, is required to a hospital dedicated, equipped, and staffed to rapidly treat such patients.

Other medical conditions are usually not as time critical and allow the prehospital provider time to assess the patient and develop a treatment plan while transporting the patient.

The major factor that brought about the recognition of the three major types of emergency patients was the development of the Advanced Cardiac Life Support (ACLS) course in the mid 1970s, the Advanced Trauma Life Support (ATLS) course in the late 1970s, and the Prehospital Trauma Life Support (PHTLS) course in the early 1980s.

The second understanding came with the recognition that not all hospitals were created equal and that some offered specialized services that would help improve patient outcome. Such specialized services include trauma care, pediatric care, hyperbaric oxygen treatment, burn care, and now cardiac and stroke care. The preferential transport of a patient needing one of these services, even if it means bypassing another closer hospital, has become a standard part of EMS delivery.

34. What is ATLS and how has it impacted EMS?

In 1976, Dr. James Styner and his family were flying in his light plane across his home state of Nebraska when the plane crashed. He and his family were transported to a local hospital emergency room. He subsequently described the poor care that they got simply because the personnel in the receiving hospital lacked the appropriate knowledge to deal with trauma victims. A group of surgeons led by Paul "Skip" Collicutt began to try to remedy this situation by developing the ATLS course. The course was developed within the Lincoln Medical Foundation (Lincoln, Nebraska). The planning process began in the summer of 1977 and the first pilot course was run in February 1978. The American College of Surgeons Committee on Trauma approved it as a national course of the ACS at the annual meeting of the American College of Surgeons/Committee on Trauma (ACS/COT) in March 1979 and the ACS Board of Regents approved it in June. The first course to train national faculty took place in Lincoln in January 1980. During the rest of that year, 376 regional and state faculty were trained across the United States.

35. Is there a prehospital equivalent to ATLS?

There are two courses that teach trauma management to prehospital providers.

Basic Trauma Life Support, now known as International Trauma Life Support (ITLS), was started by John Campbell, MD, and the Alabama branch of the American College of Emergency Physicians in 1981. PHTLS was founded by the National Association of Emergency Medical Technicians with the assistance of the ACS/COT in 1981.

36. What is the history of PHTLS?

In 1981, Norman McSwain, MD, requested that he be allowed to teach ATLS to EMS personnel; the ACS refused. Instead the ACS/COT agreed to assist the National Association of Emergency Medical Technicians in developing a specific course based on the principles of ATLS but directed to the needs of the patient before the patient arrived in the hospital. This was named the Prehospital Trauma Life Support Course. Development began immediately and prototype courses were run in 1982 and 1983 in Connecticut,

Iowa, and Louisiana under the leadership group of Jim Paturas, Rick Vomacka, Ray Bias, Gene Salassi, Jon Boyle, MD, and Joseph Dineen, MD.

37. What is the more recent history of EMS?

No discussion of history can be considered truly current. The DOT EMT and paramedic curricula were revised several times in the intervening years since their original development. Most recently, the traditional curricula have been supplanted by the development and publication of the National EMS Educations Standards and their supporting documents. Of ongoing interest is the potential for expanding the scope of a paramedic's function beyond traditional boundaries. The base for prehospital functions continues to fluctuate among private, third-service, public utility, and fire-based operations. The value of a medical director's time and input is being increasingly recognized. Almost certainly, financial considerations will be a major driving force in the future of the EMS.

References

1. Barkley JT. The Ambulance. Kiamesha Lake, NY: Load N Go Press, 1990.
2. National Emergency Medical Services Education Standards. National Highway Transportation and Safety Administration, Department of Transportation, 2009. http://www.ems.gov/pdf/811077e.pdf (Accessed March 9, 2011.)
3. Mustalish AC. Emergency medical services: Twenty years of growth and development. NY State J Med Aug: 414–410, 1986.
4. Page JO. Historical perspectives on EMS systems. In Roush WR (ed.): Principles of EMS Systems, 2nd ed. Dallas: American College of Emergency Physicians, 1994, pp 1–10.
5. Smiley DR. Overview of the EMS system. In Pons P, Cason D (eds.): Paramedic Field Care. St. Louis: Mosby, 1997, pp 4–16.
6. Stewart RD. The history of emergency medical services. In Kuehl A (ed.): EMS Medical Directors' Handbook. St. Louis: Mosby, 1989, pp. 3–6.

EMS System Design

Mike Nugent, MS

1. What is meant by "EMS system design"?
Modern emergency medical services (EMS) systems are comprised of much more than working EMS professionals, ambulances, and those in need of help. Effectively designed EMS systems bring into alignment a wide variety of EMS resources to provide a consistent, quality service to their patients. EMS systems administrators must be cognizant of the rapidly dynamic environment in which they operate. Today's EMS system design may not meet the needs of its community in the future.

2. What does the public have to do with EMS?
The public is a key component of the EMS response system because it is impossible to put trained and equipped medical providers on every street corner. Members of the public will often be bystanders or witnesses when an emergency medical condition occurs. Their ability to quickly recognize the presence of an emergency medical condition, rapidly activate the EMS system, and then begin initial lifesaving treatment is essential to improved patient outcome.

3. What are the components of a typical EMS system?
In its most simple form, an EMS system includes the following:
- recognition that an emergency medical situation exists
- a communication method to contact and activate the medical response system
- dispatch of response vehicles and personnel
- trained and equipped emergency medical response providers
- transport vehicles
- appropriate receiving destinations

4. I understand that dispatch plays a part in getting equipment moving, but are dispatch personnel actually involved in medical care?
Absolutely. In responding to prehospital emergencies, dispatchers serve as the first link in the patient care continuum. Although often overlooked, they are a critical part of the patient care team. Dispatchers perform medical triage using emergency medical dispatch by assessing the patient's needs. EMD is based on the principle that good information gathering during the dispatch phase of an emergency can better prepare responding EMS providers to deal with the situation at the scene. A trained emergency medical dispatcher will not only dispatch appropriate medical and rescue resources but also provide prearrival instructions giving bystanders, or the patients themselves, instructions on how to provide potentially lifesaving first aid on scene.

The dispatch function may be carried out by a variety of agencies, including law enforcement, fire department, EMS agency, or a separate public safety dispatch center.

5. What are the various models of EMS system design and service delivery?

- Private—may be operated as "for profit" or "not-for-profit" with providers of varying training levels; often financed by fee for service.
- Hospital-based—run by one or more hospitals.
- Municipal third service—operated by the local government or health agency, not part of the fire or police departments.
- Fire department—may use uniformed firefighters (firefighters may serve in dual role, handling fire and EMS calls or EMS calls only) or civilian EMS staff to provide basic to advanced level care; often financed by the fire department budget, although many fire departments bill patients for care and transportation.

A survey of EMS systems conducted in 2003 by the National Association of State EMS Directors (NASEMSD) and the Health Resource Services Administration (HRSA) Office of Rural Health Policy indicated that there were almost 16,000 credentialed EMS systems in the United States. Among the systems identified by the survey, 45 percent were fire-based, 6.5 percent were hospital-based, and 48.5 percent were labeled as nonfire-and nonhospital-based.

6. Is there any evidence that one service model is better than another?

No. There are a number of difficulties when evaluating the pros and cons of any service model. These difficulties include the lack of objective processes, outcome data to compare one model of service delivery or even one ambulance company to another, and adequate cost data. As a result, EMS systems frequently rely on crude measures such as numbers of personnel, numbers of ambulances, unit hour use, and response times. These are poor indicators of the quality of care delivered. Instead, patient outcome–based measures of system performance should be the standard by which EMS agencies are evaluated.

7. Are there any specialized EMS system components?

As the EMS operational climate increases in complexity, so will the required number of specialized services. Many EMS systems have specialized components to address response challenges such as tactical emergency medical services, hazardous materials response, and specialized rescue teams. Tactical medics provide immediate medical care to injured persons during a SWAT-type operation, treating them onsite or stabilizing them and extracting them from the scene. Tactical medics usually work alongside law enforcement officers. EMS hazardous materials teams possess the ability to provide patient care in potentially contaminated environments while dressed in specialized personal protective equipment. Other specialized EMS system components include bariatric service, farm rescue, high-angle rescue, and confined-space rescue. In addition, many EMS systems also have air transportation services, either fixed or rotary wing (helicopter), available.

8. What is medical direction?

The next essential part of the system is medical direction. All nonphysician EMS personnel, whether they are dispatchers, first responders, EMTs, or paramedics, should be required to operate under the supervision of a physician medical director. This is especially true of paramedics, who perform the most extensive out-of-hospital medical procedures. A knowledgeable, experienced, interested physician must be actively involved with and responsible for the medical care provided by the EMS system regardless of that system's design or structure.

EMS System Design

9. **Where do emergency departments and hospitals fit within an EMS system?**
    A major component of the EMS system is the facility or facilities that will receive patients with emergency medical conditions. The typical EMS system will include multiple hospitals with varying levels of capability and capacity within its geographical boundaries. Some facilities will have special capabilities that are recognized based on national standards, such as trauma centers, burn centers, poison control centers, regional pediatric centers, and the like. Others may have special roles assigned by the local, regional, or state EMS system, such as the responsibility to be a "base hospital" and a source of on-line medical direction for prehospital personnel.

10. **Now that all of the system components have been defined, how are they put together into a "system"?**
    There are an infinite number of ways that the various potential components can be organized into a successful EMS system. Typically, a state government EMS agency will have statutory and regulatory authority over EMS activities within the state. This office will be headed by an individual known as the state EMS director. Commonly, a physician knowledgeable in EMS will be the state EMS medical director. Many states are then subdivided into regional or local EMS areas with defined governing boards. In the absence of these regional entities, local government usually assumes the responsibility for the delivery of EMS. Although EMS system design varies, the four most prevalent models are

    - Fire-based system
    - Private system
    - Public–private partnership—often, the public sector provides first responder services while the private sector offers transportation.
    - Public utility model—some local municipalities grant a single provider a government-supported monopoly to provide all services.

    Decisions about which EMS system components to include and how to link them together usually result from a balance between medical, political, and financial considerations. Therefore, actual EMS system design is highly variable from one location to another. Regardless of these variations, all systems consist of those components described earlier: a communications method to alert and activate the EMS agency, dispatch of the responders, response to the scene of the emergency, medical care providers to begin assessment and treatment of the patient, transport of the ill or injured patients, and receiving facilities to provide ongoing care.

11. **What exactly does EMS provide to the community?**
    The EMS system enables rapid response to medical and traumatic emergencies, provides the first contact with the emergency health care delivery system, and facilitates lifesaving care. In communities where trauma systems have developed, EMS and trauma providers are interdependent, working closely within established protocols to help ensure that injured patients are transported to the most appropriate facility as quickly as possible while providing needed interventions, mostly during transport. In many communities, EMS encompasses a variety of functions, including not only response to trauma and medical emergencies but also critical care transport between health care facilities, nonemergency transport of patients between facilities or their homes, transportation services for wheelchair or other

patients requiring special vehicle accommodation, and, in some systems, transport of medical items such as blood, organs for transplant, supplies, or equipment.

12. Are all EMS systems created equal?

No. There are inherent advantages and disadvantages with each EMS system model. The type of EMS system design selected will be heavily community dependent:

(a) Fire-based EMS systems—one consideration for having an integrated fire and EMS system is the structural efficiency it brings. Firehouses are usually well positioned to respond to the local population. These structures provide a strategic location for EMS services that are stationed there as well as a place for EMS providers to rest between calls. Fire departments also possess the necessary infrastructure to manage personnel, provide training, and purchase and maintain equipment and supplies. A disadvantage to fire-based EMS is the cultural divide that may exist between EMS and fire personnel[1,2] who have differing priorities, activities, and education and the need for continuing medical education. In addition, EMS is under the leadership of the fire department, which often considers its primary mission to be fire suppression rather than medical care. Consequently, priority is often given to fire suppression at the expense of EMS in training and budget allocations.

(b) Hospital-based EMS systems—an advantage to hospital-based EMS systems is the closeness personnel frequently have with medical personnel in the emergency department and hospitals. It is often much easier for hospital-based EMS personnel to become fully immersed in emergency medicine, discuss the management and outcome of patients with physician and nursing staff, have the opportunity to observe or conduct procedures in their host institution, and attend progressive continuing education offerings. A disadvantage to hospital-based EMS services is that these services are in potential competition with other hospital departments for resources and training. In communities serviced by a number of hospital-based EMS services, competition among the various entities could translate to system inefficiency and unnecessary redundancy.

(c) Private EMS systems—private EMS systems often address some of the challenges seen in fire-based EMS systems and achieve some of the benefits of hospital-based EMS systems in that they offer dedicated personnel who are engaged in professional EMS services. A disadvantage to private EMS system delivery is in the system's profit orientation. Disputes between the municipality and private EMS contractor can be detrimental to the community being served. Certain contracts lack the necessary medical oversight for quality EMS delivery.

13. Why do different models of EMS systems exist?

For a variety of reasons, some of which can be controlled and others which cannot. Some factors that affect EMS system design include

- Geography. It is more difficult to deliver rapid, efficient care in a large, sparsely populated area than in most cities.
- Population. It may be easier to support a higher level of care in high-volume systems. Typically, greater resources and more funding are available in more populated areas.
- Timing. The development of EMS does not necessarily follow the growth of a community. Communities often expand despite the limited concurrent growth of public safety resources and

EMS System Design

services. EMS may be an afterthought to the planning process unless it is actively promoted by a stakeholder in the community.

- Politics. When service need, funding, territory, and revenue intermingle, sectors whose interests are not primarily motivated by patient care may have conflicting desires.
- Community commitment. Much time and money are needed for the community to ensure that their EMS system is of high quality. Active involvement by physicians, adequate funding including market-competitive EMS salaries, quality equipment, and a commitment to training are all requirements for quality care that must be provided by the community.

14. What is a tiered system?

A tiered EMS system delivers care at a variety of levels. For example, the first rescuer to approach a person who is in cardiac arrest might be a nearby police officer who could start cardiopulmonary resuscitation (CPR). Then, several minutes later, the local fire department might arrive and might be able to initiate basic life support measures such as CPR, oxygen administration, and automated defibrillation. Then a transporting ambulance might arrive, perhaps from a private company or from a different fire station, with paramedics who could intubate the patient and initiate advanced life support care as well as transport the victim to the hospital. Each level of care (first responder, basic life support, advanced life support) is a tier.

15. How many tiers can there be?

There is no definitive answer to this question. In some rural areas patients might be cared for by many tiers as they move toward the hospital. For instance, a county sheriff might be the first tier, followed by a volunteer rescue group. A basic life support ambulance from a nearby town might be the next tier and could start transport. The ambulance might be met on the highway by an advanced life support ambulance or aeromedical unit, which would continue care to the hospital. Alternatively, a single agency can provide response, advanced care, and transport as a single tier.

16. Is there shared responsibility or obligation between tiers?

Whether the providers belong to one agency or come from different organizations, the ultimate shared responsibility is a cooperative effort to care for the patient. Medical direction should focus all providers on a seamless continuum of patient care regardless of their position in the hierarchy of response.

17. Is there a risk in tiered systems related to transferring a patient's care?

Possibly. Patient "handoffs" increase the risk of the loss of information about the patient's complaint, mechanism of injury, or past medical history. However, an efficient EMS system will get the right type of resource (basic life support or advanced life support) to the right type of emergency at the right time and maintain seamless communication from one component of the response system to the next. Tiered systems with medical direction and oversight can achieve efficiency and deliver high-quality care to patients.

18. Given this risk, why would an EMS system have tiers? Would it not be better to have a single responding agency to eliminate the risk of handoffs?

Yes and no. A single responding agency would decrease the handoff risk of lost information. But a single-tiered system might dramatically increase response time, cost, or consumption of valuable resources.

Tiered systems work because they use resources that are close to the patient to initiate care and actively manage the transfer of care in a prudent fashion.

19. **What is the difference between fixed and dynamic deployment?**
Fixed deployment refers to having a constant number of EMS units, such as ambulances or rescue units that respond from fixed locations such as fire stations. EMS employees benefit from fixed deployment by having easy access to amenities such as sleeping quarters, kitchens, and recreation. Dynamic deployment involves having varying numbers of EMS units respond from mobile locations, strategically placed based on historical data and projected resource demand. Systems that use dynamic deployment have an easier time adapting to changing community demographics and demands for service.

20. **What is system status management?**
A concept developed by EMS system expert Jack Stout, system status management is a dynamic deployment model that attempts to match the anticipated demand for services with the supply and placement of EMS resources including vehicles and staff. Simply stated, system status management means having the right number of EMS units in the right place at the right time. Therefore, during peak periods, more EMS units are staffed and available in the ambulance dispersal system than in slow periods.

21. **What is the point of system status management?**
The assumption behind dynamic deployment is that vehicles will be strategically placed at the location where and when they are most needed. This is achieved through system status management, which involves a detailed analysis of EMS demand based on hour of the day, day of the week, month of the year, and factors such as historical call patterns and traffic-related issues.

22. **Why do all EMS systems not use system status management?**
For two simple reasons. The first is tradition. Some EMS and fire organizations have built organizations around strategically placed fixed stations. They provide constant station-based staffing. Crews work fixed shifts. During peak times they work like crazy, often traveling far from their stations; during slow times they may wait for long periods of time in the station for the next call. This tradition continues. The emotional and capital cost of changing this model would require a huge investment. Many people believe that the fixed-based model is the best model for their community, if not universally.

The second impediment is knowledge and technology. Effective system status management requires that managers of the EMS system have a firm understanding of the timing, location, and nature of its workload. These types of data, typically computerized, are not available in many EMS organizations and may be cost prohibitive to install. EMS organizations must also dedicate sufficient personnel to the continued analysis of demands for service and resource allocation.

23. **What is "unit hour utilization"?**
As applied to EMS, a unit hour refers to an EMS unit (e.g., an ambulance) that is stocked, staffed and ready to provide EMS care for one hour. Utilization is measured by the number of calls run. Unit hour utilization (quantified as the number of calls run per hour) is a tool that is used to evaluate the effectiveness of system status management. The efficient system has achieved a balance between the available unit hours and their utilization.

24. **Are there nationally accepted standardized performance metrics for EMS systems?**
Over the last decade, there has been significant progress in the development of EMS system performance indicators. The EMS Performance Measures Project, coordinated by NASEMSD in partnership with the

National Association of EMS Physicians, and supported by the National Highway Traffic Safety Administration, and HRSA, developed consensus measures of EMS performance to assist in demonstrating the system's value and define the adequate level of EMS service and preparedness for a given community. Work undertaken by the EMS Performance Measures Project in 2004 resulted in the initial development of 138 indicators of EMS performance. This list was pared down to 25 indicators in 2005 and ultimately expanded to 35 indicators on final publication in 2009. The list included system measures such as "What are the time intervals in a call?" and "What percentage of transports is conducted with red lights and sirens?" and clinical measures such as "How well was pain relieved?" The questions were defined using data elements from the National EMS Information System dataset so that results could be compared across EMS systems.

25. **What factors need to be considered in EMS resource deployment?**
    Most EMS managers see strategic resource deployment as an effective way to match demand and supply. Attention to resource deployment, effective dispatching, and workload management are critical to enhancing performance while limiting employee fatigue. The EMS manager must consider factors such as workload and how available resources can achieve a balance among coverage, response times, and crew satisfaction. Additional factors to be considered include population density, geographic density, call-demand patterns, road systems, and location of health care facilities.

26. **What are the five hallmarks for ensuring high performance when designing an EMS system?**
    (a) Accountability: EMS systems should have clearly defined performance expectations that include obtaining patient feedback and providing assurances that medical protocols reflect current standards of practice.
    (b) Independent oversight mechanism: There are numerous ways in which independent oversight can be provided to EMS systems. Strong physician participation coupled with accreditation by national independent EMS organizations can improve system operations and patient care.
    (c) Account for all service costs: EMS systems operate in a dynamic environment and require constant financial oversight. The EMS system should be accountable for ensuring it has adequate funding, its infrastructure is maintained, and that upgrades in technology, medicine, training, and vehicles are routinely contemplated and implemented.
    (d) Economic efficiency: EMS systems should use resources effectively and efficiently. The system should eliminate duplicate resources that are unnecessary, constantly strive to minimize risks to patients and employees, and deploy the right resource to the right location at the right time.
    (e) Ensure long-term high performance: EMS systems must use an assortment of strategies to assure long-term high performance. An established and active quality assurance/improvement program and consistent national benchmarking with similar EMS systems is important. In addition, performance-based contracting with managerial oversight is necessary.

Pearls and Pitfalls

1. The incorporation of system quality assurance and improvement analysis into the overall operation will allow for system modifications and redesign prior to a major crisis or system shortfall.

2. Effective EMS managers will give the patient a voice in EMS delivery and system design.
3. A standard set of measures that can be used to assess the performance of the full emergency and trauma care system within each community, particularly those that focus on patient outcome and the ability to benchmark that performance against statewide and national performance metrics, remains an elusive goal.

References

1. Davis, R. Many lives are lost across USA because emergency services fail. USA Today, July 28, 2003a:1.
2. Davis, R. The method: Measure how many victims leave the hospital alive. USA Today, July 29, 2003b:1.
3. Fitch, J. Prehospital care administration: The industry's best articles, essays, and case studies on the toughest EMS issues. San Diego, CA: JEMS Communications, 2004.
4. Institute of Medicine (IOM). Crossing the quality chasm: A new health system for the 21st century. Washington, DC: International Press, 2001.
5. Institute of Medicine (IOM). Future of emergency care: emergency medical services at the crossroads. Washington, DC: National Academies Press, 2006.
6. Kuehl AE, ed. Prehospital Systems and Medical Oversight, 2nd ed. National Association of EMS Physicians. St. Louis: Mosby Lifeline, 1994.
7. Mears, G. 2003 survey and analysis of EMS scope of practice and practice settings impacting EMS services in rural America: Executive brief and recommendations. Chapel Hill, NC: University of North Carolina at Chapel Hill, Department of Emergency Medicine, 2004.
8. Emergency Medical Services Performance Measures. Recommended attributes and indicators for system and service performance. National Highway Traffic Safety Administration, U.S. Department of Transportation, 2009 [online]. Available: http//www.ems.gov/pdf/81811211.pdf [Accessed March 9, 2010.]
9. Narad RA. Emergency medical services system design. Emerg Med Clin North Am 8:1–16, 1990.
10. National Highway Traffic Safety Administration: EMS system development: Results of the statewide EMS assessment program. Washington, DC: U.S. Government Printing Office, 1994.
11. Roush WR, McDowell RM, Pons PT. Emergency medical services systems. In Principles of EMS Systems, Roush WR, ed., pp. 11–24. Dallas: American College of Emergency Physicians, 1994.
12. Smith JE. Administration, management, and operations. In Principles of EMS Systems, Roush WR, ed., pp. 103–122. Dallas: American College of Emergency Physicians, 1994.
13. Valenzuela TD, Goldberg J, Keeley KT, et al. Computer modeling of emergency medical system performance. Ann Emerg Med 19:898–901, 1990.
14. Weigand JV. Prehospital ground transport: System structure and function. In Roush WR, ed., Principles of EMS Systems. Dallas: American College of Emergency Physicians, 1994, pp. 165–182.

The Prehospital Environment

James Robinson, Paramedic

CHAPTER 3

1. **What is the prehospital environment?**

   The prehospital environment is the emergency medical service (EMS) provider's place of business. It includes everything from the door of the ambulance bay to the border of the response area. It may include high-rise buildings, wheat fields, multimillion-dollar homes, homeless shelters, or all of the above. Anywhere an EMS may respond to a call for assistance is the prehospital environment. The prehospital environment never sleeps, and this aspect of our vocation is what demands our constant attention and state of readiness.

2. **What makes the prehospital environment so unique and so challenging?**

   The prehospital environment is fluid and unpredictable. Although there are some similarities between them, every call for service is a unique entity. Each call has its own context, pace, and players. The challenges of prehospital medicine are numerous, but EMS providers tend to thrive on the variability. In a single day, the prehospital environment can be dirty, dark, wet, and depressing or sunny, bright, joyful, and happy. From a work environment perspective, providers may work in the back of an ambulance or in a stadium full of people. The work is almost always different from day to day and varies in weather, lighting, clientele, and level of emotion, among numerous other factors. If you like challenge, EMS may be just the thing for you. Add to the constantly changing working environment the spectrum of human behavior and emotion and the practice of medicine, and you have a practical definition of the word "challenge."

3. **Why do seasoned EMS providers often say that the prehospital setting is a wealth of information?**

   The prehospital environment *is* a wealth of information and also a wealth of emotion. The challenge for the EMS provider is to be a detective, separate the information from emotion, and make the most of both in caring for patients. If a provider is compassionate, observant, attentive to detail, and puts forth the necessary effort, he or she can maximize the utility of available information in making the best decisions for the customer.

4. **Who are our "customers"?**

   This seems like an easy question to answer. In reality, EMS providers are working not just for the patient or patients in front of them, but for every other *potential* patient who lives in or visits their response area—not an insignificant obligation by any stretch of the imagination. Providing timely, competent prehospital medical care to people is part of the charge of EMS providers. Whether one is a paid professional or a volunteer, the EMS provider has customers who expect quick service with a smile whether or not the EMS provider has not eaten or slept, it is 3:00 in the morning, there is a full-blown blizzard, or there was a traumatic death on the previous call. EMS is about serving others.

5. **Of all the variables that I may encounter in the field, about which should I be most concerned?**
   The biggest factor that can destabilize a scene is the people in it. Emotion, alcohol, drugs, violence, psychiatric disorders, and many other factors influence people's behavior. The unpredictability of human behavior is the most concerning element of the prehospital environment. It challenges the personal safety of EMS providers and fosters incredible skill in interpersonal communication and "on your feet" thinking in any provider who minds its lessons.

6. **What types of calls can I expect?**
   The types of calls an EMS provider will see depend largely on their prehospital environment. It is unlikely that urban EMS providers will see farm equipment accidents. Similarly, rural providers are less likely to see injuries from gang fights. Despite the disparity of the previous examples, both can probably expect to see automobile accidents, patients with chest pain and breathing problems, and perhaps deliver a baby. The emotional climate of any call may range from horrifying to joyous. This is part of the allure of EMS.

7. **Do all EMS providers experience the same challenges?**
   Some challenges are universal—weather, lighting, 24-hour-a-day operation, routing to calls, and the like. Other challenges, however, may be EMS system specific. Urban providers may have to learn to become expedient in their care and delivery of patients to a hospital so that they can return to service for the next call. Rural providers, on the other hand, may have to learn to care for an acute patient for hours while they transport the patient to distant hospitals. Urban providers may have concerns such as extricating a patient from a subway platform, whereas rural providers may have to transport a patient by horseback or snowmobile. All challenges unique to the particular prehospital environment of the provider require different thought processes and logistical support.

8. **Are urban providers the only ones at risk for violence toward EMS providers?**
   No. Any scene has the potential to deteriorate into a dangerous one. Alcohol, drugs, psychiatric disorders, metabolic disorders, emotion, head trauma, and most other influences on behavior are not exclusive to the urban prehospital environment. It is important for all EMS providers to be responsible for their own and each other's safety. Complacency leads to troubling outcomes.

9. **Is there anything consistent about the prehospital environment?**
   The prehospital environment is consistently inconsistent. Fortunately, unpredictability makes working in EMS interesting. One area of consistency is your "office"—the ambulance. Your ambulance is your workspace, and it should be an island of comfort in a sea of uncertainty. You know where everything is and should be comfortable providing care there. There is an element of standardization and familiarity to it that makes providing care there easier than it may be elsewhere in the prehospital environment.

10. **How can I prepare to function in the prehospital environment?**
    Make sure you have taken care of the basics first, like being appropriately dressed for the occasion—sunglasses, boots, gloves, raincoat as necessary. Make sure you are mentally alert and familiar with your response area. Be mindful of potential risks to your safety, and take appropriate steps to mitigate them, such as wearing your seatbelt, wearing appropriate personal protective equipment, carrying a flashlight, and being cognizant of people's personal space. Remember to carry your radio, as it may be the only

means of contact you have if you are in distress. Most importantly, recognize the immense responsibility EMS has to help people during the worst days in their lives.

11. The prehospital environment sounds intimidating. Should I be deterred?

The prehospital environment provides a challenging, mercurial environment capable of keeping the most seasoned EMS veterans on their toes. Prospective EMS providers who appreciate diversity in their daily work, have a sense of service, and possess the traits of adaptability and ingenuity will have a rewarding experience in the prehospital environment. Although providers are not always recognized for the services they provide, prehospital emergency medicine is exciting, and the majority of providers find the work satisfying in its own right.

Pearls and Pitfalls

1. The prehospital environment includes everything within the confines of the response area, and in cases of mutual aid, everything outside the usual response area.
2. The only consistency about the prehospital environment is that it is inconsistent. This includes the weather, traffic, the scene, and the various people you will interact with at each scene.
3. The single most unpredictable component of every scene is the behavior of the people present.
4. Any scene may become confrontational or violent. Not being prepared can lead to serious injury to the responder.

Reference

1. Dernocoeur K. Streetsense: Communication, Safety and Control, 3rd ed. Redmond, WA: Laing Communications, 1996.

Prehospital Communications

CHAPTER 4

James F. Azuero and James Simpkins

1. **This chapter title is quite broad. What is covered under prehospital communications?**
   Information about various aspects of communications, including 911 systems, radio systems, emergency medical dispatch, medical dispatch protocols, and field/hospital communications.

2. **Do I need to be a radio geek to understand prehospital communications?**
   No, unless you want to understand the really technical stuff. The information presented in this section is intended to help the EMS provider understand some of the concepts used in prehospital communications. Thus, the information should give you some background for understanding how some of this works. The technical details have been summarized to allow readers to apply the concepts to their own situations.

3. **Why is dispatch referred to as the heart of the EMS system?**
   The dispatch center is the focal point for all EMS system activity. With the exception of direct field medical control (between field personnel and the base station physician) and some hospital notifications, the balance of emergency medical services is coordinated through the dispatch center—system access for the emergency caller, resource management (unit availability and positioning), response unit assignment, response monitoring and support, hospital availability, and hospital notification. The communications center is essential to and involved in virtually every part of the emergency response.

4. **What is 911?**
   It is the U.S. nationwide emergency telephone number. It was developed by the telephone utilities to allow people quick, easy access to emergency services, regardless of where they may be. It is a number that is well publicized and easily remembered. By virtue of its nationwide implementation, people needing help do not have to search for a telephone book to find a seven-digit telephone number to call for help.

5. **Will 911 work everywhere?**
   Unfortunately, no. Although most of the country has the 911 system in place, there are still some areas, mostly rural, where 911 does not work. Most of these areas are moving toward 911 service, trying to satisfy the funding and legal and political conditions that are necessary to implement an efficient service. Until a 911 system is implemented in these locations, people who need help still have to dial a seven-digit telephone number.

6. **Why is 911 better than dialing "0"?**
   Dialing "0" (for "Operator") is a good second choice if 911 does not work. The operator can connect the caller with an emergency communications center; however, it is not as efficient as 911 for a couple of reasons. First, there is an additional call and routing process, which takes time. Second, the caller may not be connected with the correct jurisdiction or service that he or she needs. Operators (or calltakers) on the 911 system, on the other hand, are trained to manage the emergency caller, quickly eliciting the information necessary to send an appropriate response.

7. What is E911?

The "E" in E911 stands for "Enhanced." The first implementations of 911 simply routed the caller to an emergency communications center. The communications center was generally determined by the location of the telephone company's central office that managed the caller's telephone prefix. (The telephone prefix is the first three digits of the seven-digit telephone number.) Telephone service areas do not follow political boundaries. Therefore, although the call was routed to an emergency communications center, it may not have been the correct one, perhaps in the "wrong" city, county, or other response jurisdiction.

"Enhanced" 911 routes the caller to the correct emergency communications center. When the call is received in the telephone company's central office, several things happen. First, the telephone company identifies the telephone number from which the call is being placed. This is referred to as ANI, or Automatic Number Identification. Many people have a similar service on their own telephones known as Caller ID.

Once identified, the phone number is matched to a database that includes the basic information—name of the responsible party, billing address, apartment or suite number, and response jurisdiction for police, fire, and EMS. This information is referred to as ALI, or Automatic Location Information. In most cases, the ALI information is the same as the telephone location. The call is then routed to the communications center responsible for that location. Thus, in the vast majority of cases, the E911 call is routed to the correct emergency communications center.

8. What if it is not the correct center?

E911 systems have the capability of transferring all the information, both ANI and ALI, to another E911 center. For example, let us assume you live in Gotham City. Your aging mother, who has a heart condition, lives in neighboring Pleasant Valley. Unfortunately, she calls *you* instead of 911 and tells you she's having a heart attack. "I'll call 911" you say, and you do. Your call is appropriately routed (for your Gotham City phone) to Gotham City—the wrong jurisdiction. Fortunately, your astute 911 calltaker recognizes the situation and transfers your call to Pleasant Valley, allowing you to talk directly to the "correct" communications center and allowing them to get the necessary information directly from you.

9. I often hear the term "peesap" around the communications center. What is it?

PSAP stands for Public Safety Answering Point. This is the initial site where 911 calls are answered. A PSAP may serve a single jurisdiction or may answer calls for multiple jurisdictions and agencies. In either case, the initial answering point is called the "primary" PSAP. If the calls are subsequently routed to other jurisdictions or agencies, those secondary answering points are referred to as "secondary" PSAPs.

10. What if I am calling for help that is needed somewhere else?

E911 can identify the location of only the calling party. It cannot identify where help is needed. It is the calltaker's responsibility to verify the location where help is needed. The calltaker cannot simply rely on the E911 information displayed automatically on the E911 terminal but must question the caller to be sure that the appropriate assistance is being sent to the right place.

11. I just got a new phone. Will E911 work for me?

Maintenance of the E911 databases across the country is an enormous task. Although the telephone companies strive to keep the databases up to date, there is occasionally a lag of a few days, although they make every effort to enter new numbers (and remove old ones) as rapidly as possible.

12. What is EMD?

EMD stands for Emergency Medical Dispatch. This is a formal program that in its most generic form is intended to help the emergency calltaker to gather as much important information as quickly as possible, determine the appropriate response level, and give instructions to the caller to provide appropriate medical assistance to the patient.

13. What information is most important to calltakers/dispatchers?

The person answering the emergency wants to gather three pieces of information as quickly as possible. It is usually gathered in this order, for the noted reasons.
1. *Event location*. The dispatcher must know where to send the unit. Even if no other information is obtained, at least someone can go to the scene to make an assessment of what is going on.
2. *Callback number*. This is really helpful in the event that the original address is incomplete or incorrect. If the responders cannot get there, they cannot provide help.
3. *Problem or nature*. Once the calltaker can assure a response to the scene, information about what is happening there will allow him or her to make a good decision regarding who to send and how to send them. The calltaker should also gather information about scene safety and any information particular to the event that will affect the responding units.

14. What safety functions do dispatchers provide?

Dispatchers/calltakers provide several safety "nets" for emergency responders. First, the calltaker will try to make some assessment of scene safety. This includes, among other things, electrical wires down at auto accidents, the presence of an assailant at scenes of violence, or wind and weather conditions in the case of hazardous materials incidents. The dispatch center will endeavor to warn the responders of impending danger. Second, the dispatcher will try to make responding units aware of other units responding to the same or nearby incidents. This is a warning to anticipate and watch for other emergency traffic to avoid accidents. Finally, dispatchers monitor on-scene times of responding units. They do this to assure the responders' safety or assistance while on scene. Most centers use a certain time period, possibly related to the type of event, as a cue. If a responder has been on the scene in excess of the allotted time, the dispatcher will attempt to contact the responders and verify their safety. If they cannot be contacted, additional personnel (usually law enforcement personnel) will be dispatched to assure their well-being.

15. Who decides which services are sent to a call?

This is essentially the calltaker's responsibility. Most EMS communications centers provide their personnel with basic guidelines or protocols to help determine an appropriate response. Certain situations, such as stabbings and assaults, require a law enforcement response in addition to the medical responders. Other situations, such as cardiac arrests, may require more personnel than those sent on the transport unit; thus, a fire unit or other support personnel may be sent. Some calls require that the a large number of advanced life support personnel be sent. Others may require only a nonemergency basic life support response. The key is the training and experience of the calltaker, whose goal is to assure an appropriate response for the patient and the safety of responding personnel.

16. How are dispatch protocols different from field protocols?

They are similar, yet different. They are similar in that they give the provider a consistent set of guidelines to apply to a given set of circumstances. They are different in that the circumstances and the information available to the provider vary dramatically. The field provider is afforded the luxury of multiple types of sensory input in evaluating a patient. The EMS calltaker has only one—hearing. The calltaker must make a decision based solely on the information presented to him over the phone. The calltaker cannot see it, cannot feel it, cannot smell it and cannot taste it. (Yes, even taste is used by the field provider.) Thus, dispatch protocols tend to be more conservative, opting for safety, expecting the worst, sending more resources rather than less in an uncertain situation. The difficult part is balancing the safe approach with the risks associated with sending too many resources.

17. What are the risks?
The risks of sending too many resources fall into two categories. First, there is the actual risk of injury or property damage. Emergency responses are dangerous and put people at risk. This includes responders, civilians, and patients who may suffer from actual, or even near-miss, vehicle accidents. The second category is more subtle. It is the risk of not having the right resource available for the real emergency. If we send too many resources to a call where they are not needed, they may not be available for the call in which they actually are needed. Other units must be dispatched from further away. What is the cost? Who pays for increased response times and possible increases in morbidity and mortality when it takes longer to get to a scene?

18. What is a "zero response time"?
"Zero response time" is a phrase used in conjunction with emergency medical dispatch (EMD) and PreArrival Instructions. A calltaker who is well trained in EMD can actually deliver care immediately to a patient by giving instructions to the caller on how to initiate care for the patient, even before response units are dispatched. This has been well documented and can even include such complicated medical procedures as cardiopulmonary resuscitation. Thus, in many situations, by instructing the caller to initiate treatment, medical care is provided to the patient with a zero response time.

19. Does EMD work all the time?
No. There are many factors that affect EMD outcomes. Even if everything goes just as it is supposed to, there are no guarantees. We have probably all heard the comment, "The procedure was a success, but the patient died." We can do every part of the EMD process correctly and still not save the patient. It is, however, the success that we are after, which will not happen unless we are willing to accept the failures too.

20. Are EMT-D and EMD the same thing?
No, they are not. EMT-D stands for Emergency Medical Techniciar—Defibrillator. This is an EMT who has received special training in the use of a cardiac defibrillator. This is a qualification for all field personnel. EMD, on the other hand, includes training and certification in the use of emergency medical dispatch protocols and procedures. This function is unique to dispatch.

21. What is "megahertz"?
A technical term used in identifying radio frequencies.

22. I have heard the terms "simplex" and "duplex" with reference to radios. What do they mean?
These terms refer to a type of radio communication. A simplex radio system is one that uses only one frequency both for transmitting and receiving communication. The obvious disadvantage of this type of system is that only one person can speak at a time. Simplex systems are now used primarily only for

situations where broadcasting a transmission is the purpose. In contrast, a duplex system uses one frequency to transmit and one frequency to receive. This kind of system allows two-way communication, much like a telephone.

23. **What does it mean when a radio system is "trunked"?**
This is a high-tech system that allows agencies to optimize the use of radio frequencies. With older technology, agencies were assigned to particular radio frequencies, and all their communications took place on those particular frequencies. Some agencies even shared the frequency with another. This generally meant one of two things: (1) Because the frequency was dedicated to a particular agency, any time that agency was not talking was "dead air." This was, in some respects, a waste of available air time on the particular frequency in a world that is using more and more forms of wireless communications. (2) One agency had to wait while another agency completed their business. This competition for air time occasionally delayed emergency communications.
"Trunked" radio is a solution to help rectify both these problems (dead air and delays). It is a fairly complicated process. Basically, the various radios in the system have the capability to function on a variety of frequencies. The radios are programmed to talk to a particular set of radios, and a computer manages frequency assignments. When one radio wants to "talk" to other radios, the computer determines which frequency is available. It then directs all the radios in the set to go to that frequency. The frequency assignment lasts only as long as the radio transmission, and the frequency is then made available for other radio sets. The reply to the original transmission may occur on the same, or more likely, a different frequency.
This is a very simple and superficial attempt at explaining trunked radio. You can probably see, however, that a computer system has the wherewithal to coordinate the communications of several groups of radios, minimizing dead air by allocating the time to live communications, and thus reducing the number of frequencies needed.

24. **What is CAD?**
CAD stands for Computer Aided Dispatch. There are many different systems in use around the country, but they all provide some common functions. They are a tool for dispatchers to use to keep track of EMS units and their status (whether available, out of service, or involved in a response). The systems keep track of call information, as defined by the agency. Most record location, callback number, type of problem, responding unit(s), relevant times, and a disposition for each call for service. Some are much more sophisticated, collecting much more information regarding individual calls. Some deal with unit positioning, response recommendations, and call loads per unit. Some systems have an integrated EMD system. Some systems have mapping capabilities, and some of those are integrated with Automatic Vehicle Location systems. Some are integrated with Mobile Data Terminals (MDTs) or Mobile Computer Terminals (MCTs) in the response units. There are far too many system designs to describe here. Each one is unique. If you have a CAD system and you really want to know more, go to your communications center and ask for a demonstration.

25. **Is CAD a good thing?**
CAD has mixed reviews. Some say that it actually lengthens the dispatch process because the calltaker has to type in all the information in the right place and in the right way, which takes too much time. They feel that the old way was better and faster. Others say that CAD allows them to ensure that the

dispatch information is accurate and complete, that there is virtually no potential for misunderstanding, and that the information can be transmitted to multiple dispatch centers simultaneously, actually improving the overall dispatch process.

26. **What does the dispatcher have to do with transport destinations?**

The transport destination for a field unit is generally determined by the field unit in conjunction with standing destination protocols and medical control personnel. There are some happenings that draw the communications center into the decision. First and perhaps most common is a change in hospital divert status. Hospitals may, for a variety of reasons, become unable to accept certain types of patients. If this happens before a transport occurs, it is the responsibility of the communications center to advise the transport unit of a divert status. This will allow the unit to change its destination in a timely manner and assure that the patient can receive proper care when it arrives.

The second situation is also quite common. By virtue of its view of "the bigger picture," the communications center is generally aware of significant events within the jurisdiction. If an event or other situation such as construction or traffic signal problems makes the preferred destination difficult or even impossible to access, the transport unit must be notified.

Finally, the communications center acts as a resource, especially in those situations in which a transport unit is unfamiliar with local destinations. This is perhaps most likely in mutual aid situations. The communications center can identify the nearest appropriate receiving facility and provide routing assistance.

27. **Do all dispatchers do the same thing?**

No. Some personnel in the dispatch center work only as calltakers. Some work only as dispatchers. Some do both. Some work only for a particular agency. Some provide services for multiple agencies. Some provide administrative support as well. The only way to know what the dispatchers in your center do is to ask.

28. **Why does the dispatcher not have better information to give me about the type of call?**

Telephone triage is a one-sense function. The only way a calltaker gets information about what is happening at a particular scene is by listening (hearing). He or she does not have the advantage of additional types of sensory input that field personnel have—sight, smell, touch, and even taste in some cases. Try to imagine what your patient "sounds" like, in most cases through the eyes and ears of a third party, an untrained, frightened caller. Complicate that situation with telephone static, slang or cultural words, and foreign language, and perhaps you can understand why what you responded to was not quite what you thought you were dispatched to.

29. **Why do dispatchers not answer the radio right away?**

Although it may seem like dispatchers have nothing to do but answer the radio, that is usually not the case. Although some centers have the resources to assign an individual to do nothing but handle radio traffic, most do not. Dispatchers have other responsibilities. Some monitor multiple radio channels, some are responsible for hospital notifications, some have administrative responsibilities, and some have to answer emergency telephone calls. If it is not an emergency, be patient. Dispatchers are listening (probably) and will get to you as soon as they can.

30. What do doctors have to do with dispatch?

Medical dispatch should have medical control, just like a field medical unit. It is important that emergency medical responses meet the standard of care for the community. This applies to both the types of resources that are sent and the way in which they are sent. It also applies to any directions that a calltaker may give to a caller or patient. The medical director for the medical dispatch center is responsible for assuring that the medical aspect of the dispatch services that are provided is appropriate.

31. Is a biophone like a telephone?

Kind of. In both cases, you use the phone to contact a particular resource to get help. With the biophone, you get a prehospital medical control person, usually based at a hospital. Even though the term includes the word "phone," it has become more broad in its definition to include both phone and radio media.

32. What is a "biocom"?

A "biocom" is essentially the radio version of a biophone. It was the term used when most field/hospital communications were accomplished via radio. That was before cellular phones. Now, with cellular communications, the majority of field/hospital communications is performed by cellphones with radio communication used as a backup.

33. What is telemetry?

Telemetry in EMS is generally the transmission of electrocardiograms (ECGs) via radio from field units to a hospital for assistance in ECG interpretation and treatment. Some systems around the country require the use of telemetry for all cardiac patients; some use it selectively for physician support in difficult situations; and some systems do not use it at all, relying on the training and judgment of field personnel. The increasing utilization of field cardiac monitors capable of high-quality 12-lead ECGs is resurrecting the use of telemetry. Quality ECGs from the field may allow for the field use of thrombolytic therapy or the prearrival activation of cardiac catheterization teams in the setting of the acute myocardial infarction.

Pearls and Pitfalls

1. Prearrival instructions start the process of medical care before help arrives on scene, including procedures such as cardiopulmonary resuscitation.
2. Dispatch protocols, procedures, and instructions should have physician oversight.
3. 911 is intended to be the nationwide emergency telephone number.
4. Enhanced 911 (E911) has the added benefit of automatically identifying the caller's telephone number and the address associated with that number.
5. Although much of the landline telephone service in the United States is covered by 911 service, many rural areas as well as cellular phone and voice-over Internet users do not have adequate access to 911 or E911.

References

1. The Associated Public Communications Officers, Inc. The associated public safety communications officers: The public safety communications standard operating procedure manual, 22nd ed. New Smyrna Beach, FL: 1990.

2. Clawson JJ. Quality assurance: A priority for medical dispatch. Emerg Med Serv 18:53–63, 1989.
3. Culley LL, Clark JJ, Eisenberg MS, et al. Dispatcher-assisted telephone CPR: Common delays and time standards for delivery. Ann Emerg Med 20:362–366, 1991.
4. Curka PA, Pepe PE, Ginger VF, et al. Emergency medical services priority dispatch. Ann Emerg Med 22:1688–1695, 1993.
5. McMillian J, Rhett JR. The Primer of Public Safety Telecommunications Systems. New Smyrna Beach, FL,: The APCO Institute, 1990.
6. Steele S. Emergency Dispatching: A Medical Communicator's Guide. Englewood Cliffs, NJ: Prentice Hall, 1993.

Destination Guidelines and Hospital Designation

CHAPTER 5

Catherine B. Custalow, MD, PhD

1. **Besides the EMT's ability to assess and treat patients, what else may have a positive effect on the patient's outcome?**
   In addition to providing the necessary treatment, based on your patient assessment(s), the choice of destination (hospital) for the patient can be a very important decision. In communities with only one hospital, the choice is easy. In EMS systems that have more than one hospital facility to choose from, the patient should be taken to the hospital that can best provide the required services based on the patient's current medical needs.

2. **I work in an EMS system that has more than one hospital located within its service area. How do I know which hospital to take my patients to?**
   Some hospitals have the ability to provide specialized services (e.g., trauma surgery, stroke care, interventional cardiac care, etc.), whereas others may not be able to provide the same services or may not have them immediately available when needed. Your EMS system should have protocols in place for identifying which hospitals have specialized services available, when those services are available, and which patients, based on your assessment, qualify for transport to those facilities directly, even if it means bypassing other, closer hospitals.

3. **Are there any national or state guidelines to help identify hospitals that provide specialized services?**
   Several organizations (such as the American Burn Association and the American College of Surgeons Committee on Trauma) have developed guidelines and recommendations that describe the equipment, facilities, and personnel that are needed to provide optimal care for victims of burn or trauma. These organizations also provide a rigorous on-site review process to verify the preparedness of the hospital that desires to be identified as a specialty care center.

4. **What factors determine whether a trauma patient should be transported emergently to a trauma center?**
   There are various organizations (such as the American College of Emergency Physicians and the American College of Surgeons) that have published prehospital triage criteria for evaluating trauma patients. Although there are minor differences among them, all the organizations agree on the key determinants for identifying patients with a high risk for serious injury. Listed below are injuries and mechanisms of injury (MOI) commonly recognized as indicators of serious injury. All patients determined to be emergent trauma patients (patients with suspected serious injuries) should be transported immediately to the highest-ranking available trauma center.

   Injuries
   Significant blunt trauma with unstable vital signs
   Penetrating trauma to head, thorax, abdomen, neck, or proximal extremities

Altered level of consciousness (mentation) or abnormal neurologic status after trauma
- Glasgow Coma Scale ≤ 13
- Seizure activity
- Sensory or motor deficit

Flail chest

Pelvic fractures

Open or suspected depressed skull fracture

Spinal cord injury with neurologic deficit

Multiple long-bone fractures

Amputation

Burns involving > 15% of total body surface area or involving face, airway

Any trauma in the presence of the following:
- History of serious medical conditions (e.g., coronary artery disease, chronic obstructive pulmonary disease, bleeding disorder, etc.)
- Age >55 years
- Hypothermia
- Burns
- Pregnancy

Mechanism of Injury (MOI)

Auto-pedestrian hit at > 20 mph or victim thrown 15 feet or more

Falls > 20 feet

Death of occupant in the same vehicle

Ejection from vehicle

Automobile accident with significant intrusion into the passenger compartment

Motorcycle accident > 20 mph or with separation of rider from bike

Significant bicycle or all-terrain vehicle impact

5. We have a level I trauma center in our EMS system's service area. Who designates it a level I trauma center and how is it different from either a level II, level III, or level IV trauma center?

Trauma facilities are designated as level I to IV (and in some states I to V) after a thorough application and review process by an organization such as the American College of Surgeons Committee on Trauma (ACS-COT) or a designated state process. Level I trauma centers must have in-house general surgery, neurosurgery, emergency medicine, and anesthesia services available 24 hours a day, as well as many other surgical and medical subspecialties on call and promptly available. Level I facilities must also have a trauma research program and active teaching programs. Level I trauma centers do not have the same research or teaching requirements and are not required to have as many subspecialties on call. Level III trauma centers must have 24-hour emergency services but are not required to have in-house surgical services available 24 hours a day. Level IV trauma centers are primarily rural hospitals that stabilize a patient in anticipation of transfer to a higher-level trauma center.

35

6. **We have two different hospitals in our EMS system service area that we deliver patients to. One of the hospitals advertises itself as a pediatric trauma center, whereas the other hospital calls itself a trauma center with pediatric commitment. What is the difference between a pediatric trauma center and a trauma center with pediatric commitment?**
   A pediatric trauma center is a children's hospital that meets level I trauma center designation criteria, with a pediatric ED, ICU, and trauma service having appropriate personnel, equipment, and facilities to meet the needs of an injured child. A trauma center with pediatric commitment is a general hospital that meets level I or II trauma center criteria for adults and has the capabilities and commitment to care for pediatric trauma patients as well as adult trauma patients.

7. **Does trauma care in rural areas differ from that in urban areas?**
   Yes. Trauma care in rural areas and other sparsely populated areas is first challenged by a decrease in available medical resources. Other challenges include the distance from the scene to the trauma care facilities, the surrounding terrain, and the occurrence of accidents in isolated and wilderness areas. Motor vehicle collisions may go unrecognized for long periods of time in sparsely populated areas. Each EMS agency should have predetermined protocols for how and where to transport patients from all locations within their jurisdiction.

8. **When should a helicopter be dispatched directly to the scene to transport a patient?**
   There are various guidelines available for the dispatching of an air medical team to a scene. An example would be the trauma patient assessed at the scene and suspected of having critical injuries. Trauma patients with critical injuries need to be transported to a level I or level II trauma center as quickly as possible. An air medical team should be dispatched, if available, when transportation time by ground to the trauma center is more than 15 minutes; when ground transport time would result in the patient getting to an appropriate facility later than if AMT is used; in wilderness areas with difficult access; or when ground ambulance access is impeded by road conditions, weather, or traffic. (See Chapter 77, Air Medical Design and Configuration, for additional information.)

9. **What are the destination guidelines for patients with extremity amputations?**
   Although most amputations are very visually impressive and attention grabbing, always address and treat life-threatening conditions before focusing on the amputation. Also, if the patient has multiple injuries, transport him or her immediately to the highest-level trauma center available. Patients with proximal finger or extremity amputations should be taken to the nearest facility with replantation capabilities. Exceptions to this destination choice may include patients with toe amputations or distal finger amputations that occur at or beyond the distal-phalangeal joint. These patients may not be candidates for replantation of the amputated part. Treat every amputated part as if it will be replanted, with urgent transport and appropriate handling of the amputated part.

10. **How are destinations assigned during a mass casualty?**
    Whenever possible, the goal of any mass casualty or multiple-patient situation is to distribute patients to all available hospitals capable of providing the needed services and avoid overloading any one hospital. Most EMS systems have protocols in place that address mass casualty and multiple-patient situations. Critical patients should be transported to and distributed among the hospitals that have the services needed to care for the patient's condition. For example, critical trauma patients should be transported to and distributed initially among the level I and level II trauma centers, whereas patients with less serious injuries should be directed to nontrauma centers.

11. **When should burn patients be taken to a hospital with a burn center?**
    Burn patients benefit greatly from transport or early transfer to hospitals with established burn centers. The following criteria may be used as guidelines in helping to determine which patients could benefit the most from treatment at an established burn center.
    - Second- or third-degree burns involving >10% of total body surface area (BSA) in patients <10 or >50 years of age
    - Burns involving >20% BSA in all age groups
    - Third-degree burns involving >5% BSA
    - Inhalation injury
    - Circumferential burns
    - High-voltage electrical burns
    - Severe chemical burns

12. **What are the guidelines for the destination of patients with medical emergencies?**
    All emergent medical patients (e.g., acute myocardial infarction, cardiac arrest, massive gastrointestinal hemorrhage, etc.) should go to the nearest hospital as a general rule. Nonemergent medical patients may go to the hospital requested by the patient, family, or private physician as long as the EMS service is capable of honoring that request. In certain metropolitan areas some hospitals have been designated cardiac hospitals or stroke hospitals. These hospitals should be considered as the appropriate destination for medical patients who appear to be having an acute myocardial infarction or stroke. Each EMS system should have specific protocols for those medical conditions that may benefit from direct transport to a designated specialty hospital.

13. **Should patients with significant carbon monoxide exposure be taken to the nearest hospital or are there specialized services necessary to treat these patients?**
    Patients with signs of significant carbon monoxide exposure that include loss of consciousness, altered mental status, seizures, and dysrhythmias, as well as those who are pregnant, should be taken directly to a hospital with a hyperbaric oxygen chamber, if possible. The only exception is the patient with burns and smoke inhalation associated with multisystem trauma who instead should go the highest level trauma center available in order to deal with the major injuries first.

14. **We have a natural clear water lake in our EMS system service area that is more than 80 feet deep. Each year the lake attracts a significant number of scuba divers during the summer months. Do destinations differ for victims of scuba-diving accidents?**
    Victims of diving accidents with symptoms suggesting air embolism or decompression sickness require treatment in a hyperbaric oxygen chamber. Whenever possible, symptomatic scuba-diving accident patients should be taken immediately to a facility with a hyperbaric oxygen chamber (see Chapter 70, Decompression Illnesses).

15. **What should I do when a hospital is on divert or ambulance bypass, particularly if I have a patient in cardiac arrest?**
    As a general rule, a hospital's divert status should be honored and the patient transported to another facility. Ideally, cardiac arrests should go to the nearest hospital, regardless of an active divert status. In

reality, if the patient has not been resuscitated in the field, there is very little likelihood of being resuscitated at the hospital. Thus, there should be little impact on the limited resources.

16. **Can a physician at the scene alter our EMS system's destination guidelines?**
    A physician at the scene should not be allowed to change the destination as determined in accordance with your EMS agency's established protocol unless the destination change is approved by the base-station (on-line) physician. In addition, if an on-scene physician wishes to intervene, the physician should be advised that he or she will need to accompany the patient in the ambulance from the scene to the hospital.

Pearls and Pitfalls

1. Patient outcome may be determined by proper choice of hospital destination.
2. Seriously injured trauma patients should be taken to a designated trauma center.
3. Helicopter aeromedical transport is a valuable and scarce resource that should be used only when absolutely necessary.
4. Be aware of unique specialty care hospitals in your community and transport patients appropriately.
5. In a disaster or mass casualty incident (MCI), do not overload any one hospital when other hospital destinations are an option.
6. Memorize and always follow your destination protocols.

References

1. Mechem CC. Emergency medical services. In Tintinalli's Emergency Medicine: A Comprehensive Study Guide, 7th ed., Tintinalli JE, Stapczynski J, Ma OJ et al, eds., pp. 1–4. New York: McGraw-Hill, 2011.
2. Stone CK, Thomas SH. Air medical transport. In Emergency Medicine: A Comprehensive Study Guide, 7th ed., Tintinalli JE, Stapczynski J, Ma OJ et al, eds., pp. 11–15. New York: McGraw-Hill, 2011.
3. Legome EL, Rosen P. General principles of trauma. In Harwood-Nuss' The Clinical Practice of Emergency Medicine, 5th ed., Wolfson AB, Hendey GW. Ling LJ, et al., eds., pp. 126–134. Philadelphia: Lippincott-Williams & Wilkins, 2010.
4. Centers for Disease Control and Prevention. Guidelines for field triage of injured patients; recommendations of the National Expert Panel on Field Triage. MMRW Recomm Rep 58(RR01):1–35, 2009.
5. Salomone JP, Pons PT. PHTLS: PreHospital Trauma Life Support, 7th ed. St. Louis: Mosby JEMS, 2011.

Documentation

CHAPTER 6

Arthur Hsieh, MA, NREMT-P

1. **Why is documentation so important? Shouldn't the quality of care I provide to my patients be the most important?**

   You are right—the best protection you have against losing a lawsuit is effective, appropriate, and timely health care. The question is, how would you, a judge, or a jury know what health care you provided one, two, even five years after the incident? It is extremely unlikely that you will recall the fine details of a case after a few days or weeks, let alone years down the road. So your ability to document your findings and treatment is critical to help you remember such events.

   There's another reason for quality documentation. As a paramedic working in an EMS system, you are the entry point into the health care continuum. Your patient will likely see many more links in this chain—the emergency department staff, physicians, and allied health professionals such as respiratory or physical therapists. Your documentation provides them with the necessary information about what transpired at the onset of the patient's care. Your documentation serves as the basis for understanding what happened.

2. **What concepts serve as the foundation to quality documentation?**

   Start with the basics of good *writing*. Following these guidelines will help you to create a quality document:

   - Use black or blue ink to document. These colors photocopy better than lighter ones.
   - *Think*. Spend a few moments reviewing your findings and treatment before you begin writing. It will help you organize your approach and save you time later on.
   - Use a consistent method of charting. If you approach your narrative the same way each time, it will become easier and faster to remember what you found and did. Several approaches are detailed as follows (see question 6).
   - Print neatly. If you are using an electronic patient care record (PCR) device this is not an issue. If, however, you do not have access to an electronic record, you will need to put pen to paper and write. Your writing should be easily readable by anyone who reviews your PCR. For most of us, that means printing in block letters, not script. Sadly, bad handwriting is not limited to physicians.
   - Spell correctly. It reduces confusion by the reader and presents you in a professional, intelligent manner.
   - Use standard English. This means complete sentences, with correct punctuation and grammar. Writing correctly will also present your documented care in a professional appearance. Use simple sentences. Avoid medical jargon or colloquial slang.
   - Proofread your work. When you are done writing, review what you wrote. Does it make sense? Does it accurately reflect what transpired on the call? If you are not sure, have a crew member or partner

review your writing for accuracy and clarity. If you need to correct what you wrote, neatly strike out your mistake with a single line and initial the strikeout.
- Close your narrative. If any space exists on the PCR after you complete your narrative, cross it out to show the reader that you are in fact done with your documentation.

3. **I just remembered something about the patient's care, but I am done with the narrative. How do I add it?**
For any addendum writing, clearly indicate the new section was added after the fact. You can do this by beginning the new section with a phrase such as "Addendum:" and initialing the section after you are done. You should also write down the date and time of the addition.

4. **How should I fill out the check box sections?**
- PCRs are often constructed of a combination of both check boxes and narrative sections.
- Fill in all check boxes. Leaving any blank may imply to the reader that you either (a) missed it, (b) did not do it, or (c) intentionally omitted it.
- If there is a section on the PCR that did not pertain to the patient's care, strike out the box or section and write "N/A" (Not Applicable) next to it.
- If you make a mistake on a check box, neatly strike out the wording and box with one line and initial the change.

5. **I might have made a mistake during my care. What do I do?**
Recognize that mistakes occur in medicine. Providing care is not an exact science; that is why it is called the "practice" of medicine. The bottom line is that it is better to document the mistake clearly rather than omitting it from the PCR. The courts are much more forgiving of an admitted mistake, compared to finding out later about an omitted mistake.

6. **There is so much information to record. How do I keep all of it organized?**
There are several formats to use when organizing medical information. Regardless of which one you select, use it consistently.

CHART format

C = **C**hief complaint—the reason EMS was summoned

H = History—(using the SAMPLE mnemonic)

    S = Sym**p**toms—(using OPQRST mnemonic)

        O: Onset—what was happening at the time of the event

        P: Provocation/Palliation—what makes the discomfort better or worse

        Q: Quality—a subjective description of the discomfort

        R: Region/radiation/related symptoms—the location of the discomfort; any extension of the discomfort; and any related symptoms

        S: Severity—how significant is the discomfort

        T: Time—how long has the event been happening

    A: Allergies to prescription or over-the-counter (OTC) medications, food, environment

    M: Medications the patient is taking (prescription, OTC, herbal)

P: Pertinent medical history

L: Last oral intake

E: Event leading up to the injury or illness

A = (Physical) **A**ssessment: using one of the following approaches:
- Head-to-toe approach
- System-by-system approach
- Primary and secondary assessment approach

R = **R**x = Treatment: following a protocol template
- Detailed listing of the treatment in accordance with the accepted protocol
- Evaluation or response to each element of treatment

T = **T**ransport and **T**ransfer (using the *TTFN* acronym)
- *T*o—who received the patient, and what facility
- *T*ime—of transfer of care to the receiving facility
- *F*luids—type and volume of any fluids received by the patient
- *N*ecessary status update—on the patient condition

SOAP(IER) format

S = **S**ubjective information: chief complaint and patient history

    S—Symptoms: (using OPQRST mnemonic)

        O—Onset

        P—Provocation/palliation

        Q—Quality

        R—Region/radiation/related symptoms

        S—Severity

        T—Time

    A—Allergies

    M—Medications

    P—Past medical history

    L—Last oral intake

    E—Event leading to injury/illness

O = **O**bjective information: physical assessment appropriate for the patient
- Head-to-toe approach
- System-by-system approach
- Primary and secondary assessment approach

A/P = **A**nalysis of assessment and **p**rotocol used for treatment

I/E = **I**mplementation of protocol and **E**valuation of treatment
- Chronological listing of treatment provided based on accepted protocol
- Evaluation or response to each element of treatment

EMS – Overview, Design, and Operations

R = Report (using the *TTFN* acronym)
- *T*o—who received the patient, and what facility
- *Ti*me—of transfer of care to the receiving facility
- *Fl*uids—type and volume of any fluids received by the patient
- *Ne*cessary status update—on the patient's condition

7. How do I record what the patient tells me?
Subjective information should be documented using the patient's words, as you cannot see the patient's symptoms directly. Using phrases such as "Patient states that…." or "Police on scene report that…" will tell the reader that you are reporting what was said to you and not directly observed. If a patient states a negative response to a question, record it in the following fashion: "Patient denies any allergies to medicine."

8. How do I record my physical findings?
Objective information should be recorded in a professional, orderly fashion using a neutral tone. Document the patient's behavior in a nonjudgmental fashion. For example, stating that the patient was "drunk" or "intoxicated" is not as accurate as "Patient has alcohol on his breath, slurred speech, and appears to have a staggering gait."

9. Can I abbreviate my documentation to save time and space?
Yes, but use only *approved* abbreviations. Using ones that you make up may be confusing to the reader. In addition the Joint Commission on Accreditation of Hospitals (JCAHO) has a list of "Do Not Use" abbreviations because they lead to confusion (Table 6.1).

10. When should I document? Can it wait until the end of the shift?
No. If you delay the documentation of the incident, you run the risk of forgetting potentially key aspects of the assessment or treatment you rendered. In addition, most EMS systems require that you leave a copy of the PCR with the patient or medical staff prior to leaving the hospital.

Pearls and Pitfalls

1. Be concise, as there is not a lot of space on the PCR to write on. Brevity is key while including all available information.
2. Check your spelling. There are several electronic medical dictionaries that can be downloaded to a personal digital assistant or smartphone. Alternatively, an old-fashioned pocket dictionary will do. Regardless, carry one to help you correctly spell medical terms.
3. Patient refusals of medical care carry the highest legal risk to the paramedic. Make sure that you clearly document that the patient:
   - was advised that the refusal of medical care or transport might result in an adverse outcome, up to and including death.
   - was advised to seek further medical care and call the EMS system at any time.
   - understood and was able to repeat back to you the warnings you just provided.

   Secure all signatures on the form that are required, such as the patient's and any bystanders.
4. If it was not written, it was not done. This is a basic tenet of patient documentation, so, if in doubt, document.

TABLE 6.1A: JCAHO "Do Not Use" List of Abbreviations*

Do Not Use	Potential Problem	Use Instead
U (unit) IU (International Unit) Q.D., QD, q.d., qd (daily)	Mistaken for "0" (zero), the number "4" (four) or "cc" Mistaken for IV (intravenous) or the number 10 (ten)	Write "unit" Write "International Unit" Write "daily"
Q.O.D., QOD, q.o.d, qod (every other day)	Mistaken for each other Period after the Q mistaken for "I" and the "O" mistaken for "I"	Write "every other day"
Trailing zero (X.0 mg)† Lack of leading zero (.X mg)	Decimal point is missed	Write X mg Write 0.X mg
MS MSO4 and MgSO4	Can mean morphine sulfate or magnesium sulfate Confused for one another	Write "morphine sulfate" Write "magnesium sulfate"

*Applies to all orders and all medication-related documentation that is handwritten (including free-text computer entry) or on preprinted forms.

†*Exception:* A "trailing zero" may be used only where required to demonstrate the level of precision of the value being reported, such as for laboratory results, imaging studies that report size of lesions, or catheter/tube sizes. It may not be used in medication orders or other medication-related documentation.

TABLE 6.1B: Additional Abbreviations, Acronyms, and Symbols** for *possible* future inclusion in the official "Do Not Use" list

Do Not Use	Potential Problem	Use Instead
> (greater than) < (less than)	Misinterpreted as the number "7" (seven) or the letter "L."	Write "greater than" Write "less than"
Abbreviations for drug names	Misinterpreted due to similar abbreviations for multiple drugs	Write drug names in full
Apothecary units	Unfamiliar to many practitioners Confused with metric units	Use metric units
@	Mistaken for the number "2"	Write "at"
cc	Mistaken for U (units) when poorly written	Write "mL" or "milliliters"
μg	Mistaken for mg (milligrams) resulting in a 1000-fold overdose	Write "mcg" or "micrograms"

*For *possible* future inclusion in the official "Do Not Use" list.

References

1. Cone DC, Kim DT, Davidson SJ. Patient-initiated refusals of prehospital care: ambulance call report documentation, patient outcome, and on-line medical command. Prehosp Disaster Med 10(1):3–9, 1995.

2. Graham, D. The Missing Protocol—A Legally Defensible Report. Ashton. MD: Clemens Publishing, 1999.
3. Joint Commission of Accreditation of Hospital Organizations. Do Not Use List. http://www.jointcommission.org/PatientSafety/DoNotUseList/accessed 3/31/07.
4. Selden BS, Schnitzer PG, Nolan FX. Medicolegal documentation of prehospital triage. Ann Emerg Med 19(5): 547–551, 1990.
5. Weaver J, Brinsfield KH, Dalphond D. Prehospital refusal-of-transport policies: Adequate legal protection? Prehosp Emerg Care 4(1 :53–56, 2000.

Medicolegal Issues

S. Scott Henderson, Esq.

CHAPTER 7

1. **Can I practice my entire career and never be sued?**
   Sure you can. Emergency medical services (EMS) personnel enjoy, by and large, a fine reputation in the community for the care and treatment they render. Especially since 9/11/01, the public recognizes the perilous nature of the types of calls to which our emergency personnel respond and, properly, respects them for that and the hazards implicit in their work environment. The public, from whom the jury will be selected to hear a given case, will most likely presume certain things that make a verdict for the defense more likely. They will acknowledge that EMS personnel are putting their lives on the line every single shift; that the mission of EMS personnel is to serve the public and to try to prevent or reduce human suffering; that, even though a bad outcome may occur, the EMS team was most likely trying its best to save lives and help the patient.

2. **If I do make a mistake, will I get sued?**
   The answer is maybe. If a blatant error is made, it is the EMS service or employer that is the most likely entity to be sued. Historically, it has been unlikely that an individual paramedic or EMT is sued in his or her personal capacity since the medical error would have occurred within the course and scope of the provider's employment and, therefore, the employer or agency would be considered responsible under the legal theory of *respondeat superior* (a Latin phrase and legal maxim that means "let the master answer for the actions of the servant"). A major reason that the employer would be sued rather than the employee is because the employer has the insurance or assets to satisfy any judgment entered as a result of a jury verdict. Most individual EMS providers do not have the "deep pockets" necessary to satisfy a judgment for a substantial negligently-caused injury to a patient. By the same token, if the EMS service is governmental, the local or regional governmental entity will also likely be named in the suit. This is not to say that an individual EMT or physician director will never be named in the suit; however, it is much less likely to occur.

3. **Sometimes the patient has a bad outcome despite my efforts. Will that get me sued?**
   The fastest way to assure that a patient or family will call a lawyer is to stop talking to them when a bad outcome occurs. Health care providers often are too busy to spend enough time to explain the unavoidability of all adverse outcomes to patients and relatives. It is human nature to attempt to avoid dealing with problems or failures and, therefore, sometimes providers "stick their heads in the sand" when a bad outcome occurs or a mistake has been made. It is important to engage the patient and the family soon after an unexpected adverse outcome, but this generally should be done by a medical director, supervisor, or risk manager. You should discuss with your supervisors and medical director just how such a situation should be handled so that, just as your system's other medical protocols, this is clear in your mind well in advance of confronting your first such event.

4. What can I do to try to prevent a lawsuit?

The simple truth is that health care providers who have the best bedside manner or people skills and keep talking to their patients even when adversity strikes have fewer lawsuits filed against them. Good bedside manner is akin to the good manners that result in smooth interpersonal interactions, causing less friction and confrontation than abrasive words or conduct. Abrasiveness communicates that the health care provider is too busy to listen and respond to the needs of the person for whom professional services are provided. Offensive behavior attracts criticism, anger, and lawsuits.

5. What else can I do to minimize my risk of being sued?

The single most important step you can take to avoid being sued is to try your best to always do what's right for the patient. The next most important step is to document your care thoroughly. Medical malpractice cases are often referred to as "records cases." This means that, from the plaintiff's lawyer's viewpoint, there must be documentary evidence of the breach of the standard of care, either in the form of a documented wrongful act or evidence of an omission. The documented wrongful act may be clear and obvious, although the lawsuit may still be hotly contested. For example, the omission is identified by a document that fails to show that a neurologic exam was performed before a patient at risk of head injury was released and not transported, for example. Remember the saying, "if it wasn't documented, it wasn't done." Although we know sometimes important things are done that do not get documented, you will make a more convincing case for the jury when the record clearly documents that the reasonable and appropriate steps that measure up to the standard of care expected for the type of call were taken.

6. How extensive should the documentation be?

Although not all care is documented, the essential information must be recorded. Do not forget to document the "pertinent positives" and the "pertinent negatives." Sometimes the pace of EMS moves so quickly that important care that was rendered does not always make it onto the chart. However, you may count on spending considerable time in deposition and in the courtroom while the plaintiff's lawyer highlights the void in the record and grills the hapless medical witness or defendant. The lawyer will resonate the phrase, "If it's not documented, it wasn't done," in the courtroom. Although a failure to document can sometimes be defended through testimony that the provider's custom, pattern, habit, and practice is to *always* perform a particular examination or test for a patient with the particular complaint at issue, a jury may view such statements as self-serving and not be persuaded.

By contrast, the medical record that is painstakingly complete and well-documented may signal a plaintiff's lawyer to decline to pursue the case. Three factors provide good reasons for declining to accept a potential medical negligence case:

1. If the history is complete, even if it is factually wrong but shows that time and effort were taken to acquire it.
2. If the physical examination is thorough and not filled with routine, stock phrases, and is instead tailored to the individual patient.
3. If the assessment and plan are reasonable given what was known or, in the exercise of the reasonable practice of medicine, what should have been known, and they meet generally accepted policies or protocols.

Medicolegal Issues

7. **What is the statute of limitations for a medical negligence case?**
   The time frame within which a medical negligence suit must be filed or else barred forever is the statute of limitations and varies from state to state. You must check the law of your own state to know the answer to this question. The statute of limitations is usually longer than your memory is clear, so it is a good medical record that will help you recall the facts, fill in the gaps in your memory, and help you the most if a lawsuit ever is filed. Disciplined, thorough recordkeeping can often demonstrate that the standard of care was met, which means that the odds of ever having to get to the issues of causation and damages are substantially less.

8. **What are the elements of a medical negligence case?**
   There are four elements to a negligence claim; duty, breach, causation, and damages. In medical negligence cases, we use a shorthand term combining duty and breach of duty and call it "standard of care violation." Thus, in medical malpractice cases, there are three legal elements to the claim. The plaintiff has the burden to prove (a) violation of the standard of care, (b) causation, and (c) injuries, losses, or damages.

9. **What constitutes a "violation of the standard of care"?**
   The issue of whether the health care provider violated the standard of care is a question of fact for a jury to decide. Generally, when a patient accepts the offer of health care delivery from a health care provider, a legal duty to provide reasonable care arises. The duty to meet the standard of care requires that the health care provider give that degree of care based upon the health care provider's knowledge, skill, training, education, and experience that any reasonable health care provider, similarly trained, would provide under the same or similar circumstances. This "reasonable health care provider" measure of appropriate conduct, in your case, is what the reasonable and prudent EMS provider would do, or not do, when confronted with what you were doing. A standard-of-care violation is proved by expert testimony. The plaintiff is required to call a person whom the court accepts as an expert in EMS care who has more than a casual familiarity with your level of training to testify that the care was substandard or did not meet the applicable standard of care for that level of training. The defense can then cross-examine the plaintiff's expert and may also call its own expert to testify that the standard of care was met—that is, the care was acceptable. If an EMS provider violates his or her own department's policies, procedures, or protocols, or national protocols when they apply, it becomes much easier and less a matter of opinion to prove the first required element of the medical negligence case—standard of care violation. Therefore, you should always follow applicable policies, procedures, and protocols as they are there for a reason—good patient care—and provide a good defense to a lawsuit.

10. **Does "standard of care" apply to prehospital providers like it does doctors and nurses?**
    Absolutely. The anatomy of a medical negligence case is the same regardless of whether the defendant is a doctor, nurse, paramedic, or emergency medical technician (EMT) The jury will be asked to determine what the reasonable health care provider with the same level of expertise would have done under the same or similar circumstances. An important point is what is meant by the phrase, "the same or similar circumstances." The answer to the question is dramatically affected by the yardstick that is used to measure the conduct. If the site of the alleged wrong is a small community, the defense will want the defendant to be held accountable to the level of care customarily provided in that community; thus, the "community standard" or the "locality rule." On the other hand, because a national standard of care

may be more clearly defined and be more stringent, the plaintiff will most likely argue that a national standard is appropriate.

The plaintiff will also argue that the national standard is appropriate if the health care provider is certified by a nationally recognized standard such as the National Registry of Emergency Medical Technicians. Consideration of this issue is important because a rural health care provider who is certified to a national standard will be held to the same standard as an urban provider who may have had the opportunity to amass much more experience and have the benefit of a more comprehensive continuing medical education program to keep skills refreshed.

11. What is causation?

Although negligence is shown when the jury is persuaded that the defendant health care provider violated the standard of care, it is not enough for the lawyer simply to show negligent conduct. Causation must be satisfied. It is necessary to demonstrate that the violation of standard of care is what caused the patient's damages. This is often where medical negligence cases are most successfully defended. For example, the patient's preexisting medical history may be responsible for the patient's injuries rather than any negligence on the part of the health care provider.

12. How hard is it to show causation?

Causation is complicated and tricky. Although there may be "cause in fact," it does not necessarily follow that the law will recognize legal cause, meaning legal liability. "Legal cause" takes one of two forms: (a) "but for" causation and (b) "substantial factor" causation.

"But for" causation means that the defendant's conduct caused the harm to the patient in a natural and probable sequence of events, the cascade of which flowed directly from the defendant's wrongful conduct and would not have occurred "but for" the defendant's culpable behavior. Simply put, the plaintiff must prove that the injuries would not have occurred but for the negligent act or omission of the defendant.

"Substantial factor" causation arises when two or more concurrent causes exist, any one of which is sufficient to bring about the damaging result. In such instances, causation is satisfied if any defendant's action or failure to act was a substantial factor in producing the harm.

The existence of caustion is a question for the jury to decide. Causation is also presented to the jury by expert witness testimony rendering the opinion that the standard-of-care violation did, indeed, cause the plaintiff's injuries by either of the methods described above. The defense attorney again has an opportunity to cross-examine the plaintiff's expert(s) and present expert testimony from his or her own expert(s) to defend against the element of causation. By way of illustration, in Colorado, the following jury instructions are given to the jury by the court for use in determining whether causation is satisfied.

9:18 Cause When Only One Cause Is Alleged—Defined
The word "cause" as used in these instructions means an act or failure to act which in natural and probable sequence produced the claimed injury. It is a cause without which the claimed injury would not have happened.

9:19 Concurrent Causes
More than one person may be responsible for causing injuries, losses or damages. If you find that the defendant was negligent and that his negligence caused injury, losses or damages to the plaintiff, it is not a defense that some third person's negligence might also have been a cause of the injuries, losses or damages.

13. What legal damages may a plaintiff recover?

It is not sufficient to simply claim that damages occurred. Actual injuries or losses must be shown, and it is these actual losses that are compensable. In other words, actual harm must exist that likely resulted from the wrongful conduct. In medical negligence cases, a plaintiff may generally recover two forms of damages; economic damages and noneconomic damages. Economic damages consist of things such as medical and rehabilitation expenses, lost wages, loss of earning capacity and out-of-pocket expenses. Noneconomic damages consist of things such as pain and suffering, emotional distress, impairment of the quality of life, grief, inconvenience, embarrassment, humiliation and loss of enjoyment of life. Physical impairment and disfigurement are also compensable damages. Punitive or exemplary damages are very rarely an issue in medical negligence cases.

14. Must the defendant prove that he or she was not negligent?

No. It is the plaintiff's obligation to prove the required elements of a lawsuit by the required level of proof in order to prevail. Medical negligence cases, also known as medical malpractice cases, are civil cases, not criminal. In criminal cases, the burden of proof requires that each of the elements consituting a crime be proved by the prosecution "beyond a reasonable doubt." In a civil case like a medical malpractice case, the burden of proof is on the plaintiff to prove each of the three elements of this negligence action "by a preponderance of the evidence." Words and phrases that connote that the preponderance of the evidence is satisfied include "likely," "probable," "more likely than not" and, in some states, "to a reasonable degree of medical probability" or "to a reasonable degree of medical certainty." These terms mean that each of the three elements of a negligence claim must be proved to the 51% standard of probability: the jury must be persuaded that the plaintiff has prevailed on each element in even a slightly more convincing way than not. The defendant prevails if the jury concludes the plaintiff failed to prove any of the required elements by a preponderance of the evidence.

15. Should a notice that I have to give a deposition frighten me?

No. Most of the time, you will just be a fact witness, but if you are a defendant, you will not have to go it alone. You would be represented by a malpractice defense attorney selected by your employer's insurance carrier who will walk you through the process and prepare you for the questions, medical issues, and factual matters that will be explored in the deposition. You will have reviewed the case and will be familiar with the records and questions regarding the care provided. Also, if you simply tell the truth, a deposition is an easy process to get through. There are three good reasons why depositions are taken during the discovery phase of a lawsuit: (a) to discover the facts and who has them, (b) to pin down the witness to hold them to the story, and (c) to assess the credibility of the witness and estimate how a jury is likely to respond to the testimony. This final analysis is particularly important when the plaintiff's lawyer deposes the defendant health care provider. The demeanor of the defendant is one part of the equation that enters into the valuation of the case and whether the case should be tried or settled. As in all aspects of life, "nice people" are generally treated better than others. An EMT or paramedic who is arrogant, self-righteous, and egotistical is an inviting target for the plaintiff's lawyer; the lawyer will try to cast him or her as uncaring, cavalier, and disrespectful to his or her patients and try to get the defendant to show those traits in front of the jury. By contrast, the plaintiff's attorney will lose credibility by trying to paint a courteous, compassionate, and soft-spoken provider as a callous person. Remember, a jury is probably going to be on your side because of the public service you provide to the community.

EMS – Overview, Design, and Operations

You just have to give them no reasons to change that point of view, so a nonconfrontational, honest, and professional demeanor will serve you well.

16. What are DNRs, living wills, and durable powers of attorney?
So-called DNRs (do-not-resuscitate orders), living wills, and durable powers of attorney are laws enacted by state legislatures; thus they vary from state to state. As a result, the appropriate statutes in a particular jurisdiction must be carefully examined. These statutes go by various names. For instance, in Colorado, the relevant statutes are (a) the Colorado Medical Treatment Decision Act, which is the living will statute and includes an approved form entitled the Declaration as to Medical or Surgical Treatment; (b) the Proxy Decision-Makers for Medical Treatment Act, which delineates the circumstances under which a person may substitute for the patient in decision making; (c) the Directive Relating to Cardiopulmonary Resuscitation, which specifies appropriate circumstances for DNRs, and (d) the Medical Durable Power of Attorney section.

17. These laws sound the same. Is there a difference?
Although they are similar in some ways, there are important differences. For example, the living will only becomes active after a patient has become incapacitated, but in many states there is a delay in that the patient must be incapacitated for a certain time before the provisions of the living will can be implemented. On the other hand, the proxy decision makers for medical treatment and the medical durable power of attorney become active immediately upon the incapacitation of the patient. Finally, the directive relating to cardiopulmonary resuscitation is active immediately upon the patient's signature.

18. What happens if state law is not followed?
Policies, procedures, and protocols guiding EMS operations must be consistent with the statutory requirements of the laws in a particular state. Failure to abide by the legislated requirements may result in negligence *per se* (meaning, "negligence in itself" or on its face) if deviation results in foreseeable harm to the patient. Negligence *per se* means that there is a presumption of negligence as a matter of law (disregarding other factual disputes) if a law is violated that is intended to protect the group of persons that includes the harmed patient and the violation is the cause of the harm.

For example, imagine the following scenario. A patient is found unconscious and in need of advanced life support. A person on the scene tells the EMS crew that the patient does not want heroic efforts and also thinks that the patient has signed a living will to that effect. The EMS crew does not insist on inspecting the living will before electing to not resuscitate. Most statutes state that health care providers may not be held liable if the document appears on its face to be validly executed. If, as in this hypothetical case, there was no inspection of the document and none, in fact, exists, the EMS crew may be found presumptively negligent and liable for the resulting harm if advanced life support was withheld.

19. What is informed consent?
Patient autonomy means that in law and ethics the patient has the right to make decisions concerning the extent of medical care that the patient will accept. The law has long recognized that patient autonomy includes the right to make "bad" medical decisions, even potentially lethal ones, as long as the patient is competent.

In 1914, Justice Benjamin Cardozo, writing for the New York State Court of Appeals, the highest court in New York, stated that "every human being of adult years and sound mind has a right to determine what shall be done with his own body, and a surgeon who performs an operation without his patient's consent commits an assault for which he is liable in damages." Actually, the wrongful conduct that was just described is a battery, but assault and battery have been muddled for years. The point is that wrongful, actionable conduct occurs by any contact with a patient's body without the patient's consent, and the health care provider becomes responsible for *any* damages. This is of great concern because a medical procedure can be done without negligence and with all reasonable care, but the health care provider remains liable for even unforeseen, untoward reactions and even known risks of the procedure.

20. What is actually required to obtain informed consent?

Four things must be shown. The health care provider must convey to the patient (a) the ailment, (b) the treatment or procedure that is being suggested, (c) alternatives to treatment, and (d) the risks associated with treatment and nontreatment, all in simple language the patient can understand. The patient must be informed of this information to the extent a reasonable health care provider would under the same or similar circumstances.

21. How do these legal issues apply to prehospital providers in the field?

Any patient you are going to treat must give permission for that treatment. The problem in EMS is that many patients are unable to give consent, either because of their emergency or other confounding factors such as intoxication. In an emergency situation, it is important to determine whether delay would endanger the patient, whether a careful health care provider would do the same as the defendant, and whether the patient was unable to consent. If so, the health care provider may proceed under the concept of "implied consent," meaning that most people would want to receive appropriate medical care; therefore, consent is implied and the provider can treat the patient. In the second case, the intoxicated patient may not be competent to give consent. Legal capacity to consent or refuse is not the same as medical capacity to consent or refuse. The patient need not be legally adjudicated as incompetent for patient rights to be disregarded in the emergency medical setting. An example is alcohol impairment. In 1993, the Rhode Island Supreme Court examined this issue and held that a patient's intoxication may render the patient incapable of giving informed consent and, in an emergency, a health care provider may dispense with obtaining the patient's informed consent.

22. How do issues of consent apply to patients who refuse care?

Just as the medical caregiver must obtain informed consent to treat a patient, informed refusal must also be obtained if the patient decides to refuse care. Thus, any competent adult may refuse medical services, but the provider must explain the potential ramifications of the decision and be sure the patient understands the risks. Again, all of this must be accomplished using plain, simple language that the patient can understand. By the same token, the patient must be competent in order to refuse care. An intoxicated patient would be considered incompetent and unable to refuse medical care until the intoxicant wore off.

23. How do issues of consent apply to minors?

A minor's medical capacity to accept or refuse treatment is a thorny area for EMS providers and varies among the states. In general, a minor has recognized legal impediments; a minor cannot enter into a contract and generally cannot vote, but can a minor consent or refuse medical treatment? Kansas held in 1970 that there is a difference between a legal and a medical capacity. The Kansas Supreme Court held that a minor can verbally consent to medical treatment. Tennessee followed the same reasoning in

1987. The cases are fact specific, and the EMS provider needs to know the law concerning a minor's capacity to accept or refuse medical treatment for the state in which he or she practices.

24. What is a HIPAA violation and can I be sued for it?

The Health Insurance Portability and Accountability Act of 1996 (HIPAA) is a federal statute enacted by Congress. It is complicated and difficult to understand. HIPAA was created in order to "combat waste, fraud, and abuse in health insurance and health care delivery." However, Congress neither expressly provided for nor implied any private rights of action to enforce HIPAA. In EMS, we most frequently see the issue of HIPAA arise in the context of the release of personal health information. That is, a valid HIPAA-compliant release authorization must be executed by the patient or his representative before medical records or protected health information may be disclosed to anyone. The important issue for EMS health care providers is that HIPAA does not provide a basis for a lawsuit but merely provides an "enforcement mechanism for the Secretary of Health and Human Services" to enforce the act. Therefore, a prehospital provider cannot be sued for a violation of HIPAA.

A different issue, however, is legal exposure for violation of the right of privacy from disclosure of protected health information without a valid HIPAA release authorization. Such an event may occur very simply and without bad intention. For example, if private information slips into conversation intended to reassure another person, such as a friend of the patient who comes to the waiting room out of concern for the patient, a violation occurs. If the patient learns of the disclosure, the provider may be liable for consequent damages.

There are a number of different claims for violation of the right of privacy. One form is a claim for invasion of privacy by public disclosure of private facts. Protected health information contains private facts about a patient that may not legally be disclosed without an executed release authorization, which is one purpose underlying HIPAA.

In Colorado and probably other jurisdictions, the pertinent parts of the jury instruction to determine whether the defendant health care provider is liable for invasion of privacy by public disclosure of private facts of a patient would look something like this:

1. The defendant made a statement about the plaintiff's medical condition to someone.
2. The plaintiff's medical condition was private.
3. A reasonable person would find the disclosure of plaintiff's medical condition very offensive.
4. At the time of the disclosure, the defendant knew or should have known that the fact or facts disclosed were private.
5. As a result of the disclosure, the plaintiff suffered injuries, losses, or damages.

The damages for this tort include economic and noneconomic damages as outlined in the discussion of question 13.

Thus, the message here is to treat your patient's private health information with the respect and privacy it and your patient deserve.

25. What about EMTALA?

EMTALA is the Emergency Medical Treatment and Active Labor Act of 1986. It was enacted by Congress to restrict "patient dumping," especially of the indigent and underinsured, but it is applicable to all patients you will confront in prehospital care and in interhospital transfers. Only a hospital is subject to an action under EMTALA; no other person or entity is. See *Eberhardt v. City of Los Angeles*, 62 F.3d 1253, 1256-57 (9th Cir. 1995). EMTALA was enacted to prevent hospitals from "dumping" patients that they could treat but who could not pay for services. See generally, 131 Cong. Rec. 28568-28570. There are two basic principles required by hospitals subject to EMTALA (i.e., any hospital that accepts federal funds, even one Medicare patient/payment). First, the hospital must provide for an appropriate medical screening examination to determine whether or not an emergency medical condition exists. Second, if a patient at a hospital has an emergency medical condition that has not been stabilized, the hospital may not transfer the patient unless certain conditions are met. Those conditions may take two forms. One is that the patient, or person responsible for the patient and acting on the patient's behalf, requests transfer to another facility; this must be done in writing and after being informed of the hospital's obligations under EMTALA. The second form, and most common, is when a physician at the transferring hospital determines that the risks of transfer are outweighed by the benefits reasonably expected to be provided at the receiving hospital; this determination must be documented by the transferring physician in a signed certification. An "appropriate transfer" is defined by the statute as a transfer "in which the transferring hospital provides the medical treatment within its capacity which minimizes the risks to the individual's health."

For the prehospital provider responding to an inter-hospital transfer this means that, in addition to the patient, you should be sure to transport the appropriate paperwork to include the written request for transfer and consent that has been signed by the patient or the patient's representative, or the transferring physician's signed certification.

Two important and interesting cases are worth mentioning in reference to EMTALA. In *Johnson v. University of Chicago Hospitals*, 982 F. 2d 230 (7th Cir. 1992), an ambulance transporting an infant in cardiopulmonary arrest was diverted from University of Chicago Hospital to a more distant hospital because the diverting hospital's Pediatric Intensive Care Unit was full. The court decided there was no EMTALA violation where the hospital lacked the capacity to treat and diverted the ambulance while it was en route.

In *Arrington v. Wong*, 237 F.3d 1066 (9 th Cir. 2001), a security guard who arrived at work extremely short of breath was transported from the scene en route to Queen's Medical Center, the closest receiving medical facility. While en route, the ambulance contacted the Queen's Emergency Department via radio. Dr. Wong, the base station ED physician, asked the paramedic crew who the patient's doctor was. The crew responded that the patient was a Tripler Army Medical Center patient, a destination further away than Queen's, but also informed Dr. Wong that the patient was in severe respiratory distress and "we thought we'd come to a close facility." Dr. Wong said, "I think it would be okay to go to Tripler." The ambulance crew understood that as being diverted by the Queen's ED base physician to Tripler and took him there. The patient was pronounced dead at Tripler about a half-hour after arrival. The defendants in the lawsuit included Dr. Wong, Queen's Medical Center, the City and County of Honolulu (which operated the EMS system), and its paramedic crew named individually for their actions within the course and scope of their employment. The Ninth Circuit Court of Appeals cited the Department of Health and Human Services regulation interpreting EMTALA's phrase "comes to the emergency department." The regulation clarifies the meaning and implementation of the statute and instructs that if ambulance personnel contact the hospital to inform the hospital that they want to transport the individual to the hospital for examination and treatment, the hospital may not deny the patient access to the hospital unless the hospital "is in diversionary status." Being on diversionary status is defined as when the hospital does not have the staff or facilities to accept any additional emergency patients. The court also cited the *Johnson v. University of Chicago Hospital* case in its analysis and conclusion that divert status is critical to whether an EMTALA violation has occurred.

Operationally, this means that if the hospital is on divert status, you may be diverted to an alternative destination as directed. If a hospital that has an emergency department is not on divert status, the hospital may not refuse to accept a patient for an appropriate screening examination.

26. What is the key to avoiding lawsuits?

Provide good care, good documentation, and be nice to your patients. These maxims will not prevent you from getting sued if you make a mistake, but they will make it less likely.

Pearls and Pitfalls

1. Be nice to your patients. Medical providers of all types who are nice tend to be sued less often.
2. Most cases take several years before they end up in court. Your documentation will be the primary source of information about what did or did not transpire. Be complete.
3. If you did not document it, you did not do it.
4. Consent for or refusal of treatment both require that you explain the medical problem, your treatment, alternatives to treatment, and the risks of your treatment or from refusing treatment in simple language the patient can understand.
5. In order for the plaintiff to win a case against you, you must have violated the standard of care and that violation resulted in an injury to the patient.
6. Under EMTALA, a transporting ambulance may be diverted away from a hospital's emergency department only when that hospital is formally on divert status.

References

1. Ayres RJ Jr. Legal considerations in prehospital care. Emerg Med Clin North Am 11:853–868, 1993.
2. Frew SA. Emergency medical services legal issues for the emergency physician. Emerg Med Clin North Am 8:41–56, 1990.
3. Goldberg RJ, Zautcke JL, Koenigsberg MD, et al. A review of prehospital care litigation in a large metropolitan EMS system. Ann Emerg Med 19:557–561, 1990.
4. Selden BS, Schnitzer PG, Nolan FX. Medicolegal documentation of prehospital triage. Ann Emerg Med 19:547–551, 1990.
5. Shanaberger CJ. Case law involving base-station contact. Prehosp Disaster Med 10:75–81, 1995.
6. Siegel DM. Consent and refusal of treatment. Emerg Med Clin North Am 11:833–840, 1993.
7. Sullivan DJ. Minors and emergency medicine. Emerg Med Clin North Am 11:841–852, 1993.
8. Wood CL. Historical perspectives on law, medical malpractice, and the concept of negligence. Emerg Med Clin North Am 11:819–832, 1993.
9. Nicholson, WC. Emergency Response and Emergency Management Law: Cases and Materials. Springfield, IL: Charles C. Thomas, 2003.

10. American Academy of Orthopedic Surgeons. EMS and the Law (EMS Continuing Education Series). Burlington, MA: Jones & Bartlett Learning, 2003.
11. HIPAA. Health Insurance Portability and Accountability Act. Public Law No. 104-191, 110 Stat. 1936 (1996) and is codified primarily in Titles 18, 26 and 42 of the United States Code.
12. EMTALA; Emergency Medical Treatment and Active Labor Act of 1986; codified at 42 U.S.C. Sec. 1395dd, as implemented by 42 C.F.R. Sec 489.24
13. Relevant cases in reference to HIPAA and EMTALA:
    Eberhardt v. City of Los Angeles, 62 F.3d 1253, 1256-57 (9th Cir. 1995)
    Johnson v. University of Chicago Hospitals, 982 F. 2d 230 (7th Cir. 1992)
    Arrington v. Wong, 237 F.3d 1066 (9th Cir. 2001)
    Repp v. Anadarko Municipal Hospital, 43 F.3d 519. (10th Cir. 1994)
    Ingram v. Muskogee Regional Medical Center, 235 F.3d 550 (10th Cir. 2000)
    Means v. Independent Life & Accident Insurance Company, 963 F.Supp. 1131, 1135 (M.D. La. 1997)
    Acara v. Banks, 470 F.3d 569 (5th Cir. 2006)
    Barnes v. Glennon, 2006 WL 2811821, at 6 (N.D.N.Y. 2006)
    Slue v. New York University Medical Center, 409 F. Supp.2d 349, 373 (S.D.N.Y. 2006)
    Munoz v. Island Fin. Corp., 364 F.Supp.2d 131 (D.P.R. 2005)
    Association of American Physicians and Surgeons, Inc. v. United States Department of Health and Human Services, 224 F.Supp.2d 1115 (S.D. Tex. 2002).
    Doe v. High-Tech Institute, Inc., 972 P.2d 1060 (Colo. App. 1998).
    St. Anthony Hospital v. U.S. Dept. of H.H.S , 309 F.3d 680 (10th Cir. 2002)
14. Examples of relevant jury instructions:
    C.J.I. 4th, 9:18 Cause When Only One Cause Is Alleged—Defined
    C.J.I. 4th, 9:19 Concurrent Causes—Defined
    C.J.I. 4th, 28:5 Invasion of Privacy by Public Disclosure of Private Facts
    15. Relevant websites:
    www.medlaw.com
    www.pwwemslaw.com

Author's note: The author would like to thank Michael J. Turner, Esq. for his assistance in the preparation of this material.

Emergency Vehicle Operation

Bob Loop

1. **Isn't speed of the essence when responding to emergency medical calls?**
   EMS providers are constantly responding to life-and-death situations. Under such pressure, they can become obsessed with the need to travel at the utmost speed, disregarding their safety and the safety of other drivers. In reality, however, less than 10% of the calls turn out to be life-threatening cases. Emergency responses, therefore, usually turn out to be more dangerous to the responders than the nature of the emergency to the patient. In addition, recent research indicates that emergency responses save little time in the overall scheme of the emergency call, time easily recovered with good scene management skills.

2. **Why is emergency vehicle operations (EVO) training necessary?**
   Most EMS providers believe that they face the greatest personal risk while dealing with calls such as shootings, stabbings, and gang fights. However, the greatest risk for injury actually comes from the potential for emergency vehicle crashes. More EMS providers are killed and injured in such accidents than in any other type of prehospital event. Appropriate EVO driver education can significantly decrease the risk of injury during EVO.

3. **Besides decreasing the risk of injury, is there another reason to obtain bona fide EVO training?**
   With the increasingly litigious society in which EMS providers find themselves performing, there is an increased risk of personal liability if you are found responsible for a crash that occurs while you are operating an emergency vehicle. Substantial case law demonstrates that operators of emergency vehicles can be held liable for criminal and civil damages for their actions when judged responsible for an accident.

4. **Why isn't a generic defensive driving class sufficient for emergency vehicle drivers?**
   The average defensive driving course is good for the average driver, but anyone who must navigate a five-ton emergency vehicle through heavy traffic at high speed must be a much more skillful driver. Emergency vehicle drivers must understand the physical dynamics of their vehicle, such as its tires and its load transfer properties. The emergency vehicle driver *must* know the limits of the vehicle. The average driving class is inadequate for teaching these crucial skills to the emergency driver.

5. **What do EVO courses cover?**
   All emergency vehicle operators should enroll in a sanctioned emergency vehicle operations course (EVOC), which includes performance training and evaluation on a driving range. The best EVOC programs allow students to drive their emergency vehicles on a closed course at 100% capability to experience what the vehicle can and cannot do on the street. Emergency vehicle drivers who learn the limits of both themselves and their vehicles in a controlled setting are much more conservative and therefore much safer drivers.

Reasons to Obtain Emergency Vehicle Driver Training
1. Reduce emergency vehicle accidents
2. Reduce risk of personal injury
3. Reduce liability
4. Increase level of attention
5. Create greater driver maturity
6. Create greater emotional control
7. Reduce stress level
8. Increase decision-making skill
9. Improve vehicle control skills for on-duty driving
10. Improve vehicle control skills for off-duty driving

6. What is one of the most frequent complaints made by the public to supervisors of EMS agencies?
That the emergency vehicle violated one or more traffic laws. The greatest number of citizen contacts with EMS occur while citizens are driving their own vehicle and are confronted by an emergency vehicle responding to an emergency call. Therefore, it is easy to understand why a significant number of complaints are related to driving. It is difficult for other drivers to understand the complexities of driving an emergency vehicle. Emergency vehicle operators must realize the great scrutiny they are under and always drive with due regard for the safety of all other drivers.

7. What are the psychological aspects related to driving an emergency vehicle?
Because of the great risk of accidents, a mature attitude, coupled with sound judgment and 100% concentration, are important psychological attributes of a good emergency vehicle operator.

8. Is there an "onboard computer" and how does it work?
Your brain is the onboard computer, receiving data in the form of visual, audio, and tactile sensations. This information is processed rapidly by your brain, and your driving actions and reactions are produced. Approximately 90% of the input your brain needs for driving comes from vision. Most of the remaining 10% comes from tactile senses—"feeling" the weight transfer of the vehicle. A small portion comes from auditory input.

9. What are the components of vision?
Visual acuity, focal vision, peripheral vision, and depth perception.

10. How does visual acuity affect driving ability?
Visual acuity is defined as the ability of either eye to differentiate small space intervals in the discrimination of form. Because most input from driving comes visually, high acuity is critical for safe emergency vehicle operations. Visual acuity can be affected by the amount of ambient light and age of the driver. Thus, driving at night impairs acuity and, as a driver ages, macular degeneration of the retinas is more pronounced, also impairing acuity.

11. What is focal vision?
Also referred to as central vision, focal vision is the portion of the visual field you are specifically looking at. The focal visual field accounts for only 3–5% of the total field of vision. Drivers who use only their focal

EMS – Overview, Design, and Operations

vision to drive are using a limited amount of their available ability to see. Such drivers are referred to as having tunnel vision. An emergency vehicle driver must learn to use his or her total field of vision.

12. What is peripheral vision and why is it important?
Peripheral vision allows a person to perceive objects to either side of one's focal vision. Because the periphery of the retinas contain fewer nerve endings, images perceived through peripheral vision are not well defined. You can demonstrate this by holding your hands out to both sides while looking straight ahead. You can see your hands but cannot count your fingers. Peripheral vision is important to the emergency vehicle driver. If you learn to use your peripheral vision effectively, you gain valuable reaction time while clearing an intersection, for example, because you can perceive movement of approaching vehicles more quickly. You cannot tell what kind of vehicle it is until you look more directly at it, but you know a vehicle is approaching.

13. What is depth perception and why is it the most important component of vision for emergency vehicle driving?
When both eyes are open, the brain is able to compute the relative position of objects in the visual field. This ability to judge this "spatial depth" of objects is crucial for a driver. Depth perception allows the driver to determine if there is room to maneuver the vehicle through lanes and spaces as well as distance from objects. Emergency vehicle accident statistics show that a significant number of crashes are "vehicle dimension" incidents, in which the driver attempted to enter too small a space. Good depth perception requires good vision.

14. How can I improve my vision?
Visual improvement has been demonstrated through the use of a five-step method developed by three scientists. Practicing the components of this method, the Smith-Cummins-Sherman Visual Development System, allows a person to enhance his visual awareness and field of vision.

Smith-Cummins-Sherman Visual Development System

1. Aim high in steering: Keep your vehicle centered in your path by glancing well ahead at the roadway.
2. Get the big picture: Continually scan the unfolding traffic scene as you drive. Systematically scan all around your vehicle, especially your blind spots.
3. Keep your eyes moving: Never fix your focal vision on any one area.
4. Always have an escape: "Scan & Plan" to react to traffic changes.
5. Make sure they see you: Just because your emergency warning equipment is on does not mean other drivers know you are there. Always be alert for clues to wrong moves by other drivers.

15. What concerns do I need to have about night driving?
Most drivers believe that the only difference between day and night driving is that headlights are used at night. This misconception causes them to drive at night as they do in the daylight, a misconception that is all too often fatal. Visual difficulties begin at dusk as the eyes are forced to adapt to changing light levels, impaired color perception, deeper shadows, and headlights from approaching cars. With full darkness, normal driving cues are lost, acuity and depth perception are impaired, field of vision narrows, and sight distance decreases. All of these factors add up to an enormously increased risk during night driving.

Emergency Vehicle Operation

16. How do I maximize my ability to drive safely at night?
Wear corrective lenses if you need them. Be as well rested as possible. Increase your stopping cushion and reduce your speed. Know the range of your headlights so that you do not overdrive your sight distance. Good vehicle preparation is also crucial: clean all windows inside and out to reduce glare.

17. What is "load transfer"?
Also known as weight transfer, load transfer is a physical event that occurs in a vehicle whenever a "control action" is applied by the driver. This principle is best understood by imagining that the vehicle is balanced on a fulcrum placed under the center of the chassis. Whenever the driver applies a control action (i.e., turning the steering wheel, applying the brakes, or stepping on the accelerator), the weight of the vehicle shifts on this fulcrum, transferring the load around to different wheels. Anyone who has ever ridden in the back compartment of an ambulance is well acquainted with load transfer.

18. What does load transfer have to do with driving?
It is not so much the actual transfer of weight that affects driving dynamics but the fact that load transfer affects the size of the contact patch of the tires on the vehicle with the roadway. As the weight of the vehicle transfers toward one of its corners or sides, the amount of weight on the corresponding tire(s) increases. As a result, the tire's area of contact with the road surface gets larger while the contact patches of the tires on the other side of the vehicle get smaller. These changes in contact patch size can affect handling and control of the vehicle. Proper load transfer management maintains maximum contact patch size, allowing the greatest control. A good driver must learn to minimize load transfer if optimal vehicle control is to be maintained.

19. Why does an emergency vehicle have greater amounts of load transfer than the average passenger car?
An ambulance or rescue vehicle is much heavier and has a higher center of gravity than the average vehicle. These design characteristics add to the magnitude of the load transfer that occurs under maneuvering, which increases the chance of losing control. Excessive load transfer causes tires to lock up more easily under braking and lose traction while cornering, causing a loss of vehicle control.

20. How can load transfer be controlled?
Smooth and gentle control actions will minimize load transfer and allow optimal control of the vehicle. Many emergency vehicles are equipped with diesel engines that have an incredible amount of compression. Suddenly taking your foot off the accelerator of this engine simulates a tap on the brakes, creating increased load transfer. Sudden turns cause tremendous load transfer and should be avoided. One maneuver in particular to avoid is braking and cornering simultaneously. Braking should be done "in line" before entering any curves or corners. The old adage of "brake and accelerate as if there was an eggshell between your foot and pedal" has real merit. Remember that when you are driving to the limit of adhesion of the tires with the road, any increase in load transfer is an invitation to disaster. Gentle control actions on the steering wheel, accelerator, and brake pedal will allow the greatest control.

21. Are there other design characteristics of the typical emergency vehicle that can create handling problems?
Any vehicle that has dual rear wheels has twice as many tires in back as in front, giving twice as much traction to the rear of the vehicle than the front. This creates a distinct handling problem called

understeer. In an understeering vehicle attempting to negotiate a corner or curve, the front tires lose traction with the road surface before the rear tires, forcing the front end of the vehicle to "push" out in the opposite direction the vehicle is attempting to travel. Understeer is controlled by good throttle control. Slightly lifting off the accelerator will scrub some speed off the vehicle and allow the front tires to regain traction and track around the turn.

22. **Which is more dangerous, emergency driving in an urban or a rural area?**
Each setting has its own unique dangers. Urban areas have higher traffic volumes, more pedestrians, and higher call volumes. Rural emergency responses expose the driver to large animals in the roadway, less light, and less adequate road conditions. Rural and urban responders must be just as vigilant as the other.

23. **What weather conditions increase the risk for an emergency vehicle?**
Rain, snow, and ice have the result of reducing a driver's vision, reducing control, and increasing stopping distance. These impairments are magnified for the emergency driver because the vehicle is heavier and more difficult to control under normal driving conditions. One must be even more conservative when driving in adverse conditions.

24. **What are the secrets to driving in rain?**
Driving conditions are always worst during the initial minutes of a rainstorm as the road grime floats on the water in the roadway. Brakes get wet, impairing stopping ability, and heavy rain impairs visibility. Reduce your speed and increase the cushion between other drivers. Be wary of hydroplaning, which can occur in an emergency vehicle just as with any other vehicle. Be prepared to react to the subsequent control loss by reducing speed.

25. **How do I know when there is enough water on the road to create hydroplaning?**
It takes as little as $1/16$ in. of water on the roadway to cause hydroplaning, reducing your ability to steer and stop. With that amount of water, reflections from other vehicles' brakelights and headlights are visible on the road and tires will leave a visible wake.

26. **What are some secrets to driving on snow and ice?**
In winter conditions, bridges and shaded areas freeze first and melt last. Because any sudden control actions can cause you to lose control due to the increased load transfer of the emergency vehicle, speed reduction and gentle control input is essential. Increase the following distance from other vehicles. One extremely helpful tip when attempting to stop on icy roads is to slip the transmission into neutral, removing the engine compression from the load transfer equation.

27. **What is the most common mistake made by both civilian and emergency vehicle drivers that creates an accident?**
When a driver, including the emergency vehicle driver, gets in a bad situation, the most common mistake is to lock up the brakes of the vehicle. Once the brakes are locked, tiny balls of rubber tear loose from the tires. Essentially the vehicle "floats" on these rubber marbles, causing it to travel in the direction it was headed at the instant the brakes locked up. The resultant loss of directional control often causes the vehicle to strike whatever the driver was attempting to avoid. One of the fundamental driving skills taught in EVOC is appropriate use of emergency braking techniques. A properly trained emergency vehicle driver can evade almost all impending collisions because this panic braking and control loss will not occur.

Emergency Vehicle Operation

28. Can a vehicle with an antilock braking system (ABS) stop in a shorter distance than a vehicle with standard brakes?
No. The only road surface on which ABS brakes can stop the vehicle more quickly is on gravel. The advantage of ABS brakes is that they will not lock up under maximum braking input, allowing the tires to maintain rolling friction and enabling the driver to still maneuver the vehicle. On an emergency vehicle with a standard braking system, a driver can simulate ABS brakes with use of a technique called threshold braking.

29. What is threshold braking?
Application of the maximum braking input while still allowing the tires to keep rolling, thereby maintaining vehicle control. It requires lots of practice and a skillful driver who can feel load transfer and listen for the characteristic sound made by tires at the limit of their adhesion. During an emergency stop, the driver applies maximum pressure to the brake pedal. Just before a tire loses traction (i.e., its "point of incipient skid"), a high-pitched whining sound is produced. When that sound is heard, the driver must "flare" his toes on the brake pedal, bleeding a small amount of hydraulic pressure off the brakes, thereby allowing the tires to keep rolling. This technique allows maximum braking ability while preserving steering control.

30. What is brake fade?
Buildup of heat in the braking system impairs braking ability and can dramatically increase pedal force requirements. During responses, heat is generated by the heavy use of brakes and can affect the composition of the brake component material. In a vehicle with drum brakes, this can cause formation of a layer of superheated gas molecules to build up between the brake drum and brake shoes, preventing contact. The brake pedal gets soft and stopping ability is impaired. In extreme cases, the brakes can simply disappear. In a vehicle with disc brakes, excessive heat can be generated in the brake pads, which then transfers into the brake fluid through the calipers. The brake fluid can actually boil, at which time all braking is lost.

31. What should I do if brake fade occurs?
If the brakes fade while en route to a call, minimize your speed and use of brakes. If the brakes are lost completely, the only option is to terminate your response. Assuming you arrive at the scene and the brake fade is due to excessive drum and shoe heat, cooling will occur while you are attending to the call. Once you load the patient to begin transport, the brakes should be functional again, but the vehicle should be serviced as soon as possible. If brake fade is due to boiling of the brake fluid, steam will be generated in the brake lines and it is unlikely that the brakes will recover with cooling. The vehicle should be removed from service immediately.

32. Are turns and curves of concern?
Remember that the laws of physics impose limits on your cornering ability. Centrifugal force quadruples as speed doubles; therefore, there is a maximum speed for each curve. The tighter the curve, the slower the speed must be. In addition, the design characteristics of a heavy emergency vehicle increase the amount of load transfer that occurs while maneuvering. A good emergency driver must know the limit of the vehicle, especially as it relates to cornering speed.

33. How should I negotiate turns and curves?
First, brake to the proper speed before entering the turn. Because braking distance quadruples as speed doubles, any hard braking at high speed should be done "in-line," with the vehicle traveling in a straight

line. This will minimize lateral load transfer. Then position the vehicle for entry as far outside the lane as you can, using as much road as possible. By noting the inside point of the road edge, establish an apex (the lowest point of the turn), driving low across it while maintaining your speed. Now exit high from the curve, again using as much road as possible. This is called high-low-high cornering and it allows you to maintain a higher speed through the corner with less load transfer. Finally, as you reach the apex of the turn, accelerate gently, transferring some of the load off the front tires, allowing them to track more efficiently around the turn.

34. **What are the types of skids and how do I recover from them?**
Three types of skids are involved with driving: the braking skid, the cornering skid, and the power skid. The power skid cannot occur in a heavy emergency vehicle because the engine cannot produce enough power to spin the tires. Braking skids, however, are common because of the panic braking applied by many emergency vehicle drivers. Recovery from a braking skid is easy—get off the brakes, thereby recovering rolling friction and regaining control. A cornering skid occurs when too much speed is carried into a turn. Usually the front tires will lose traction first, creating an understeer situation. Applying the brakes makes a cornering skid worse due to increased load transfer. Recovery is accomplished by easing off the accelerator and avoiding braking.

35. **What are some of the most dangerous situations for an emergency vehicle?**
Intersections account for more than half of the accidents involving emergency vehicles. Blind intersections are the worst because oncoming lateral traffic cannot be seen. The most perilous situation occurs when an emergency vehicle is attempting to negotiate a red light at an intersection of multilane roads. "Green" traffic in some of the lanes crossing your path will stop, leaving an "open lane" with a green light for opposing traffic. This is a setup for disaster: a driver in the gridlocked cars behind the stopped "green" traffic will not see or hear your emergency equipment, become frustrated by the stopped cars on a green light, and blast through the open lane. Maneuvering near large trucks and buses is risky since it is practically impossible for them to stop or turn suddenly. You must develop respect for them since they physically cannot pull over and yield like other cars.

36. **What is the "warning process"?**
The process by which other drivers become aware of and respond to an emergency vehicle. The three components of the process are detection, recognition, and response, and they are integral to one another. The better the emergency equipment is and the better it is maintained, the sooner the vehicle is detected by other drivers, giving them maximum time to recognize the vehicle and respond appropriately.

37. **What color of emergency lights should an emergency vehicle have?**
Most sources recommend red and blue lights since red is more readily detected in daylight and blue is more readily detected at night. Many agencies also use white. The real key to visibility is to have very bright lights of different colors and lots of patterns of light.

38. **What kind of audible warning devices should the vehicle have?**
The average sound level of normal street traffic is 90 decibels. The siren should generate at least 120 decibels to be heard over normal street traffic, but that alone is not enough to be heard by all drivers. Because human hearing is quite effective in identifying changes in pitch and tone, the key to being heard is to continually vary the siren settings while responding.

39. Where can I learn more about emergency driving classes?
Contact your state EMS office for listings of EVOC courses. Most local police agencies will have listings of available programs. The National Safety Council also has developed an EVOC program.

Pearls and Pitfalls

1. Responding to a call at high speeds is much less important than many EMTs understand, as very few calls involve a life-threatening emergency.
2. Motor vehicle collisions involving ambulances are a source of significant injury to and occasionally death of EMTs.
3. Most crashes involving ambulances occur on dry pavement in daylight hours.
4. Learning how to drive an ambulance safely is of great importance as the increased mass of the vehicle makes its handling different than the EMT's automobile.

References

1. Abbott T. Training Program for Driving Instructors. Colorado Springs, CO, Paragon School of Driving.
2. Bondurant B, Blakemore J. Bob Bondurant on High Performance Driving. Motorbooks International Publishers & Wholesalers, 1993.
3. Federal Emergency Management Agency. United States Fire Administration Emergency Driver Training Manual.
4. Greenwald J. Driving Yourself Sane. Health 4:88–89, 1994.
5. Rice B, Coxon K, Carle L, et al. DHHPD Driving Performance Standards, Policies, and Procedures. Denver, DHPD, 1981–1997.

Public and Media Relations

Will Chapleau, EMT-P, RN, TNS

CHAPTER 9

1. **Should I wait for the media to call me for information on a story?**
   No. Prehospital personnel perform hundreds of thousands of life-saving acts every year. Unfortunately, most of the media coverage occurs when there is a perceived miscue or mistake. Emergency incidents provoke interest in everyone. They are exciting, humanistic, and have a great impact on patient outcomes. When positive events occur, make sure the appropriate media are notified. It is essential that the public understand the caring, competency, and readiness of those individuals who are available to respond at a moment's notice within their communities.

2. **How do I get the media to respond to me?**
   Start out by letting the media know about interesting activities going on in your department. Once you have their attention, make sure to let them know that you are available as a resource on related topics. Once you are perceived as a reliable source for information, you are more likely to get their attention when you have something to report.

3. **Should everyone in the department be briefed about an incident so they all will communicate the information consistently?**
   Inquiries about incidents should be handled in accordance with a department policy that all personnel are trained to follow. It is important that a single consistent message goes out. To ensure positive and informative communications, planning and training provide the best chance of compliance with requests for assistance and our best chance at maintaining a positive reaction to our story.

4. **Can anyone in the organization deal with the media?**
   It is ideal to have designated spokespersons for the media. A spokesperson must be available 24 hours a day for the initial break into media coverage. If the incident will be in the news longer than four or five days, departmental meetings should occur to brief staff members.

5. **What are some tips for speaking with reporters?**
   An interview with a reporter is not a conversation with a professional peer. It takes practice to conduct an interview that will satisfy you. Reporters are not trained in the practice of prehospital medicine just as you are not educated as a reporter. Reporters generally have an angle that they are looking at. Once the interview is over, you are at the mercy of the reporter and the editor. The important facts should be stated at the beginning of an interview because most editors will cut from the end of the story first. The usual interview will last about 5 minutes; a sit-down, scheduled interview as much as 20 minutes. However, only 15–30 seconds will be used and your statements will be sliced into "bites" with the reporter choosing "gem" statements and then narrating between video and audio segues. Consider this and prepare for the interview. Do not make statements that have not been thoroughly thought out and discussed among your staff or superiors and do not speculate or offer opinions.

Public and Media Relations

6. **What are the advantages and disadvantages of having a public information officer (PIO)?**

   The advantage to having a PIO is the opportunity to have a trained individual or individuals who are knowledgeable in department policy and possess media relations skills. This way, the best chance of relaying concise, clear, and productive messages is ensured. Most police and fire departments and now hospitals have designated PIOs who are the only individuals permitted to address the media. Using the department head or chief as the PIO initially demonstrates that the top person in the department is actively involved in the incident and clearly speaks for the agency.

   The potential pitfall to the use of a PIO is the delay in communications while waiting for the PIO to be available, the possibility of the PIO not having complete information to comment on, and the potential for a narrower picture influenced by personal bias. A PIO who serves as a relay between the department and the media may lose credibility if he or she does not have the operational knowledge or is not allowed to speak to nearly all matters for the department. If the PIO must constantly "track down that information and get back to you," aggressive reporters will find other sources to extract information that may not be the opinion of the department.

   It is important to understand the positives and negatives to monitor the performance of any PIO program.

7. **What should I be aware of and always do in an interview?**

   (a) Be aware of whether the interview is being conducted for radio, television, or print.

   (b) Be pleasant and positive. It is important to show human compassion and warmth in times of crisis.

   (c) Challenge misinformation. If a question is asked based on inaccurate information, do not answer the question. Correct the premise immediately without restating the question.

   (d) Slow down if you get angry. Take a deep breath and gather your thoughts.

   (e) End statements definitively. Reporters tend to keep the microphone aimed your way. This may cause you to make off-the-cuff or unprepared statements. This technique makes the interviewee feel as if there is something else he or she should say. The result of these spontaneous comments may end up as sound bites.

   (f) Speak plainly and direct your comments to the lay public. Avoid using industry jargon that the general public will not understand.

   (g) Tell the truth. Give accurate and factual information. If you are uncertain of the facts, say so.

   (h) Be candid and direct, especially on television. Deal with what's on peoples' minds, what frightens them. Sometimes there are no good answers.

   (i) Draw on your personal experiences to illustrate your point and use analogies to explain difficult technical situations.

   (j) Cite outside experts on prevailing industry standards or practices. Communities constantly compare themselves to one another.

8. **What should I avoid doing during an interview?**

   Do not:

   (a) be hostile, sarcastic, or confrontational.

   (b) consider the interview a conversation. Everything is on the record.

   (c) overload your message with complex or technical data.

(d) personally attack other organizations or competitors.
(e) answer a question with "no comment."
(f) attempt to cover up a mistake or mislead the media. Reporters are professionals who make their living extracting information and judging people's characters.
(g) theorize, speculate, hypothesize, or agree with a reporter who does so.
(h) interfere with any legitimate duties of the media
(i) offer opinion and conjecture. Stick with the facts and science.
(k) be condescending or talk down to reporters.
(l) defensive when challenged. Breathe deep, pause, and answer.
(m) interfere with reporters doing their job on-scene if they are acting appropriately and are safe.

9. **What are some tips for videotaped interviews?**
   (a) Be prepared and proactive. Communicate key messages.
   (b) Turn negatives into positives. This requires practice.
   (c) Think in terms of "sound bites." Try to deliver definitive answers lasting 7–10 seconds.
   (d) Let the microphone be the reporter's concern. Unusable audiotape is the reporter's or photographer's fault, not yours. It is the media's responsibility to assure proper sound levels are in place prior to the interview. Speak in your normal tone.
   (e) Always look directly at the reporter, not the camera. Watch others being interviewed and notice the difference between a well-seasoned interviewee and a novice.
   (f) Use a handout or media kit. Fax it to the assignment editor the day before the interview. This may educate and inspire the reporter to ask questions relative to the specific issues.

Pearls and Pitfalls

1. Be prepared for your interview.
2. Think about your answer to the reporter's question before you actually give the answer.
3. Think in terms of "sound bites" but be careful what you say.
4. Answer the question you are asked and do not offer additional unasked for information.
5. Having a PIO serve as the official spokesperson for your agency allows a trained individual to interact with the media.

References

1. Paine and Associates. Presented at The American Ambulance Association, Nashville, TN, November 1994.
2. On dealing with people like us—Dealing with reporters. New Mexico Business Journal September 2001http://findarticles.com/p/articles/mi_m5092/is_7_25/ai_78550749/?tag=content;col1 Accessed October 21, 2011.
3. Grunig JE, Hunt T. Managing Public Relations. New York: Holt, Rinehart and Winston, 1984. ISBN 0-03-058337-3 4. Cultip S. The Unseen Power. Public Relations, A History. Hillsdale, NJ: Erlbaum Associates, 1994. ISBN 0-8058-1464-7.

CHAPTER 10

Ethics in EMS

Jean Abbott, MD, MH, and Kelly Bookman, MD

1. **What is the difference between ethics and the law?**
   Ethics is the systemic study and analysis of right and wrong behavior. It examines the frameworks for determining how a person should act, either professionally or personally. The law codifies rules of "right" action and the consequences for conduct that a society feels are wrong. Legal "rules" generally align with what is moral or ethical, but they can be inadequate in many difficult issues. Some situations simply have not been addressed by the law; in others, the rigidity of laws may be at odds with individual dilemmas. Thus, laws may not always reflect ethical behavior.

2. **What is your duty to the patient as a prehospital provider?**
   You have a professional duty to respond to requests for assistance and to provide care regardless of patient income or social position. Care must not be limited unfairly to any specific group or class of people. The EMS provider has a duty to be appropriately trained and skilled and to both know and provide the community-defined "standard of care."

3. **What is your duty to yourself? How do you manage your personal risk for scene safety or infection protection?**
   Prehospital care providers have no duty to place themselves at serious personal risk in order to care for a patient. Self-preservation can be justified because it is a natural instinct that professionalism does not abolish and because the EMS provider is a valuable societal resource that should not be frivolously endangered. The health care team must be protected first because there will be no one to care for the ill and injured if care providers are lost.

4. **What is informed consent? Presumed consent? Emergency exception?**
   A person may not be touched without their consent. *Informed consent* requires that the health care provider explain to the patient the common risks and benefits of treatment as well as the potential complications from the lack of treatment. Although the standard of obtaining explicit consent is a goal in medical treatment, the EMS system often relies on *presumed consent*, where permission to touch and treat is implied by the act of requesting help from the EMS system. The *emergency exception* presumes that consent is provided if the patient is unable to express it because of illness or injury. Emergency exception is invoked when intervention is necessary to protect the seriously ill or life-threatened patients who cannot give consent as a result of their injury or illness or who may not be competent to refuse care.

5. **Who can refuse care?**
   Patients with decision-making capacity (DMC) may refuse care. Adult patients are presumed to have DMC. We usually assume DMC if the patient agrees to our treatments. When the patient refuses standard treatments, however, he or she must be assessed to assure that he or she can demonstrate understanding of the illness or injury, recognize the risks of refusal, and be able to explain why he/she is choosing something different. The refusal needs to be free and voluntary. The complexities of such a conversation

often are beyond the time limits and scope of assessment of EMS personnel. If a patient does not clearly demonstrate DMC, he/she should be transported, even if he/she objects. Communication with medical control will help to make these determinations. Note that patients with severe psychiatric disease—which may render them "incompetent" in the eyes of the law—may still retain DMC for some medical care decisions.

6. **From whom should the EMS provider withhold life sustaining treatments?**
There are medical indications for withholding (not starting) interventions. These include decapitation, dependent lividity, and obvious fatal injuries. In many jurisdictions, formal protocols for withholding resuscitation or stopping it have been developed (e.g., asystole with no response to initial treatment). Legal indications for withholding treatments near the end of life include various written forms of Advance Directives (ADs), including CPR Directives, DNAR (Do Not Attempt Resuscitation) forms, POLST (physician orders for life-sustaining treatment) paradigm state-based orders or wishes expressed through other formal documents. In addition, a legally designated Medical Durable Power of Attorney (MD-POA) is authorized to speak for the patient. A few local EMS agencies have also developed guidelines for withholding resuscitation from terminally ill patients on verbal instruction from family or caregiver.
In each case, the goal is to ensure that withholding treatment reflects the informed wishes of the patient. EMS providers must know the policies and official forms of AD requests valid in your state or EMS system. These AD documents have become increasingly common methods of expressing patient wishes to avoid unwanted resuscitation at the end of life. Many nursing home systems require explicit documentation of wishes regarding resuscitation from all their residents. Such written directives should always be brought to the hospital with the patient. Handwritten orders, tattoos, or other informal documents indicating "No Resuscitation" cannot be honored by EMS providers. Finally, it should always be remembered that every patient has the right to change their mind and rescind ADs or DNARs.

7. **Can you honor verbal requests to withhold resuscitation from family?**
Verbal requests from relatives generally cannot be accepted unless they come from a person with a formal MD-POA. Alternative nonwritten means of limiting resuscitation would be phone communication with the patient's primary physician or with hospice personnel attending the patient. If there is any doubt about the legitimacy or authority of a request to withhold treatment, treatment should be initiated.

8. **What do you do if you initiate treatment and then discover an Advance Directive?**
Despite good literature describing the ethical equality of withholding and withdrawing treatments, prehospital providers should continue treatments, once initiated, and transport the patient. When in doubt, contact a medical base for a change in treatment plan. Transport can be helpful in that it will allow the hospital team to sort out the next appropriate step—even if the best outcome is eventually determined to be withdrawal of undesired treatments in the emergency department or after admission.

9. **What does futility mean? Should futility or nonbeneficial treatment decisions be made in the field?**
"Futility" is a term used to describe medical treatment that has no likelihood of benefiting the patient. This judgment is difficult to make in an emergency situation. The context of the emergency is usually either not known, or known incompletely, and medical futility often hinges not just on the patient's medical condition but also on knowing the patient's goals and values. Only strict physiologic criteria, such as decapitation or lividity, should be applied when determining prehospital futile care.

Ethics in EMS

10. **What does "hospice" mean? How do you manage these patients?**
    Hospice care is a comprehensive management approach to care chosen by patients to maximize quality of life in the last months of living. It is palliative in nature, focusing on providing comfort in instances where cure is not possible. An EMS response may and should be available to all persons, including terminally ill patients. EMS is most often activated when hospice patients suddenly deteriorate or symptoms arise that overwhelm their caregiver. These calls are appropriate, even though hospice systems try to be available to teach and support their clients with end-of-life emergencies. During transport, hospice patients should be made comfortable with oxygen, positioning, suctioning, and other low-burden measures. Invasive interventions (such as IVs) should generally be avoided except when it is necessary to provide such comfort measures as analgesia. The EMS provider may need to be guided by hospice attendants, ADs, or family to clarify what help is wanted.

11. **Should you physically restrain violent patients?**
    Although it is sometimes unavoidable, forcibly restraining combative patients may distort your role as a medical professional. Patients will see you as a security guard and may not trust you as a care provider. You should ask for police assistance when you or the patient cannot safely engage in an interaction needed to promote medical care.

12. **What if honoring a patient's wishes challenges your personal values?**
    The ethical standard for the health care professional requires that the EMS provider put the patient's interests and needs over their own, as long as such care does not seriously jeopardize their own physical safety. You are not required to provide nonbeneficial treatment, to do anything that would injure a patient or a bystander, or to help the patient kill him or herself. You should be comfortable, however, with the standard treatments that are within your scope of practice and offer these to all patients in whom they are appropriate.

13. **What is patient confidentiality? When can it be broken?**
    All information obtained by EMS personnel should be considered confidential and treated as such. Information should only be given to those directly involved in patient care. Deidentified information can be used for quality assurance and training purposes.

14. **What is the ethical justification for triage in mass casualty/disaster situations?**
    In a disaster situation, medical resources are scarce, and the EMS provider is obligated to maximize provision of medical interventions to as many patients as possible. This ethic assures that the greatest good will be delivered to the greatest number of people in a mass casualty situation. The maximum "good" is achieved through the formal process of triage (rapid evaluation of patients), which focuses resources and skills on patients who are most critical but in whom simple interventions can save lives, and the recognition that death is fairly likely in a subgroup of patients who might be able to be saved if they were the sole patient that the EMS system was encountering. Patients with ambulatory injuries that are not life threatening also receive delayed attention because their injuries can be managed satisfactorily at a later time when more resources are available.

References

1. Becker LJ, Yeargin K, Rea TD, Owens M, Eisenberg MS. Resuscitation of residents with do not resuscitate orders in long–term care facilities. Prehosp Emerg Care 7: 303–306, 2003.

2. Citko J, Moss AH, Carley M, Tolle S. The national POLST paradigm initiative, 2nd ed. #178. J Palliat Med 214: 241–242, 2011.
3. Heilicser G, Stocking C, Siegler M. Ethical dilemmas in emergency medical services: The perspective of the emergency medical technician. Ann Emerg Med 27:239–243, 1996.
4. Iserson KV. Bioethical dilemmas in emergency medicine and prehospital care. In Monagle JF, Thomasma DC, eds. Health Care Ethics: Critical Issues for the 21st Century. Gaithersburg MD: Aspen Publishers, Inc., 1998.
5. Iserson K, Sanders A, Mathieu D, eds. Ethics in Emergency Medicine, 2nd ed. Tucson, AZ: Galen Press, Ltd., 1995.
6. Kellermann A, Lynn J. Withholding resuscitation in prehospital care. Ann Intern Med 144: 692–693, 2006.
7. Marco CA, Schears RM. Prehospital resuscitation practices: A survey of prehospital providers. J Emerg Med 24: 101–106, 2003.
8. NAEMSP Ethics Committee. Ethical challenges in emergency medical services. Prehosp Disaster Med Apr–Jun;8(2):179–182, 1993.
9. Sabatino CP. Survey of state EMS–DNR laws and protocols. J Law Med Ethics; 27: 297–315, 1999.
10. Sanders AB. Futility in resuscitation from cardiac arrest: role of out–of–hospital healthcare professionals. J Emerg Med 24: 87–88, 2003.
11. Schears RM, Marco CA, Iserson KV. "Do not attempt resuscitation" orders in the out–of–hospital setting. ACEP Policy resource and education paper. Ann Emerg Med 44: 68–70, 2004.
12. Schmidt TA, Hickman SE, Tolle SW, Brooks HS. The physician orders for life–sustaining treatment program: Oregon emergency medical technicians' practical experiences and attitudes. J Am Geriatr Soc 52(9):1430–1434, 2004.
13. Stone S, Lowenstein SR, McClung CD, Colwell CD, Abbott J. Paramedic knowledge, attitudes and training in end–of–life care. J Prehosp Disaster Med Nov–Dec;24(6):529–534, 2009.

Medical Direction

Chapter 11
Medical Direction—Overview 73
Marilyn Gifford, MD, FACEP

Chapter 12
On-Line Medical Direction 79
Christopher B. Colwell, MD, FACEP

Chapter 13
Off-Line Medical Direction 83
Carl J. Bonnett, MD, and Jason M. Liu, MD, MPH

Chapter 14
Continuous Quality Improvement 89
Robert Swor, DO, FACEP

Medical Direction—Overview

Marilyn Gifford, MD, FACEP

1. **What is an Emergency Medical Services system?**
   As described in *The EMS Agenda for the Future*, it is an organized, integrated program that allows for, and provides to an individual in need of acute medical assistance, the means to access and enter the health care delivery system in a timely manner.

2. **Why does an Emergency Medical Services system need medical direction?**
   An EMS system by definition is involved with the practice of medicine. Only physicians are licensed to practice medicine. The system needs physician input, oversight, and coordination from a medical director to optimize the overall plan for the entire system. Coordination of the many components of an EMS system ideally requires a physician capable of understanding the prehospital care of patients and the intricacies of guiding that care with the unified effort of many different participants. There are some small rural basic life support systems that function without medical direction, but most of those would benefit from physician involvement, and advanced life support systems must have a medical director.

   Additionally, in this day and age, the local EMS system is the same system used for disaster response, terrorism response, or hazardous material incident response. This makes it even more important to use the expertise of a physician in planning and directing the system response to any eventuality.

3. **What organizations are part of an EMS system and how many require medical direction?**
   EMS systems are structured in a wide variety of ways and the organizations and agencies delivering that service vary significantly.

   The local fire department may function with first responders, basic emergency medical technicians (EMTs), or paramedics. It may respond with a private ambulance service or it may be the transporting agency.

   Volunteer or private ambulance services are often the entire EMS system in rural areas and sometimes the contracted responder or transporting service in urban and suburban settings.

   Some communities use a third city service that provides paramedic response and transport with a parallel structure to police and fire services. This service is often based within the health agency of the city or community.

   The communication or dispatch system is the means of receiving, prioritizing, and providing verbal assistance to callers with emergencies while dispatching appropriate vehicles and personnel to involved locations with instructions and information updated to responding vehicles. The dispatch system may be based within the agency responsible for response and transport, or it may be located in a communications center or in the police or fire department.

   Receiving facilities are hospitals or specialty care centers set up to communicate with prehospital personnel and prepared to care for arriving emergency patients. Ideally these facilities will also be involved in education, case review, and providing opportunities for practical skills training/practice for prehospital providers.

Medical Direction

Mutual aid services agreements with surrounding services to the local EMS agency are essential, as it is recognized that no one or two agencies can handle every conceivable emergency. Regardless of the size of the primary agency, all agencies should have additional written agreements with those adjacent agencies that are most likely to be needed.

Finally, there should be an EMS lead agency to serve as an administrative body to direct and coordinate all components of the system. The lead agency may exist within local government or may be established as an independent council with authority to manage the system.

All of the foregoing components need medical direction.

4. Why do state-licensed paramedics need a medical director or physician advisor?

Because the practice of medicine in most states is restricted to physicians, the extension of medical care in the field requires a physician to accept responsibility for the acts of each paramedic and, in many states, each basic EMT.

5. What is the difference between on-line and off-line medical direction?

On-line (or concurrent) medical direction is the direction given to the paramedic by the physician (most often an emergency physician) on the radio or phone while the paramedic is on the scene or en route to a hospital with a patient. Off-line medical direction is the direction provided by a medical director who plans and evaluates the prehospital care by reviewing and recommending equipment and medications to be used, protocols to be followed, and continuing education necessary to maintain skills.

6. What are the important agencies and organizations that are involved with EMS?

This list is not exhaustive.

Federal agencies:

- The Federal Emergency Management Agency (FEMA) coordinates the federal government's role in preparing for, preventing, mitigating the effects of, responding to, and recovering from all domestic disasters whether natural or man-made, including acts of terror.
- The National Highway Traffic Safety Administration's (NHTSA) mission is to save lives, prevent injuries, and reduce economic costs due to road traffic crashes through education, research, safety standards, and enforcement activity. The Office of Emergency Medical Services, which is within the agency, supports national EMS system development.
- The National Disaster Medical System (NDMS) is a federally coordinated system that augments the nation's medical response capability.
- The Federal Interagency Committee on Emergency Medical Services (FICEMS) is a committee charged with coordinating the various federal agencies that interface with state, local, and tribal EMS agencies.

National organizations involved in EMS activities:

- American Academy of Orthopedic Surgeons (AAOS)
- American Academy of Pediatrics (AAP)
- American Ambulance Association (AAA)
- American Burn Association (ABA)
- American College of Cardiology (ACC)
- American College of Emergency Physicians (ACEP)
- American College of Osteopathic Emergency Physicians (ACOEP)
- American College of Surgeons (ACS)

Medical Direction—Overview

- American Heart Association (AHA)
- American Medical Association (AMA)
- American Red Cross (ARC)
- American Trauma Society (ATS)
- Association of Air Medical Services (AAMS)
- Emergency Nurses Association (ENA)
- International Association of Emergency Managers (IAEM)
- International Association of EMS Chiefs
- International Association of Fire Chiefs (IAFC)
- International Association of Fire Fighters (IAFF)
- National Association for Search and Rescue (NASAR)
- National Association for EMS Educators (NAEMSE)
- National Association of EMS Physicians (NAEMSP)
- National Association of Emergency Medical Technicians (NAEMT)
- National Association of State EMS Directors (NASEMSD)
- National EMS Pilots Association (NEMSPA)
- National Flight Paramedics Association (NFPA)
- National Safety Council (NSC)
- Society for Academic Emergency Medicine (SAEM)
- Society for Critical Care Medicine (SCCM)

National accrediting agencies:
- American Board of Emergency Medicine (ABEM)
- American Osteopathic Board of Emergency Medicine (AOBEM)
- Commission on Accreditation of Allied Health (CAAHEP)

Education programs:
- Commission on Accreditation of Ambulance Services (CAAS)
- Commission on Accreditation of Medical Transport Services (CAMTS)
- Committee on Accreditation of Educational Programs for the EMS Professional (COAEMSP) (works with CAAHEP)
- Continuing Education Coordinating Board for EMS (CECBEMS)
- Joint Commission (JC)
- National Registry for Emergency Medical Technicians (NREMT)

7. **Why are there so many organizations involved in EMS?**
There are numerous organizations because EMS grew up in such a haphazard way. There were no generally accepted or standardized ways of providing emergency medical care to patients; as a result, each community had to figure out what worked for them. This is why there are some fire services supplying EMS, some police services, and some ambulance services. There are first responders, EMTs, paramedics, nurses, and even physicians involved in providing EMS care. These organizations assist different services, different levels of service, and different aspects of patient care (e.g., trauma, cardiac, and pediatric).

Medical Direction

8. What are the requirements to become an EMS medical director?

Although there are no nationally recognized requirements, ACEP delineates both *essential* and *desirable* selection criteria.

Essential criteria include the following:
1. License to practice medicine or osteopathy.
2. Familiarity with the design and operation of out-of-hospital EMS systems.
3. Experience or training in the out-of-hospital emergency care of the acutely ill or injured patient.
4. Experience or training in medical direction of out-of-hospital emergency units.
5. Active participation in the management of the acutely ill or injured patient.
6. Experience or training in the instruction of out-of-hospital personnel.
7. Experience or training in the EMS quality improvement process.
8. Knowledge of EMS laws and regulations.
9. Knowledge of EMS dispatch and communications.
10. Knowledge of local mass casualty and disaster plans.

Desirable criteria include the following:
1. Board certification in emergency medicine.
2. Fellowship training in EMS.

9. What are the responsibilities of an EMS medical director?

The authority and responsibility of the EMS medical director will vary by locale, but the primary skills necessary for a successful EMS medical director are communication, communication, communication. It does not matter what great clinician accepts the job if he or she is not able to effectively communicate with politicians, business professionals, mothers, fathers, firefighters, surgeons, cardiologists, dispatchers, police, and the county coroner—it will be an uphill battle.

The primary responsibility of those communication skills is to represent the patient *always* in discussions, planning, reviewing, or preparing. What is best for the patient has to become the mantra of the EMS system—and it has traditionally been the physician who maintains that focus.

10. What resources are available to help assure a quality training program, quality paramedics, and a quality ambulance company?

The national accrediting agencies listed previously can assist with this goal. CAAHEP reviews and accredits nearly 2000 educational programs in 19 health science occupations including paramedic training sites. As the national EMS certification organization, NREMT provides a valid, uniform process to assess the knowledge and skills required for competent practice required by EMS professionals. CAAS was established to encourage and promote quality patient care in America's medical transportation system. However, all of these organizations are unable to evaluate the dedication, quality of work, and caring manner necessary for a great system. The medical director must be personally involved to assess the character, work ethics, personal conscience, and clinical care of personnel involved in the system.

Medical Direction—Overview

11. What are the seven levels of out-of-hospital care providers?
Emergency medical dispatch, emergency medical responder (formerly first responder), emergency medical technician (formerly emergency medical technician—basic), emergency medical technician—intermediate, paramedic, and advanced paramedic, as well as flight nurses.

12. What is an emergency medical dispatcher program?
EMDs are trained through a standard program that includes use of pre-arrival interrogation and instruction cards or computer programs designed to aid emergency victims before the arrival of emergency medical responders, EMTs, or paramedics. The second portion of their job is dispatching of appropriate assistance, which requires knowledge of available units, geography, proximity, and whether emergency medical responders, EMTs, or paramedic units are required. The enhanced 911 system and computer-assisted dispatch systems have made many decisions easier and more routine. These programs should have medical oversight as well, and that may involve a separate physician from the EMS system medical director.

13. What are treatment protocols?
Treatment protocols are specific, written guidelines that describe a general approach to common presenting conditions. Without a standard approach to common medical conditions the responder could be left guessing as to the right way something should be done in any particular system. No one can be held to a standard if there is none.

14. How do treatment protocols differ from standing orders?
Standing orders are specific authorizations to perform procedures or administer medications in clearly defined circumstances. Standing orders should be signed by the medical director who is ordering the procedure or medication. These orders can be followed in standard situations without the need for a physician on the radio providing direction or permission.

15. Describe destination policies.
In any EMS system the medical director should determine where certain critical or high-risk patients should be transported according to the resources available in a given community. The lay public is not expected to know, for instance, which hospital has the pediatric critical care capabilities or which has the highest level trauma capabilities.

16. Are all paramedic training programs the same?
No. Paramedic programs have varied tremendously in the number of hours they require of their students. There has been increased adherence to recommended standards, however, as accreditation has become available through CAAHEP. Programs have also been upgraded after NHTSA's publication of the *National EMS Education Agenda for the Future: A Systems Approach*. Physician involvement in overseeing the paramedic educational program can help ensure the overall quality of the education and training.

Pearls and Pitfalls

1. The primary skill needed for a successful EMS medical director is communication.
2. All aspects of the EMS system including EMT education, medical dispatching, and all medical care should be under the oversight of a qualified EMS physician.

Medical Direction

3. Although many organizations are involved in EMS locally and nationally, none are able to directly evaluate the overall quality and caring provided by an EMS system and its people.
4. The EMS medical director must be actively involved in assessing and evaluating the care provided by the EMS system and its employees, not just serve as a signature rubber stamp.

References

1. Brennan JA, Krohmer JR (eds.). Principles of EMS Systems. 3rd ed. American College of Emergency Physicians. Sudbury, MA: Jones and Bartlett, 2006
2. Kuehl AE (ed.). Prehospital Systems and Medical Oversight. 3rd ed. Dubuque, IA: Kendall/Hunt, 2009.
3. E.M.S. Agenda for the Future. National Highway Traffic Safety Administration, U.S Department of Transportation and Health Resources and Services Administration, U.S. Department of Health and Human Services, 1996.
4. National EMS Education Agenda for the Future: A Systems Approach. National Highway Traffic Safety Administration, U.S Department of Transportation and U.S. Department of Health and Human Services, 2000.

On-Line Medical Direction

Christopher B. Colwell, MD, FACEP

1. **What is meant by on-line medical direction?**
   On-line medical direction (OLMD), also referred to as medical control, on-line medical command, or real-time medical control, is the process by which emergency medical services (EMS) providers receive physician directives contemporaneously with the care of patients encountered in the out-of-hospital setting. Treatment protocols are usually initiated based on a patient's symptoms or complaints, such as shortness of breath or chest pain. After assessment has been completed, the initiation or continuation of treatment is discussed with a physician. The physician and EMS providers decide on the best treatment plan given the patient's complaints, physical assessment findings, current situation, and treatment modalities available. OLMD can be accomplished by a variety of methods, including radio, traditional telephone (land line), cellular telephone, or direct contact (on-scene).

2. **Is there an alternative to OLMD?**
   Yes. Some EMS systems, whether because of topography, high patient volume, or unavailability of OLMD physicians, use a standing-order protocol system for patient care. This type of patient treatment procedure allows the EMS providers to initiate treatment based on either the patient's complaint or symptoms without contemporaneous contact with a physician. Implicit in this type of EMS patient care paradigm is a vigorous quality management program that ensures the timely review of the patient care record to determine if the patient care is timely and appropriate given the presenting complaints or symptoms. Many EMS systems now use a system that combines liberal "standing" orders where much of the prehospital treatment occurs without direct physician contact or before contact is made. These systems then make OLMD available for when treatments fall outside of protocol or additional input or consultation is warranted.

3. **Does OLMD always involve contact with a physician?**
   In most instances, yes; however, there are some medical direction systems that allow nurses or other advanced life support EMS providers to provide OLMD in a delegated fashion. A physician needs to be in close proximity, either physically or by immediate communication, in the event of the need to change treatment protocols or if the patient falls outside of specific treatment protocols.

4. **Why are most EMS systems designed around the OLMD model?**
   Currently, in most states, EMS providers function under the direct supervision of a physician when they are caring for patients. Although certified and appropriately credentialed, EMS providers are not licensed to practice medicine. The EMS system medical director and the OLMD physician delegate certain functions to the EMS providers to effect patient care in the out-of-hospital arena. This stems from the recognition that for some medical and surgical conditions, such as acute myocardial infarction and multisystem traumatic injuries, early medical care may improve patient outcome.

Medical Direction

5. **Can OLMD play a role when dealing with the patient who is refusing transport?**
   Yes. The patient's voice on a recorded line, speaking with the physician, can be a very valuable means of documenting the refusal of care and ensuring the appropriateness of the refusal. Online communication alone may not be adequate, however, and a written nontransport worksheet or run report should be considered in addition to involvement of OLMD.

6. **Can OLMD play a role in reducing the number of patients refusing transport?**
   Yes. Under appropriate circumstances, in particular when the paramedic believes the patient should be transported to an emergency department but the patient is competent and refusing, having a physician speak with the patient is associated with more patients agreeing to be transported. This process can be time consuming, however.

7. **Do only advanced life support EMS personnel require OLMD?**
   No. Although only advanced life support (ALS) EMS providers are required to contact OLMD for patient care issues because of the nature of the treatment modalities and pharmacotherapy in some systems, others use OLMD for basic life support (BLS) providers as well. With the expanding scope of practice of BLS providers in some parts of the country, including defibrillation, intravenous line placement, and some medication use, OLMD for BLS may make sense. For the same reason, OLMD for intermediate providers is used in many systems as well.

8. **Does contacting OLMD delay treatment?**
   In some cases, yes. There will always be unavoidable delays encountered in out-of-hospital medicine. For instance, the time between receiving a call for assistance and dispatching an ambulance, the time to respond, and the time to access OLMD are all unavoidable. Most EMS systems, however, do not require OLMD for those therapies such as defibrillation and airway management that are life saving, time critical, and routinely done by ALS providers. Administration of other treatments beyond those that are immediately life saving will require contact with a physician. It is not uncommon for EMS systems that require OLMD to have built in a standing-order treatment plan in the event of communication failure for life-saving interventions previously described or to begin routine ALS therapy such as oxygen administration, establishment of intravenous access, or provision of first-line advanced cardiac life support drugs.

9. **What is the configuration of a successful OLMD?**
   Each EMS system must design an OLMD system that meets its unique needs for the care of patients. Some systems have every emergency department within the EMS system prepared for OLMD, whereas others limit the number and type of physicians who provide OLMD. In communities that have a sufficient number of qualified and interested physicians, the solution may be to share the responsibility. In other communities, EMS-knowledgeable physicians might be scarce, requiring the EMS medical director to develop an on-call list of physicians who are available to the EMS providers. Some systems use a finite number of emergency physicians who are mobile, respond to assist EMS providers in the care of patients, and provide OLMD for all patients regardless of the hospital destination. Other systems have a stationary physician in a medical command center who provides OLMD for the entire system. There are services that function on a combined standing order and OLMD system, with the OLMD shared among the receiving hospital emergency departments. Still others have a single base station with a small group of EM physicians providing OLMD.

10. Do physicians receive training in OLMD?

Not universally, no. In some states the EMS statutes require that physicians who provide OLMD complete a Base Station Medical Command Course. Other states have required this training specifically for those physicians who have not been trained in emergency medicine. All emergency medicine residency programs are required to provide EMS education to their physicians in training. While some variability exists between the residency programs with regard to the quality of this training, OLMD is almost uniformly taught with opportunities for supervised experience. Important to any OLMD program will be involvement of trained physicians with specific interest and experience in EMS and prehospital care. Some systems don't have physicians giving the OLMD, and even those that do may not have physicians trained in emergency medicine. It is very important for prehospital providers to be aware of who is giving their OLMD.

11. What is the advantage of OLMD?

The single most important advantage is the ability to combine or change treatment protocols for patients with complicated medical or surgical problems. The EMS provider, by presenting the salient features of the patient's presenting complaint and the physical assessment, can use the physician's more extensive medical training to help sort out the best treatment approach. Often, a physician on the radio or the telephone, who is in a more controlled environment, will think of alternative potential causes for the patient's complaints or symptoms and offer suggestions for management. In addition, the OLMD physician may suggest using established out-of-hospital medications in a nontraditional fashion, such as nitroglycerin for hypertensive emergencies rather than only for patients with chest pain. OLMD, therefore, can also become an educational venue for the EMS system. The OLMD physician can speak directly to the patient in those instances when the patient is refusing care and often can convince the patient to accept EMS transport to a hospital. The OLMD physician can also assist the EMT in assessing the competency of a patient who is refusing care. The transmission of timely patient-related information and establishing the responsibility of the physician for the patient are benefits of OLMD as well. Another distinct advantage of OLMD is the opportunity for concurrent quality management of patient care.

12. Are there any disadvantages to OLMD?

There is no obvious measurable or apparent disadvantage to OLMD. The criticism most often heard, however, is that there is no clear difference in patient outcome for patients who receive OLMD compared with patients who do not. Consequently, opponents of OLMD support the notion that OLMD is time consuming and takes EMS providers away from patient care. They feel that standing-order EMS systems deliver comparable patient care. From a system standpoint, the only potential disadvantage to OLMD is that sufficient resources are necessary to fulfill the demand for service. The EMS system must have a community of willing and able physicians to assume this important responsibility.

Pearls and Pitfalls

1. OLMD can play a role in getting reluctant patients to agree to be transported, when appropriate.
2. In some situations, OLMD can add to times spent at scenes.
3. Not all those giving OLMD will be the same level of provider or have the same training.
4. There are a variety of ways to successfully implement OLMD.
5. Most successful systems will have a mix of standing orders and OLMD.

References

1. Braun O. Direct medical control. In Kuehl AE (ed.): Prehospital Systems and Medical Oversight, 2nd ed. St. Louis: Mosby, pp. 196–216, 1994.
2. Paris PM, Roth R, Verdile VP (eds.). Prehospital Medical Direction: The Art of On-line Medical Direction. St. Louis, Mosby, 1996.
3. Roush WR. Medical accountability. In Roush WR (ed.): Principles of EMS Systems, 2nd ed. Dallas, American College of Emergency Physicians, 1994, pp. 227–244.
4. Wuerz, RC, Swope, GE, Holliman, CJ, Vazquez-de Miguel, G. On-line medical direction: A prospective study. *Prehospital Disaster Med* 10(3):174, 1995.
5. Krentz, MJ, Wainscott, MP. Medical accountability. Emerg Med Clin North Am 8(1):17, 1990.
6. Hoyt BT, Norton RL. Online medical control and initial refusal of care: does it help to talk with the patient? Acad Emerg Med 8(7):725, 2001.
7. Tortella, BJ, Lavery RF, Cody RP, Doran, J. Physician medical direction and advanced life support in the United States. Acad Emerg Med 2(4):274, 1995.
8. Rottman, SJ Schriger, DL, Charlop, G, et al. On-line medical control versus protocol-based prehospital care. Ann Emerg Med 30(1):62, 1997.
9. Benitez, FL, Pepe, PE. Role of the physician in prehospital management of trauma: North American perspective. Curr Opin Crit Care 8(6):551, 2002.
10. Stone, RM, Seaman, KG, Bissell, RA. A statewide study of EMS oversight: Medical director characteristics and involvement compared with national guidelines. Prehosp Emerg Care 4(4):345, 2000.
11. Stuhmiller, CF, Cudnik, MT, Sundheim, SM, et al. Adequacy of online medical command communication and emergency medical services documentation of informed refusals. Acad Emerg Med 12(10):970, 2005.
12. Gratton, MC, Bethke, RA, Watson, WA, Gaddis, GM. Effect of standing orders on paramedic scene time for trauma patients. Ann Emerg Med 20(12):1306, 1991.

Off-Line Medical Direction

Carl J. Bonnett, MD, and Jason M. Liu, MD, MPH

1. **What is medical direction?**
   Medical direction describes the spectrum of activities provided by a physician to ensure that an emergency medical services (EMS) agency provides appropriate patient care. The physician provides the professional expertise to help ensure that EMS agencies recruit and train qualified personnel who then practice high-quality prehospital medicine. Other terms that have been used to refer to medical direction include "medical control," "medical command," or "physician direction."

2. **Is a "medical director" the same thing as a "physician advisor?"**
   Partly because the field of emergency medicine was in its infancy at the time, there was little meaningful physician oversight as many original EMS systems were developing. In fact, the 1973 Emergency Medical Services Act, in describing the fifteen core building blocks of EMS, included aspects such as training, personnel, and communications, but did not even mention physician oversight. Some services developed a culture where physician involvement played a minimal role. These services tended to use the term "physician advisor," implying that the physician was solely a subject matter expert to consult (or ignore) as needed. Modern EMS systems utilize a medical director. A "medical director" has the ability to define the medical standards which a service will uphold, based on the best current scientific evidence.

3. **"Advisor", "Director"—aren't we just playing games with semantics?**
   In a word, no. In many states emergency medical technicians (EMTs) are required to have a physician medical director who oversees their medical care. Being a medical director implies that the physician overseeing a system is playing a proactive role in ensuring the highest level of care to its patients. It also implies that the physician has the authority to remove or modify medical protocols as appropriate.

4. **Any physician can be an EMS medical director, right?**
   In most jurisdictions, legally, any licensed physician can be an EMS medical director. However, EMS has become a very specialized field. The idea of just placing anyone with a medical degree in the role of medical director is no longer considered acceptable. Table 13.1 describes a number of essential and desirable characteristics that have been proposed by the American College of Emergency Physicians and the National Association of EMS Physicians.

5. **What is off-line medical direction?**
   Off-line medical direction (also known as indirect medical oversight) consists of all the guidelines, protocols, and policies that the medical director and leadership of the EMS agency create to give EMTs direction on how to deliver care. It also includes all of the educational and review processes needed to ensure adherence to these policies and procedures. Off-line direction is different from on-line medical direction, where EMTs speak directly with a physician or designee while they are caring for a patient.

Medical Direction

TABLE 13.1: American College of Emergency Physicians Recommended Characteristics of an EMS Medical Director

Essential
1. Licensed to practice medicine or osteopathy
2. Familiarity with the design and operation of out-of-hospital EMS systems
3. Experience or training in the out-of-hospital emergency care of the acutely ill or injured patient
4. Experience or training in medical direction of out-of-hospital emergency units
5. Active participation or experience in emergency department management of the acutely ill or injured patient
6. Experience or training in the instruction of out-of-hospital personnel
7. Experience or training in the EMS improvement process
8. Knowledge of EMS laws and regulations
9. Knowledge of EMS dispatch and communications
10. Knowledge of local mass casualty and disaster plans including preparation for responding to terrorism and weapons of mass destruction

Desirable
1. Board certification in emergency medicine by the American Board of Emergency Medicine or the American Board of Osteopathic Emergency Medicine
2. EMS fellowship training
3. Completion of an EMS Medical Directors training course

6. What does off-line medical direction encompass?

Off-line medical direction is made up of two main categories of responsibilities—prospective and retrospective. The prospective elements include everything that must be defined before an ambulance ever takes to the street, such as standards for EMTs and the protocols that they must follow (Table 13.2). The retrospective components include all the things that a medical director must do after a patient encounter to respond to problems and improve patient care (Table 13.3).

7. I keep hearing about the QRI process. What is that?

These are critical components of the retrospective elements of medical direction. QRI stands for Quality Review and Improvement. This involves reviewing cases to ensure that protocols are being followed correctly. For instance, one may use the QRI process to see if aspirin is being given to all patients with suspected cardiac chest pain. Quality improvement is exactly what it sounds—finding ways to improve the delivery of patient care once the review process has found a deficiency. An example would be looking at methods to increase the percentage of cases where aspirin is given to patients with suspected cardiac chest pain.

8. Doesn't the federal government come up with protocols for everyone to use?

No, there are no mandated "national protocols." A number of textbooks and national EMS organizations have published "model" protocols that can be used as templates to prepare policies and protocols tailored

TABLE 13.2: Off-line Medical Control: Prospective Components

1. Define medical standards for hiring new EMTs
2. Establish protocols and define the scope of practice for EMTs
3. Ensure compliance with applicable governmental regulations
4. Establish and oversee training programs
5. Oversee EMT continuing education compliance
6. Oversee new equipment programs and ensure appropriate training for agency personnel
7. Develop dispatch and response protocols
8. Liaison with the local EMS and hospital community
9. Authorize and train online physicians
10. Serve as an advocate for EMS in the legislative process
11. Ensure that agency mutual aid programs and disaster plans are developed and trained on

TABLE 13.3 : Off-line Medical Control: Retrospective Components

1. Conduct quality assurance and quality improvement programs
2. Perform counseling and remedial training with individual EMTs as appropriate
3. Investigate and respond to complaints from the public or other agencies and institutions

to a specific locale. A few states have statewide protocols that must be used by all EMS agencies within the state.

9. Does the federal government then have any input into EMS agencies?

The National Highway Traffic Safety Administration (NHTSA) released a standardized curriculum for EMT training, as well as an "EMS Agenda for the Future." Laws regulating EMS vary from state to state. Although the law does not require anyone to adhere to NHTSA standards, many state and local governments and EMS agencies have adopted them. One area where the federal government can exert a direct influence is in the area of disaster preparedness. If an agency receives federal funding (either directly or indirectly through a state or local government), it may be required to be compliant with the National Incident Management System (NIMS) or other federal guidelines. The NIMS allows rescuers from multiple agencies and organizations to integrate themselves into a unified response operation. Even if a given agency is not receiving any federal funding, the EMS medical director should have an understanding of NIMS, as this will be the organizational response system that agencies and municipalities will be using during future disasters.

10. Do protocols have to follow national medical guidelines such as Advanced Cardiac Life Support (ACLS) or Pediatric Advanced Life Support (PALS)?

Regulations concerning EMS are developed on a state by state basis, so there are no federal regulations mandating the use of such national medical guidelines in local protocols. That said, if an agency decides

Medical Direction

to veer too far from these guidelines, the medical director should make sure there is a good evidence-based reason to do so.

11. **How can a system make sure its protocols fall within a reasonable standard of care?**
    The "standard of care" for medicine has traditionally been defined in terms of what is reasonable in a given community. In other words, the standard of care may vary slightly from one area to the next. It is the medical director's responsibility to determine what the local standards are, and that the protocols are consistent with them. One strategy that can be adopted is for the medical directors of all local EMS agencies to meet regularly and agree on a certain basic set of protocols. That way, by definition, each agency is practicing at the community standard. For example, in the Denver metro area, the majority of local agencies' medical directors participate in the Denver Metropolitan EMS Medical Directors organization. Since the group's inception in the early 1990s, it has been able to create the Denver Metropolitan EMS Protocols. Each agency is free to make modifications as it chooses, but most base their practice on the core protocols developed by the group.

12. **Do we need both on-line and off-line medical direction?**
    Theoretically, no. There are some EMS systems that only operate with off-line medical direction, and have no provisions for real-time, direct communication with a physician. It is also theoretically possible to have an EMS system with only on-line direction. However, this would be impractical, as it would mean an EMT would not be able to do anything without direct contact with a physician at all times. One should realize that on-line and off-line medical direction are complementary and work together toward a common goal. Using both on-line and off-line direction allows an EMS agency to maximize the quality of patient care.

13. **Does off-line medical direction apply to all EMS providers?**
    Yes, for the reasons mentioned in the last question. All systems should have at least a basic set of protocols and procedures that give their providers a framework within which to practice.

14. **What situations mandate a switch to on-line medical direction?**
    Most EMS systems define in their protocols specific situations that warrant on-line direction. Many systems, for example, require physician or nurse contact for high-risk procedures such as cricothyroidotomy or patient refusal of care. Most systems also encourage providers to request on-line direction when an issue seems to go beyond the standard protocols. Prehospital providers should view medical control physicians as a resource to be accessed any time they perceive the situation to be out of the ordinary, overly complicated, or high risk.

15. **What happens if on-line medical direction cannot be established?**
    This is a very real possibility, especially in rural areas or areas that experience severe weather. It could also occur in times of disaster when communication systems fail. This situation should be clearly addressed in the agency's policies. In some jurisdictions, there may be legal requirements that stipulate what a provider can do in such a situation. If the prehospital provider cannot make on-line contact, and the situation is truly beyond the scope of the protocols, then the provider will have to use his or her best judgment. Prehospital providers must be encouraged to do what is best for their patients. This is why off-line medical direction is so important—having qualified, thoughtful, well-trained EMS personnel using sound protocols monitored with quality assurance mechanisms will maximize the quality of the care delivered.

Off-Line Medical Direction

16. **If on-line medical orders contradict off-line medical direction, which takes priority?**
   One of the responsibilities of the medical director is to ensure that any and all physicians who are serving as on-line ("base") physicians understand EMS operations, know the system protocols, and are qualified and willing to provide on-line direction. If this is the case, then orders given by the base physician are given with knowledge of the off-line protocols and for a reason. As such, they should take precedence over off-line standing orders. If the order is in clear violation of protocols or beyond the provider's legal scope of practice, the provider will have to make a judgment and do what is best for the patient. Depending on the gravity of the situation, the prehospital provider may refer the matter to the EMS medical director.

17. **What if a physician arrives at the scene? Do they supersede off-line medical direction?**
   This is often an uncomfortable and complex situation. Just because someone is a physician does not mean he or she is adept at providing emergency care, understands the nuances of prehospital care, or knows the local protocols. Depending on the situation, an on-scene physician may be more of a liability than an asset. An EMS system's protocols and policies should address this situation ahead of time. If there is any question, on-line medical direction should be requested, which would then take precedence. Unless the physician and his or her capabilities are well known to the prehospital provider, the best course of action will usually be to thank the on-scene physician for his or her assistance and politely, but firmly, take charge of the patient and initiate care and transport using system protocols.

18. **What about during disasters? Don't you need all the help you can get?**
   One could argue that during a disaster is when unsolicited help can cause the *most* problems. As mentioned earlier, most physicians who are not involved in emergency medicine are unfamiliar with prehospital medicine (many emergency physicians are unfamiliar with EMS). It is likely that they are even less comfortable with working in a disaster environment. Disaster scenes require a defined chain of command and, with the concurrent implementation of an incident command system (ICS), physicians who self dispatch may not know how to (or may not want to) work within an ICS structure. They also will not have the training or protective equipment to work at a potentially dangerous scene.

19. **Does patient preference or managed care requirements supersede off-line medical direction?**
   This can also be a challenging situation. EMS systems which operate in a competitive marketplace or that are under contract are often affected by this issue. System policies and protocols should address this. In truly emergent situations, the EMT should always transport to the closest, most appropriate hospital. The patient may not have an appreciation of the differences between the resources of each hospital, and may not be able to make an informed decision. That being said, patient autonomy and customer service should be a foundation of any EMS system. If taking a patient to the hospital of his or her choice does not affect care or overly tax the system, then the patient's request should be honored.

20. **What happens if what the EMT thinks is best for the patient is in conflict with the protocols?**
   All medical providers are charged with acting in the patient's bests interest at all times. Occasionally, a situation may arise that has been inappropriately or inadequately addressed by standing protocols. The first action should be to obtain on-line medical control. If that is not possible, the prehospital provider must ultimately act in the best interest of the patient. It is important, however, that EMS providers

Medical Direction

understand the significance and consequences of breaking protocol and be held accountable for their actions under their systems' policies, as well as local law.

Pearls and Pitfalls

1. Off-line medical direction involves physician oversight of those medical elements of the EMS system that must be in place before the ambulance and EMTs respond to a call as well as those components that must occur after the call to ensure that quality health care was provided.
2. The off-line medical director should be a physician knowledgeable about EMS and actively involved in the EMS system and agency delivering care. A medical director in name only is not acceptable.
3. Protocols should be in place in the event a physician arrives on scene and desires to initiate care in place of the responding EMS providers.
4. EMS systems should have protocols in place to deal with managed care issues such as choice of destination.

References

1. Stewart RD. History of EMS: Foundation of a system... Building Blocks and Bridges. In Brennan JA, Krohmer JR, (eds.): Principles of EMS Systems. 3rd ed., Dallas, TX: American College of Emergency Physicians, pp. 2-16, 2005.
2. Swor RA. Medical oversight and accountability. In Brennan JA, Krohmer JR, (eds.): Principles of EMS Systems. 3rd ed., Dallas, TX: American College of Emergency Physicians, pp. 64-73, 2005.
3. Racht EM. Indirect medical oversight. In Kuehl AE (ed.): Prehospital Systems and Medical Oversight. 3rd ed., Dubuque, IA: Kendall/Hunt, pp. 308–317, 2002.
4. Post C, Treiber M. History. In Kuehl AE (ed.): Prehospital Systems and Medical Oversight. 3rd ed., Dubuque, IA: Kendall/Hunt, pp. 3–19, 2002.
5. National Association of EMS Physicians Position Paper: Physician Medical Direction in EMS. NAEMSP Website. Available at: http://www.naemsp.org/pdf/physicianmedical.pdf. Accessed April 30, 2011.
6. Medical Direction of Emergency Medical Services Policy Resource Education Paper. American College of Emergency Physicians. Available at: http://www.acep.org/Content.aspx?id=29570&terms=medical%20direction. Accessed April 30, 2011.
7. National Incident Management System Integration Center Website. Federal Emergency Management Agency. Available at: http://www.fema.gov/emergency/nims/index.shtm. Accessed April 30, 2011.
8. NIMS Compliance Requirements for Local Emergency Planning Committees Fact Sheet. Federal Emergency Management Agency. Available at: http://www.fema.gov/pdf/emergency/nims/lepc_fs.pdf. Accessed April 30, 2011.
9. Unsolicited Medical Personnel Volunteering at Disaster Scenes: A Joint Position Paper From the National Association of EMS Physicians and the American College of Emergency Physicians. NAEMSP Website. Available at: http://www.naemsp.org/pdf/unsolmedper.pdf. Accessed April 30, 2011.
Direction of out-of-hospital care at the scene of medical emergencies. Position Paper from the American College of Emergency Physicians. Available at http://www.acep.org/Content.aspx?id=29170&terms=medical%20direction Accessed April 30, 2011

Continuous Quality Improvement

CHAPTER 14

Robert Swor, DO, FACEP

1. **What is quality?**
   The American Heritage Dictionary defines quality as a "grade of excellence," but quality has been described in a variety of ways. There is no single uniform definition. Ultimately, quality has been defined functionally. Joseph Juran, one of the leaders of the quality movement, describes it as "fitness for use." Others have expressed a more global statement, "We know it when we see it." Virtually all authors agree that quality is what the customers say it is. Ultimately, the definition of quality in health care is subjective, based on both the science of medicine and the accepted art of medical practice.

2. **Why do I need quality?**
   Our patients and communities demand and expect quality health care. As health care providers, we strive to supply services that are consistent, high quality and continuously improved. A less philosophic but no less important reason to pursue quality is that the payers for health care are increasingly demanding accounting for the enormous amount of money spent on health care. Payers (insurers, governments) are under intense pressure to reduce health care costs. This translates into demands on the health care and EMS systems for increased efficiency and demonstration that there is significant value for the care rendered relative to the funds allocated for it. The Center for Medicare and Medicaid Services (CMS) has now initiated a "Pay for Performance" program that financially rewards hospitals that provide certain aspects of care that are in accordance with evidence-based standards for selected clinical entities. The current focus on quality health care has primarily been driven by economic issues.

3. **What is quality assurance?**
   Quality assurance (QA) implies a warranty of quality and a demonstration by the medical community that efforts are in place to review medical care and assure its appropriateness. Its initial emphasis was on individual accountability, therefore emphasizing individual responsibility for "errors." This approach has pervaded medical quality efforts and has perhaps had an adverse impact on efforts to improve quality. Basically, QA requires a feedback loop involving monitoring (audits, incident reports), assessment, action, reevaluation, and follow-up. QA efforts are outcome oriented, which is an area of intense interest in the era of health care reform. Similarly, QA recognizes that medical practice is an art as well as a science and that review of care by other practitioners in the field (peer review) is a crucial aspect of evaluating care.

4. **Why are some people threatened by quality assurance?**
   Historically, QA was perceived as a method of finding the patterns of individual mistakes, and indeed, there is a focus on individual accountability. Its remedy, focusing on improvement or "reeducation" of the individual, although not intended, was viewed as a form of punishment. Practitioners in EMS and in health care at large were at risk of supplying quality data that could point to themselves as a "problem," or as not participating in QA activities.

Medical Direction

Despite well-intended efforts to improve the quality of services, QA programs were often not well supported by the members of organizations. The results of the individual-oriented process were data of suspect quality, poor support for findings of QA activities, and a general decrease in morale despite honest efforts to improve the care within an organization. Not all EMS QA efforts had these results, but significant care and skill were required to prevent QA from becoming a punitive exercise rather than one to improve quality. QA was also crafted as an "add-on" program to many EMS programs, the responsibility of a QA office or individual. The data collection, reviews, and results were all obtained and assessed separately from the rest of an organization. Predictably, there was little support for the findings.

A final reason that QA has been viewed with concern by EMS professionals is that because the focus of QA was on identifying outliers, most of the time, energy, and effort was focused on the vast majority of providers that were, by definition, providing appropriate care within an acceptable standard range.

5. **What is continuous quality improvement?**
   Continuous quality improvement (CQI) focuses not on the individual workers but on the system. A fundamental concept of QI is that a *system* is responsible for most errors (85%) in a given process and that individual errors are far less common than errors in fundamental processes. If processes are improved, efficient, and support individuals, it follows that people's performance and the services delivered (i.e., quality) will improve.

6. **What is a process? What are some examples?**
   A process is the means by which things get done, the steps in getting from point A to point B. A number of different activities in EMS may be thought of as processes: patient flow, information flow, and equipment flow. All require a number of steps to reach the necessary endpoint. For example, a man collapses with chest pain, and his wife calls 911. EMS responds by sending out the necessary first-response personnel and higher-level providers with equipment necessary for the emergency. Radio communications with an appropriate physician are in place, and the patient is transported to the facility able to care for that person's condition. Delivering health care to this patient involves screening the call, deploying the appropriate vehicle, getting to the patient, starting medical intervention with previously established standing protocols or direct medical oversight, communication of vital patient care data to the hospital, and the preparation of the appropriate facility and personnel to care for the individual patient. The various steps in this pathway can be thought of as the processes of the system.

7. **What is the difference between QA and CQI?**
   Retrospective reviews, outcome data evaluations, and peer reviews are all a standard part of QA activities. They are limited, however, in their ability to generate genuine system improvements.
   CQI, in theory, is broader in focus and uses descriptive and analytic methods to improve the processes of EMS organizations. Its implementation requires the participation of a broad cross-section of organizational members. It requires that efforts to improve quality be integrated into the daily functions of an organization and be funded just as other primary processes. In the EMS model, data collection and process evaluation would be viewed as integral components of care delivery, just as dispatch, rapid response, and treatment are integral components.
   A fundamental difference of QI is a broad focus on customer service, defining both external customers (patients) and internal customers (hospitals, physicians, and emergency departments). This view identifies

front-line personnel as key customers as well; thus paramedics are customers of the dispatcher, and the role of the dispatcher is to make sure that the customers' needs are met. The QI efforts would focus on improving the service to that customer.

8. **What are the costs of quality care?**
Not only do we want to deliver quality care to our patients, we need to do it cost effectively. There is a price to be paid for QI in the short run; however, improvements in efficiency can make CQI pay for itself in the long term.

The initial costs of quality improvement are significant. Time, energy, and leadership are required to conceive and develop QI programs. Resources, including technical training and support for staff and investment in data systems, are required. Finally, QI efforts must become a part of the workers' responsibilities, so that part of the time is focused not only on performing work, but also on helping improve the processes of that work. There is abundant literature in manufacturing, service, and medical sectors that document that quality efforts often result in decreased cost through enhanced efficiency, increased benefit through improved clinical care, or increased revenue through perceived improvements in clinical service.

9. **Who should perform CQI?**
W. Edwards Deming, known for quality management, identifies the front-line workers as key. Those individuals have the most intimate and "profound knowledge" of the processes that they perform. Accordingly, they are best able to identify the barriers to quality processes and to suggest data to be collected or solutions to be attempted. The provision of out-of-hospital emergency care is a team effort, so CQI should be a team effort. Provider peer review is invaluable. Physician input is also important, because EMS is patient care. Administrators must also be committed to CQI for it to succeed. They not only must participate in quality activities, such as QI teams, but must also provide such resources as staff and computer support, data collection expertise, and personnel. Finally, the leadership of the organization must be willing to support the decisions reached by front-line providers if they conform to parameters developed by the leadership.

10. **How do I start?**
To work to improve quality, there must be a commitment to a new approach to attaining quality. The role of leadership moves from a traditional "top-down" management style to one of devolving control of decisions to front-line personnel within defined parameters. In EMS, the role of front-line workers moves from just providing care to a more active role in QI activities, including assessment and problem solving. The use of multidisciplinary QI teams, which use QI methods and tools, are the heart of QI problem solving.

11. **What are the components of CQI?**
Juran identified three components of CQI.
    1. *Quality planning*—"getting it right the first time."
        - Determine who the customers are. EMS customers are not only patients and their families (external customers) but also individuals working within the system (internal customers).
        - Determine the needs of the customers. This process varies with n each portion of the organization but identifies and drives which products and processes are of key importance and require

attention. The simplest approach to this issue is to identify the customers and ask them to identify their needs.
- Develop product features that respond to customer needs.
- Develop processes that are able to produce the features.
- Transfer the resulting plans to the operating forces to test and improve those processes.

2. *Quality control*—minimize fluctuations so that the system is stable.
    - Evaluate actual product performance. The instruments for its measurement are varied and may range from sophisticated control charts to simple patient surveys.
    - Develop product goals and compare actual performance to product goals.
    - Act on the difference.

3. *Quality improvement*—to facilitate QI, one needs to identify simple "winning" projects that are necessary improvements but that utilize QI methods to demonstrate their ability to impact change. The selection of such a project is crucial. It must be relevant to caregivers, measurable, relatively frequent, and a process thought to be able to be improved. The data to be collected have to be well defined (or at least measurable), consistently documented, easily retrievable, and able to be analyzed.

12. What outcomes do I measure?

While quality patient care appears to be a readily agreed-upon outcome, there is little consensus in the literature defining what the attributes of that quality are. The most commonly accepted definition of an improved outcome is an increased rate of survival after a life-threatening event. Generally, outcomes may be defined more broadly to include a variety of changes in the patient's health status. These include the six Ds:

Death:	Did the patient survive to hospital discharge?
Disease:	Underlying illness and morbidity.
Disability:	Was there a better functional patient outcome because of patient care rendered? Examples might include a patient immobilized on a backboard after an accident who had a cervical spine fracture but sustained no spinal cord injury, or a patient who did not require an ICU bed or mechanical ventilation because of field treatment for congestive heart failure.
Discomfort:	Relief of patient's symptoms.
Dissatisfaction:	Is the patient satisfied with service rendered?
Destitution:	Did treatment decrease costs of patient care to the patient, the payer, or society as a whole?

In a survey of paramedics in the Pittsburgh, Pennsylvania, EMS system, Myles Greenberg asked them to identify what they thought were the attributes of quality and how they should be measured. In addition to patient outcome and symptomatic improvement, a number of other parameters were identified including patient satisfaction; provider satisfaction; educational, supervisory, and equipment quality; employee turnover rates; and other measures. These factors could be measured using survey tools, which although not completely objective, can be used in a reproducible fashion.

13. What is a model of CQI in EMS care?

The model most commonly applied to EMS is survival after an out-of-hospital cardiac arrest. This clinical entity is particularly attractive as an outcome measure for a number of reasons:

1. It addresses a clearly definable clinical entity, sudden cardiac death.
2. Treatment is standardized (advanced cardiac life support, ACLS).
3. Advanced life support (ALS) has been shown definitely to improve outcome.
4. Survival is time dependent.
5. It has a clearly definable outcome (dead or alive).
6. Data definitions are also now more standardized (Utstein templates).
7. A wealth of literature exists to serve as a benchmark for comparison with other systems.

All these factors allow a system to use cardiac arrest as a measure of structural components (response), process (is care rendered consistent with existing ACLS protocols?), and outcome (survival to hospital discharge). There are also many limitations of this method of evaluation. Cardiac arrest cases comprise only a small percentage of a system's care. Mortality is high, with survival rates varying from 1–30% depending on case definitions and system studied. Access to hospital outcome data is not consistently available, although death certificates are public documents. An EMS system may not have a large enough number of cardiac arrests from which to derive useful information. All these factors make cardiac arrest survival data useful and identify it as only one parameter of many that may be used to assess system performance.

Other measures of patient survival are more difficult to obtain. Difficulties encountered include standardizing clinical entities for comparison (e.g., multiple-trauma patients or myocardial infarction patients) and adjusting for confounders such as age or preexisting illnesses. Injuries may be identified and classified using the Abbreviated Injury Score (AIS-90) and the Injury Severity Score (ISS), which are standardized scoring systems quantifying the severity of a given patient's injuries. The ISS, in combination with the Revised Trauma Score (RTS), which identifies a patient's initial physiologic status (vital signs), have been used by many authors to calculate a probability of survival (P_s). A comparison of P_s with patients' actual outcome has been suggested to be a measure in aggregate of a trauma system's care relative to what should be expected. This methodology (Trauma Score–Injury Severity Score, TRISS) has come under increasing question in the trauma literature. Trauma systems routinely collect inpatient data that may be used as part of an EMS system's quality activities.

Multiple other parameters may be used to evaluate an EMS system's care. There has been a great deal of literature assessing endotracheal intubation and emergency airway management. This literature suggests that this topic should be closely scrutinized by EMS agencies.

EMS leaders identify patients that refuse care as a potential source of treatment error and legal entanglements. EMS systems should include some structured review of these cases as well.

As EMS systems implement new technologies, such as 12-lead EKGs, digital capnography, and others, they must also evaluate how these technologies are implemented and how they improve the quality of EMS patient care. Integrated evaluations, such as clinical accuracy of EKG diagnosis of acute myocardial infarction and impact on door to reperfusion time, are also important parameters for system evaluation.

Medical Direction

14. What tools do I use?
Descriptive Tools
- Process flowcharts are a graphic representation of the sequential steps in the process and reveal bottlenecks in flow. Critical evaluation of policies and processes are crucial components of a QI program.
- Fishbone (cause-and-effect or Ishikawa) diagrams categorize and display in groups theories about how and why processes fail. The groups may be internal customers, external customers, supplies, the work environment, or policies and protocols for work.

Data Collection and Display Tools
- Check sheets are used for collection and quantification of data.
- Histograms illustrate the frequency distribution of a process.
- Trends charts display the changes in process over time.
- Pareto charts are histograms graphing the frequency of defects from greatest to least, drawing attention to the former.
- Statistical or control charts show the variability of data around its mean.

Opinion-Gathering Tools
- *Nominals*—gather opinions from groups to identify theories regarding a given issue or potential solutions to a problem.
- *Brainstorming*—a method by which thoughts may be generated on a given topic to identify potential approaches to problem solving or problem identification.

15. What is the scope of its application?
EMS is patient care, and anything that touches on patient care is within the scope of CQI—personnel, equipment, and all factors influencing the processes of getting the ill and injured patient appropriate care. Personnel issues encompass recruitment, retention, training, certification, continuing education, and recertification. Equipment issues include purchasing and maintenance of items such as vehicles, radios, and defibrillators. Communication issues include access to 911, postdispatch instructions, and communication equipment on ambulances, in hospitals, and at the communications center. Treatments rendered include not only whether performance was up to standard but also include documentation and reporting. Medical oversight, both direct radio control and indirect standing protocols, are within this scope. Looking at the system as a whole, there is an interrelationship between EMS agencies (e.g., who provides the primary and secondary response; who does the transports) and the hospitals (e.g., for the time patient and EMTs spend at the triage area).

An important component of a system's QI activities includes evaluation of prospective or structural elements including developing standards for the system and its providers and ensuring that providers are appropriate, equipped, trained, and educated to provide emergency care. This methodology is similar to that of hospitals, which require documentation of qualifications prior to a physician being able to practice and perform procedures within the hospital.

16. What happens now that we've started QI?
Is CQI work ever finished? CQI is a continuous process. Although a project may be completed, the system needs to be constantly reviewed.

Continuous Quality Improvement

17. What are some examples of CQI in health care?

CQI is being implemented in a variety of health care environments. Applications may be operational (decreasing the time to admit a patient to a bed), fiscal (decreasing the time to send a bill upon patient discharge), or clinical (decreasing the time to thrombolytic therapy for myocardial infarction patients or decreasing the rate of medication errors).

18. What are some examples of CQI in EMS?

System status management (SSM) is a success story of CQI in EMS. Here, the deployment of ambulances is strategic in both time and location. Typically, implementing this sort of process is the result of a leadership initiative to meet the needs of customers (faster response). The process is evaluated, data are gathered, and the process is improved by changes in system structure.

A variety of other QI applications are being tested in EMS. Some agencies are working with teams to facilitate ambulance turnaround in emergency departments. State EMS agencies have applied QI methods to effect more rapid turnaround of licensure applications. Many agencies work with hospitals to facilitate the process of identifying acute MI patients and their time to reperfusion. Pinellas County, Florida, and Tucson, Arizona, reported using QI methods to address drownings in their community.

19. Are quality activities actually research?

CQI and research projects have many elements in common. Research advances medical knowledge and sets the standards for medical care, whereas CQI involves improving the care currently delivered to meet these ever-increasing standards. In addition, research is for publication, whereas CQI is confidential. Both are disciplined, analytic approaches to evaluation and to improving patient care.

20. Would lawyers be interested?

If the purpose of QI activities is to identify areas for improvement, it is clear that the potential exists to identify and document problems that could potentially be used in lawsuits against the organization. To prevent this and to encourage health care entities (including EMS providers), most states have enacted statutes that give protection from discovery to QI activities provided those activities have appropriate safeguards and follow specified processes. There are two fundamental legal issues: confidentiality and liability.

Practical Steps to Enhance Confidentiality

1. EMS organizations need to research and be cognizant of state and federal statutes governing their QI activities.
2. CQI needs to be organized, with the bylaws of the EMS organizations specifying who and what constitute QI activities.
3. The data to be collected should be prospectively identified for the purposes of CQI.
4. Documents generated do not identify patient or provider and are marked confidential and distributed only to people involved in CQI.

Practical Steps to Reduce Risk of Liability

1. Follow CQI bylaws so that review activities are seen as official.
2. The CQI process should not be used for any other purpose than to improve patient care.
3. Preserve the confidentiality of CQI records.

Pearls and Pitfalls

1. It is far easier to evaluate an agency, person, or process than to be the object of that evaluation.
2. When someone or something is being assessed, they should be informed that the assessment is being performed.
3. Do not publicly distribute results or findings to others without distributing the information internally and giving those involved the opportunity to address identified or perceived errors or shortcomings first.
4. Lead by example; evaluate items or processes that may be under the control of leadership first, rather than evaluating front-line personnel.
5. Protect each entity's dignity, using blinded data for comparison.
6. Use QI activities to evaluate, identify, and celebrate positive accomplishments, as well as identifying errors and shortcomings.
7. Ask for front-line providers' input first. In addition to being inclusive, front-line providers' perspective is invaluable, described by Deming as profound knowledge.

References

1. AMA Council of Medical Services. Guidelines for quality assurance. JAMA 259:2572–2573, 1988.
2. Berwick DM, Godfrey AB, Roessner J. Curing Health Care: New Strategies for Quality Improvement. San Francisco: Jossey-Bass, 1990.
3. Crosby P. Quality Is Free: The Art of Making Quality Certain. New York: McGraw-Hill, 1979.
4. Donabedian A. Promoting quality through evaluating the process of patient care. Med Care 6:181–202, 1968.
5. Donabedian A. The quality of care: How can it be assessed? JAMA 260:1743–1748, 1988.
6. Kritchevsky S, Simmons BP. Continuous quality improvement: Concepts and applications for physician care. JAMA 266:1817–1823, 1991.
7. Shackford SR, Hollinsworth-Fridlund P, McArdle M, Eastman AB: Assuring quality in a trauma system—The medical audit committee: Composition, cost and results. J Trauma 27:866–875, 1987.
8. Holroyd B, Knoop R, Kallsen G. Medical control, quality assurance in prehospital care. JAMA 256:1027–1031, 1986.
9. Kohn LT, Corrigan JM, Molla S (eds.). To Err Is Human: Building a Safer Health System. Committee on Quality of Health Care in America. Washington, DC: Institute of Medicine National Academy Press, 1999.
10. Institutes of Medicine. To Err Is Human. Washington, DC: National Academies Press, pp. 2000.
11. Swor RA, Pirrallo RG. Improving Quality in EMS. Dubuque, IA: Kendall Hunt Publishers, 2005.
12. Harrawood D, Gunderson M, Fravels S, et al. Drowning prevention: A case study in EMS epidemiology. J Emerg Med Serv 19:34–41 1994.
13. Greenberg, Myles D. et al. Quality indicators for out-of-hospital emergency medical services: The paramedics' perspective. Prehosp Emerg Care 1:23–27, 1997.
14. Mainz J. Developing evidence-based clinical indicators: A state of the art methods primer. Int J Qual Health Care 15(Suppl 1):i5–i11, 2003.
15. Maio RF, Garrison HG, Spaite DW, et al. Emergency medical services outcomes project I (EMSOP I): prioritizing conditions for outcomes research. Ann Emerg Med Apr;33(4):423–432, 1999.
16. Cannon CP, Gibson CM, Lambrew CT, et al. Relationship of symptom-onset-to-balloon time and door-to-balloon time with mortality in patients undergoing angioplasty for acute myocardial infarction. JAMA 283(22):2941–2947, 2000.

17. Knight S, Olson LM, Cook LJ, Mann NC, Corneli HM, Dean JM. Against all advice: An analysis of out-of-hospital refusals of care. Ann Emerg Med Nov;42(5):689–696, 2003.
18. Jacobs I, Nadkarni V, and the ILCOR Task Force on Cardiac Arrest and Cardiopulmonary Resuscitation Outcomes. Cardiac Arrest and Cardiopulmonary Resuscitation Outcome Reports. Update and Simplification of the Utstein Templates for Resuscitation Registries: A Statement for Healthcare Professionals from a Task Force of the International Liaison Committee for Resuscitation. Circulation 110:3385–3397, 2004.
19. Wang H, et al. Recommended guidelines for uniform reporting of data from out-of-hospital airway management: Position statement of the National Association of EMS Physicians. Prehosp Emerg Care 8:58–72, 2004.

Personal Safety and Wellness

SECTION III

Chapter 15
Well-Being of the EMS Provider   101
Debra Cason, RN, MS, EMT-P

Chapter 16
Scene Safety   108
James Robinson, Paramedic

Chapter 17
Infectious Diseases Exposures   114
Connie S. Price, MD

Chapter 18
Critical Incident Stress   122
Philip Rach, MS, NREMT-P

Well-Being of the EMS Provider

CHAPTER 15

Debra Cason, RN, MS, EMT-P

1. **What constitutes a healthy individual?**
   A healthy individual is more than a person who is free from disease. Health involves various dimensions of wellness including physical, emotional, intellectual, social, and spiritual wellness. Optimal health requires a balanced, well-rounded individual who understands his or her body and mind and works to promote a high quality of wellness to improve lifespan and happiness.

2. **How are EMS providers at risk for a less-than-healthy lifestyle?**
   EMS providers inherently have various risks, some of which include the following: long and stressful work hours, driving and being the occupant of a vehicle that frequently is traveling at high speed, working in dangerous environments and situations, physically demanding work, watching and being part of human suffering and human inhumanity to each other, working around death and dying, exposure to infectious disease, and working with sometimes violent and impaired patients. Additionally, if the EMS provider is not careful, the work can contribute to poor nutrition, ineffective sleep patterns, sedentary lifestyle, poor methods of dealing with stress, and inattention to safety concerns.

3. **How do EMS providers compare in occupational fatalities to other public safety personnel?**
   According to B. J. Maguire and colleagues in a study published in 2002, EMS workers have a fatality rate of 12.7 per million workers annually, which compares to 14.2 for police, and 16.5 for firefighters during the same time period. However, in occupational issues related to transportation, EMS workers have a 9.6 fatality rate per 100,000 workers, police have 6.3, and firefighters have 4.5 fatality rate per 100,000. The general public has a fatality rate of 2.0 per 100,000 related to transportation. In this study, EMS personnel transportation related fatalities were as a vehicle driver or passenger (either in the front or in the back with a patient), struck by a moving vehicle, or involved in a helicopter crash.

4. **What are the leading causes of death in the United States?**
   Heart disease remains the leading cause of death today for all ages, with cancer following as the second leading cause of death. These two causes of death are responsible for two thirds of all deaths. Both heart disease and cancer are caused in part by lifestyle choices. Although the current average life expectancy in the United States is 78 years old, deaths that occur before age 65 years of age can be prevented 83% of the time by healthy lifestyle choices.

5. **What is the leading cause of preventable death?**
   Cigarette smoking is the number one cause of preventable deaths in the United States. Cigarette smoking causes cardiovascular diseases such as hypertension; heart disease; stroke; cancers in the lungs, stomach, bladder, cervix, esophagus, and pancreas; and respiratory diseases such as emphysema and chronic bronchitis. Tobacco-related deaths number more than 400,000 per year and also impact those who do not smoke. Nonsmokers exposed to tobacco smoke have an increased risk for cardiovascular disease and lung

cancer. Children who are exposed to cigarette smoke have higher rates of respiratory infections, allergies, and asthma.

6. **What successful strategies are available for individuals who would like to quit smoking?**
Evidence shows that it is never too late to quit smoking and that whenever a person quits smoking, it positively impacts their health. Factors that are associated with successful smoking cessation are (1) environmental changes, (2) substitute behaviors such as exercising or reading, (3) support through family, friends or a group, (4) stress management counseling, (5) medications such as nicotine replacement therapy, and 6) identifying and managing triggers.

7. **Are smokeless tobacco products also detrimental to one's health?**
Chewing tobacco and snuff are smokeless tobaccos and contain 28 cancer-causing agents. They can lead to nicotine addiction and adolescents who use these products are more likely to smoke cigarettes. For these reasons, smokeless tobacco is not a safe substitute to smoking tobacco.

8. **How do I decrease my risk for cardiovascular disease?**
Besides tobacco use, the factors that contribute to cardiovascular disease are high blood cholesterol, high blood pressure, obesity, and physical inactivity. Although heredity, age, and being a male are all risk factors for the development of cardiac disease, one must focus on controllable and modifiable prevention factors. Stress and how an individual responds to stress may also contribute to cardiac disease development as well as high alcohol intake.

A high cholesterol level is one risk factor that can be identified and usually managed. Individuals should have their cholesterol level measured at least once every 5 years after the age of 20 years. The lipoprotein profile measures low-density lipoprotein cholesterol (LDL or "bad cholesterol"), high-density lipoprotein cholesterol (HDL or "good cholesterol"), as well as triglycerides (free fatty acids), which are fats in the blood from excess sugars. Total cholesterol is also included in the profile. Interpretation of the lipoprotein profile is identified in Tables 15.1–15.4.

TABLE 15.1: LDL Cholesterol Values and Interpretations

LDL (bad) Cholesterol Value (mg/dl)	LDL (bad) Cholesterol Interpretation
Less than 100	Optimal
100–129	Near optimal
130–159	Borderline high
160–189	High
190 and above	Very high

TABLE 15-2: HDL Cholesterol Values and Interpretation

HDL (good) Cholesterol Value (mg/dl)	HDL (good) Cholesterol Interpretation
60 and above	Optimal; low risk of heart disease
Less than 40 in men	Low; considered to be a risk factor for heart disease
Less than 50 in women	

TABLE 15.3: Triglyceride Values and Interpretation

Triglyceride Value (mg/dl)	Triglyceride Interpretation
Less than 150	Normal
150–199	Borderline high
200–499	High
500 or higher	Very high

TABLE 15.4: Total Cholesterol Values and Interpretation

Total Cholesterol (mg/dl)	Interpretation
Less than 200	Desirable
200–239	Borderline high
240 and above	High

9. **What can be done about undesirable cholesterol levels?**
   LDL cholesterol can be decreased by losing body fat, significantly decreasing fat intake, exercise, and medication such as statin drugs.
   HDL cholesterol is primarily determined by genetics; however, there are methods to increase the "good cholesterol." A regular aerobic exercise program, weight control, smoking cessation, and medications help to increase HDL and lower cardiac disease risk. Triglyceride levels can usually be decreased by eliminating sweets and alcohol in the diet and losing weight.

10. **What physical fitness activities are important for health and wellness?**
    Health-related physical fitness includes cardiovascular endurance, muscle strength and endurance, muscle flexibility, and body composition. In addition to reducing stress, anxiety, and depression, physical activity and conditioning prevents injuries from lifting and moving and decreases cardiovascular disease risk.
    Cardiovascular endurance is probably the most important element of physical fitness, as it promotes efficiency of the cardiovascular system. Prolonged exercise enables the heart, lungs, and blood vessels to nourish muscles. In order for the body to acquire these effects, this cardiovascular endurance exercise should be done three to five times a week for 30 minutes of continuous vigorous aerobic activity. The target heart rate during this activity should be at 50–80% of an individual's heart rate reserve. This is estimated at 134–180 beats per minute for a 20-year-old person.
    Muscle-strengthening exercise is important for daily activities such as sitting, walking, lifting and carrying, and enjoying sports and recreational activities. Muscle strength lessens the risk for injuries, which is important for EMS providers. Muscular strength is improved and also maintained by resistance exercise such as free weights, weight machines, and use of resistance tubes.
    Muscle endurance exercise is important for good posture and injury prevention as an individual repeats movements without fatigue. These are characteristics that are desirable in the EMS workplace as well as in sports and recreation. Weight machines and free weights used repetitively with increased resistance build muscular strength and endurance.

Personal Safety and Wellness

Muscular flexibility is not always given its fair share of importance in exercise regimes but it is another important component to enhance the quality of life. Muscular flexibility is the ability of the joint to move easily through the full range of motion. This ability can prevent injury, particularly when sudden and strenuous moves are needed. Additionally, back problems can often be traced to inflexible and weak muscles, a high risk issue for EMS personnel.

11. **What is body composition?**
Body composition refers to the percent of body fat versus lean body mass. Obesity is associated with serious health problems including cardiovascular disease, diabetes, hypertension, high cholesterol, and blood clots that contribute to strokes and pulmonary embolism. Assessment of body composition can be accomplished by measuring skinfold thickness and girth, hydrostatic or underwater weighing, or bioelectric impedance. Many workout facilities have these methods available.

12. **Are there ways to decrease the risk of getting cancer?**
Absolutely! Cancer is greatly feared for many reasons and individuals can take steps to prevent it. Diet, exercise, and avoidance of smoking or tobacco are three major ways to prevent cancer. A diet to help prevent cancer would be high in fruits and vegetables, fiber, vitamins A and C, and low in fat. Antioxidant foods such as berries, broccoli, tomatoes, red grapes, garlic, spinach, tea, carrots, beans, russet potatoes, and whole grain foods can help prevent cancer and lower blood pressure. Obesity causes the body to produce more hormones such as estrogen and insulin and these substances circulating in the body can stimulate cancer growth. Alcohol should be consumed in moderation only. Additionally, excessive sun exposure is a major contributor to skin cancers.

13. **Are screening tests for cancer effective in early detection?**
Early detection through periodic cancer screening tests is essential to control or cure cancer. Premature deaths from cancer that could have been avoided through screening vary from 3% to 35%, depending on the location of the cancer and the screening methods. Additionally, screening may reduce cancer hospitalization, as treatment for earlier-stage cancers typically requires less aggressive intervention than that for more advanced-stage cancers. Table 15.5 provides the screening guidelines for individuals without symptoms.

14. **What cancer warning signs should prompt a person to see a doctor?**
Being aware and alert to cancer warning signs can mean early detection and a better outcome.
- Lung cancer is often signaled by hoarseness, a chronic cough, or persistent pain in the chest.
- Difficulty urinating, painful urination, and blood in the urine are warning signs of prostate or bladder cancer.
- A lump in the testicle is often the first warning sign of testicular cancer, which means the disease has progressed significantly.
- Pancreatic cancer is signaled by pain in the abdomen or lower back, jaundice, weight and appetite loss, nausea, and weakness.
- Blood in the stool can signal colon or rectal cancer.
- Esophagus and stomach cancer warning signs include a two-week or longer duration of indigestion, blood in the stool, vomiting, and rapid weight loss.
- Changes in a mole or skin sore are a warning sign of skin cancer. A wart that is asymmetrical, bigger than a pencil eraser, more than one color, an uneven shape, or bleeds or crusts needs to be evaluated by a dermatologist for melanoma, a deadly skin cancer.

TABLE 15.5: Screening Guidelines for Individuals without Symptoms

Cancer Site	Screening Tool	Frequency	Age to Begin Screening	Risk Factor to Alter Beginning Age or Increase Screening Intervals
Breast	Self-exam	Monthly	20	Family history, genetic tendency, history of breast cancer
Breast	Mammogram	Yearly	40	Family history, genetic tendency, history of breast cancer
Colon and rectum	Fecal occult blood test	Yearly	50	Family history
Colon and rectum	Flexible sigmoidoscopy or colonoscopy	Every 5–10 years	50	Family history
Prostate	PSA blood test	Yearly	45–50	African American men, family history
Prostate	Digital rectal exam	Yearly	45–50	African American men, family history
Uterus	Pap smear	Yearly	21 or 3 years after vaginal intercourse begins	HIV infection, weak immune system

- Irregular or abnormal vaginal bleeding is a warning sign for ovarian, cervical, or endometrial cancer.
- Jaundice, fever, nausea, and liver tenderness signal liver cancer.
- An enlarged lymph gland is the first sign of lymphoma, cancer of the lymph system. Other signs of lymphoma may be fever, back or abdominal pain, night fever, unexplained weight loss, and nausea and vomiting.
- Thyroid cancer may have a lump in the neck, difficulty swallowing, choking, and persistent hoarseness.
- Leukemia warning signs include fatigue, paleness, night sweats, repeated infections, nosebleeds, bone and joint pain, and easy bruising.

Being aware of one's body and body changes is a key to early detection and intervention of cancer.

15. **How do sleep and sleep patterns impact the health and well-being of EMS providers?**
    EMS providers have job responsibilities that frequently require them to be awake and alert when their bodies are meant to sleep. This interference with normal circadian rhythms can certainly create problems. Shift work is defined as a variety of work schedules that change, whether they are 8- or 12-hour shifts

TABLE 15.6: Potential Impact of Shift Work

Hypertension	Increased risk of accidents
Cardiovascular disease	Increased sleep disorders
Obesity	Greater use of health care
Increased indigestion and heartburn	Increased consumption of caffeine
Increased triglycerides	Interference with social life
Impaired glucose tolerance	Increased psychological problems

or two to three shifts in a row, with or without weekends. An extended shift such as 24 hours or straight night or evening shifts have many issues in common with these changing work schedules.

Several conditions and diseases have been associated with shift work including the list in Table 15.6.

16. How can the problems associated with shift work and long hours be lessened?

For the individual who must work rotating shifts, there are several strategies to help lessen the problems of the necessary work schedule. Regular eating patterns and meal times should be maintained as much as possible and greasy foods and junk foods avoided. Individuals who work afternoons and evenings should have their largest meal at midday. Those who work night time shifts should eat small meals during the shift with a moderate breakfast so they do not get hungry during the day while they are asleep. As much as possible, meals should be relaxing and allow for digestion time.

In addition to meal strategies, sleep should be on a set schedule. Different patterns of sleep working around the shift should be tried to see how the individual responds to the sleep. Family and friends should be aware and sensitive to sleep needs and a dark, quiet, and cool place to sleep is important. A time of quiet relaxation with muscle relaxation and breathing techniques before sleep time are recommended. If sleep is delayed once in bed, reading or soothing music should be considered.

17. How does stress manifest itself?

Stress impacts individuals in different ways. Some people do not like to admit they are stressed and fail to recognize its symptoms. Identifying stress is the first step in managing it. Some common symptoms of stress include headaches, neck and shoulder aches, grinding teeth, insomnia, nervous tics such as finger tapping or jiggling keys, fatigue, depression, impotence, anger, hostility, stomach pain, poor concentration, pacing, restlessness, loss of sex drive, acne, high blood pressure, increased or decreased appetite, stuttering, and others. Stress stimulates the sympathetic nervous system which activates catecholamines (hormones) that cause the "flight or fight" mechanism. This mechanism is necessary for the body to respond to severe stress. Physical manifestations include increased heart rate and blood pressure, increased blood sugar, increased blood flow to muscles and brain, increased oxygen use, and an increase in general awareness.

18. What are some effective stress-reduction strategies?

There are healthy stress reduction techniques other than yelling, abusing alcohol or drugs, breaking things, kicking the dog or child or spouse, or hiding in front of the computer for hours. The combined strategies of managing the body, mind, heart, and spirit can be more successful in reducing stress than any single technique. The reader will not be surprised that stress reduction includes healthy eating and exercise. Eliminating fats, simple sugars, caffeine, and alcohol in the diet as well as consuming complex carbohydrates and lots of water are healthy eating habits that can reduce stress. Regular, vigorous exercise, meditation, music relaxation therapy, and communication with a personal support system are additional stress-reduction habits. Many resources are available on stress and stress reduction through an Internet search or at the public library or bookstore.

Pearls and Pitfalls

1. A healthy mind and body are of critical importance to EMS providers, as they should first take care of themselves in order to care for others and role model a healthy lifestyle.
2. EMS providers must have a heightened awareness of safety issues at all times as occupational risk, particularly related to vehicles, is very high.
3. Cigarette smoking and tobacco use are the number one preventable risk factors for illness and disease.
4. With the many health risk factors associated with EMS, a healthy diet and regular exercise should be mainstays of the provider's lifestyle.
5. Periodic cancer screening as prescribed can assist in early detection and more effective treatment and cure of this much-feared disease.

References

1. American Cancer Society. Cancer Facts and Figures 2007. Atlanta, GA: www.cancer.gov/cancertopics/pdq/screening/overview/, accessed May 31, 2011.
2. American Heart Association: Risk Factors and Coronary Heart Disease. www.americanheart.org/presenter.jhtml?identifier=4726/, accessed May 31, 2011.
3. The Link between Lifestyle and Cancer. http://www.sciencedaily.com/releases/2007/12/071207120839.htm, accessed May 31, 2011.
4. Centers for Chronic Disease Prevention and Health Promotion. Smokeless Tobacco Fact Sheet. http://www.cdc.gov/tobacco/basic_information/smokeless/index.htm, accessed May 31, 2011.
5. Centers for Disease Control, National Institute for Occupational Safety and Health. Overtime and Extended Work Shifts: Recent Findings on Illnesses, Injuries and Health Behaviors. Publication number 2004-143. http://www.cdc.gov/niosh/docs/2004-143/, accessed May 31, 2011.
6. Hoeger, WWK, Hoeger, SA. Principles and Labs for Fitness and Wellness. Belmont, CA: Thomson Wadsworth, 2005.
7. Hoeger, WKW, Hoeger, SA. Lifetime Physical Fitness and Wellness. 8th ed.. Belmont, CA: Thomson Wadsworth, 2005.
8. Hopson, JL, Hopson, EH, Dyar, JT. Burnout to Balance, EMS Stress. Upper Saddle River, NJ: Prentice Hall, 2001.
9. Maguire, BJ, Hunting, KL, Smith, GS, Levick, NR. Occupational fatalities in emergency medical services: A hidden crisis. Ann Emerg Med 40:6, 2002.
10. Mikolaj, AA. Stress Management for the Emergency Care Provider. Upper Saddle River, NJ: Prentice Hall, 2004.
11. Robinson, D, Kish, CP. Core Concepts in Advanced Practice Nursing. Philadelphia: Mosby, 2001.

Scene Safety

James Robinson, Paramedic

1. **I am an EMS provider. Who would want to hurt me?**
   The environment in which EMS providers function is unpredictable and dynamic. Patients, family members, and bystanders all have the potential to pose a threat to responders. Contrary to what may seem to be common sense, EMS providers are not always welcomed with open arms. Alcohol, illicit drugs, gang activity, domestic violence, mutual combatants, psychiatric issues, head trauma, or metabolic disorders may make otherwise reasonable and rational people act violently. There is also the uniform. In the "heat" of an incident all uniforms tend to look alike. People who may have animosity toward police officers or other uniformed services may perceive EMS in the same light and behave accordingly. There is increasing concern about the potential for specific targeting of EMS providers. In today's society, with the growing threat of terrorism, the prospect of secondary improvised explosive devices targeted at EMS providers and other emergency workers is a grim but real one.

2. **The police will always protect me, right?**
   Although police take the role of protecting EMS providers seriously, they will not always be requested, nor will they respond on every call for EMS service. When they do co-respond, the extent of the police cover may be a lone officer. It is imperative that EMS providers be responsible for their own safety at all times. Although the presence of police cover does improve EMS provider safety, it does not mean a scene is safe. Any scene may deteriorate, and EMS providers must remain constantly vigilant about their personal safety.

3. **What are the most perilous calls?**
   One of the common misconceptions is that the most dangerous calls are shootings and stabbing scenes. In fact, these calls may present little risk simply because most perpetrators leave the scene after committing their crime. Calls that probably hold the greatest risk involve alcohol, drugs, and psychiatric patients because the behavior of patients and bystanders is unpredictable. Domestic violence calls are also very unpredictable; more police officers are killed or injured on domestic violence calls than on any other type of call.

4. **Can I control every scene?**
   The perception that one can "control" a scene is arguably overly optimistic. Perhaps a more realistic concept is scene *management*. It is possible to manage many of the variables of an EMS call, but it is impossible to control them all. There are things that are absolutely out of our control such as weather, or the width of a staircase for egress, and things that are manageable, such as bystanders on a scene, or lighting. The misconception that EMS providers can control every scene is dangerous and can lead to untoward events. Being adaptable and being a problem solver are prerequisites for all successful EMS providers.

Scene Safety

5. What is the best tool I have to ensure my safety?
Situational, or global, awareness—the ability to see the big picture. The term is derived from military pilots who fly combat missions. To ensure survival, a pilot in combat must be aware of everything going on around the aircraft at all times. We can draw a direct analogy between the pilot in combat and an EMS call. To be safe, EMS providers must be aware of the big picture on every scene. Unfortunately, many EMS providers fall prey to "tunnel vision." Focusing solely on the patient, to the exclusion of everything else around them, is perilous to providers. As mundane as an EMS call may seem, it is important to always maintain global awareness. It is also important for EMS providers to look out for each other. Because EMS providers work in teams, it is important that when one member of the team is focusing primarily on the patient, the other(s) maintain global awareness.

6. How do I learn global awareness?
As with any other skill, practice and reinforcement lead to success. Global awareness is linked in many ways to the provider's comfort level with patient assessment and care. As expertise grows, providers' thought processes become more automatic, allowing them to improve global awareness and see the context of the call in its entirety more easily. Because of this, it is even more important for inexperienced EMS providers to make global awareness a conscious thought process. To begin with, practice anticipating and identifying potential safety hazards as you arrive at the scene and sizing up the entire situation as you approach. Successful mental imaging will improve this skill, and it will become a conditioned response. It is important to assess the situation initially, and then reassess, reassess, reassess. Successful global awareness requires continual scanning since scenes are constantly changing. A scene that was initially safe may not remain so. One must keep that "mental searchlight" moving and assess all of the environmental variables: the patient, the patient's family, the bystanders, and the physical setting. Early identification of changes in scene dynamics will maximize your safety by allowing you to recognize a scene that is dangerous or deteriorating.

7. So, when do I have to start worrying about my safety?
The time prior to making patient contact poses safety risks in addition to the scene itself. Getting to a scene may actually be one of the more dangerous elements of an EMS call. It is important to ensure your safe arrival by safe vehicle operation and the use of seatbelts. When you arrive at a scene, you are guaranteed to become the focus of the neighborhood's attention; everything you do will be under a microscope. No one in EMS likes to perform for crowds. When approaching any scene, particularly those that are potentially high risk, consider shutting down the emergency lights and sirens several blocks away to allow for a discreet arrival. This will enable you to survey the scene before announcing your presence. Choose a strategic parking location that will provide a safe approach to the scene and a quick exit should the need arise. Approach houses and doors from the side instead of directly from the front. During the approach, scan for any signs of danger and listen for sounds that may be clues to safety hazards—yelling and screaming, barking dogs, and the like.

8. Shouldn't I just wait for the police before entering a high-risk scene?
Many EMS systems have policies that direct their personnel to wait for police to secure a violent scene before entering. The problem with this is that it is often difficult to determine whether or not a scene is high risk prior to arriving and this type of policy ignores the fact that the most hazardous calls can start out innocently and deteriorate rapidly. It is vitally important for EMS providers to

Personal Safety and Wellness

maintain global awareness and make the best possible decisions about whether or not to enter a scene. Just because the dispatched nature or priority sounds innocuous does not mean that there are not potential dangers. Attention to changes in elements of a scene and scene dynamics are keys to minimizing risks.

9. **Are there any red flags that can help me identify potential danger?**
   A dark house at night, an open door, and signs of violence such as blood and broken glass and furniture may be indicators of an unsafe scene. Traffic zooming by in close proximity, unusual smells, hallways with one way in and out are others. These types of findings should raise red flags in your head, but probably will not if you are not being globally aware. The "fight or flight" response is universal. When something does not "feel" right, increase your awareness and trust your instincts. With patients, bystanders, and family members, look for signs of hostility such as body language, tone of voice, and level of animation. Scan the environment for any type of potential weapon, and a way out. Do not let yourself be cut off from your egress when you can avoid it.

10. **What is the lion-tamer theory?**
    It is one of the most effective techniques for controlling a high-risk patient or a high-risk scene. The lion tamer at a circus enters the large cage and then watches as the lions and tigers are brought into this cage one by one. By bringing these dangerous cats into the cage, the lion tamer establishes a psychological advantage over the animals. The lion tamer will *never* go into the lion's cage, because it's the lion's home, a place where the lion has an instinctive psychological advantage. Problem patients maintain a similar advantage when we enter their "cage." By moving such a patient quickly into our cage, the ambulance, or by simply moving them out of their environment, we can reverse this psychological edge.

11. **What is the best way to manage a scene to keep yourself safe?**
    The variability of EMS scenes makes algorithmic management of them difficult. A good start on any scene, however, is to enter with confidence, and actively manage it. Patients—like dogs—can smell fear. If the people on a scene sense weakness or indecision, any semblance of control you may have will soon be lost. Conversely, confident management and delegation quietly tell everyone on the scene that you are the person in charge. It is important to pick out the key players in the crowd as well. Enlisting them in your efforts may be the best thing you can do, by making allies out of potential enemies. It is important to maintain your empathy and inform the people on the scene what is going on, as much as the patient's rights to privacy will allow.

12. **What are the red flags signaling that a patient may become violent?**
    You must learn to read not only the scene but also your patients by observing their body language and verbal comments. Common forms of aggressive body language include the boxer's stance, where the patient "squares off" to fight. Another form is a stance taken when one is feeling threatened, called blading; the patient will turn at an angle toward you, "blading his body." The "1000 yard stare," where the patient is "looking right through you," is seen when a patient is mentally preparing to fight—the calm before the storm. Any patient showing obvious anxiety and lots of agitated motor activity is also at high risk for becoming violent. You may observe "target glancing," with the patient stealing furtive glances at the trauma scissors on your belt or the door. This patient is telegraphing his intention to grab

your scissors or try to escape. Verbal cues, with the patient screaming or using pressured speech, also can help to predict violent behavior.

13. What is the best way to approach a patient who may become violent?
Any patient may become violent, and almost everyone dislikes intrusions into his or her personal space. Intoxicated or psychiatric patients are especially prone to violence if you approach them too quickly and violate their personal space. With all patients, it is important to telegraph your intentions, either expressly by verbally forewarning them, or subtly by waiting for acquiescence to a slow, deliberate movement toward their personal space. Informing patients of your intentions will prevent an unwanted response to your actions. If a patient seems safe to contact, approach slowly from an angle instead of from directly in front. Make eye contact with the patient, and when possible, at eye level with the patient. Take care not to put yourself in a compromised position where you can be pushed, punched, and kicked while interviewing the patient or performing an exam.

14. How do I verbally control problem patients?
Most potentially violent patients can be controlled verbally. Set the proper tone for the call by being cooperative. Be empathetic, and portray an understanding of the patient's points of view. Being verbally aggressive with these patients is counterproductive and will often escalate them to violence. Make an effort to give the patient options—even if they are limited—instead of ultimatums, and allow them to make a choice. Be an advocate for them while directing them to the outcome you are looking for.

15. Which patients do I need to restrain?
Anyone who is violent needs to be restrained, and anyone who you feel is going to become violent probably needs to be. It is also important to restrain acutely ill or injured patients who require a lot of interventions. Many of these decisions will be driven by department policy or medical protocol, but as long as the reasons are legitimate and well documented, provider judgment will usually be defensible. It is important to remember that the decision to restrain a patient may constitute a deprivation of a civil liberty, and that it is not a decision to be made haphazardly. Patient and crew safety come first, and using this as a guideline will serve you well. It may take up to six people to restrain an extremely violent patient. Have a team approach, with each member of the team assigned to restraining a certain portion of the patient. Four-point restraints, at a minimum, are recommended. Chemical restraint with intravenous or intramuscular sedation is an adjunct to consider if patients pose a risk to providers or themselves.

16. Do I need to search my patients?
Any patient that you think may pose a threat to you needs to be searched. A search for weapons should be incorporated into the physical assessment of any patient. If you are not comfortable performing a search, ask a police officer to do it. Remember to search the patient's belongings if you feel it is necessary, as well as those of any other person you allow to ride in the ambulance with the patient. Your ambulance needs to be a weapons-free environment. Being in the back of a 10-foot by 15-foot box with a person who has a weapon is a less than advantageous position to be in. Patients should be separated from purses, backpacks, pocket knives, knitting needles, lighters, and the like during transport, and reunited with them at the hospital. Most patients will understand the reasons for this, as long as you frame it in the context of overall safety.

Personal Safety and Wellness

17. Do I need to wear concealed body armor?

The decision to invest in concealed bullet-resistant body armor is a personal one. Most employers do not fund the purchase, which can cost $300–$500. Many EMS providers, like most police officers, would never work without their vests. Although the risk of EMS providers being shot may be low, soft body armor provides some protection from blunt injury such as kicks, punches, and automobile crashes. More than one EMS provider has been saved by a trauma plate in the front of a ballistic vest when the steering wheel was pushed into their chests during a motor vehicle crash. Some more modern versions of soft body armor are puncture and slash resistant as well, protecting from sharp objects and blades. Body armor may also keep you warmer in the winter.

18. What's the greatest danger the prehospital provider will face in the field?

Exposure to infectious diseases. Always take appropriate precautions to avoid any potential exposure, and always wear gloves and protective eyewear. Mask and gowns should be donned situationally.

19. Besides the personal risk from violence, are there other safety concerns?

There are always risks beyond the obvious threat of violence. Be careful when attending to motor vehicle accident victims in active traffic lanes. Strategic parking of the ambulance is important on such scenes. Be aware of terrain when approaching scenes. Slipping on ice, or falling into a hole, will not help you help your patient. Back injury from lifting patients is one of the most common injuries to EMS providers. Be sure to use proper body mechanics when lifting, and solicit extra help when necessary. Most EMS agencies do not have restraint systems for the EMS provider attending to the patient during transport. Be sure to limit standing up in the back, and, unless you are performing a procedure or an assessment, try to remain seated and seat belted. When you are unbelted, try to maintain three points of contact with the ambulance.

Pearls and Pitfalls

1. All aspects of the EMS call, including the response, the scene, and the transport, provide potential hazards to the EMS responder.
2. Focusing only on the patient and failing to maintain a global awareness of what is happening on the scene can lead to unexpected and potentially serious consequences and injury to the unwary EMS responder.
3. One of the best ways to help control a potentially high-risk patient or scene is to move the patient into your environment – the ambulance.
4. It is essential to know and recognize the physical and verbal clues that signal that a patient or bystander may become violent.
5. The greatest danger that an EMS responder will face on every scene is infectious disease exposure.

References

1. Dernocoeur K. Streetsense: Communications, Safety, and Control. Bowie, MD: Brady, 1985.
2. Mizell LR Jr. Streetsense for Women: How to Stay Safe in a Violent World. New York: Berkley Books, 1993.
3. Remsberg C. The Tactical Edge: Surviving High Risk Patrol. Northbrook, IL: Calibre Press, 1986.

4. Thompson GS, Jenkins JB. Verbal Judo: The Gentle Art of Persuasion. New York: Quill Publishing, 1993.
5. Whitfield RG. Dealing with violence. Int J Offender Ther Comp Criminol 26:255–262, 1982.
6. Winfree L, Williams L. Call security: The effects of fear and public image on staff-security contacts in a public hospital. J Police Sci Admin 13:310–329, 1985.
7. Klein G. Sources of Power: How People Make Decisions. Cambridge, MA: MIT Press, 1998.
8. Shiller R. Street Control: Survival and Scene Management for EMS Professionals. Denver, CO: 1999.
9. Shea, T. CSM Restraint Guidelines: A Guide. Denver, CO: 2005

Infectious Diseases Exposures

Connie S. Price, MD

CHAPTER 17

1. **What are pathogens and communicable diseases, and how are they transmitted?**
   Pathogens are microorganisms that cause disease; pathogens include viruses, bacteria, fungi, protozoa, multicellular parasites, or even proteinaceous particles (prions). Communicable diseases are infections that can be transmitted from one person or species to another by transfer of a pathogen through one or more of several different mechanisms. In the prehospital setting, infectious diseases are most commonly spread through direct contact with an individual, contact with the bodily fluids of infected individuals, or with objects that the infected individual has contaminated. Some examples of specific infections and their mode of transmission are shown in the following table:

Mechanism	Infectious Disease Example
Aerosolization of small droplet nuclei suspended in air	Tuberculosis
Aerosolization of large droplets within 3 feet of direct line of droplets	Bacterial meningitis, influenza, pertussis
Direct contact with body fluids	Sexually transmitted diseases
Direct contact with contaminated surfaces or hands	Common cold, multidrug-resistant bacteria (e.g., MRSA), influenza
Ingestion of contaminated food or water	Cholera, food poisoning
Direct penetration of skin	Strongyloidiasis
Vector (e.g., mosquito)	Malaria, West Nile virus

2. **Are prehospital personnel at higher risk for infections?**
   Health care workers who provide direct patient care are at greater risk for diseases that can be transmitted human to human. Not all infectious diseases are efficiently transmitted this way. Zoonoses such as Q fever, tularemia, anthrax, and many of the viral hemorrhagic fevers are typically spread efficiently from animals to humans but inefficiently spread from human to human. Infections such as malaria and West Nile virus require the presence of their mosquito vectors. Diseases transmitted solely by sexual activity (gonorrhea, chlamydia) do not pose much risk to the prehospital provider. Diseases transmitted by ingestion of contaminated food can often be transmitted by inadvertently ingesting contaminated stool.

3. **But cannot modern medicine treat and cure these infections?**
   Only some. That's why this chapter is so important. Some diseases such as hepatitis B, hepatitis C, and human immunodeficiency virus, and even some strains of tuberculosis, can only be curtailed

with treatment and eventually may cause significant morbidity and even death. Prevention is primary!

4. **What is personal protective equipment and how does it help prevent the spread of infection?**
Personal protective equipment (PPE) is any type of specialized clothing, barrier product, or breathing (respiratory) device used to protect workers from serious injuries or illnesses while doing their jobs. Examples include devices such as surgical gowns, gloves, masks, and respirators that act as a barrier between infectious materials and the skin, mouth, nose, or eyes (mucous membranes). Proper use of PPE by workers involved in patient care aids infection control because it helps protect wearers against infection or contamination from blood, body fluids, or respiratory secretions; reduces the chance that health care workers will infect or contaminate patients or coworkers; and reduces the chance of transmitting infections from one person to another.

5. **What types of masks should be used in patient care?**
Surgical masks help protect against microorganisms, body fluids, and large particles in the air and are designed to cover the mouth and nose loosely. Masks also help prevent exposure to the wearer's saliva and respiratory secretions. The masks are not sized for individual fit and are made of soft materials that are more comfortable to wear than other types of masks. Choose a surgical mask to help protect yourself if you may be splattered by someone else's body fluids (such as blood, respiratory secretions, vomit, urine, or feces) or help protect others if you are caring for an open wound or if you are sick.
In addition to all of the protection offered by surgical masks, N95 respirators are masks that are designed to protect against small droplets of respiratory fluids and other airborne particles. These respirators fit closely to form a tight seal over the mouth and nose and must be adjusted to your face through fit testing to provide intended effectiveness. Choose a surgical N95 respirator to provide the same protections as a surgical mask AND to help protect yourself if you will be exposed to very small particles (e.g., fine aerosolized droplets) such as those produced by coughing or for caring for persons with known or suspected pulmonary and laryngeal tuberculosis or other airborne diseases.

6. **When do prehospital personnel need to use PPE?**
As part of standard precautions (formerly universal precautions), the health care worker assumes that every patient potentially has a communicable disease, and he or she wears appropriate PPE for the situation. This is important because it is not always possible to know from the history, appearance, or examination whether or not a patient has a communicable disease. Standard precautions apply to blood, all body fluids, secretions, and excretions (except sweat), nonintact skin, and mucous membranes.
- Latex or plastic gloves are recommended for all potential exposures to bodily fluids, including blood and open wounds, or when handling hazardous materials.
- Use protective eyewear when splashes to the face are possible.
- Use surgical gowns to cover your trunk, arms, legs, and clothing when you may be splattered by someone else's body fluids (such as blood, respiratory secretions, vomit, urine, or feces).
- Use surgical masks to protect the oral mucous membranes during splash settings as well as to filter potentially infectious droplets from patients suspected of having a disease spread by large respiratory droplets.

Personal Safety and Wellness

- Use N95 masks for patients who are suspected of having a communicable respiratory disease spread by the airborne route (such as tuberculosis), or when performing high-risk aerosol-generating procedures on patients with respiratory infections.

7. **What are transmission-based precautions?**
   In addition to standard precautions, there are three types of additional precautions—airborne, droplet, and contact—which are based on the mode of transmission, also known as transmission-based precautions. (See the following table.)

Type of Precaution	Examples of Diseases	Special Factors
Airborne	■ Tuberculosis ■ Measles ■ Chicken pox ■ Smallpox ■ SARS	■ Tell the receiving facility that the patient will require a negative-pressure private room. ■ Wear NIOSH-certified N95 mask for patient care. ■ If possible, the patient should wear a surgical mask during transport. ■ Set air conditioning or heating of the transport vehicle to nonrecirculating mode or open the vehicle windows if possible. ■ Disinfect vehicle after transport.
Droplet	■ Influenza ■ Whooping cough ■ Mumps	■ Private (or separate) room upon arrival to the receiving facility or separate at least 3 feet from other patients. ■ Wear surgical mask when working within 3 feet of a patient. ■ If possible, the patient should wear a surgical mask during transport. ■ Disinfect vehicle after transport.
Contact	■ VRE ■ MRSA ■ lice ■ scabies ■ RSV ■ Impetigo ■ Smallpox	■ Private (or separate) room upon arrival to the receiving facility. ■ Wear gown and gloves for patient contact. ■ Limit movements and transport of the patient. ■ Use dedicated patient care equipment when possible. ■ Disinfect vehicle after transport.

NIOSH = National Institute of Occupational Safety and Health. SARS = Severe acute respiratory syndrome. VRE = vancomycin-resistant enterococcus. MRSA = methicillin-resistant *Staphylococcus aureus*. RSV = respiratory syncytial virus.

Always maintain a high index of suspicion for communicable diseases. When in doubt, isolate the patient. Hand hygiene should always be performed before and after patient contact and after removal of personal protective equipment (e.g., gowns, gloves, masks). If a patient being transferred has known active

TB or is highly suspected of such, the transferring facility should notify prehospital staff on transport. This knowledge should also be communicated to the receiving facility, preferably before arrival, so that airborne isolation rooms can be arranged.

8. **What clues may indicate that a patient has a communicable disease?**
Often there are none, but in some cases, "classic" signs and symptoms may be present:
- Tuberculosis (TB)—Persistent cough >3 weeks, cough productive of bloody sputum, fever, night sweats, weight loss, and previous exposure to TB. Groups at highest risk include immigrants from countries with a high prevalence of TB. Other risk groups include the homeless, incarcerated, or institutionalized patients.
- Pertussis (whooping cough)—Persistent hacking nonproductive cough, most often pediatric patients.
- Meningitis—Fever, stiff neck, or neck pain; muscle aches; rash on extremities; "flulike" syndrome.
- Hepatitis—Fever, nausea, jaundice (yellowing of the skin), fatigue.
- HIV/AIDS—This depends on the stage of illness. Acute illness may manifest with symptoms of fatigue, fever, rash, lymphadenopathy, and weight loss. Later in the course of the illness, evidence of the immunocompromised state such as thrush may be present. As with hepatitis B and C, HIV occurs more frequently but not always in high-risk groups such as intravenous drug abusers, homosexuals, bisexuals, heterosexual exposure to high-risk partners, or maternal-neonatal exposure.
- MRSA—Any skin abscess or similar lesion that resembles a spider bite, draining wound, or pus. Now common in the community without known risk factors.

9. **What are the principles of universal respiratory etiquette and why is this important for prehospital personnel?**
In response to the severe acute respiratory syndrome (SARS) outbreak that resulted in disproportionate numbers of health care worker illness and death, in October 2003, the Centers for Disease Control and Prevention (CDC) issued draft documents to assist health care personnel in preparedness for a possible reemergence of SARS or other emerging infection spread by respiratory droplets. The assumption is that every person with a respiratory illness is a potential source of serious respiratory infection that can be transmitted to others. This represents a paradigm shift in preventing disease in daily medical practice and includes the use of surgical or procedure masks by health care personnel during the evaluation of any patient with respiratory symptoms, and, when possible, to provide surgical masks to all patients with symptoms of a respiratory illness with instructions on the proper mask use and disposal. For patients who cannot wear a surgical mask, provide tissues to cover their nose and mouth when coughing or sneezing. Continue to use droplet precautions to manage patients with respiratory symptoms until it is determined that the cause of symptoms is not communicable. Triage staff should consider wearing surgical masks during respiratory infection season or remain behind Plexiglas barriers. Keeping a distance of at least 3 feet from symptomatic patients is recommended until a private room or cubicle is available. Good ventilation is also important, as is access to hand hygiene. These measures will minimize the transmission of respiratory illness, even without knowing whether the specific infectious agent is SARS coronavirus, H5N1 influenza virus, common cold virus, or seasonal influenza virus.

10. **What additional precautions are recommended for prehospital personnel caring for avian/H5N1 influenza patients or other highly lethal infectious diseases that are potentially airborne transmitted?**
    These principles may apply to H5N1 influenza and many other infectious diseases transmitted by the airborne route, and include:
    - Following universal respiratory etiquette principles
    - Observing standard precautions for patient care and for handling waste
    - Use of full barrier (contact) precautions when caring for potentially communicable patients
    - Unless lifesaving, avoiding aerosol-generating procedures (suctioning, positive pressure ventilation)
    - Optimizing air exchange in the transport vehicle, ideally with separate compartments for the driver and the patient/provider
    - Notifying the receiving facility of a potentially infectious patient
    - Cleaning and disinfecting the vehicle and reusable patient care items after patient transport

11. **How is TB transmitted and what are the risks to prehospital personnel?**
    TB is an airborne illness caused by a bacterium, *Mycobacterium tuberculosis*. It is generally a pulmonary disease but may also affect other organs such as the kidneys, lymph nodes, vertebrae, or adrenal glands. It is spread by the airborne route from a coughing or sneezing patient with active pulmonary or laryngeal disease. Proper drug treatment may contain a primary infection within scar tissue and make the disease inactive. Reactivation of the disease can occur in immunosuppressed patients, such as those with AIDS, cancer, or advancing age. The drug arsenal against TB is limited to five or six primary drugs. Recent development of multidrug resistant (MDR) TB and extremely drug-resistant TB (XDR-TB) has been seen. Infection with TB can be lethal, particularly strains with drug resistance, so the utmost attention must be paid to protective mask wearing, especially particulate (N95) respirators, when transporting high-risk patients.

12. **How are hepatitis B and hepatitis C transmitted, and what is the course of these diseases?**
    Hepatitis B virus (HBV) and hepatitis C virus (HCV) are organisms transmitted by blood or by sexual contact. Both viruses cause inflammation of the liver in the acute phase of infection and sometimes cause long-term effects. Hepatitis can also be caused by food (hepatitis A) or by chemical toxicity (alcohol). Up to 50–75% of transmitted cases of HBV or HCV will be minimally symptomatic (or asymptomatic). Of those with acute HBV, 5–10% will develop chronic hepatitis, cirrhosis (scarring of the liver), or liver cancer; 25% of minimally symptomatic "carriers" will develop some of these long-term effects. HCV infection will produce such long-term effects in 20–60% of cases. Currently, HBV infection can be prevented with the hepatitis B vaccine, which is usually provided free of charge by employers. No such vaccine for HCV currently exists.

13. **How is AIDS transmitted, and what is the course of disease?**
    The acquired immunodeficiency syndrome (AIDS) is caused by the human immunodeficiency virus and is transmitted by blood or by sexual contact. Infection with the virus causes a disease spectrum ranging from asymptomatic infection to AIDS. AIDS generally develops 3 to 8 years after HIV infection as the virus decreases the ability of the body's immune system to fight infection. Specific illnesses seen with

Infectious Diseases Exposures

AIDS (thrush, pneumocystis pneumonia, Kaposi's sarcoma) are fought off quite well by people with competent immune systems. Recent breakthroughs in drug therapy have markedly decreased the progression of HIV and AIDS, but a cure for the disease remains elusive.

14. How can occupational exposures be prevented?

Many needle sticks and other cuts can be prevented by using safer techniques such as:
- Never recapping needles
- Disposing of used needles in puncture-resistant sharps disposal containers
- Using medical devices with safety features designed to prevent injuries
- Using appropriate barriers such as gloves, eye and face protection, or gowns when contact with blood is expected can prevent many exposures to the eyes, nose, mouth, or skin

15. What should I do if I am exposed to a patient's blood?

- Immediately following an exposure to blood:
    - Wash needle sticks and cuts with soap and water
    - Flush splashes to the nose, mouth, or skin with water
    - Irrigate eyes with clean water, saline, or sterile irrigants
- No scientific evidence shows that using antiseptics or squeezing the wound will reduce the risk of transmission of a blood-borne pathogen. Using a caustic agent such as bleach is not recommended.
- Report the exposure to the department responsible for managing exposures (e.g., occupational health, infection control). Prompt reporting is essential because, in some cases, postexposure treatment may be recommended and it should be started as soon as possible. Discuss the possible risks of acquiring HBV, HCV, and HIV and the need for postexposure treatment with the provider managing your exposure. You should have already received hepatitis B vaccine, which is extremely safe and effective in preventing HBV infection.

16. What is the risk of infection after an occupational exposure?

- HBV—Healthcare personnel who have received hepatitis B vaccine and developed immunity to the virus are at virtually no risk for infection. For a susceptible person, the risk from a single needlestick or cut exposure to HBV-infected blood ranges from 6-30% and depends on the hepatitis B e antigen (HBeAg) status of the source individual. HBeAg-positive patients are more likely to transmit HBV than those who are HBeAg negative. Although there is a risk for HBV infection from exposures of mucous membranes or nonintact skin, there is no known risk for HBV infection from exposure to intact skin.
- HCV—The average risk for infection after a needlestick or cut exposure to HCV-infected blood is approximately 1.8%. The risk following a blood exposure to the eye, nose, or mouth is unknown, but is believed to be very small; however, HCV infection from blood splash to the eye has been reported. There also has been a report of HCV transmission that may have resulted from exposure to non-intact skin, but there is no known risk from exposure to intact skin.
- HIV—The average risk of HIV infection after a needlestick or cut exposure to HIV-infected blood is 0.3% The risk after exposure of the eye, nose, or mouth to HIV-infected blood is estimated to be, on average, 0.1%. The risk after exposure of non-intact skin to HIV-infected blood is estimated to be less

than 0.1%. A small amount of blood on intact skin probably poses no risk at all. There have been no documented cases of HIV transmission due to an exposure involving a small amount of blood on intact skin (a few drops of blood on skin for a short period of time).

17. **Are prehospital personnel at risk for getting meningitis if they take care of someone with the disease?**
Fortunately, the bacteria and viruses that cause meningitis are not spread by casual contact or by simply breathing the air where a person with meningitis has been. However, certain forms of bacterial meningitis—particularly *Neisseria meningitidis* (also called meningococcal meningitis) or *Haemophilus influenzae* type b (Hib)—are spread to those directly exposed to the patient's oral secretions (e.g., through kissing, mouth-to-mouth resuscitation, endotracheal intubation, or endotracheal tube management). If PPE such as surgical masks are routinely used for contact with respiratory secretions, this is usually adequate to prevent exposure. Accidental exposure in personnel who qualify as close contacts of persons with meningitis caused by *N. meningitidis* should receive antibiotics to prevent them from getting the disease. Even though there is a meningococcal vaccine, it cannot prevent all types of the disease. Because the rate of secondary disease for close contacts is highest during the first few days after onset of disease in the primary patient, antimicrobial chemoprophylaxis should be administered as soon as possible (ideally within 24 hours after the case is identified). Conversely, chemoprophylaxis administered >14 days after onset of illness in the index case patient is probably of limited or no value. Usually a single dose of ciprofloxacin or ceftriaxone, or two doses of rifampin provide adequate protection against disease after a high-risk exposure. Antibiotics for contacts of a person with Hib meningitis are no longer recommended if all contacts 4 years of age or younger are fully vaccinated against Hib, as the vaccine is very effective.

Pearls and Pitfalls

1. Prehospital personnel are at risk for airborne and blood-borne human to human transmission of pathogens.
2. PPE such as gloves, goggles (eye protection), mask, and gown should be used at all times.
3. When airborne transmission is suspected, a mask should be placed on the patient.
4. The most important way to prevent spread of health care-associated infections in the prehospital setting is through hand hygiene.
5. A properly fitted N95 respirator mask should be used in special situations such as suspected TB or SARS.
6. Those closely exposed to a patient with meningococcal or Haemophilus meningitis should receive antibiotic prophylaxis.
7. The greatest danger to prehospital personnel is from needlesticks and contact with blood and body fluids.
8. Report all occupational exposures immediately after thorough soap and water cleansing of skin or irrigation of mucous membranes (eye or mouth).

References

1. World Health Organization. Avian Influenza, Including Influenza A (H5N1), in Humans: WHO Interim Infection Control Guidelines for Health Care Facilities (10 May 2007).

2. Barillo DJ. Infection control. In Pons PT, Cason D (eds.), Paramedic Field Care: A Complaint-Based Approach, pp. 131–144. St. Louis: Mosby, 1997.
3. Centers for Disease Control and Prevention. Guideline for Hand Hygiene in Health-Care Settings. MMWR 51:1–44, 2002.
4. Centers for Disease Control and Prevention. Guidelines for preventing the transmission of *Mycobacterium tuberculosis* in health-care settings. MMWR 54(RR-17), 2005.
5. Centers for Disease Control and Prevention. Control and prevention of meningococcal disease and control and prevention of serogroup C meningococcal disease: Evaluation and management of suspected outbreaks: Recommendations of the Advisory Committee on Immunization Practices (ACIP). MMWR 46(RR-5), February 14, 1997.
6. Centers for Disease Control and Prevention. Exposure to blood: What healthcare personnel need to know. Information from the Centers for Disease Control and Prevention, National Center for Infectious Diseases, Division of Healthcare Quality Promotion, Division of Viral Hepatitis. Updated July 2003. http://www.cdc.gov/ncidod/dhqp/pdf/bbp/Exp_to_Blood.pdf [Accessed April 8, 2007. Page last modified December 17, 2003].
7. Garner J. Guideline for isolation precautions in hospitals. Infect Control Hosp Epidemiol 17:53–80, 1996.
8. Centers for Disease Control and Prevention. Respiratory Hygiene/Cough Etiquette in Healthcare Settings. http://www.cdc.gov/flu/professionals/infectioncontrol/resphygiene.htm [Page last modified December 17, 2003] [accessed April 8, 2007].
9. Sehulster L, Chinn R. Guidelines for environmental infection control in health-care facilities. Recommendations of CDC and the Healthcare Infection Control Practices Advisory Committee (HCPAC). MMWR;52:1–42, 2003.
10. Seto WH, Tsang D, Yung RW, et al. Effectiveness of precautions against droplets and contact in prevention of nosocomial transmission of severe acute respiratory syndrome (SARS). Lancet 361:1519–1520, 2003.
11. Williams WW. The Hospital Infection Control Practices Advisory Committee guideline for infection control in healthcare personnel. Infect Control Hosp Epidemiol 19:407–463, 1998.
12. Centers for Disease Control and Prevention. Updated U.S. Public Health Service guidelines for the management of occupational exposures to HBV, HCV, and HIV and recommendations for postexposure prophylaxis. June 29 50(RR-11):1–42, 2001.
13. Centers for Disease Control and Prevention. Updated U.S. Public Health Service guidelines for the management of occupational exposures to HIV and recommendations for postexposure prophylaxis. MMWR September 30 54(RR09):1–17, 2005.

Critical Incident Stress

Philip Rach, MS, NREMT-P

CHAPTER 18

1. **What is a critical incident?**
   Critical incidents are events with significant emotional impact that overwhelm the usual coping mechanisms of the individual or group. Critical incidents tend to occur suddenly and are outside the range of normal human experience. Emergency responders are typically in the "right place at the right time" to encounter these profound traumatic events. These incidents may cause a "crisis" where one's psychological homeostasis is disrupted.

2. **I've been in this business a long time, and I've seen a lot. I've always been able to handle it, so why can't everyone else do the same?**
   This is a two-part question. First, we all have different tolerance levels for stress. Several types of stress may affect emergency responders, which we shall address shortly. Some individuals may go their entire careers without experiencing a particularly stressful or distressing call or event. However, studies have shown that approximately 85% of emergency personnel have experienced acute stress reactions after working in one or more situations that meet the criteria of a critical incident. Approximately 2–4% of personnel may experience longer-term, more profound effects on their lives. Recently, there has been a growing realization that some of the things that emergency responders thought did not bother them were merely buried deep in a mental file drawer. Sometimes those files pop out later with worse effects than originally felt. Interviews with Korean War medics revealed recurrence of symptoms from critical incidents as long as 50 years after the end of the war. What we experience is rarely truly forgotten. The important point is to deal with the event or situation effectively at the time, rather than postpone the inevitable.

3. **Why is critical incident stress suddenly such a big deal?**
   This is largely a matter of perspective. The critical incident stress "movement" officially began in 1983 with the publication of an article on the subject by Dr. Jeffrey T. Mitchell.[5] Emergency responders began to realize and acknowledge that some events are critical incidents, and personnel deserve to learn methods to effectively cope with the aftermath. The proof of the perceived need lies in the development of over 300 critical incident stress management teams throughout the United States and teams in numerous other countries. Emergency responders from all specialities have adopted the critical incident stress management philosophy.

4. **I have heard it said that emergency responders may be victims of things they experience in their profession. How can that be? Are not the victims the people to whom we respond?**
   There are three categories of victims:
   - Primary victims—individuals most directly affected by a traumatic event, usually considered the direct or immediate victims of accidents, disasters, and nonaccidental trauma.
   - Secondary victims—observers of the immediate traumatic effects on the primary victims (e.g., emergency responders, witnesses).

- Tertiary victims—individuals indirectly affected by the traumatic event, either by later exposure to the traumatic scene or to the primary or secondary victims (e.g., family members of the initial victims, emergency responders, etc.).

Critical incident stress management services, as discussed in this chapter, are focused on the emergency responder and the emergency responder's family. The critical incident stress process over the past decade has clearly demonstrated that these individuals and groups do become victims and deserve rapid and timely psychological assistance.

5. **What is the difference between the everyday stress we experience in our lives and critical incident stress?**

Good question. We are inundated daily with talk of stress in the workplace, schools, families, and society. Many of us have probably tuned out the talk of stress and stress management. When everyone else is stressed, who wants to hear about it? Our everyday stress level is affected by many factors, events, and people in our lives. Our stress level may go up and down frequently or rapidly, like springtime temperatures, or our stress level may remain fairly high (or fairly low) for long periods, depending on what is going on in our lives. Various factors have been shown to directly affect the stress level, including:

- Emotions, thoughts, and beliefs
- Psychosocial causes such as adaptation, frustration, overload, and deprivation
- Bioecological stressors, including biorhythms, eating and drinking habits, drugs, noise pollution, and climate and altitude
- Personality causes, such as self-perception, patterns of behavior, anxious personality type, and the need for control
- Occupational stress and stressors

Critical incident stress (CIS), on the other hand, is usually incident specific. Alternately, multiple incidents of lesser psychological impact may occur in rapid succession or in close time proximity to cause an acute stress reaction.

6. **Is stress like caffeine? Most of us need it to get us going in the morning.**

Yes, most of us do need a little stress in our lives to get us going and keep us mentally sharp. Not all stress is bad. The positive, productive aspect of stress is called eustress. Eustress enhances health, performance, and productivity. It provides motivation, overcomes lethargy, and facilitates coping. For any individual, at any particular moment, there is an optimal level of stress, however. When stress becomes negative and debilitating, harmful distress ensues. Distress interferes with normal psychological homeostasis. The key to staying on the right side of stress is learning to recognize the signs of distress when they occur in ourselves and others.

7. **Are critical incidents just the major ones like plane crashes, building collapses, and large-scale natural disasters?**

Early discussion of critical incident stress highlighted experiences of emergency responders following disasters such as plane crashes; natural disasters, including hurricanes and tornados; building collapses; mass murder scenes; and other large-scale responses. The nature and enormity of these events helped bring to light both the short- and long-term effects of stress on rescue personnel. Many emergency responders still equate critical incidents with the Big One. However, the vast majority of critical incidents occur when the incident is on a much smaller scale but is extraordinary for one or more reasons. Examples of critical incidents include:

- Serious injury or death of a coworker in the line of duty
- Suicide of a coworker
- Death of a civilian as a result of emergency service operations
- Mass casualty incidents resulting in serious injury or death
- Death or serious injury to a child
- Responding to calls when the victim is known to the emergency service worker
- Threat to the safety of the responders (i.e., hostage or sniper situation, hazardous materials, or other threat to personal safety)
- Situations with excessive media interest or criticism
- Loss of a patient following prolonged rescue or resuscitation efforts
- Personal identification with the victim or circumstances
- Incidents in which the sights and sounds are particularly distressing

This list of critical incidents is not exhaustive. A variety of circumstances may combine to produce acute stress reactions in responders, including a high cummulative stress level, which may trigger a crisis response to a seemingly lesser incident. Emergency responders may experience a crisis to virtually any call, based on many factors. If someone reacts to an incident, it is important to understand that the incident, for whatever reason, triggered a crisis response in the rescuer. This crisis is best dealt with soon after the crisis response.

8. Is this stress stuff all in your head? Can't you just think or talk yourself out of it if you really want to?

Stress *is* all in your head. Or at least the stress response *starts* in your head. The cortex of the brain receives input from the senses and interprets the data at both the conscious and subconscious levels. The midbrain and limbic system are stimulated, which adds emotional interpretation, such as fear or anger. When a stressor is identified, the hypothalamus is activated, initiating a chain reaction resulting in stimulation of both the sympathetic and parasympathetic nervous systems. Stress hormones, including epinephrine, norepinephrine, cortisol, and aldosterone are released. Once the stress response is initiated, arousal continues until the stress products are absorbed. Because the process operates at both the conscious and subconscious levels, your conscious mind may say "Don't sweat it" but your subconscious may not agree. Guess who wins?

9. I hear a lot about burnout in our profession. What is burnout and how does it happen?

Burnout is an overused, and frequently misused, term that refers to cumulative stress reaction. This phenomenon is usually caused by several factors causing low level, but frequent, stress responses. Factors may encompass every aspect of one's life. For instance, a difficult time in one's personal life may suddenly make minor job stressors seem much more stressful. A high chronic level of stress often exists. The individual's coping mechanisms and ability to adapt to a changing environment may be slow to respond or inadequate. The onset of cummulative stress reaction may be insidious, developing over months or years. The syndrome is characterized by physical and emotional exhaustion and negative, cynical attitudes. The quality of the individual's life and the ability to enjoy family, friends, and social life is decreased. Job performance eventually declines, physical illness and work absences increase, and emotional distress becomes more apparent. Other symptoms may include substance and alcohol abuse, disillusionment, apathy, withdrawal, chronic irritability and anger, disrespectful attitudes towards others, and an increase in interpersonal conflict. Resolution of cumulative stress reaction is many times complex and requires psychological and career counseling.

10. **Do emergency responders have certain personality characteristics that make us immune to critical incident stress?**

    We like to think we are immune to critical incident stress, but we are not. We all have certain personality characteristics that we either brought to the job or developed on the job. Either way, there are characteristics that are common among emergency responders. Each factor can produce a positive effect or can actually increase one's stress level. Characteristics of emergency responders include:

    - Having a strong need to be in control
    - Taking risks, being action oriented (easily bored)
    - Being detail oriented
    - Being idealistic
    - Being dedicated and loyal
    - Suppressing emotions

    Although these personality characteristics may help us to cope with cumulative and critical incident stress, they do not make us immune. Knowledge of how our personal characteristics work for, or against, us helps us to recognize those times we may need additional support.

11. **By admitting that I am occasionally affected by critical incidents, doesn't that mean I am crazy or have posttraumatic stress disorder?**

    The answer to both is no. You are having normal reactions to abnormal situations. Emergency responders may routinely be called to some pretty awful scenes and situations, *but this does not mean they are normal life events.* Emergency responders are in a unique situation to be routinely exposed to great human misery, tragedy, and suffering. A protective shell and coping mechanisms develop, but they may not always be adequate to protect you from what you encounter on your job. Developing a crisis based on these events is quite normal. However, one should not think of being in crisis as a normal state. Efforts should be made to restore psychological homeostasis.

    Posttraumatic stress disorder (PTSD) is a formally recognized psychological disorder that may result from exposure to a traumatic event, an event outside the range of normal human experience. This diagnostic label includes specific criteria in four areas: the traumatic event, reexperiencing the event, avoidance and numbing reactions, and symptoms of increased arousal. The term "PTSD" is often used casually, and erroneously, to refer to any exposure to a psychologically traumatic event. PTSD is a complicated diagnosis that can only be made by a competent mental health professional. Critical incident stress management is a process designed to prevent the development of PTSD through early, and effective, intervention.

12. **Why can't I just forget about what happened? Why do I need to drag it all up again by talking about it? It seems to me that the less said, the better.**

    "Reveal and heal" is the watchword here. Remember the subconscious mind mentioned earlier? The subconscious stores what happens to us in greater detail than the conscious mind does. You may think

Personal Safety and Wellness

it is past, or "filed," but all the details are waiting in your stored memory. Sometimes, out of nowhere, with a single unintentional key stroke, the entire event from years earlier is back.

Jeffrey Mitchell and George Everly identified several possible mechanisms of action of critical incident stress debriefings (CISD), including early intervention; the opportunity for catharsis or venting; the opportunity to verbalize the traumatic event; behavioral and psychological structure of the critical incident stress debriefings; group support; peer support; stress education; and opportunity for follow-up.[8] The chance to ventilate emotions and verbalize specific traumatic elements is a key concept. Mitchell and Everly explored numerous studies documenting the importance and efficacy of early effective intervention with individuals and groups who have experienced traumatic events. Reduction of stress arousal and improved immune system functioning result from release of emotions. Suppression of emotions leads to increased anxiety and depression over time.

13. What is the difference between CISD and critical incident stress management (CISM)?

CISD refers to only one of the interventions involved in the critical incident stress management (CISM) process. A CISD is a structured group meeting between personnel directly involved in a critical incident and a CISM team. A debriefing is a confidential, nonevaluative discussion of the involvement, thoughts, reactions, and feelings resulting from the incident. The formal debriefing allows for ventilation of feelings by the responders and an assessment by a CISM team mental health professional and other CISM team members of the intensity of the stress response. A debriefing provides support, reassurance, and education. It stimulates mobilization of individual and group resources and allows the design of a plan of action, if needed. Formal debriefings have both psychological and educational components. Debriefings accelerate recovery in normal people who are having normal reactions to abnormal events. Other CISM interventions include:

- Preincident education
- On-scene support services
- Demobilizations
- Defusings
- Family and significant other support programs
- One-on-one crisis intervention
- Stress management and trauma management education programs
- Follow-up programs

14. How do I know when I or one of my coworkers are experiencing the effects of critical incident stress?

Evaluation of the need for CISM services may be obvious, as in the case of a line of duty death. However, more often indications for CISM services may be less clear. Here are some questions you may consider in making an evaluation.

- How many individuals are affected, one or many?
- What reactions or symptoms are being reported by participants in the event? Continuation of symptoms of acute or delayed stress reactions or intensification of symptoms are key indicators for interventions. Acute stress reactions may include physical, cognitive, emotional, and behavioral signs and signals. Common physical reactions include: fatigue and exhaustion; gastrointestinal upset,

elevated blood pressure and heart rate; and headaches and muscle aches or twitches. Cognitive reactions involve poor concentration and attention span, memory problems, poor problem solving, nightmares, and intrusive images. Emotional reactions may appear as anxiety, guilt, grief, denial, loss of emotional control, depression, inappropriate emotional response, apprehension, feeling overwhelmed, intense anger, and irritability. Behavioral reactions include change in activity, withdrawal, emotional outbursts, change in usual communications, loss or increase in appetite, alcohol consumption, inability to rest, antisocial acts, hyperalert to environment, intensified startle reflex, pacing, and erratic movements.

- Has there been a change in the behavior or affect of the participants in the event? Only debrief events that require debriefing. Do not dilute the process by debriefing events that do not have significant emotional impact.

15. **How important is prior education in making CISM interventions more effective?**
Preeducation about critical incident stress debriefings can make the debriefings much more effective. Understanding the debriefing process, objectives and methods will help all participants have a positive debriefing experience. Preincident education about the nature of the stress response, possible reactions, and appropriate management techniques raises the level of awareness of emergency responders.
Education should help to dispel the "it's all in your head" myth, but most education materials available to EMT and paramedic students fall far short of being truly helpful in the area of cumulative and CIS. As we learn about critical incidents in paramedic class, we are often quizzed on the types of calls that should or should not cause a crisis situation. This gives EMS personnel the impression that they really should not react to many types of calls. This may lead to repressed emotions and an unwillingness to seek help. Educating individuals on the difficulties of cumulative and critical incident stress is often completely overlooked in our educational process.
Education makes us more aware of our resources, and when to activate or use those resources, including a CISM team. Emergency responders are action-oriented individuals; providing management techniques for acute stress reactions can be extremely beneficial in both the short- and long-term.

16. **What can and/or should be done when the effects of critical incident stress are recognized?**
The menu of CISM interventions was listed earlier. The appropriate intervention will depend on the incident and the amount of time elapsed. For example, in a large mass casualty situation, the CISM team should be called to the scene to assist in psychological support of personnel. If the event is prolonged, a series of demobilizations should be organized. Debriefings should be scheduled following on-scene response and involvement. Follow-up services should be available to all personnel. Debriefings for significant others would be appropriate.
For other, smaller scale events, a defusing the same day of the incident is beneficial. If scheduling a defusing is not possible, consider a debriefing within 24–72 hours. A one-on-one discussion may be needed if only one individual is affected. Consult with your local CISM team for the most appropriate interventions. Table 18.1 shows recommended timing of different interventions.

17. **What is the difference between a debriefing and a defusing?**
The format of a debriefing was described in the answer to question 13. The formal debriefing is ideally scheduled within 24–72 hours following the critical incident. This provides a normalizing period and an

TABLE 18.1: Critical Incident Stress Management (CISM): The Core Components

	Intervention	Timing	Activation	Goal	Format
1.	Pre-crisis preparation	Pre-crisis phase	Crisis anticipation	Set expectations. Improve coping. Stress management.	Groups/Organization
2 a.	Demobilizations & staff consultation (rescuers)	Shift disengagement	Event driven	To inform and consult, allow psychological decompression. Stress management.	Large groups/Organizations
2 b.	Crisis Management Briefing (CMB) (civilians, schools, business)	Anytime post-crisis			
3.	Defusing	Post-crisis (within 12 hours)	Usually symptom driven	Symptom mitigation. Possible closure. Triage.	Small groups
4.	Critical Incident Stress Debriefing (CISD)	Post-crisis (1 to 10 days; 3-4 weeks mass disasters)	Usually symptom driven, can be event driven	Facilitate psychological closure. Stress mitigation. Triage.	Small groups
5.	Individual crisis intervention (1:1)	Anytime, anywhere	Symptom driven	Symptom mitigation. Return to function, if possible. Referral, if needed.	Individuals
6 a.	Family CISM	Anytime	Either symptom driven or event driven	Foster support, communications. Symptom mitigation. Closure, if possible. Referral, if needed.	Families/Organizations
6 b.	Organizational consultation				
7.	Follow-up/Referral	Anytime	Usually symptom driven	Assess mental status. Access higher level of care, if needed.	Individual/Family

(Adapted from: Everly and Mitchell, 1999. Critical Incident Stress Management (CISM): A New Era and Standard of Care in Crisis Intervention. International Journal of Emergency Mental Health. Ellicott City, MD: Chevron Publishing. Used with permission.)

opportunity to internally process the experience. It also affords an opportunity to invite all emergency and health care personnel involved in the call to the debriefing. One of the unique advantages of this inclusive approach is the opportunity to share information and generate support within the group.

The defusing is a small group intervention following a traumatic event. Defusings differ from debriefings in timing and number of individuals involved in the group. Defusing is held the day of the incident before the personnel leave their duty shift. The immediacy of the defusing allows for early ventilation and education on anticipated effects of the stress response. Due to the close proximity to the traumatic event, personnel may not have yet had an opportunity to assess the depth or degree of potential reactions. However, evidence suggests that immediate intervention may be more beneficial than waiting for a later debriefing. Rapid scheduling of a defusing may make it impossible for all personnel involved to attend the defusing. A defusing may eliminate the need for a debriefing or a debriefing may be an important CIS management component. These decisions should be made between the requesting personnel and the CISM team.

18. **Just what happens in a CISD? Is it the same as a critique of the call?**

Critiques and psychological debriefings are opposites. The critique focuses on the cognitive: what went right, what went wrong, what we will do next time. The critique is meant to be a logical, thoughtful evaluation of events. The psychological debriefing consists of seven phases and is structured to transition from the cognitive to the emotional level, returning to the cognitive plane. The phases of a formal debriefing include introduction, fact phase, thought phase, reaction phase, symptom phase, teaching phase, and reentry. The appropriately run debriefing should steer participants away from critique and evaluation to a safe expression of thoughts, reactions, and feelings. All group members must respect the expressions and feelings of others. Material divulged in a debriefing may not be used outside the session by other members of the group (command personnel, peers, or CISM team members).

Debriefings are intended for personnel that were directly involved with the incident and not to include family members, supervisors or other tertiary individuals who were not directly involved with the incident. Debriefings are not individual counseling sessions, should not be incorporated with other training, and should not be mistaken for psychotherapy.

Successful debriefings should include:

- Well-trained, experienced, and skilled providers
- Adherence to established standards of practice
- Application to homogenous groups who have had roughly the same exposure to a traumatic event and under circumstances in which the traumatic event is at least under control if not fully completed
- Application in appropriate circumstances
- Realistic goals to achieve with the CISD
- Application of the CISD within the context of the comprehensive and multitactical package called CISM

19. **I know that occasionally a call affects me. But I do not take my work home and I keep my family insulated from the distressing things I encounter on the job. There really is not any need to bother them with that side of the job, is there?**

Most of us would like to think that we can compartmentalize our lives and leave work at work and home at home. The reality is that the subconscious is always with us. We are all a sum of our parts and experiences, which we carry around with us. Consider who knows you best. Is it not the family and other loved ones who are the first to spot when something is amiss with you? When you show signs of distress, be assured that those closest to you will notice. Unless they have information to the contrary, what or who will they consider is causing the problem? Correct. Your loved ones will assume the problem is with them or with your relationship. They may feel you are distancing yourself for some reason other than your effort to leave work behind. The best approach is open communication. Discuss how to handle these situations *before* traumatic events occur.

Discuss with your spouse or significant other what you are willing to share and how much they are willing to hear. Talk about your needs and usual style; for example, do you typically withdraw, seek comfort, talk, or keep silent? Help them to understand that, perhaps, discussing things with someone who's "been there" is much more beneficial. You have a stressful job. Understand that the job stress translates to your family and plan for how you can handle the stress as a family. Many EMT, paramedic, and firefighter training programs have educational sessions with families and loved ones to discuss the stressful characteristics of our field. Many offer counseling for family members.

20. **There isn't any hurry to have a CISM intervention, is there? There are so many things to do following most calls, can't the CISM part just wait? Shouldn't we do our critique first?**

CISM is a preventative strategy aimed at preventing or mitigating traumatic stress syndromes. Early intervention is crucial. Same-day interventions, such as defusings, have proven to be extremely effective in decreasing the level of acute distress in emergency responders. The analogy is early attention to a physical wound. Proper early wound management leads to primary healing with minimal discomfort and disability. Delayed treatment often results in infection and other complications that may end in scarring, continued discomfort, and even disability.

Emergency responders are trained to continually evaluate their performance and response. Critique and continuous quality improvement activities are important processes. Following critical incidents, however, psychological debriefing should occur *before* a critique. The debriefing process allows emergency responders to deal with the emotional impact and aftermath of the event. The critique or evaluation that is scheduled at a later date following a debriefing will be more constructive, objective, and beneficial to the individuals and the organization.

21. **Will the same approach to providing CIS services work for all situations? Is there a difference about interventions for a disaster versus a fatality of a child, for example?**

Experience has taught us that all types of critical incidents are not the same and different approaches to interventions are needed. Each situation requires careful assessment of the most appropriate response. The usual approach of defusings and debriefings may be inappropriate, or even counterproductive, in the disaster situation requiring long-term disaster recovery efforts. This is especially true if the emergency responders were also primary victims, as in the case of a natural disaster such as a hurricane or flood. Event stressors for disaster workers may include: the type of disaster; continued threat of recurrence; personal loss or injury; continued exposure to traumatic stimuli; and mission failure or human error. Consultation with an experienced CISM team is essential in structuring appropriate CISM disaster intervention strategies.

22. **Is CISM just another name for therapy? I do not feel like I need therapy. Well, at least not most of the time.**
    By now it should be clear that CISM interventions are preventive strategies and not therapy. A key concept in the CISM model is to avoid doing therapy. The CISM process focuses on a specific work-related incident, or accumulation of incidents, that created an acute stress response in the emergency providers. CISM focuses on returning the individuals and group to their previous level of functioning, protecting them from further psychological harm, and preventing further harmful reactions. The CISM process was developed for the psychologically healthy to assist them in maintaining and enjoying that state.
23. **I have heard that we have a regional CISM team. What is it and what does it do?**
    The CISM team is normally a multidisciplinary, multijurisdictional, regional team of volunteers trained in all aspects of the CISM process. The core team members include mental health professionals, EMS personnel, law enforcement officers, firefighters, and health care personnel (nursing and other health care providers). Other disciplines involved may include chaplains, dispatchers, search and rescue personnel, ski patrol, corrections officers, victims' advocates, and other specialty personnel in the region. The CISM team is trained to provide all interventions discussed in this chapter. The team may be part of a larger state or regional organization and may also be registered with the International Critical Incident Stress Foundation (ICISF). For more information, contact the ICISF at 410-750-9600.
24. **Do we really need to use a CISM team? Can't we just take care of things "in-house"?**
    One form of CISM intervention is called the initial discussion. Emergency responders are encouraged to use their work group to explore their initial thoughts, reactions, and feelings regarding troublesome calls. This is often all that is needed in a supportive environment that encourages open sharing of feelings. The initial discussion can be accomplished "in house" without outside facilitation. The difficulty with initial in-house discussions is that they are frequently facilitated by shift supervisors or other administrative staff. Too often the initial discussion is ineffective based upon prior personality or work conflict with the informal facilitator who is not skilled in the process of a CISD. It is usually beneficial to bring in a team from outside the organization to provide defusings or formal debriefings. Experience has demonstrated that the most effective debriefings and defusings are inclusive of all personnel involved in the incident and facilitated by an experienced, outside CISM team. Participants generally experience a higher level of trust and confidence in a regional team. There is little to no concern about how information in the debriefing or defusing will be used or if it will become part of an internal investigation or critique. Using CISM team members who are not familiar with incident personnel is psychologically protective for both the team and the impacted personnel.
25. **You know, this call did not seem to bother me, but it sure seems to have hit some of my coworkers hard. What can I do to help them?**
    Peer support is an extremely important component of the critical incident stress management process. The most important part of peer support is listening. Frequently emergency responders are reluctant to offer assistance or support to distressed coworkers because "I don't know what to say." The key is to say little, listen a lot, and allow the individual his or her feelings. It is okay to feel angry, sad, frightened, overwhelmed, or depressed. Validate feelings as normal. Do not try to talk individuals out of feeling the way they feel. Be sure that they understand that you accept their feelings and that your opinion of them will not change based on their crisis. Do not give pat advice such as, "It will be okay, try not to think

about it," "You'll get over this," or "I know just how you feel." As a supporter, ask yourself this question: "What would help me the most if I were in that person's position?" If only one individual seems to be affected by the call, spend time one on one. If you are uncomfortable in that role or feel unprepared, find another coworker to provide peer support. If several of your team members have been impacted, contact your local CISM team.

26. I believe in the CISM process, but administration sure does not seem to. What can I do to help convince them it is needed?

Preincident education provides an excellent opportunity to educate administrative personnel on the effects and costs of critical incident stress. A well-prepared presentation on the topic can illustrate the potential costs to an emergency responder team and organization. Even administrative personnel who have "been there, done that, and it never bothered me" can be made to realize that critical incident stress can result in increased sick time, decreased productivity, increased mistakes and errors, increased on-the-job injuries, and ultimately increased turnover in personnel. Each of these effects is costly for an organization. Turnover is very expensive in any industry with extensive training and experience requirements, such as emergency services. Aside from financial motivation, attention to psychological well being should be the concern of every employer.

27. Okay, so if I attend debriefings and defusings, that will take care of all the stress in my life, right?

There is no simple solution. The issue of stress in all spheres of our lives is complex. Critical incident stress debriefings and defusings are only part of the answer. A regular stress management program and attention to diet, exercise, and outside interests are musts. Developing and maintaining a strong and supportive social network provides ongoing support. Tending to important relationships in our lives with spouses, significant others, children, parents, and others close to us is essential. Tending to relationships includes striving to improve our communications and becoming more open and sharing. Recognition of both acute and chronic stressors in our lives allows us to develop appropriate ways of dealing with stress on a long-term basis. Evaluate your current methods of coping with stress. Are they healthy and helpful? Or are they self-damaging and destructive? Stress management and mitigation is an ongoing process. Most of all, find ways to enjoy your life, your job, and your family.

Pearls and Pitfalls

1. Critical incident stress typically involves an event that produces large numbers of casualties or a particularly horrific injury.
2. A critical stress response may also result from the accumulation of multiple, seemingly small stresses.
3. A critical stress response can manifest itself in a variety of physical, emotional, and behavioral ways.
4. Critical incident stress management involves a variety of techniques and should be tailored to the specific event.
5. Telling a coworker suffering from critical incident stress that they "will be ok" or to "just suck it up" are not appropriate stress management techniques.
6. Critical incident management is not psychological therapy; it is designed to help prevent the need for psychological therapy.

References

1. Bisson JL, Jenkins P, Alexander J, Bannister C. Randomized controlled trial of psychological debriefings for victims of acute burn trauma. Br J Psychiatry 171:78–81, 1997.
2. Bledsoe BE. Critical incident stress management (CISM): Benefit or risk for emergency responders. Prehosp Emerg Care 7(2):272–279, 2003.
3. Everly GS Jr. (ed.): Innovations in Disaster and Trauma Psychology, Vol. 1: Applications in Emergency Services and Disaster Response. Ellicott City, MD: Chevron, 1995.
4. Everly GS. Five principles of crisis intervention: Reducing the risk of premature crisis intervention. Int J Ment Health 2(1):1–4, 1994.
5. Everly GS Jr., Mitchell JT. (1999). Critical Incident Stress Management (CISM). A New Era and Standard of Care in Crisis Intervention. Ellicott City, MD: Chevron, 1999.
6. Girdano D, Everly G Jr., Dusek D: Controlling Stress and Tension: A Holistic Approach, 4th ed. Englewood Cliffs, NJ: Prentice Hall, 1993.
5. Mitchell JT, When disaster strikes ... The critical incident stress debriefing process. JEMS 8(1):36–39, 1983.
7. Mitchell JT, Bray G. Emergency Services Stress: Guidelines for Preserving the Health and Careers of Emergency Services Personnel. Ellicott City, MD: Chevron, 1990.
8. Mitchell JT, Everly GS Jr. Critical Incident Stress Debriefing: An Operations Manual for the Prevention of Traumatic Stress among Emergency Services and Disaster Workers. Ellicott City, MD: Chevron, 1994.
9. Mitchell JT. Crisis Intervention and CISM: A Research Summary. Ellicott City, MD: International Critical Incident Stress Foundation, 2003.

Disasters, Mass Casualty Incidents, and Mass Gatherings

SECTION IV

Chapter 19
Incident Management   137
Christopher B. Colwell, MD, FACEP

Chapter 20
Disasters and Mass Casualty Incidents   146
Jon Krohmer, MD

Chapter 21
Small-Scale Multiple Casualty Incidents   152
Nita Ham, EMT-P

Chapter 22
Weapons of Mass Destruction—Chemical   158
Stephen V. Cantrill, MD

Chapter 23
Biological Terrorism   163
Edward Eitzen, MD, MPH, COL, USA (Retired)

Chapter 24
Weapons of Mass Destruction—Radiologic   174
Jonathan Burstein, MD, and Evan Bloom, MD, MPH

Chapter 25
Weapons of Mass Destruction—Explosives   180
Stephen J. Wolf, MD

Chapter 26
Mass Gatherings   186
Jedd Roe, MD, MBA, FACEP

Incident Management

CHAPTER 19

Christopher B. Colwell, MD, FACEP

1. **What is an incident?**
   An incident is anything out of the ordinary day-to-day activities that necessitates a response. Examples can include disasters, disease outbreaks, special events, or conferences (Figure 19.1).
2. **What is a disaster?**
   A disaster is any situation that overwhelms the ability of local resources to respond and manage that incident. It is not necessarily based on the size of the event but on the ability and resources a community has to respond to it. A situation that is a disaster in one area might not necessarily qualify as a disaster in another with different resources available. Incident management will be affected, in part, by whether or not that particular incident is a disaster for that area or not.
3. **What are the critical features of incident management?**
   Organization, communication, identification, cooperation, and coordination.

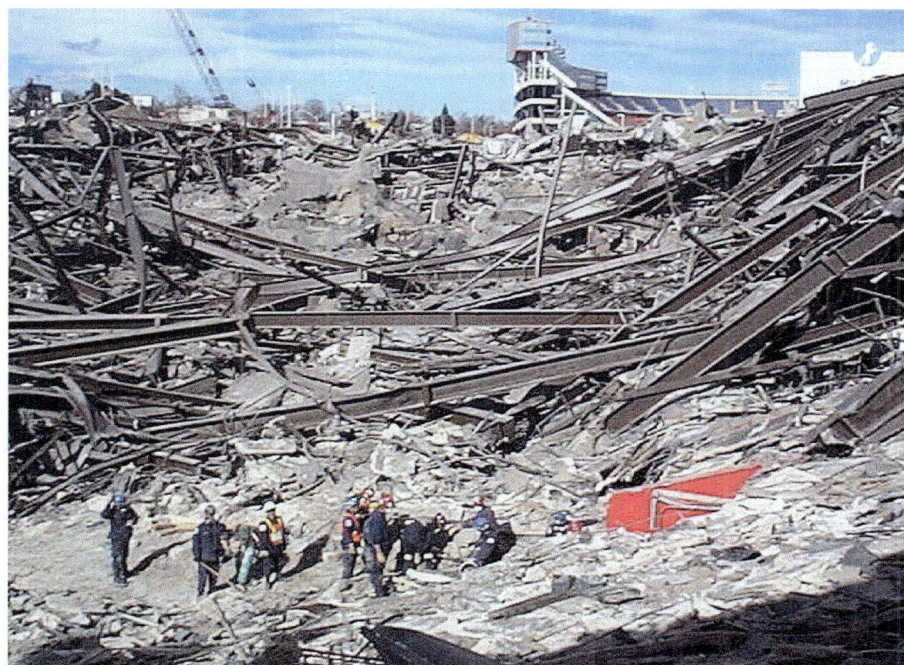

FIGURE 19.1 Incident management is an important component of any incident such as a building collapse.

Disasters, Mass Casualty Incidents, and Mass Gatherings

4. **What have published studies identified as the weakest link in mass casualty incident responses?**

   Communication! Difficulties with communication have been identified in essentially every critique of the management of major incidents. The lack of communication on the part of the responders, the inability to communicate, and disruptions in communication have all been identified as problems, both at the scene and at hospitals. Lack of communication often occurs when responders do not know or think about who needs to have key information, or clear responsibility for this communication is not arranged in advance. Agencies that use different methods of communication may be unable to communicate with each other when multiple agencies respond to an incident. Even in situations where similar methods are used, such as 800-MHz radio systems, plans need to be in place identifying what channel should be used for what incident. Disruptions in communication can also occur when volume overwhelms capacity or batteries run out.

5. **What are the problems related to identification of personnel in incident management?**

   Personnel identification is often cited as a challenge at incident scenes.

   Often, large numbers of people, both in terms of professional responders as well as volunteers, will descend on a scene in an effort to assist. Credentialing and identification of responders is crucial so that those individuals who are needed at the scene can gain access and those who are not part of the organized response can be gathered and used in roles better suited to their abilities.

   In addition, it is not uncommon to have a large number of responders performing a variety of roles at a scene, and identifying key personnel in the midst of large groups of people in various uniforms can be difficult (Figure 19.2). Brightly colored vests with clearly labeled roles written on them have been

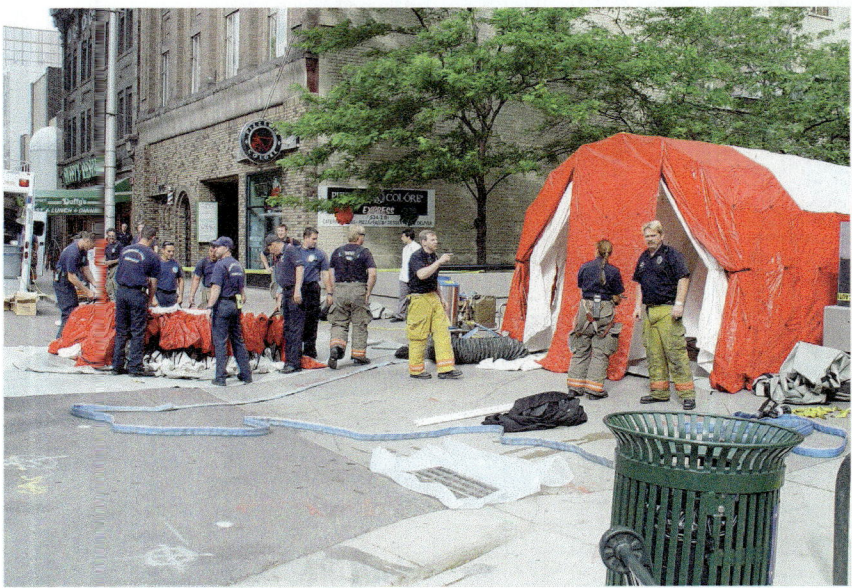

FIGURE 19.2 Personnel identification and roles and responsibilities are difficult to ascertain at scenes where multiple individuals all wearing the same or similar uniforms are found.

Incident Management

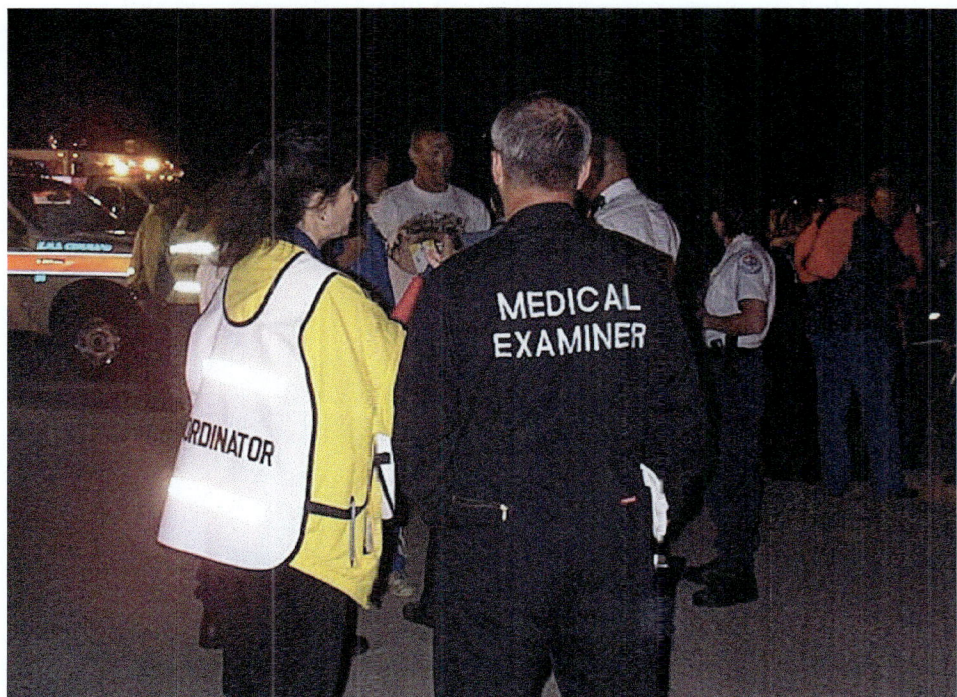

FIGURE 19.3 Labeled vests or other clearly visible identification helps to ascertain the roles of responders to a scene.

advocated as a way to help identify key individuals both at the scene of an incident as well at the hospital (Figure 19.3).

6. **How does coordination impact the management of personnel in an incident?**
   One of the major benefits of good scene coordination will be felt at the hospital. When triage and transport from an incident are not well coordinated, the result is often the transfer of the disaster from the scene of the incident to the hospital, which can negatively impact patient care. A coordinated effort at the scene to distribute patients appropriately to all available hospitals so as not to overwhelm any one particular hospital will result in better patient care for all. In communities in which there is only one hospital option to transport to, good coordination can ensure the patients with the greatest need are transported first, perhaps even keeping some victims at a scene for longer periods of time so the receiving hospital is not overwhelmed. While in most situations, the individual prehospital provider will make the determination as to the appropriate destination for their patient, a centralized, coordinated effort from the scene may be more appropriate for proper incident management.

7. **How can organization be accomplished at the scene of an incident?**
   Plan ahead. Although it may not be possible to be prepared for everything, we can often be better prepared for predictable problems. Implementation of a command post, resources for both victims and providers, and dealing with the media are just some of the areas often identified at incident scenes that can be

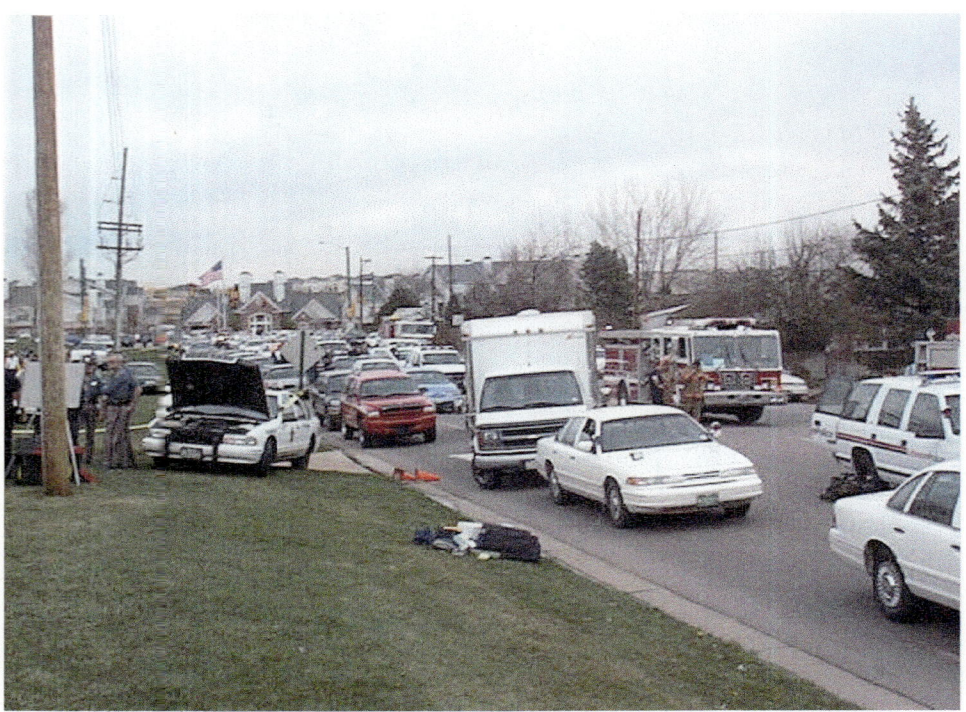

FIGURE 19.4 Unorganized vehicle response to a scene can lead to difficulties in subsequent ingress and egress.

organized to some degree before an incident even occurs. One common problem at the scene of an incident is how to organize all the vehicles that arrive at the scene (Figure 19.4). Responders will arrive in various different vehicles and will often try to get as close to the incident as possible before getting out of the vehicle and proceeding on foot. A well-organized scene will include plans to direct certain vehicles to where they can be of use while ensuring that all others are directed to a location where they will not be a hindrance (Figure 19.5). Ingress and egress routes can be obstructed when too many vehicles are brought too close to a scene.

8. **Instead of worrying about incident management, why don't we just deal with the first patient we find, transport to the nearest hospital, and get back to the scene to help?**
Although this is a common practice at many incident scenes, the result is often that the disaster is simply transported from the scene to the nearest hospital. That hospital is often quickly overwhelmed and will be less able to care for the victims transported there. Accurate triage and a coordinated transport effort from the scene are critical to preventing this transplantation of the disaster. Studies have indicated better outcomes with good, organized incident management where there is a coordinated effort made by those in charge of the incident. Although not as well studied, good incident management very likely affects not only the immediate morbidity and mortality of the victims, but also the management at the hospital.

Incident Management

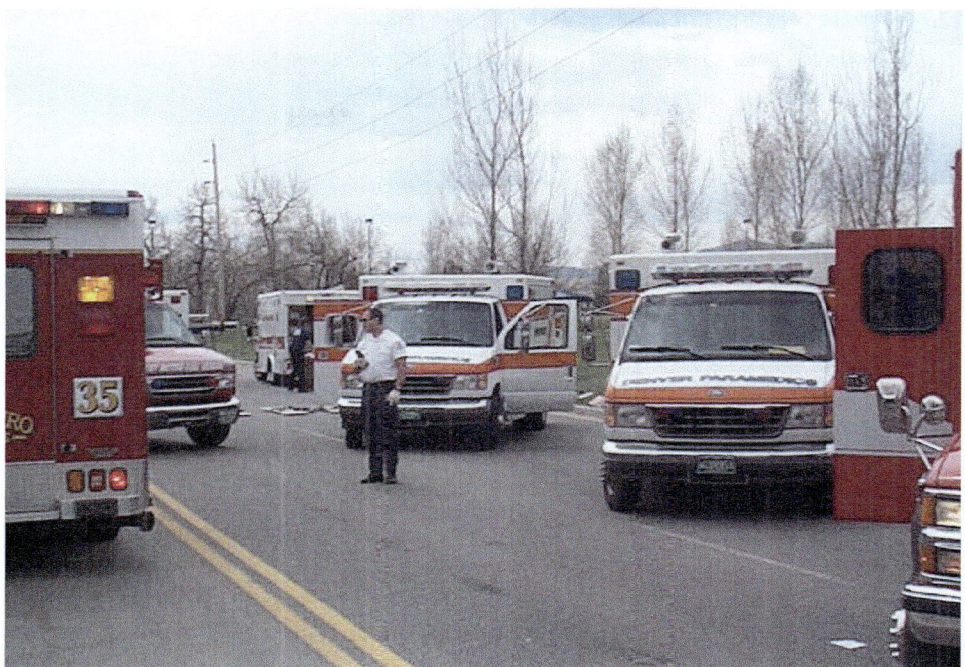

FIGURE 19.5 Planned vehicle response into a scene with an organized approach to placement can provide easy ingress and egress from a disaster scene.

9. **What is the Incident Command System?**
   The Incident Command System (ICS) is a standardized management structure that provides command, control, and organization of personnel and resources at an incident scene. ICS provides a framework within which emergency response organizations, including health care institutions, can work in concert with appropriate local, state, and federal agencies. Use of ICS allows multiple agencies to work more effectively together by providing common structure, terminology, and descriptions that all can understand and use. The National Incident Management System (NIMS) standardizes the ICS structure to be used by EMS agencies, fire-rescue, law enforcement, and hospitals in an effort to enhance response coordination at all levels and for all types of incidents. NIMS mandates when the ICS structure is to be used. For incidents involving multiple local agencies or any federal resources, an ICS is mandated.

10. **What is ICS not?**
    ICS is **not** a means to wrestle control or authority away from agencies or departments that participate in emergency response. It is not decision making by committee or a system that is only used by the fire department. What the ICS does do is allow for greater efficiency, better coordination, and more effective communication at the scene of an incident.

11. **Describe the ICS standardized structure.**
    ICS recognizes that every incident, regardless of the type, nature or size, requires five key functions to be accomplished: incident command, planning, logistics and supply, operations, and finance.

12. **What are the responsibilities of each of these functions?**
    - Incident command—has overall responsibility for the management of the incident
    - Planning—determines what is needed to manage the incident
    - Logistics—knows where to get what is needed to manage the incident
    - Operations—uses what is needed to manage the event
    - Finance—pays for it all

13. **How many people do I need to have to implement the ICS?**
    The answer is "it depends." In a small incident, one individual will serve as the incident commander and can often perform many or all of the other four functions. As the incident gets larger, separate individuals will be assigned to perform the required functions. One of the important points about ICS is that most of the necessary roles and functions have been anticipated and are built into the ICS structure. Each position has a detailed job action sheet that describes the role and responsibilities of that position.

14. **How and where did ICS originate?**
    ICS began in the fire service during the 1970s when large wildfires in California necessitated the response by numerous firefighting agencies from all over the country. It was rapidly discovered that each agency brought its own administrative structure, communication system, and internal language leading to significant difficulty coordinating response among these diverse groups. ICS was developed to bring uniformity to the response process and has since been expanded to now include law enforcement, EMS, health care agencies, and the federal government.

15. **Is there a role for a physician at the scene of an incident?**
    Yes, but it should be a physician familiar with prehospital medicine, incident management (including ICS), and the prehospital agency (or agencies) involved in the incident. Physicians can bring knowledge of local hospital capabilities and assistance with triage, destination, and other decision making that can prove very valuable at the scene of an incident. If the physician is not familiar with the EMS agency, local protocols, and incident management, however, the potential value is reduced.

16. **Do the principles of incident management apply to a hospital?**
    Yes. In most situations where a major incident has occurred, hospitals, especially the closest hospital to the incident, become as chaotic as the scene itself. There are many reasons for this, including the disaster being simply moved to the hospital, many well-intentioned volunteers showing up at the emergency department wanting to help (this occurs at the scene as well), and the fact that although this incident is occurring, normal patient traffic through the emergency department and hospital continues to occur as well. Therefore, using an ICS structure at the hospital can help to organize the hospital as well.

17. **How do I organize the patient care at an incident?**
    One of the most important aspects of managing and organizing patients at the scene of a major incident is using a triage system to categorize patients based upon the extent of their injuries and the likelihood of survival. The triage category is then used to prioritize patients for transport and care. Several different triage systems exist and a commonly used one will be described below.

18. **What are the triage categories in MCIs?**
    There are basically four categories which are Red, Yellow, Green and Black.

- *Red (immediate)* is assigned to any patient who, given available care, has a reasonable chance of survival but without care has a markedly diminished chance of survival. These patients will receive the highest priority for treatment and transport. A gunshot wound to the abdomen might be a good example of a patient who would fall into the red category.
- *Yellow (delayed)* is assigned to any patient whose injuries will not lead to significant morbidity or mortality if they do not receive immediate care BUT clearly will need medical management at a hospital. Most fractures may fall into this category.
- *Green (minor)*, or so-called walking wounded, is assigned to any patient whose injuries are not anticipated to result in significant morbidity while they wait for treatment and transport of red and yellow patients. In many cases, patients triaged to the green category may not even need to go to a hospital for management of their injuries.
- *Black (dead/dying, or expectant)* would be any patient felt to be mortally wounded or dead. In a true disaster, where resources are overwhelmed, patients not breathing on their own should be triaged as black. Some triage systems will categorize the dead as black and the expectant victims as gray or dark blue. By doing so, once all of the red and yellow patients are dealt with, the expectant patients can be easily identified and reevaluated to see if any are still alive. Those who have not expired will require transport to the hospital.

19. Describe the simple triage and rapid transport triage system.

The simple triage and rapid transport (START) system is designed to triage a patient in about 30 seconds. The provider evaluates the patient for respiratory rate, presence or absence of a pulse, and mental status and, based on these findings, determines which category to triage the patient to. For patients with no respiratory rate but with a pulse, basic airway maneuvers and insertion of an oropharyngeal airway (OPA) are performed. If spontaneous breathing results, the patient is triaged to Immediate, if not, to Expectant. Table 19.1 describes the START triage system. This is commonly used to determine which patients should be triaged to which category.

TABLE 19.1: Start Triage

Red (immediate)	Respirations: >30 *or* radial pulse not present *or* unable to follow simple commands	Highest priority for treatment and transport
Yellow (delayed)	Respirations <30 *or* radial pulse present *or* able to follow simple commands but unable to ambulate without assistance	Will need to go to the hospital but can wait for those in the red category to be transported
Green (minor)	Respirations <30 *and* radial pulse is present *and* able to follow simple commands and ambulate without assistance	Patients may not need to go to the hospital. If they do, can often be transported in large groups, perhaps even in a bus
Black (dead/dying or expectant)	Respirations are absent. Head tilt and insertion of OPA does not result in a spontaneous respiratory effort	Should be reevaluated as soon as possible for any evidence that they may be salvageable

20. What is critical incident stress management?

Critical incident stress management (CISM) is a system designed to help providers deal with incident-related stress. This stress is a normal response to abnormal circumstances. Especially trained teams of peer counselors and mental health workers can provide a number of essential services to providers following an incident. These services can include stress education, peer support, wellness programs, and follow-up services. Critical incident stress debriefing is a function of CISM that uses specific techniques to aid providers in the recovery from a stressful incident.

Pearls and Pitfalls

1. A disaster is any situation that overwhelms a community's ability to respond to it.
2. The weakest link in MCI responses is most commonly communication.
3. Communication methods should be arranged in advance ensuring access for those that will need it.
4. Cell phone systems may be overwhelmed, rendering these phones useless during an incident.
5. Clear identification of critical individuals and their roles is essential at the scene of an incident.
6. Organize the vehicles that will arrive at the scene of an incident or to the hospital to prevent difficulties in ingress and egress.
7. Triage all patients before initiating treatment and transport when possible.
8. Do not simply rush the first/next patient found to the nearest hospital. Transport will need to have a coordinated approach.
9. Everyone at the scene of an incident, or at a hospital receiving patients from an incident, should be familiar with ICS.
10. Physicians can play an important role in incident management when properly trained and familiar with local protocols.
11. Principles of incident management apply to hospitals as well as at the scene.
12. An organized scene response will help to prevent the transfer of the disaster from the scene to the closest hospital.

References

1. Kenar L, Karayilanoglu T. Prehospital management and medical intervention after a chemical attack. Emerg Med J 21(1):84, 2004.
2. Aylwin CJ, Konig TC, Brennan NW, et al. Reduction in critical mortality in urban mass casualty incidents: Analysis of triage, surge, and resource use after the London bombings on July 7, 2005. Lancet 368(9554):2218, 2006.
3. Feldman MJ, Lukins JL, Verbeek RP, et al. Half-a-million strong: The emergency medical services response to a single-day, mass-gathering event. Prehosp Disaster Med 19(4):287, 2004.
4. Einav S, Feigenberg Z, Weissman C, et al. Evacuation priorities in mass casualty terror-related events: Implications for contingency planning. Ann Surg 239(3):304, 2004.
5. Rodoplu U, Arnold JL, Tokyay R, et al. Mass-casualty terrorist bombings in Istanbul, Turkey, November 2003: Report of the events and the prehospital response. Prehosp Disaster Med 19(2):133, 2004.
6. Lockey DJ, Mackenzie R, Redhead J, et al. London bombings July 2005: The immediate pre-hospital medical response. Resuscitation 66(2):ix, 2005.

7. Ashkenazi I, Kessel B, Khashan T, et al. Precision of in-hospital triage in mass-casualty incidents after terror attacks. Prehosp Disaster Med 21(1):20, 2006.
8. Gutierrez de Ceballos JP, Turegano Fuertes F, Perez Diaz D, et al. Casualties treated at the closest hospital in the Madrid, March 11, terrorist bombings. Crit Care Med 33(1 Suppl):S107, 2005.
9. Hayes BE, Dahlen RD, Pratt FD, Sullivan RM. A prehospital approach to multiple-victim incidents. Ann Emerg Med 15:458, 1986.
10. Helling TS, Nelson PW, Moore BT, et al. Is trauma centre care helpful for less severely injured patients? Injury 36(11):1293, 2005.
11. Sola JE, Scherer LR, Haller JA, et al: Criteria of cost-effective pediatric trauma triage: Prehospital evaluation and distribution of injured children. J Pediatr Surg 29(6):738, 1994.
12. Spaite DW, Criss EA. Medical Oversight and Disaster Management. In Markovchick VJ, Pons PT (eds.), Emergency Medicine Secrets, 4th ed. Philadelphia: Mosby, 2006.

Disasters and Mass Casualty Incidents

CHAPTER 20

Jon Krohmer, MD

1. **What is a disaster?**
    A disaster is any situation that disrupts normal community function; it overwhelms the community's ability to respond to the situation and threatens the safety, property, or health or lives of the citizens. It may stress the area's ability to provide public health resources, utilities, communications, food, shelter, and clothing. A disaster also may involve more injuries than the local emergency medical services (EMS) system or local hospitals can care for. However, not all disasters result in injuries or illnesses.

2. **How is a mass casualty incident different from a disaster?**
    A mass casualty incident (MCI) is any situation in which multiple patients with injuries or illness occur from a single event. Several events occurring simultaneously or a large MCI may qualify as a medical disaster. Although an MCI technically is any situation involving more than one patient, most systems do not consider it an MCI until there are more than 5–10 patients. When these situations require more resources than are immediately available to provide the necessary care, a disaster plan may need to be activated. MCIs are sometimes called medical disasters.
    An individual incident may be both a disaster and an MCI, but it does not always have to be both. For example, a flood may affect a large geographic area and displace many people from their homes while destroying farms, homes, stores, and utilities. Such a situation could easily qualify as a disaster. However, without a large number of injuries or illnesses, it would not qualify as an MCI. Similarly, a motor vehicle collision involving a school bus and a small van that injures 18 people with varying degrees of severity would be an EMS MCI requiring many prehospital resources and possibly requiring the activation of the EMS disaster plan. However, a disaster response is unnecessary if the area hospitals are able to adequately care for all of the patients. Many of the components of a disaster plan will be used in smaller MCIs; the principles are the same, but the magnitude of the response will vary depending on the size of the event and the availability of local medical resources. The effects of the hurricanes in the Gulf coast in the fall of 2005 were examples of both a disaster and mass casualty events—the infrastructure of the community was destroyed and there were large numbers of injuries and medical needs in the population.
    With the focus on greater planning for events of terrorism or very large-scale natural events, the concept of "mass casualty" has also been introduced. Such an incident would produce huge numbers of patients and may require an altered standard of medical care.

3. **What are examples of disaster situations?**
    Natural disasters include hurricanes, tornadoes, floods, earthquakes, tsunamis, severe winter storms, and volcanic eruptions. Disasters made by humans are airplane, train, or motor vehicle crashes, industrial explosions, fires, and hazardous materials incidents such as chemical spills and radiation leaks. Events caused by humans may also be related to acts of terrorism from biological, chemical, explosive, radiological, or nuclear events. It is possible that natural and human-caused events may occur at the same time, as when a tornado causes a hazardous materials incident.

Disasters and Mass Casualty Incidents

4. **Why is it important to understand the principles of MCIs and disasters?**
   Most emergency care personnel, including emergency medical technicians, paramedics, emergency physicians, and nurses, will find themselves in situations in which they will need to handle MCI situations. Many will never have to handle situations such as a plane or train crash, but the principles of the response to both the MCI and the larger disaster (mass casualty) are the same.

5. **How is the focus of medical care during an MCI different from the routine daily focus of medical care?**
   During daily medical care, there are a limited number of persons for whom care must be provided and providers can therefore commit a large level of very intensive resources to each of those patients. During an MCI, however, many persons require care, and that care must be provided with relatively limited resources. The goal of care during an MCI is to provide the greatest amount of good for the greatest number of potentially survivable victims. This change in philosophy (e.g. not trying to resuscitate someone in cardiac arrest or intubating someone with a fatal head injury) is often difficult for emergency medical personnel to adopt in disaster situations.

6. **Who should participate on the disaster management team?**
   Representatives from all groups who will be providing services during the disaster: the local, state, or national government, police, fire services, EMS, hospitals, utilities, and public works departments, emergency management, Red Cross, social services, and mental health services. All of these representatives will be responsible for coordinating the activities of the respective disciplines to ensure that the needed services are provided to the community. Representatives should work together to develop a response plan to use in the event of a disaster working within the emergency management structure of the area.

7. **Why is it important to develop a disaster response plan?**
   To ensure successful response to a disaster, which depends on the coordination of the activities of many agencies, including the government and public and private organizations. Plans must be developed prior to the incident to ensure that (1) lines of authority are established, (2) appropriate communications will occur, and (3) all agencies and personnel will understand their areas of responsibility. The plan should include a risk analysis of potential disaster-producing factors, such as chemical plants, nuclear power plants, busy airports, and train routes. A survey of available resources also should be made. The disaster plan should structure response activities as closely as possible to normal daily operations.
   Once the plan has been developed, it is important to regularly conduct disaster exercises to test the plan so that everyone involved understands what is expected of them during a disaster response.

8. **What are the four phases of a disaster response?**
   Activation, implementation, mitigation, and recovery.

9. **Describe the activation phase of a disaster response.**
   The activation phase includes the initial notification that an incident has occurred, the response to the incident, and the establishment of the command structure. The first responders should quickly assess the scene to ensure that their safety and the safety of other responders is maintained. They must then determine the nature and magnitude of the event, an estimated number of victims, and an idea of the resources that will be needed to handle the situation. This information must be communicated to the dispatch center or medical command facility to initiate the remainder of the response. Additionally, a command structure must be established to assure proper coordination, communication, and use of resources.

10. What are the components of the implementation phase?
The implementation phase initially involves a search for victims and rescue, which is usually provided by the fire department or specially trained search and rescue teams. This is followed by triage and beginning stabilization and transport of victims to hospitals.

11. What does the mitigation phase involve?
The hazards are controlled, and treatment is provided to patients. Treatment provided at the scene is generally limited to airway, breathing, and circulation issues and immobilizing patients for transport to hospitals. The purpose is to provide care to preserve life and function. Occasionally, if there is a delay in transporting patients from the site, additional treatment may begin in the field. Sometimes, trained medical teams from the hospital may assist with medical care as long as they are integrated into the structure of the response system as part of the planning process and are appropriately trained to function in the out-of-hospital environment.

12. What happens during the recovery phase?
Responders leave the scene and return to normal operations. They restock equipment and supplies. A debriefing session should be held to review the response to the event, to determine if the disaster plan must be modified and to address any psychological issues that rescuers or victims may be experiencing. Also, displaced persons are sheltered until they can find other places to live or return to their homes.

13. Explain the command structure of a disaster response.
The command structure most commonly used in the United States is called the incident command system (ICS) or incident management system (IMS). This concept was developed in the fire service to outline a structure for coordinating all activities that occur during a major incident. It is routinely used in the fire service and has been found useful and easily adaptable to MCI and disaster responses. The federal government has now formally adopted the National Incident Management System (NIMS) as the national model for response planning. Federal, state, and local organizations are required to comply with the NIMS to be eligible for the federal Homeland Security Grant Program.
Under the ICS, one person assumes overall responsibility for coordinating the activities of the response. The role of incident commander frequently is filled by the fire chief, although in terrorist events, that role may be filled by someone in law enforcement. All of the functions that must occur during the response are then assigned to others to coordinate, but they report to and are responsible to the incident commander. The various functions are referred to as sections. EMS personnel generally are responsible only for the medical aspects of the response and fall under the operations section. Establishing this type of structure allows for an established chain of command and authority and for an effective span of control.

14. What is the triage process?
Triage is a process of prioritizing patient care based on the severity of the injury or illness, the patient's prognosis, and the availability of resources. The goal of triage is to identify the patients in greatest need of immediate medical attention and arrange for that treatment with the currently available resources. The concept of triage is best represented by Charles Dickens' phrase: "The needs of the many outweigh the needs of the few."
Triage should be started as soon as possible by the most trained medical person available. It is a rapid survey to determine the number of victims, any hazards to victims and rescuers, and what additional resources are needed.

15. Why is triage so important?

When faced with many persons who are injured or ill but with limited resources to care for them, the rescuers must decide which patients have the best chance of survival and should be taken care of quickly with the available resources. This may mean that some patients will not get the care they need and may not survive. Triage decisions are the most critical decisions that medical personnel make during an MCI. Recent planning for mass casualty situations acknowledges the concept of an altered level of care in those situations compared with the care that persons would receive were a mass casualty situation not existing. This concept is an extension of small-scale triage but reflects that, in mass casualty events, the same resources as are available for routine, daily care will not be available – thus an "altered" level of care is available to patients.

16. How does triage affect treatment and transport of patients?

The triage category determines how quickly a patient receives treatment in the field and how rapidly he or she is transported to the hospital. Triage is a continuous process that is repeated when patients are prepared for transport and when they arrive at the hospital. Triage is repeated because the patient's condition may improve with treatment or may deteriorate.

17. What does "triage category" mean?

A patient who is assessed during triage is assigned to an urgency category based on the severity of the injury or illness. The most common scheme uses four categories: immediate, delayed, minimal, and expectant. Patients in the *immediate* category have injuries or illnesses that require immediate care for life-threatening situations but have a high likelihood of surviving if the situations are corrected. *Delayed* category situations can be treated within hours to days without an expectation of significant deterioration or morbidity. *Minimal* conditions generally can be treated by the patient or require minimal medical care. Patients who are declared *expectant* have such severe injuries that they will likely die in spite of aggressive medical care or because an adequate level of care is not possible ("altered standard"); if resources allow, they should receive comfort measures.

18. What are triage tags?

Triage tags are sometimes used to identify the patient's triage category to other rescuers. The most commonly used tags are color-coded to identify the patient's category immediate (red), delayed (yellow), minimal (green), and expectant or dead (black). Once the patient is triaged, the tag is attached to the patient. Many people do not believe that triage tags work well during a disaster. Some people simply place a piece of colored tape on the patient's forehead to identify the triage category. Whether tags or tape are used, some method of identifying the patient's triage category should be used.

19. How do I perform triage?

There are a number of different triage systems available for use by prehospital providers. These systems include simple triage and rapid treatment (START) triage, JumpSTART triage for pediatric patients, MASS triage, the Sacco Triage Method, SALT triage, and various physiologic and injury-based approaches. None of these triage systems has been demonstrated to be superior to any of the other methods. What is clearly important is that EMS systems have a triage process that they use and that the prehospital providers be knowledgeable in its application.

20. Is it important to have doctors and nurses on the scene?

There is no concrete answer. Generally, care can be provided quite well by EMS personnel. Occasionally, it may be necessary or helpful for physicians and nurses to assist with patient care in the field. This is particularly important if significantly advanced care, such as limb amputation, is needed. Additionally, if there will be a long delay before transport, physicians and nurses can further stabilize patients at the scene, freeing up prehospital providers to perform transport, until there are adequate resources that they can be transported. In situations in which hospital personnel do respond to the scene, they must be very knowledgeable about providing medical care out of the hospital.

21. How do the responders communicate with each other?

Although communication is very important during a disaster response, it is the factor that often causes the most problems.

Many people must be able to communicate with each other, whether by radio, telephone, or in person. The incident commander must be able to talk with those coordinating the various sections, including EMS personnel. The EMS coordinator must communicate with those coordinating triage, treatment, and transportation as well as with the medical control facility or hospital coordinating center. The transportation coordinator also must communicate with hospitals or the coordinating center.

However, with so many people needing to talk with each other, radio frequencies can become overcrowded. Aggravating that situation is the fact that many different agencies are responding to the event; the agencies often have individual frequencies, which makes it impossible to communicate between agencies. Land-line telephones and cellular circuits are often tied up with disaster-related activities—from disaster responders as well as citizens using the phones to get information. There are several initiatives ongoing to try to coordinate reponders' ability to communicate, to create "interoperable" communications systems.

22. How can such problems be overcome?

Responders should try to talk face to face with each other when possible. When dedicated radio frequencies are available, they can be used effectively. The use of messengers and amateur radio operators also can be effective. Information can be shared using bullhorns in relatively controlled areas. Disaster responders are starting to use computers for communications.

23. When the radios are busy, how can EMS personnel call the hospital to discuss patients and receive medical care orders?

Usually, in disaster situations, there is little communication between the EMS personnel and the hospitals. Much more emphasis is placed on the personnel taking care of patients by standing orders in the protocols. It is important, however, to inform hospitals of the number and severity of casualities that they will be receving to allow them to adequately prepare for the influx of patients.

24. Once the transport of patients begins, how are victims assigned to receiving hospitals?

This component of MCI management is often overlooked. The common tendency is for the transporting personnel to want to bring the patient to the closest hospital so they can quickly turn around to get the next patient. Before too long, the MCI has been transferred from the disaster site to the closest hospital. Part of any disaster plan is appropriate distribution of patients and hospital destination assignments. Victims in the *immediate* category should be transported to trauma centers. Patients with less severe injuries can be taken to nontrauma centers. Although dispersing patients to multiple hospitals will entail longer transport times, care will generally be improved by not overwhelming one facility.

Assigning patients to specific receiving facilities is the responsibility of the transportation officer. Those assignments should be based on the needs of the patients and the available resources of receiving facilities. Many EMS systems are now using computer (Web-based) resources to survey and catalog available hospital resources in real-time.

25. How should I deal with the media at the disaster site?

The media can be very important and helpful during a disaster. Initially, the media can provide public information about the situation, announcing potential hazards and educating the public about evacuation routes if necessary. The media, if given proper information, can inform the community about health care issues and threats. They can announce to medical personnel the need to return to hospitals or other care facilities. A public information officer should be identified whose responsibility is to regularly provide the media with reliable and accurate information. The media will not go away; they should be used constructively.

Pearls and Pitfalls

1. The definition of what constitutes a disaster is relative to the size and available resources within the impacted community.
2. Failure to implement an incident management structure at a disaster or MCI only serves to prolong the confusion and complicate the response.
3. Communications problems are a common difficulty at disasters and MCIs. Intra- and interagency communications plans should be developed and tested before a major incident.
4. Medical care at a disaster or MCI is guided by the concept of doing the most good for the largest number of patients.
5. Hospital personnel who respond to a scene should be knowledgeable and trained in providing care in the prehospital setting.

References

1. Doyle CJ. Mass casualty incident. Integration with prehospital care. Emerg Med Clin North Am 8:163–175, 1990.
2. Morres CA, Burkle FM, Lillibridge SR. Disaster medicine. Emerg Med Clin North Am 14(2):267–480, 1996.
3. Tintinalli J (ed.). Disaster preparedness—Section 2. Emergency Medicine. A Comprehensive Study Guide, 6th ed. New York: McGraw-Hill, 2003.
4. Noji EK. Natural disaster management—Chap 67. In Auerbach PS (ed.): Wilderness Medicine, 4th ed. St. Louis: Mosby, 2001.
5. Reed SB. Natural and human-made hazards: Mitigation and management issues. In Auerbach PS (ed.). Wilderness Medicine, 4th ed. St. Louis: Mosby, 2001.
6. Schultz CH, Koenig KL, Noji EK. A medical disaster response to reduce immediate mortality after an earthquake. N Engl J Med 334:438–444, 1996.
7. Waeckerle JF. Disaster planning and response. N Engl J Med 324:815–821, 1991.
8. Altered Standards of Care in Mass Casualty Events: Bioterrorism and Other Public Health Emergencies. AHRQ Publication No. 05-0043, April 2005. Agency for Healthcare Research and Quality, Rockville, MD. http://www.ahrq.gov/research/altstand/
9. National Incident Management System (NIMS), FEMA, US Department of Homeland Security, http://www.fema.gov/emergency/nims/index.shtm

Small-Scale Multiple Casualty Incidents

Nita Ham, EMT-P

CHAPTER 21

1. **What is a multiple casualty incident?**
   A multiple casualty incident (MCI) is a situation in which the number of patients initially overwhelms the ability of the EMS response team to care for them. An MCI usually does not cover a large geographic area, but may cause a sudden redirection of many (or most) available resources. This could be a motor vehicle accident (MVA) with as few as three patients (depending on the resources available in a community) or an airliner crash with hundreds of patients.

2. **What is a small-scale MCI?**
   A small-scale MCI refers to an incident that will tax the ability of the EMS responders in a given community to respond to the event with the resources immediately available but is not so large that assistance from the state or federal government will be needed. Mutual aid from adjacent communities may well be a component of the effort. Generally, a small-scale incident will be managed within a relatively short period of time (a few hours), be geographically contained, and stress the local community but not beyond.

3. **What are some common types of calls that create small-scale incidents with multiple casualties?**
   Motor vehicle crashes are most common, by a large margin. Building fires, especially large apartment buildings, can create multiple patients, along with other unique management problems. Hazardous material exposures can produce large numbers of patients as well. Also, the specter of domestic terrorism with the potential for significant numbers of casualties must be acknowledged. A thorough understanding of the unique problems encountered with the various scenarios will enable you to anticipate and respond to each MCI.

4. **How is an MCI different from a "usual" or "routine" EMS response?**
   In most "usual" or "routine" responses, you generally have more responders than you have patients. The majority of EMS responses involve a single patient and a single ambulance, with a minimum of two EMS personnel. However, with an MCI, you will have more patients than medical personnel, and scene assessment and management priorities are different. When multiple ambulances are required to respond to the same incident, the dynamics of scene control must change, too.

5. **How do I prepare to adequately manage an MCI?**
   Training is the key to being prepared for an MCI. Having a response plan and ensuring all team members are familiar with the plan is critically important. If the plan includes infrequently used protocols or equipment, or expects personnel to change their usual roles or behaviors, confusion can easily result if the plan is not reviewed and practiced on a regular basis.
   In most situations, multiple casualty incidents also result in multiagency responses. The more responders on a scene, the greater the opportunity for confusion and conflict, especially when personnel from the

responding agencies do not routinely work together and do not understand each other's roles and responsibilities. Agencies that will likely respond together should also dedicate time to develop a mutual response plan. Another key to a successfully managed MCI is a "teamwork" attitude between agencies developed through regularly scheduled joint training exercises and drills. Joint training exercises can be "tabletop" or "paper" exercises in which agency personnel meet and talk through a plan. Tabletop exercises should then be followed by practical exercises and drills to increase response efficiency and allow the opportunity to correct any deficiencies that may be identified.

6. **What goes into the planning effort?**
Planning an MCI response involves an organized approach to anticipating extraordinary events in advance of their occurrence. Planning activities include, but are not limited to, risk assessment, resource identification, and a communications plan. Risk assessment, also sometimes referred to as hazard vulnerability analysis, is the process of evaluating what kind of multiple casualty incidents are likely to happen in a given area. Although response plans should be designed to be effective in any type of situation, planning for the most likely events prepares everyone for the most likely eventuality. Historical data may prove to be very beneficial in planning for future events.

Because most MCIs initially tax available resources, resource identification is an important part of planning. Resources include people, equipment, vehicles, and information.

"People" resources can include on-duty public safety personnel from the surrounding area, off-duty personnel available to return to duty, and specialty teams such as confined space rescue, hazardous materials, or clergy and mental health teams available for emotional support.

Identifying sources for equipment, and ensuring the equipment is functional at all times, is an important part of the planning process. A process for access to the equipment in the event of an MCI or for activating mutual aid agreements is crucial. Unfortunately, embarrassing stories circulate periodically about stocked-and-ready MCI equipment and vehicles sitting unused because no one had access or could locate the keys.

A communications plan is absolutely necessary to ensure that adequate communications resources are assigned to the MCI operation and that all responding agencies are able to talk to one another during the event. This plan may include a communications center supervisor who immediately dedicates channels and personnel as necessary to the MCI.

7. **Do I need to implement incident command or unified command for a small-scale MCI?**
Absolutely. The standard for the coordination of any significant event, regardless of size, is incident command. If multiple agencies are involved in the incident response, then unified command is also appropriate. Unified command places commanders from each agency in one location, with each agency receiving reports from their own personnel. The unified command team keeps each other informed about the progress of the response and has the ability to exchange information, make decisions, and communicate necessary information with their own personnel, reducing the chances for confusion or disagreements between agency personnel on the scene.

8. **Why can't I apply my usual EMS disaster plan to a small-scale MCI?**
Most communities have some sort of disaster plan, but those plans are designed to respond to a large-scale disaster and are usually complicated and not designed to be practically applied to a small-scale MCI. Typically, "disaster" plans address the large-scale event that covers a wide geographic area and involves damage to community infrastructure. Examples include natural disasters such as hurricanes or

tornadoes or terrorist attacks where roads, homes, hospitals, and other aspects of the infrastructure are impacted. In these cases, the community will take the initial action but outside resources and assistance will be needed to assist the community.

9. **Will the time of day an incident occurs affect the management of an MCI?**
In many EMS systems, available resources vary based on the time of day, especially in agencies that use system status management that tailors staffing to the usual daily demand for service. It may take longer to get additional ambulances to the scene in the middle of the night, there may be fewer staffed vehicles, and they may be on other calls or responding from more distant locations. The time of day will also affect the ability of responders to get to the scene based on traffic patterns. In addition, motor vehicle crashes or other situations block main thoroughfares and limit access by EMS. Rerouting often delays the arrival of needed resources.

10. **What is triage?**
Triage is the process of sorting and prioritizing patients. By definition, an MCI or disaster has more patients than medical responders, so the first responders to the scene should begin by systematically determining how many patients are present, the severity of their injuries, and what level of care is needed for each. The goal is to provide the most care to the most number of casualties without expending limited resources on patients who have little likelihood of surviving. This is different than the "usual" triage EMS responders perform routinely. When the number of victims from an incident is limited, the EMT generally will find the sickest individual and then dedicate all of their effort and resources at treating the life-threatening problems. In an MCI, where the number of victims exceeds the available resources, such efforts will only lead to additional mortality.

There are many types of triage systems, but the basic priority levels in most systems are the same:

(a) Highest priority (immediate)—patients with the most serious life-threatening injuries but who have a reasonable likelihood of survival,

(b) Second priority (delayed)—patients with significant but not immediate life-threatening injuries,

(c) Lowest priority (minimal or minor)—patients with injuries that can wait for treatment, sometimes referred to as the "walking wounded,"

(d) No priority (dead or expectant)—patients that are obviously dead, in cardiac arrest, or have injuries incompatible with life.

11. **Are all triage systems the same?**
No, all triage systems are not the same. Therefore, it is necessary that each responder understand the system that is used by their service and is ready to use the system if they find themselves participating in triage during a mass casualty incident.

12. **What is meant by first in, last out?**
This is a concept regarding the first ambulance to arrive at the scene of an MCI. The initial responding ambulance needs to perform a number of essential functions before the process of providing patient care is initiated. The crew should perform a survey of the scene, determine the approximate numbers of patients, determine medical resource or other specialized needs, notify the communication center of their findings and the need to implement the MCI plan, assume medical command, and then and only then begin the process of patient triage. By taking these actions, the first crew on the scene will be choreographing the entire EMS response to the scene. If the first ambulance simply grabs a couple of

patients and immediately transports them, not only does this cause a control vacuum at the scene, but subsequent EMS crews will have to come in and perform the necessary tasks. Therefore, the first crew to arrive is often the last one to leave.

13. **What are some common types of errors made at the scene of a small-scale multicasualty incident?**

    There are a number of common problems that are encountered at the scene of an MCI. One problem is failure of the initial responding EMS crew to establish strong scene control. The initial minutes of an MCI response are crucial to success. If control is not established immediately before additional crews begin to arrive, a "control vacuum" will occur, creating chaos at the scene. More problems occur if incoming EMS crews do not follow the direction of the scene commander, essentially "freelancing" their own scene management. This causes a breakdown in scene control. Another frequent problem is the failure to identify and rapidly contain the patients involved in an incident. A classic example is a multiple vehicle crash with injured passengers wandering around the scene, making it easy to overlook patients during the initial scene survey. Patients must, therefore, be rapidly identified and sequestered on any MCI scene.

14. **What unique problems will I encounter with an MCI involving motor vehicles?**

    Scene safety is a priority at the scene of a motor vehicle crash. EMS crews may be the first public safety agency to arrive and should focus on strategic parking of their own vehicle, wearing proper safety equipment, and containing any ambulatory patients in a safe location for evaluation. Patient containment is difficult because of the natural tendency for patients to wander around the scene. The initial EMS crew must rapidly determine how many occupants were in each vehicle so that they can determine resource needs.

    Rescue vehicle gridlock is a concern, as there will usually be multiple fire trucks, police cars, ambulances, and tow trucks at the scene. Strategic parking is important, therefore, with appropriate concern given to ingress and egress for other ambulances.

    Another problem occurs when patients are trapped in vehicles and require extrication. When extrication is necessary, personnel on the scene should defer to the appropriately trained and equipped responders. Usually, the goal is to transport the worst injuries first. Unfortunately, critically injured patients from a motor vehicle crash may be the last ones transported, due to the delay in extrication. This must be taken into account when setting up receiving emergency departments so they know to reserve their critical care rooms for the more seriously injured patients still to come.

15. **What unique problems should I anticipate at a structure fire with multiple casualties?**

    Scene safety is the priority for all responders. The fire department is usually the lead agency in charge at a fire scene, and all rescue and fire suppression operations are the responsibility of fire department personnel. Incident and unified command will allow for coordinated activities of the various agencies on scene and communication with each other. As patients are rescued from the building, information can be provided to the EMS commander and EMS personnel can prepare to receive and evaluate patients. An important thing to keep in mind about fire scenes is the potential for multiple self-evacuation points from the building. If medical providers are stationed on only one side of the building without anticipating patients fleeing the building from other exits, patients can be missed.

    Another common problem is that people with smoke inhalation do not always exhibit symptoms immediately; in fact, symptoms may take hours to evolve. Therefore, anyone who has inhaled smoke must receive a thorough assessment and must be educated about the possibility of worsening symptoms if allowed to refuse care initially.

People trapped in a burning building will do anything to escape from the fire, even jumping from the roof of a multistory building. You must anticipate major injuries from such falls along with burns and smoke inhalation.

16. How should I handle a multiple casualty scene resulting from violence, such as shootings or stabbings?

Violent scenes, even those with obviously injured patients, are the responsibility of law enforcement to initially contain and control, particularly if the scene is not stable and the potential exists for additional injuries. Many law enforcement agencies have specialty teams trained in entering and taking control of the scene. Once again, a unified incident command structure will allow information to be provided to each agency commander as the scene evolves. Once individual sections of the scene are secured, patients can be evacuated to a safe location for proper assessment, treatment, and transport.

17. What should I consider if I encounter a large number of patients with a similar illness such as vomiting and diarrhea?

Rescuer safety is of particular importance. All personnel should don personal protective gear to ensure they reduce the chance of contact with the source of any potential contaminants or any potentially contaminated body fluids. Although personal protection and patient care are the primary goals of the EMS responders, consideration should also be given to the source of the illness. Large groups of patients with the same illness have likely come in contact with the same source, such as food contamination. However, medical personnel should be alert to the possibility of intentional contamination as well as viral outbreaks that could become a public health concern. Personnel should be familiar with reporting mechanisms through local Public Health Departments to allow for early recognition and notification in the event of a public health emergency.

18. When should I contact medical control?

As soon as you determine that you are dealing with an MCI, notification of medical control should be considered. The sooner the receiving hospital(s) receive word of the incident and the likelihood of multiple incoming patients, the better prepared they will be. The initial call can be a simple setup advising about the potential for multiple casualties and generally does not require great detail about the types of injuries. Once the scene has been completely triaged, medical control can be updated as needed.

19. What are the responsibilities of the incoming ambulances?

It is critical that additional arriving crews receive as much information about the scene as possible. The first arriving crew should advise the communications center of the situation on the scene and provide as much information as possible regarding approach to the scene by other responders. As soon as incident command can be established, the incident commander can work directly with the communications center to provide additional information regarding the number of vehicles needed at the scene and staging locations for those vehicles. The communications center is usually responsible for relaying information to all of the incoming crews, which assists in organization of resources on the scene and reduces radio traffic.

It is important that all personnel responding to the scene follow the direction of incident command and resist the temptation to wander around or "freelance" once on the scene. Coordination on the scene is extremely important, and all personnel should work within their assigned areas.

Small-Scale Multiple Casualty Incidents

20. Should I request or expect a separate radio channel be designated for the MCI?

Most EMS agencies have tactical frequencies available for use during MCIs or other major incidents. Some MCIs may require little radio traffic, whereas others can be quite radio intensive. The decision to move the MCI to its own channel should be made by the person in charge at the scene if the need arises. This can also be done at the request of the dispatcher if normal operations cannot be performed on the same channel. However, an organized communication plan should be part of the planning phase.

21. What should I consider regarding distribution of patients to hospital emergency departments?

Early notification and reasonable distribution of patients from the scene to appropriate facilities is critical to the best outcome for the patients. A dedicated individual in the communications center may be very helpful by calling hospital emergency departments to advise them of the situation and getting available bed counts from each facility.

Emergency Department (ED) personnel may have to activate their own MCI. Outlying hospitals and EMS services may need to be notified to prepare to move patients from the local hospital to other facilities once they have been stabilized.

Pearls and Pitfalls

1. The most important action the first arriving EMS crew can take is to size up the situation in terms of numbers of casualties and resource needs and then communicate that information to the dispatch center.
2. EMS crew safety is of paramount importance at the scene of any MCI, especially when hazardous materials or weapons of mass destruction are potentially involved.
3. Early notification of hospital EDs is essential in order to prepare for incoming casualties.
4. Incoming resources should be certain to follow the direction of the incident commander and stage themselves at the staging point for future task assignment.
5. Incident command should be implemented at all multiple casualty and multiagency incidents, regardless of size.

References

1. McSwain, Norman E. Jr., Paturas, James L., eds., Emergency preparedness The Basic EMT: Comprehensive Prehospital Patient Care, 2nd ed., p. 774. St. Louis: Mosby 2003.
2. NAEMT. PHTLS Prehospital Trauma Life Support, Scene Assessment, Chapter 4, 7th ed., p. 87–108. St. Louis: Mosby, 2011.
3. NAEMT. Disaster management, Chapter 18, PHTLS Prehospital Trauma Life Support, 7th ed., p. 461–466. St. Louis: Mosby, 2011.
4. Moore, RE., Commanding the vehicle rescue incident, Chapter 5. In Vehicle Rescue and Extrication, 2nd ed., p. 167. St. Louis: Mosby, 2003.
5. Emergency Management Institute. Introduction to the National Incident Management System (IS-700). Washington, DC: Federal Emergency Management Agency, http://training.fema.gov/EMIWeb/is/is700a.asp Accessed October 25, 2011.

Weapons of Mass Destruction—Chemical

CHAPTER 22

Stephen V. Cantrill, MD

1. **What are the classes of chemical agents and specific agents usually considered as potential weapons of mass destruction?**
   The major classes of chemical agents that are conventionally considered as potential weapons of mass destruction include nerve agents, vesicants (blister agents), pulmonary toxicants, and cyanide. The nerve agent class includes sarin, tabun, soman, and VX. Vesicants include sulfur mustard and Lewisite. Phosgene, chlorine, and ammonia make up the class of pulmonary toxicants. Cyanide agents include hydrogen cyanide and cyanogen chloride.

2. **Why do we sometimes see chemical agents referred to by two character names?**
   Two-character names for chemical agents are those assigned by the military but that may be used in civilian literature as well. The following table shows the common names of chemical agents that have two-letter military designations:

Two-Letter Military Designation	Common Name	Agent Class
GA	Tabun	Nerve agent
GB	Sarin	Nerve agent
GD	Soman	Nerve agent
VX	VX	Nerve agent
HD	Sulfur mustard	Vesicant
HL	Lewisite	Vesicant
CG	Phosgene	Pulmonary toxicant
AC	Hydrogen cyanide (hydrocyanic acid)	Cyanide
CK	Cyanogen chloride	Cyanide

3. **Chemical agents seem so deadly; how can anyone survive?**
   Although potentially lethal, patients who present after exposure to chemical weapons of mass destruction with vital signs stand an excellent chance of survival if they receive appropriate care. As an example, the sarin release in Tokyo produced approximately 5500 victims but only 12 deaths. Through proper knowledge and training, we can increase any victim's chances for survival.

4. **Nerve agents are similar to what class of chemicals that we may encounter in the civilian world?**
   Nerve agents are very similar to organophosphate pesticides (such as malathion, diazinon, etc.), the toxic effects of which are sometimes seen from accidental spills or exposures, ingestions, or farm pesticide incidents.

Weapons of Mass Destruction—Chemical

5. What are the major manifestations of nerve agent exposure?

Nerve agents, as a group, act by inhibiting acetylcholinesterase at the neurosynaptic junction, causing unmitigated stimulation of the distal nerve, gland, or muscle. The nature and extent of the symptoms will depend on the dose and nature of the exposure. Symptoms and findings may include salivation (drooling), lacrimation (tearing), rhinorrhea (runny nose), eye pain, dim vision, urination, defecation, gastrointestinal distress (nausea), emesis, shortness of breath, bronchospasm, coma, seizures, and apnea. Many of the presenting symptoms can be easily remembered by the acronym SLUDGE:

> **S**alivation (drooling)
> **L**acrimation (tearing)
> **U**rination
> **D**efecation
> **G**astrointestinal distress
> **E**mesis (vomiting)

6. How may the presentation of exposure to vapor nerve agents differ from exposure to liquid nerve agents?

The onset of symptoms will be significantly faster with vapor (e.g., sarin) exposure than with liquid (e.g., VX) exposure. The onset of the vapor effects will be in seconds, peaking within minutes (e.g., 5 minutes or so). There will be no late onset of symptoms. With mild liquid exposure, symptoms may be delayed for as long as 18 hours and may be limited to the body location of exposure (with muscle fasciculations and localized diaphoresis); eye findings may not be present.

7. What are the mainstays of treatment for exposure to nerve agents?

Two drugs comprise the major method for treating patients symptomatic from nerve agent exposure: atropine and pralidoxime (also known as 2-PAM). The atropine should be administered first (2 mg IM in an adult) to relieve the bronchoconstriction and excess secretions. This can then be followed by pralidoxime (1 gm IM or IV in an adult) to help speed long-term recovery. The atropine may be repeated, as necessary, up to a dose of 20 mg in an adult.

8. What is a Mark I autoinjector?

The Mark I autoinjector is a device that contains premeasured doses of atropine (2 mg) and pralidoxime (600 mg) packaged in units that allow simple, accurate, rapid drug administration (Figure 22.1). These units

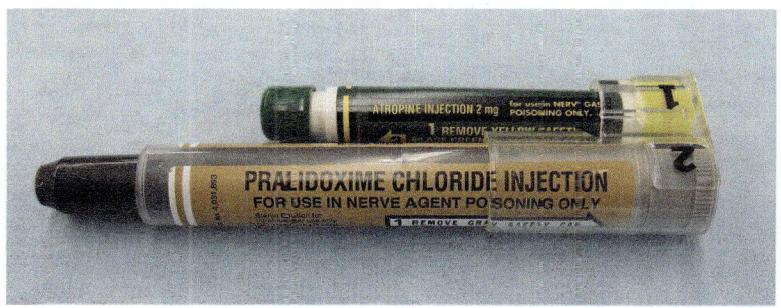

FIGURE 22.1 Mark I Autoinjector: The atropine-containing unit is labeled "1"; the pralidoxime unit, "2"

each contain a needle that fires out of the tip of the device when pressed against the leg. The pressurized medication is then forced through the needle into the surrounding tissue over about a 10 second period. These units, originally developed for military use, are now available to civilian medical personnel.

9. **I have been hearing the term "Duodote™." What is that all about?**
   The Mark I autoinjector kits which contained two separate autoinjectors, one each of atropine and pralidoxime, are gradually being replaced with an autoinjector called Duodote™. The Duodote™ autoinjector contains both the atropine and pralidoxime in a single device (Figure 22.2).

10. **How do I use the Mark I or Duodote™ autoinjector?**
    To use a Mark I autoinjector:
    - Remove the #1 (atropine) medication unit from the safety clip, using care to not touch the colored tip (which will trigger the needle)
    - Holding the unit like a pen, place the colored end against the thickest part of the thigh
    - Press the injector firmly against the thigh, which will cause the needle to spring from the unit into the surrounding tissue and force the medication from the unit
    - Hold in place for 10 seconds, then remove and discard
    - Massage the area of injection
    - Repeat with the second unit (pralidoxime)

    If the Duodote™ device is provided, the steps are the same as for the Mark I kit except that only a single device is used.

11. **How can I become a secondary victim from a nerve agent incident?**
    It's easy:
    (a) Lack of situational awareness: park your response vehicle too close or downwind from a possible nerve gas release scene; enter a room where multiple people are drooling, vomiting, and seizing without proper personal protective equipment
    (b) Provide care to contaminated victims without appropriate personal protective equipment or first decontaminating the victims. (In the Tokyo sarin attack, 10 percent of the first responders became secondary victims.)

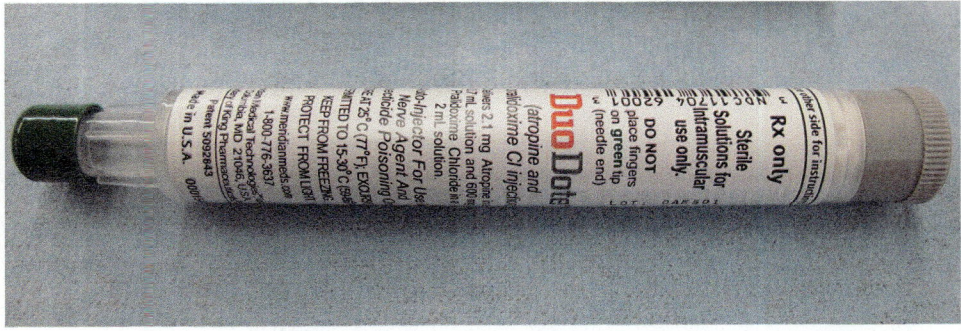

FIGURE 22.2 Duodote autoinjector containing both atropine and pralidoxime in one device.

12. What are blister agents and what is the initial treatment for exposure to these agents?
Blister agents (sulfur mustard and Lewisite) are vesicants that represent a threat both in liquid and vapor form. They quickly bind to human tissue, eventually causing cellular death. They can have a major effect on the skin, initially causing erythema then progressing to vesicles that coalesce into blisters and bullae. These agents may also cause significant injury to the eyes and the lining of the airway. Significant exposures may be fatal because of systemic toxicity particularly to the bone marrow (sulfur mustard). Symptoms may take hours to develop after a sulfur mustard exposure but will develop immediately after Lewisite exposure. Initial treatment consists of immediate and rapid decontamination of the eyes and skin of the victim with special attention to the risk of cross-contamination to the rescuer. Other treatment is supportive, with intubation, if necessary.

13. What are the common aspects of exposure to pulmonary toxicants?
Pulmonary toxicants include phosgene, chlorine, and ammonia. These may cause a severe life-threatening injury after inhalation. Initial symptoms may include cough, shortness of breath, and irritation of the eyes and airway, although some symptoms may be delayed for up to 72 hours after exposure, particularly with phosgene. Treatment includes removal from the source of exposure, decontamination, and supportive care, including intubation and positive pressure ventilation, if necessary.

14. What are the different types of gaseous cyanide that could be used in a chemical incident?
There are two: hydrogen cyanide (chemical formula HCN) and cyanogen chloride (chemical formula CNCl).

15. How does cyanide affect the body?
Both forms of cyanide are cellular poisons that disable the cell's ability to metabolize oxygen necessary to create energy and keep the cell alive. This means that oxygen is not extracted from the blood, leading to bright-red venous blood and a profound metabolic acidosis without cyanosis. Exposure to low concentrations may result in gradual onset of symptoms of headache, weakness, lightheadedness, and ataxia. With high concentrations, rapid onset of seizures, rigidity, respiratory depression, and cardiac arrest may be seen.

16. Is the bitter-almond smell of hydrogen cyanide a reliable test?
No. The nose should never be considered as a detection device. Only about 50 percent of the population is capable of smelling the bitter-almond fragrance of hydrogen cyanide. Cyanogen chloride reportedly has a pungent, biting odor but is often masked by its irritation of the nose and respiratory tract.

17. How should cyanide exposure be treated in the field?
Field treatment consists of safe removal of the patient from the area of exposure followed by decontamination by removal of clothing and a washdown. Securing airway, breathing, and circulation should then be accomplished, but mouth breathing should not be performed, as the patient will continue to exhale cyanide. The patient should be provided with 100 percent oxygen and transported. If available, hydroxocobalamin (Cyanokit), an injectable form of vitamin B12 may be administered in the field, which will take up the cyanide, rendering it harmless.

18. What is the definitive treatment for cyanide exposure?
Definitive treatment of cyanide poisoning includes administration of hydroxocobalamin (as mentioned above) or administration of amyl or sodium nitrite (to free up the cyanide from the cells),

followed by sodium thiosulfate to form thiocyanate, a nontoxic compound that is then excreted in the urine.

Pearls and Pitfalls

1. The potential diagnosis of possible nerve agent exposure must be made by situational assessment (multiple casualties with similar symptoms, common time or location factors) and evaluation of the patient's presenting symptoms.
2. Treatment of nerve agent poisoning may require huge doses of atropine, as much as 10–20 mg, sometimes even more.
3. Failure to recognize the situation or to use appropriate personal protective equipment may cause you to become a secondary victim of a chemical agent.
4. Mouth-to-mouth breathing must be avoided for the purpose of rescuer safety after exposure to pulmonary toxicants and cyanide.

References

1. Centers for Disease Control and Prevention. Sulfur mustard. Available at www.bt.cdc.gov/agent/sulfurmustard/index.asp (accessed 5/1/11)
2. Centers for Disease Control and Prevention. Choking/lung/pulmonary agents. Available at www.bt.cdc.gov/agent/pulmonary (accessed 5/1/11)
3. Chemical Casualty Care Division, USAMRICD. Medical Management of Chemical Casualties Handbook, 3rd ed. Aberdeen Proving Ground, MD, 2000.
4. FDA. FDA approves drug to treat cyanide poisoning. Available at www.fda.gov/bbs/topics/NEWS/2006/NEW01531.html (accessed 3/20/07)
5. Holstege CP, Kirk M, Sidell FR. Chemical warfare. Nerve agent poisoning. Crit Care Clin Oct; 13(4):923–942, 1997.
6. Nakajima T, Sato S, Morita H, Yanagisawa N. Sarin poisoning of a rescue team in the Matsumoto sarin incident in Japan. Occup Environ Med 1997 Oct; 54(10):697–701.
7. Okumura T, Takasu N, Ishimatsu S, et al. Report on 640 victims of the Tokyo subway sarin attack. Ann Emerg Med Aug; 28(2):129–135, 1996.
8. Sidell FR, Borak J. Chemical warfare agents: II. Nerve agents. Ann Emerg Med Jul; 21(7):865–871, 1992.
9. Sidell FR, Takafuji ET, Franz DR (eds.): Medical Aspects of Chemical and Biological Warfare. Washington, DC: Office of the Surgeon General, 1997.
10. Tokuda Y, Kikuchi M, Takahashi O. Prehospital management of sarin nerve gas terrorism in urban settings: 10 years of progress after the Tokyo subway sarin attack. Resuscitation Feb; 68(2):193–202, 2006.

Biological Terrorism

Edward Eitzen, MD, MPH, COL, USA (Retired)

CHAPTER 23

1. **Isn't the threat of biological terrorism overblown?**
   It really depends on what kind of biological attack one is talking about. The type of attack that would kill hundreds of thousands in a major city, although within the realm of possibility, is unlikely. There are technical challenges and adverse meteorological conditions that make this type of event difficult to carry out, even by a sophisticated and determined group of perpetrators. However, biological attacks are not unprecedented, as the anthrax attacks of autumn 2001, and the Rajneeshee Cult attacks in Oregon in 1984 attest. Although many "experts" worry about engineered biological agents that can evade vaccine-induced immunity or are resistant to multiple antibiotics, far more likely are attacks using classical biological threats that are not completely resistant to treatment. Many of the key biological threat agents may be readily available in the environment, infect animals, and may relatively easily be produced or cultivated. Many people have the education and training necessary to become a biological terrorist. Finally, Mother Nature herself may be the most likely "bioterrorist," as history reveals that emerging natural infections in new localities are much more common events than intentional terrorist attacks (West Nile fever, SARS, H1N1, and avian influenza are just a few recent examples. We must be prepared for either, however.

2. **What are the biological agents we should worry the most about?**
   There are many lists of biological threat agents. Probably the best known is the Centers for Disease Control and Prevention (CDC) select agent list, which includes categories A, B, and C agents, A agents being considered the greatest threats. Category A agents include *Bacillus anthracis*, or anthrax, *Variola major*, or smallpox, botulinum toxins derived from *Clostridium botulinum* bacteria, *Yersinia pestis*, or plague, *Franciscella tularensis*, or tularemia, and viral hemorrhagic fever (VHF) agents such as Ebola and Marburg viruses. These agents are on the "A list" for a combination of reasons, including lethality, rapidity of illness, potential for concentration and weaponization, availability, person-to-person spread of disease (smallpox, plague, and viral hemorrhagic fevers), and difficulty of diagnosis and treatment. In addition, most of the A list agents have been weaponized in the past at one time or another by former nation-state–sponsored bioweapons programs (the former Soviet Union, the United States, and Iraq included). However, it should be emphasized that the armamentarium of the biological terrorist is only limited by his or her ingenuity and imagination—historically biological attackers have used *Salmonella* species, *Shigella*, ricin toxin, glanders, *Brucella*, and other agents. In order of concern, most experts would list smallpox and anthrax first, botulinum toxins and plague second, and tularemia and VHFs third.

3. **What are the indicators of an intentional biological attack as opposed to a natural epidemic?**
   There are several epidemiological indicators and clues that might indicate an intentional biological attack including:

- high disease attack rate, especially if in a discrete population such as those living in a given geographic area or those working in a particular setting, especially a setting a terrorist might consider a target (such as a government building, for example)
- a disease outbreak unusual for a given geographic area, such as Ebola occurring in Washington, DC, or occurring at an unusual time of year
- high morbidity and mortality
- unusual routes of exposure, such as the airborne route for diseases that occur naturally by a different route of exposure
- a disease entity that fails to respond to standard therapy for that type of disease—such as community-acquired pneumonias that are unusually severe and don't respond to standard treatment
- a single case of disease by an unlikely agent—such as smallpox, which no longer occurs naturally
- disease occurring in an unusual age group for that disease or syndrome
- multiple disease outbreaks with the same pathogen in noncontiguous areas, or multiple epidemics with different pathogens presenting simultaneously
- sentinel animal disease outbreaks or simultaneous or temporally related outbreaks of human and animal disease; and
- intelligence indicating an attack, claims by terrorist groups, or discovery of a weapon or means of spreading a biological agent. Some of these factors may indicate an outbreak of naturally emerging infectious disease as well, but a high index of suspicion for biological terrorism should be maintained if any of these are present until proven otherwise.

4. **Which agents of biological terrorism may be spread person to person or nosocomially? Which are not spread person to person?**

Of the key agents of bioterrorism, smallpox, plague, and the viral hemorrhagic fevers can be spread from person to person. Smallpox is spread by airborne and respiratory droplet primarily, although the lesions can be infective by contact. Plague may be spread by respiratory droplets from person to person in a bioterrorism event, and by the flea vector in natural bubonic disease. The viral hemorrhagic fevers Ebola and Marburg are generally spread from person to person by direct contact with patients or deceased individuals and their secretions, including blood and body fluids. Anthrax, tularemia, and botulism are not spread from person to person typically, although cutaneous anthrax can theoretically be spread by direct skin to skin contact.

5. **For bioterrorism agents that are spread from person to person, how can I protect myself?**

Most important is observing standard precautions with all patients and taking care not to be exposed to blood and certain other body fluids. Good handwashing, wearing gloves and other protective equipment, and avoiding needle sticks form the basis of standard precautions. Standard precautions are required for patients with anthrax, tularemia, and botulinum intoxication. Further protection is necessary when some bioterrorism agents are suspected: if smallpox is suspected, then airborne precautions must be undertaken; if pneumonic plague is suspected, droplet precautions must be taken; if viral hemorrhagic fever is suspected, then contact precautions must be observed, and consideration should be strongly given toward observing airborne precautions, as rare instances of airborne spread from person to person have been apparently observed. Definitions and information on isolation precautions can be found at http://www.cdc.gov/hicpac/2007IP/2007isolationPrecautions.html.

Biological Terrorism

6. **If I am already exposed to a biological terrorism agent, are there any measures that can be taken to avoid becoming a casualty?**
   For most bioterrorism agent exposures the answer is yes. Unimmunized persons exposed to smallpox can be immunized with smallpox vaccine up to 3–5 days after exposure and may still be either protected from illness, or have a milder version of the illness. Persons exposed to anthrax either environmentally or in the attack itself (anthrax is not spread person to person) may be given antibiotics for 45–60 days postexposure to prevent spore germination; the addition of three doses of anthrax vaccine to this regimen may shorten the length of time antibiotics are needed, but antibiotics should be given a minimum of 30–45 days even with postexposure use of anthrax vaccine. Persons exposed to plague and tularemia but who are not yet ill can be treated with antibiotics such as doxycycline. Persons exposed to viral hemorrhagic fevers (VHFs) such as Lassa fever, HFRS (hemorrhagic fever with renal syndrome caused by hantaviruses), CCHF (Crimean–Congo hemorrhagic fever), or Rift Valley fever (RVF) might be treated with the antiviral drug ribavirin, which has limited availability and must be administered under an investigational new drug protocol. Certain VHFs such as Ebola and Marburg do not respond to ribavirin. Patients exposed to botulinum toxin(s) in an attack could theoretically be treated with botulinum antitoxins prior to onset of symptoms while the toxin is still circulating; however, practically it would be very difficult to identify such patients and because of limited supplies of antitoxins, patients would likely be treated shortly after onset of symptoms to try to stop progression of paralysis.

7. **What are the signs and symptoms of anthrax?**
   There are three typical forms of anthrax depending on the route of exposure: cutaneous anthrax, gastrointestinal (or pharyngeal) anthrax, and inhalational anthrax. The form that would be most expected after an aerosol bioterrorism attack would be the inhalational form. After a 1–6 day incubation period, inhalational anthrax signs and symptoms begin with a prodrome featuring fever, malaise, and fatigue, which may last for 24–48 hours. A nonproductive cough and vague chest discomfort may also be present during this period. This prodrome may be followed by symptomatic improvement for 2–3 days, or may progress directly to the abrupt onset of severe respiratory distress with dyspnea, stridor, diaphoresis, and cyanosis. Bacteremia, septic shock, metastatic infection (meningitis in approximately half of cases), and death usually follow within 24–36 hours. It was once thought that once symptoms of inhalational anthrax appear, treatment would almost invariably be ineffective; however, in the anthrax attacks of autumn 2001, over half of clinically ill patients with inhalational anthrax survived with agressive and intensive care, including respiratory support, antibiotics, and intensive supportive care.

8. **What are the signs and symptoms of smallpox?**
   After aerosol exposure, the incubation period for smallpox averages 12 days, with a range of 7–19 days. This is followed by abrupt onset of clinical manifestations marked by systemic toxicity with prominent malaise, high fever, rigors, vomiting, headache, prostration, and backache; 15% of patients develop delirium. Approximately 10% of light-skinned patients exhibit an erythematous rash during this phase. Two to 3 days later, ulcers of the oropharynx and tongue appear concomitantly with a discrete rash about the face, hands, and forearms. The mucous membrane ulcerative lesions shed infectious oropharyngeal secretions in the first few days of the eruptive illness. These respiratory secretions are the most important but not the sole means of virus transmission to contacts. After eruptions on the lower extremities, the rash spreads centrally to the trunk over the next week. Lesions quickly progress from macules to papules and

eventually to pustular vesicles and finally to umbilicated pustules. Lesions are more abundant on the extremities and face, and this centrifugal distribution is an important diagnostic feature. In distinct contrast to varicella (chickenpox), lesions on various segments of the body remain generally synchronous in their stage of development, whereas varicella lesions erupt in "crops," are at different stages of development simultaneously, and are more abundant on the trunk than the extremities (centripetal distribution). In the second week after onset of smallpox, the pustules form scabs that leave depressed depigmented scars on healing. Although variola titers in the throat, conjunctiva, and urine diminish with time, virus can readily be recovered from scabs throughout convalescence. Therefore, patients should be isolated and considered infectious until all scabs separate.

9. **What are the signs and symptoms of botulinum intoxication?**

   The onset of symptoms of botulism usually occurs from 12–36 hours after exposure but can vary according to the amount of toxin absorbed and the route of exposure (oral versus inhaled). Unlike other bioterrorism agents, botulinum is not a very stable aerosol weapon; thus, an attack with this agent may in fact be food borne. Cranial nerve palsies are prominent signs early, with eye symptoms such as blurred vision due to dilated pupils, double vision, ptosis, and photophobia, in addition to other cranial nerve signs such as dysarthria, dysphonia, and dysphagia. Flaccid skeletal muscle paralysis follows, in a symmetrical, descending, and progressive manner. Collapse and obstruction of the upper airway may occur due to weakness of the oropharyngeal musculature. As the descending motor weakness soon involves the diaphragm and accessory muscles of respiration, respiratory failure may occur abruptly. Progression from onset of symptoms to respiratory failure has occurred in as little as 24 hours in cases of severe botulinum intoxication. Typical anticholinergic signs and symptoms manifest the autonomic effects of botulism: dry mouth, ileus, constipation, and urinary retention. Nausea and vomiting may occur as nonspecific sequelae of an ileus. Dilated pupils (mydriasis) are seen in approximately 50% of cases. Sensory symptoms usually do not occur. Botulinum toxins do not cross the blood/brain barrier and do not cause central nervous system manifestations, thus patients remain alert even when skeletal muscles are paralyzed.

10. **What are the signs and symptoms of plague?**

    There are three major clinical forms of plague: bubonic, septicemic, and pneumonic. The form most often associated with natural, flea-borne disease is the bubonic form (swollen infected lymph nodes). The expected form of disease after a bioterrorism attack (inhalation of infective aerosols) would be the pneumonic (lung) form. Pneumonic plague begins with sudden onset of symptoms after an incubation period of 1–6 days. Signs and symptoms include high fever, chills, headache, malaise, followed by cough (often with hemoptysis), progressing rapidly to dyspnea, stridor, cyanosis, and death. Gastrointestinal symptoms are also often present. Death results from respiratory failure, circulatory collapse, and a bleeding diathesis. Bubonic plague is characterized by swollen painful lymph nodes called buboes (often in the inguinal area), high fever, and malaise. Bubonic plague may progress spontaneously to the septicemic form (septic shock, thrombosis, disseminated intravascular coagulation) or to the pneumonic form. Pneumonic plague may also progress to the septicemic form. Plague meningitis is also possible although less frequent than occurs with anthrax.

11. **What are the signs and symptoms of tularemia?**

    After an incubation period of 3–6 days (with a range of 1–21 days, probably dose dependent), onset of disease is usually acute. Tularemia typically appears in several forms, which can generally be categorized as either typhoidal or ulceroglandular. In humans, as few as 10–50 organisms will cause disease if inhaled or injected intradermally, whereas approximately 10^8 organisms are required with oral challenge. The form of tularemia most likely to be associated with a bioterrorism attack is typhoidal (septicemic) tularemia, which occurs mainly after inhalation of infectious aerosols. The disease manifests as a nonspecific syndrome consisting of abrupt onset of fever (38–40°C), headache, malaise, myalgias, and prostration; but unlike most other forms of tularemia disease, it presents without lymphadenopathy. Occasionally patients will present with nausea, vomiting, diarrhea, or abdominal pain. Case fatality rates are approximately 35% in untreated naturally acquired typhoidal cases. Mortality is higher if pneumonia is present. Mortality is less than 5% in treated cases overall. Survivors of untreated tularemia may have symptoms which persist for weeks or, less often, months, with progressive debilitation.

12. **What are the signs and symptoms of viral hemorrhagic fevers (VHFs)?**
   Diseases classified as VHFs are diverse in clinical presentation. Mortality may range from very high (50–90%) in Ebola and Marburg disease to less than 5% in Rift Valley fever (RVF). In their most severe form, these diseases manifest as the VHF syndrome, with capillary leak, severe bleeding diathesis, and hemodynamic compromise leading to hypotension and shock. Early symptoms of VHF are nondescript in most cases, consisting of fever and constitutional symptoms such as malaise, myalcias, and headache. This constellation of findings is difficult to discern from any number of viral, bacterial, or parasitic diseases (note the clinical descriptions of plague, tularemia, and anthrax above). Disseminated intravascular coagulation (DIC) is thought to underlie the hemorrhagic features of Rift Valley, Marburg, and Ebola fevers; but in most VHFs, the etiology of the coagulopathy is multifactorial (e.g., hepatic damage, consumptive coagulopathy, and primary bone marrow dysfunction). Why some infected persons develop full-blown VHF while others do not remains unresolved. Virulence of the infecting agent clearly plays a large role. The VHF syndrome occurs in a majority of patients manifesting disease from filoviruses (Ebola and Marburg), CCHF, and the South American hemorrhagic fever viruses (Junín, Machupo, Guanarito, Sabia), whereas it occurs in a small minority of patients with dengue, RVF, and Lassa fever. The reasons for variation among patients infected with the same virus are still unknown but probably stem from a complex interplay of virus–host interactions.

13. **Is a patient already clinically ill with a bioterrorism agent automatically going to die, or is there therapy that may be life saving even after onset of clinical symptoms?**
   In many cases, patients already clinically ill with bioterrorism related illness may still be saved. Although all of these agents can cause very severe disease and death, sometimes rapidly, there are treatment modalities available that may slow or even reverse the progression of disease in some cases. Many of these therapies are stored in the nation's Strategic National (Pharmaceutical) Stockpile (SNS). For the bacterial diseases such as anthrax, plague, and tularemia, a variety of antibiotics are stockpiled. Efforts are also being made to develop alternative treatments (other than antibiotics) as adjunctive therapies for these bacterial illnesses, particularly anthrax. For botulinum intoxication, several different antitoxins are available which can be used once clinical signs of botulism are apparent. For the viral illnesses, antiviral therapies are also under research and development. The SNS also includes supportive care modalities such as IV fluids, IV administration equipment, and ventilators.

14. **How important is decontamination in a bioterrorism event?**
   It really depends on the event and the biological agent used and how much time has elapsed. Most biological agents will be inactivated over time, usually hours to days, when in the exposed external

environment by natural ultraviolet radiation (even anthrax spores). In more sheltered environments or indoors, agents can persist longer and spores may persist almost indefinitely in the right environments. As seen in the 2001 anthrax attacks, some individuals may be more susceptible to lower doses of a biological agent such as anthrax, even in the absence of gross contamination. Therefore, with certain agents such as anthrax, maximal decontamination is very important, and there may not be any completely "safe" level of residual spores. Blood and certain body fluids of patients with viral hemorrhagic fevers are also very hazardous and must be decontaminated on surfaces immediately to avoid exposure. For most patients exposed to a biological aerosol, contamination of skin and clothing will not be that significant, and may even be no longer present after a several day incubation period— removal and discarding of clothing and soap and water decontamination of skin surfaces should be sufficient unless very gross contamination is present. A complete discussion of biological decontamination issues is beyond the scope of this chapter and can be found in several of the references listed at the end of this chapter.

15. **What are the most important principles (based on and modified from the "Ten Commandments of Biological Defense," first postulated by Dr. Ted Cieslak) for prehospital care providers and first receivers in the management of casualties from a biological terrorism attack?**

   (a) **Maintain a high index of suspicion.** In the case of chemical or conventional warfare and terrorism, victims would likely succumb in close temporal and geographic proximity to a dispersal or explosive device. Complicating the identification of a biological attack, however, is the fact that biological agents typically possess inherent incubation periods. These incubation periods, typically hours, days, or even weeks long, permit the wide dispersion of victims (in both time and distance) prior to developing symptoms and signs of illness. Moreover, they make it likely that the "first responder" to a biological attack would not be the traditional first responder—fire, police, paramedics and EMTs—but rather primary care physicians, emergency department personnel, and public health officials. In such circumstances, the maintenance of a healthy 'index of suspicion' is imperative. The best chance we have, still, to detect an unusual biological event, natural or unnatural, is the astute clinician, first responder, laboratory, or public health professional who says: "there's something unusual going on here," even when they don't know the exact nature of the event or illness.

   (b) **Protect yourself.** Before medical personnel approach a potential biological casualty, they must first take steps to protect themselves. These steps may involve a combination of physical, pharmaceutical, and immunologic forms of protection. Wearing an N95 (or even a simple surgical) mask will afford some respiratory protection against biological agents. Pharmaceutical protection refers, in general, to the pre- and/or postexposure administration of antibiotics when exposure is either anticipated or known after the fact. Immunologic protection principally involves active vaccination and refers mainly to preexposure protection against anthrax and smallpox, where available.

   (c) **Assess the patient.** This initial assessment is somewhat analogous to the primary survey of advanced trauma life support management. As such, airway adequacy should be assessed and breathing and circulation problems addressed before attention is given to specific management. The initial assessment is conducted before decontamination is accomplished and thus should be brief. Historical information of potential interest to the clinician should also be gathered if possible: it might include information about clusters of illnesses among family, friends, and coworkers; the presence of unusual munitions or dispersal devices, recent food and water sources, vector exposures, travel and immunization histories, and occupational duties and exposures. The physical exam at this point should concentrate on the pulmonary, circulatory, neurological, and muscular systems as well as unusual dermatologic findings.

(d) **Decontaminate as appropriate.** As discussed above, the incubation period of biological agents makes it unlikely that victims of a bioweapons attack will present for medical care until hours to days afterward. At that point, and depending upon the mode of exposure, the need for decontamination may be minimal or nonexistent. In those cases where decontamination is warranted, simple soap and water showering or bathing will almost always suffice. Routine use of caustic substances, such as sodium hypochlorite or bleach, especially on human skin, is rarely warranted after a biological attack.

(e) **Practice good infection control.** Standard precautions provide adequate protection against most infectious diseases, including those potentially employed in a biological attack. Anthrax, tularemia, brucellosis, glanders, Q fever, Venezuelan equine encephalitis, and toxin-mediated diseases are not generally contagious, and victims can be safely managed using standard precautions. Such precautions should be familiar to all first responders and other clinicians. In addition to standard precautions, one of three forms of transmission-based precautions is warranted with smallpox, plague, and the viral hemorrhagic fevers. Smallpox victims should be cared for using "airborne precautions" (including, ideally, a HEPA-filtered mask). Pneumonic plague warrants the use of "droplet precautions" (which include, among other measures, the wearing of a simple surgical mask), and certain viral hemorrhagic fevers require "contact precautions." The CDC website and several of the listed references go into great detail on infection control precautions.

(f) **Alert the proper authorities.** One of the major tenets of proper response to a suspected biological attack is to notify the proper authorities, both health and law-enforcement authorities. Note that such notification should be immediate upon **suspicion** of an attack, not confirmation. Suspicion may be engendered by only one case of an unusual disease, or by clusters of disease that are suspected to be unnatural in origin. Reporting suspicions to local law enforcement and the Federal Bureau of Investigation should be simultaneous with informing proper health officials. In the field this may mean informing medical control of the possibility of bioterrorism; in the hospital it usually means contacting infection control professionals immediately and reporting suspicious cases to local or regional health department officials in a very timely manner. In the United States, larger cities often have their own health departments. In most other areas, the county health department represents the lowest echelon health jurisdiction. In some rural areas, practitioners would access the state health department directly. Once alerted, local and regional health authorities are normally well versed on the mechanisms for requesting additional support from health officials at higher jurisdictions. Each practitioner should have a point of contact with such agencies and should be familiar with mechanisms for contacting them before a crisis arises. Hospital and local/regional clinical laboratories should also be notified. This will enable laboratory personnel to take proper precautions when handling specimens and will also permit the optimal use of specialized facilities and appropriate diagnostic modalities for suspected bioterrorism related causes. Timeliness cannot be stressed greatly enough—the ability to respond effectively to a bioterrorism attack may be measured in hours, and the quicker that response can be triggered, the greater is the chance of mobilizing resources and saving lives.

(g) **Assist in the epidemiologic investigation and manage the psychological consequences.** All health care providers must have a basic understanding of epidemiological principles. Even under austere conditions, a rudimentary epidemiologic investigation may assist in diagnosis and in the discovery of additional bioweapons victims. Clinicians should, at the very least, query patients about illness onset and symptoms, potential exposures, ill family members or coworkers, place of work and residence, food/water sources, seeing unusual munitions or spray devices, and vector exposures; plus develop an ongoing listing of potential cases. Early discovery of clinical cases might help to identify those exposed but not yet ill and permit postexposure prophylaxis, thereby avoiding excess morbidity and mortality in the victims. Public health officials would normally conduct more elaborate epidemiologic investigations and should be contacted **as soon as one suspects the possibility** of a biological attack. Veterinarians should be queried as to the presence of coexistent animal disease which may also be attack related.

In addition to implementing specific diagnostic evaluations and medical countermeasures and initiating an epidemiologic investigation, the provider must be prepared to address the psychological effects of a known, suspected, or feared biological terrorism event. An actual exposure to a bioterrorism agent (or the threat of such exposure) can provoke fear and anxiety in the population, and may result in overwhelming numbers of patients seeking medical evaluation and treatment. Many of these will likely have unexplained symptoms and many may demand antibiotics, antitoxins, and other therapies, all of which may be in limted supply. Anxiety-provoked symptoms and signs, as well as the side effects of postexposure antibiotic prophylaxis, may suggest prodromal disease due to biological-agent exposure and pose challenges in differential diagnosis. This "behavioral contagion" is best prevented and managed by good, proactive, risk communication from health and government authorities. Such communication, at a minimum, should include a realistic assessment of the risk of exposure, information about the resulting disease, and what to do and who to contact for suspected exposure. Risk communication must be timely, accurate, consistent, and well coordinated. It must be planned in advance to be effective. Every jurisdiction should have a well-thought-out risk communication plan that has been practiced and exercised before an event occurs. Similarly, plans must be in place (and must also have been exercised) to rapidly deploy resources for the initial evaluation and administration of postexposure prophylaxis, to proactively develop patient and contact tracing and vaccine screening tools, to access stockpiled vaccines and medications, and to identify and prepare local facilities and health care teams for the care of mass casualties.

(h) **Maintain Proficiency.** Fortunately, the threat of bioterrorism has remained a theoretical one for most communities and medical personnel. However, it is extremely important that first responders and primary and emergency care providers maintain awareness and proficiency in dealing with this low-probability, but potentially high-consequence problem. This can be done, in part, by availing oneself of several comprehensive resources. The CDC's bioterrorism response website (http://www.bt.cdc.gov/bioterrorism/) and the US Army Medical Research Institute of Infectious Diseases

(USAMRIID) web site (www.usamriid.army.mil) all provide a wealth of excellent information; the USAMRIID site includes the full text of USAMRIID's *Medical Management of Biological Casualties Handbook*. Numerous satellite television broadcasts sponsored by USAMRIID, as well as other video resources, provide in-depth discussion and training in medical biodefense and emerging infectious diseases. CD-ROM training aids are also available. Continuing medical education programs provided by medical specialty organizations such as the American Medical Association, the American Nurses Association, the Emergency Nurses Association and the American College of Emergency Physicians are ongoing, and some state and local medical associations also provide training to health care providers licensed in their jurisdictions. Frontline medical personnel, once aware of the threat and educated on how to deal with the situation, must ensure that other personnel in their organizations receive training as well. It is only through ongoing education and training that personnel will be ready to deal effectively with biological terrorism should it occur. We owe our families, our communities, and our society such preparedness.

Pearls and Pitfalls

1. The most important preventative measure that a field provider can take is to use standard infection precautions. Use appropriate personal protective equipment on both yourself and the patient.
2. All patients with respiratory symptoms should be treated as potentially infectious and have a mask placed on them.
3. Decontamination is generally not necessary in a biologic weapons attack except for obvious powder exposure.
4. Most victims of a biologic attack will present days after their exposure with a flulike syndrome and then progress to more serious illness.

References

1. Woods J, Darling R, Dembek Z, Carr B, Ceislak T, Lawlor J, Lttrell A, Kortepeter M, Rebert N, Stanek S, Martin J. Medical Management of Biological Casualties Handbook, 6th ed. Frederick, MD: US Army Medical Research Institute of Infectious Diseases, April 2005.
2. Eitzen EM. Testimony before the Permanent Subcommittee on Investigations, Govermental Affairs Committee, US Senate, on the Threat of Use of Biological Warfare by Terrorists in the United States, October 31, 1995.
3. Franz DR, Jahrling PB, Friedlander AM, McClain DJ, Hoover DL, et al. Clinical recognition and management of patients exposed to biological warfare agents. JAMA 278;399–411, 1997.
4. Pile JC, Malone JD, Eitzen EM, Friedlander AM. Anthrax as a Potential Biological Warfare Agent. Arch Intern Med. 1998; 158: 429-434.
5. McGovern TW, Christopher GW, Eitzen EM Jr. Cutaneous manifestations of biological warfare and related threat agents. *Arch Dermatol.* 1999: 135: 311–322.
6. Franz DR, Jahrling PB, Friedlander AM, McClain DJ, Hoover DL, Clinical recognition and management of patients exposed to biological warfare agents. In Biological Weapons: Limiting the Threat. Lederberg J (ed.) BSCIA Studies in International Security. Cambridge, MA: MIT/Harvard University Press, 1999.
7. Inglesby TV, Henderson DA, Bartlett JG, Ascher MS, Eitzen EM, et al. Anthrax as a biological weapon: medical and public health management. Consensus statement of the working group on civilian biodefense. JAMA 281: 1735–1745, 1999.

8. Henderson DA, Inglesby TV, Bartlett JG, Ascher MS, Eitzen EM, et al. Smallpox as a biological weapon: Medical and public health management. Consensus statement of the working group on civilian biodefense. JAMA 281: 2127–2137, 1999.
9. Army FM 8-284, Treatment of Biological Warfare Casualties, Department of the Army, Fort Sam Houston, TX:. US Army Medical Department Center and School.
10. Henretig F, Cieslak T, Madsen J, Eitzen E, Fleisher G. The emergency department response to incidents of biological and chemical terrorism. In Textbook of Pediatric Emergency Medicine, Fleisher GR, Ludwig S, eds., 4th ed. Philadelphia: Lippincott Williams & Wilkins, 2000.
11. Cieslak T, Eitzen EM. Clinical and epidemiological principles of anthrax. Proceedings of the National Symposium on Bioterrorism, February, Emerg Infect Dis 1999:5(4), 1999.
12. Eitzen, EM Jr. Education is the key to defense against bioterrorism. Ann Emerg Med 34:221–223, 1999.
13. Cieslak T, Christopher G, Eitzen EM Jr. The "slammer": Isolation and biocontainment of patients exposed to biosafety level 4 (BSL-4) Pathogens. Abstract, Meeting of the Infectious Disease Society of America, Philadelphia, PA, November 1999.
14. White SR, Eitzen EM. Hazardous materials exposure. In Tintinalli JE et al., Stapczynski JS, Kelen GD, eds.: Emergency Medicine: A Comprehensive Study Guide, 5th ed., pp. 1201–1214. New York: McGraw-Hill, 2000.
15. Macintyre AC, Christopher GW, Eitzen EM, et al. Weapons of mass destruction events with contaminated casualties: Effective planning for healthcare facilities. JAMA 283:242–249, 2000.
16. Hawley RJ, Eitzen EM. Protection against biological warfare agents. In Disinfection, Sterilization, and Preservation, Block SS, ed. 5th ed. Philadelphia: Lippincott Williams & Wilkins, 2000.
17. Inglesby TV, Henderson DA, Bartlett JG, Ascher MS, Eitzen EM, et al. Plague as a Biological Weapon: Medical and Public Health Management. Consensus Statement of the Working Group on Civilian Biodefense. JAMA 2000; 283: 2281-2290.
18. Cieslak TJ, Christopher GW, Kortepeter MG, Rowe JR, Pavlin JA, Culpepper RC, Eitzen EM Jr. Immunization Against Potential Biological Warfare Agents. Clinical Infectious Disease 2000;30(6):843–50.
19. Cieslak TJ, Eitzen EM Jr. Bioterrorism: Agents of concern. J Public Health Manag Pract 6(4):19–29, 2000.
20. Cieslak TJ, Rowe JR, Kortepeter MG, Madsen JM, Newmark J et al. A field-expedient algorithmic approach to the clinical management of chemical and biological casualties. Mil Med 165(9):659–662, 2000.
21. Hawley RJ, Eitzen EM. Bioterrorism and biological safety. In Biological Safety: Principles and Practices, Fleming DO, Hunt DL, eds., 3rd ed. Washington, DC: ASM Press, 2000.
22. Kortepeter MG, Cieslak TJ, Eitzen EM. Bioterrorism. Special report. J Environ Health, January/February:21–24, 2001.
23. Kortepeter M, Christopher G, Cieslak T, Culpepper R, Darling R, et al. Medical Management of Biological Casualties Handbook, 4th ed. Frederick, MD: U.S. Army Medical Research Institute of Infectious Diseases, February 2001.
24. Dennis DT, Inglesby TV, Henderson DA, Bartlett JG, Ascher MS, et al. Tularemia as a biological weapon: Medical and public health management. Consensus Statement of the Working Group on Civilian Biodefense. JAMA 285:2763–2773, 2001.
25. Arnon SS, Schechter R, Inglesby TV, Henderson DA, Bartlett JG, et al. Botulinum toxin as a biological weapon: Medical and public health management. Consensus Statement of the Working Group on Civilian Biodefense. JAMA 285(8):1059–1070, 2001.
26. Franz DR, Jahrling PB, McClain DJ, Hoover DL, Byrne WR, et al. Clinical recognition and management of patients exposed to biological warfare agents. Clin Lab Med 21(3):435–473, 2001.
27. Inglesby TV, O'Toole T, Henderson DA, Bartlett JG, Ascher MS, et al. Anthrax as a biological weapon, 2002: Updated recommendations for management. Consensus Statement of the Working Group on Civilian Biodefense. JAMA 287(17):2235–2252, 2002.

28. Borio L, Inglesby T, Peters CJ, Schmaljohn AL, Hughes JM, et al. Hemorrhagic fever viruses as biological weapons: Medical and public health management. Consensus Statement of the Working Group on Civilian Biodefense. JAMA 287(18):2391–2405, 2002.
29. Darling RG, Mothershead JL, Waeckerle JF, Eitzen EM, eds. Bioterrorism. Emerg Med Clin North America, May 20(2), 2002. Eitzen E Jr. Contributor. In Henderson DA, Inglesby TV, O'Toole TO, eds. Bioterrorism: Guidelines for Medical and Public Health Management. Chicago: AMA Press, 2002.
30. Jones J, Terndrup TE, Franz DR, Eitzen EM. Future challenges in preparing for and responding to bioterrorism events. Emerg Med Clin North Am May;20(2):501–524, 2002.
31. Cieslak TJ, Eitzen EM Jr. Anthrax. In Conn's Current Therapy 2004, 56th ed., pp. 124–127, Rakel RE, Bope ET, eds. New York: Elsevier, 2004.

Weapons of Mass Destruction—Radiologic

CHAPTER 24

Jonathan Burstein, MD, and Evan Bloom, MD, MPH

1. **What is radiation?**
   Radiation is energy that comes from a source and travels through space or through some material. The radiation released from a nuclear disaster or terrorist event falls into the category of ionizing radiation, so named because it can produce charged particles (ions) in matter. Ionizing radiation is released by unstable atoms that release energy or mass in order to reach a stable state; the chemicals that release them are called "radioactive."

2. **What are the types of ionizing radiation?**
   There are four major types of ionizing radiation: alpha particles, beta particles, gamma rays, and neutrons.

3. **What are alpha particles?**
   Alpha particles are comprised of two protons and two neutrons. These particles typically only travel short distances from their emitting source and can be stopped by minimal shielding (such as a piece of paper or skin).

4. **If alpha particles are so easily stopped, why are they a danger?**
   The primary risk from this type of radiation is from internal contamination either through ingestion, inhalation, or wound contamination; in such circumstances, the heavy particles do direct damage to tissue with which they are in contact.

5. **What are beta particles?**
   Beta particles are comprised of electrons, which are much smaller and higher in energy than alpha particles. These particles can travel a moderate distance from their emitting source and can penetrate to the growth layer of the skin, causing cellular damage and tissue injury. These particles require more robust shielding material to be stopped (such as steel or thick wood).

6. **What about gamma radiation?**
   Gamma rays are comprised of photons, and act similarly to conventional X-rays. These photons carry great energy and can penetrate deeply, with the potential for a large amount of tissue and organ damage. Very dense material is required to shield against gamma rays, such as thick concrete or lead.

7. **What are neutrons?**
   Neutrons are just that, neutrons from the nucleus of an atom. These particles are also deeply penetrating and can cause significant tissue damage. Very thick lead or concrete is required for shielding from these particles.

8. **What are the types of radiation injury?**
   There are four types of radiation injury:
   (a) **Localized exposure:** This is caused by direct handling of radioactive sources. Damage is generally localized to the area of contact and systemic symptoms either do not occur or are not nearly as severe

as whole body exposure. The injury itself will appear as a burn, which is very similar to a thermal burn except that it will likely appear several days after the original exposure. Treat this burn as any other with pain control, clean dressings, and infectious precautions.

(b) Whole-body exposure (external irradiation): This occurs when the whole body is exposed to an external radiation source. The effects of that radiation are dose dependent. The first symptoms of organ or tissue injury may begin to manifest within hours from the time of exposure or may not begin for days. Generally, the higher the dose of radiation, the sooner the initial symptoms will be manifested. It is important to remember that the patient is not radioactive and that no precautions need to be taken when interacting with this person.

(c) Contamination: This involves an exposure to some form of ionizing radiation that results in particles of radioactive material being deposited on or inside the body. Therefore, this person may be carrying radioactive particles on their body or clothing in open wounds or may have ingested or inhaled radioactive materials. These people must undergo a decontamination process before interacting with those who are not contaminated.

(d) Incorporation: This situation occurs when radioactive material has been taken up by cells, tissues, or organs of the body. Contamination necessarily occurs as a precursor to incorporation.

9. **What are the basic principles of protection from ionizing radiation?**
The amount of radiation exposure an individual is subject to depends on three factors.

Time: The shorter amount of time a person is exposed to ionizing radiation, the less damage is caused by that radiation.

Distance: The farther one is from the emission source of the radiation, the less damage the radiation will cause.

Shielding: The more appropriate the shielding for the type of ion zinc radiation being emitted, the less damage that radiation will cause.

10. **What is "risk perception" and how does it apply to a radiologic incident?**
As defined by Slovic in his article on risk perception, two factors significantly increase general fear: (a) "Threat," which particularly has characteristics of being uncontrollable, potentially fatal, and with adverse outcomes that cannot be easily managed or reduced, and (b) "Observability," which encompasses a person's inability to sense exposure to a threat and the possibility of delayed effects of that threat. A nuclear disaster, or a nuclear terrorist event, encompasses both of these fear factors, greatly elevating the apprehension surrounding any form of nuclear incident. Radiation is an uncontrollable, potentially fatal threat that is essentially invisible and that has delayed effect.

11. **What types of methods may be used to carry out a moderate to large-scale nuclear or radiologic terrorist attack?**
Use of radiologic agents in a terrorist attack may fall into one of several delivery methods.

(a) Nuclear bomb: The fabrication of a nuclear weapon requires scientific expertise, procurement of highly secure nuclear materials, and great care and time taken in producing the weapon. Although the likelihood of developing a weapons-grade nuclear weapon is small, less expertise is required and material is more readily obtained to create a low-level nuclear weapon (0.01–10 kiloton explosive force).

(b) Radiologic dispersion device (RDD): This involves the use of an explosive device to disperse low-level radioactive material, likely in solid or powdered form. The area of exposure is unlikely to be large, and would depend on the energy of the conventional explosive, the geography of where the explosion occurred, and the environmental conditions at the time of the explosion. Although less likely, an RDD may also use other delivery methods such as an aerosol or spray.

(c) Radiologic exposure device (RED): This involves the clandestine placement of a nonexplosive radiation source or device that will expose those near it to radiation.

(d) Nuclear power plant or spent fuel rod storage facility attack: Although there have been many media reports discussing the possibility of a nuclear plant attack, this scenario is unlikely to occur. These facilities are well protected with both armed guards and many security checkpoints. An attack from the air is possible, but reactor cores are sealed in large concrete and steel domes that are resistant to very large forces. In fact, a 1988 test involving flying an unmanned airplane at 480 mph into a 3.6-m concrete test wall resulted in only a few centimeters of penetration into the wall. Less secured are large depositories for spent nuclear fuel cells, but considering the small amount of nuclear material that is still left in these spent cells, the risk of radiation exposure to the surrounding population is minimal. The psychologic consequences and subsequent health care system use after such an attack, however, will likely be very significant.

12. What are the aspects of a nuclear weapon detonation that may cause injury or illness?

The initial force of the nuclear detonation, the type of ionizing radiation involved, and the distance of the victim from the detonation site are the main factors in the determination of morbidity and mortality. Secondary factors that will affect subsequent injury and illness are the surrounding environment (e.g., are there tall buildings that assist with radiation containment, current weather, and wind patterns?).

13. What actions should be taken during the response to a radiologic attack/disaster?

Once the release of nuclear materials has been confirmed, immediate communication of this fact should be relayed to local and federal emergency management officials. Coordination of communication should be facilitated between local response officials and regional emergency management centers. First responders should be equipped with proper protective equipment including personal radiologic dosimeters, and as soon as is possible from local radiation readings, an estimated area of contamination should be established. Local weather patterns and wind speed/direction should be immediately assessed as this will be a major determining factor of the size and location of subsequent radioactive fallout. Staging and decontamination sites should be established out of the radioactive zones and upwind from the fallout area. The weather should be constantly monitored as staging areas may have to be moved on very short notice due to change in local atmospheric and wind direction.

14. What types of injuries are expected at the site of a nuclear attack/exposure?

Types of injury caused by a nuclear weapon detonation will depend on the size of the weapon detonated and on the proximity of the victim to the detonation location. Generally, injuries suffered immediately after the detonation of a nuclear device will be standard blast injuries and burns.

The blast wave consists of two parts: (a) a shock wave of high pressure and (b) the blast wind. The shock wave damages organs, particularly at air–fluid interfaces (tympanic membrane rupture, pulmonary trauma, intestinal rupture, etc.), and the blast wind often propels surrounding shrapnel into victims causing blunt and penetrating injuries.

Weapons of Mass Destruction—Radiologic

A moderate or large nuclear detonation will cause thermal injury due to immediate flash or flame burns as well as due to the ensuing firestorm. These injuries should be treated as would any standard burn but should be washed of any possible radioactive ash or debris to minimize radioactive contamination. Finally, radiation produced by the detonation of a nuclear weapon will cause delayed illness and injury. Radiation exposure may be immediate from primary ionizing radiation exposure at the detonation itself, but many more will be affected by subsequent radioactive fallout over a more extended period of time.

15. **How should you treat the initial victims from a nuclear attack/exposure?**

    If the patient is very ill or has a life-threatening injury, he or she should be assumed to be contaminated and should be taken to a local hospital. If time permits, all patients who are possibly contaminated should be appropriately decontaminated prior to definitive treatment. If a large number of patients exist, on-scene decontamination will likely not be possible, and less injured or uninjured patients should be removed to a location upwind of the radiation release/fallout. Decontamination staff should use universal precautions and wear gowns and gloves to appropriately dispose of all of the patient's clothing in self-contained bags. N95 masks or similar respiratory protection may prevent rescuers from ingesting or inhaling radioactive particles from victims. Victims should wash all skin surfaces to remove topical radioactive particles, particularly paying attention to higher risk areas of hair and perspiration (head, armpits, groin).

    Hospitals should be notified as soon as possible of a possible nuclear event and of the likelihood of receiving contaminated patients. Those patients with life-threatening injuries should be transported to a hospital immediately regardless of field decontamination. Those victims complaining of nausea/vomiting should be transported to a hospital for assessment of radiation exposure, but effort should be made to transport these patients to alternate facilities that are not caring for victims receiving the severely ill and victims with traumatic injuries.

16. **How should you protect yourself during a rescue response for a nuclear attack/exposure?**

    Universal precautions should be used by all health care workers. If working in the contaminated zone, the health care provider should be provided with a radiologic dosimeter to keep track of personal radiation exposure so as not to expose oneself to dangerous levels of radiation. Those in active areas of radiation/fallout should refrain from eating/drinking any possibly contaminated food or drink to avoid internal contamination.

    Initially, use of SCBA and encapsulated chemical-resistant suits may be appropriate when it is unknown whether there has been chemical/biological contamination along with the release of radioactive materials. Once it is established that there is only radioactive danger and no biologic/chemical agent release, health care responders should use gowns/disposable suits, gloves, N95 masks if available, and eye shields while decontaminating patients for their own protection.

17. **What is acute radiation syndrome (ARS) and what are its symptoms?**

    The symptoms and subsequent outcome of acute radiation syndrome and radiation sickness depend directly on the amount of ionizing radiation absorbed. ARS is the result of cell death in hematopoietic (blood cell-producing), gastrointestinal, and neurovascular tissues. ARS is generally described as having four stages:

(a) *Prodromal*—onset is minutes to days after exposure and consists of nausea, vomiting, anorexia, and possibly diarrhea.
(b) *Latent* stage—during this stage, the victim will generally feel well for hours to days.
(c) *Manifest illness*—dose-dependent, ranging from slight bone marrow depression to dehydration, electrolyte imbalance, hemorrhage, infection, cerebral edema, seizures, and death.
(d) *Recovery*– this stage includes the resolution of the acute radiation symptoms but includes delayed health effects of ionizing radiation including cancer, cataracts, growth and mental retardation, and genetic effects.

18. **What are the dose-related symptoms of radiation?**

0.05 gray(Gy)	No symptoms
0.5 Gy	Minor decreases in white blood cell counts in some people
1 Gy	Nausea/vomiting in 10% of people within 48 hours of exposure
2 Gy	Nausea/vomiting in 50% of people within 24 hours, marked decrease in white blood cell count
4 Gy	Nausea/vomiting in 90% of people within 12 hours, diarrhea in 10% within 8 hours, 50% mortality if no medical treatment
6 Gy	100% mortality within 30 days without medical treatment
10 Gy	Maximal survivable dose with best medical care available
>10–30 Gy	Nausea/vomiting in <5 minutes, likely death in 2–3 weeks
>30 Gy	Central nervous system damage, death in 24–72 hours

19. **Where should victims be taken for treatment?**
Tertiary care centers/trauma centers should be used for the seriously/critically injured, but local hospitals should have capacity for those less injured with low radiation exposure or low level thermal burns/low level trauma.

Pearls and Pitfalls

1. Removing clothing of contaminated victims eliminates approximately 90% of contamination.
2. If available, use radiation detectors that can identify what type of radioactive elements were released, as this will guide medical treatment and prophylaxis for the majority of the exposed population.
3. Accurate communication is critical. If addressing the public or media, make sure that the information you are providing is accurate, up to date, and consistent with the information being provided by emergency management leaders.
4. Patient care comes first. If a patient is seriously injured or ill, treat the patient, and equipment and vehicle decontamination can come later. There is no reason for not treating an ill patient in a timely fashion due to fear of contamination.
5. All health care providers dealing with victims of a radiologic incident should take appropriate precautions (use universal precautions, take potassium iodide pills in the event of an iodine[131] release, check your personal dosimeter frequently to accurately monitor the cumulative radiation exposure).

References

1. Slovic P. Perception of risk. Science 236:280–285, 1987.
2. Barnett DJ, Parker CL, Blodgett DW, et al. Understanding radiologic and nuclear terrorism as public health threats: Preparedness and response perspectives. J Nucl Med 47:1653–1661, 2006.
3. Mettler F, Voelz G. Major radiation exposure—What to expect and how to respond. N Engl J Med 346:1554–1561, 2002.
4. Chapin DM, Cohen KP, Davis WK, et al. Nuclear power plants and their fuel as terrorist targets. Science 397:1997–1999, 2002.
5. Depalma RG, Burris DG, Champion HR, et al. Blast injuries. N Engl J Med 352:1335–1342, 2005.
6. Gusev I, Guskova AK, Mettler FA Jr, eds. Medical Management of Radiation Accidents, 2nd ed. Boca Raton, FL: CRC Press, 2001.
7. Schleipman AR, Gerbaudo VH, Castronovo FP Jr. Radiation disaster response: Preparation and simulation experience at an academic medical center. J Nucl Med Technol Mar 32(1):22–27, 2004.

Weapons of Mass Destruction—Explosives

Stephen J. Wolf, MD

CHAPTER 25

1. **What are common sources of blast injury?**
   - Industrial accidents
   - Utility accidents
   - Military explosions
   - Terrorist explosions
   - Fireworks
   - Land mines

2. **Name the two classes of explosives and give examples.**
   - Low-order explosives (e.g., petroleum and gunpowders)
   - High-order explosives (e.g., nitroglycerin, dynamite, plastic (C-4), ammonium nitrate/fuel oil (ANFO), trinitrotoluene (TNT))

3. **Describe the difference between low- and high-order explosives.**
   High-order explosives generate a supersonic blast overpressure wave, whereas low-order ones generate a subsonic pressure wave. High-order explosives are much more likely to cause injury due to the blast pressure wave itself that low-order explosives cannot produce.

4. **What are IEDs?**
   Improvised explosive devices (IEDs), as opposed to military manufactured devices, are devices that are "homemade" or used outside of their intended purpose to cause harm and destruction.

5. **What is done to increase the damage and lethality of IEDs?**
   IEDs are often combined with nails or other solid objects to generate a greater shrapnel effect. Additionally, they can be laced with chemicals or radioactive materials to contaminate the scene.

6. **What are the four types of blast injury? Describe them.**
   - Primary blast injury occurs as a direct result of the blast overpressure wave damaging tissue in the body.
   - Secondary blast injury occurs as a result of objects, either shrapnel or environmental, being thrown by the blast overpressure wave or blast winds into the victim. These injuries may result in penetrating or blunt forces and are managed as such.
   - Tertiary blast injury occurs as a result of the victim being thrown by the blast overpressure wave or blast winds into an object relatively fixed in space. These injuries are typically blunt but may be either penetrating or blunt forces, and are managed as such.
   - Miscellaneous or quaternary blast injury occurs as a result of the explosion and are not otherwise categorized as primary, secondary, or tertiary blast injury.

7. **What are the main types of miscellaneous blast injury?**
   - Thermal injury
   - Smoke inhalation injury
   - Toxic inhalant injury (carbon monoxide and cyanide poisoning)
   - Chemical exposures
   - Radiation injury

8. **What is a blast overpressure wave?**
   A blast overpressure wave is the pressure wave generated by the rapid exothermic conversion of a liquid or solid explosive material to a gas. This pressure wave spreads out radially from the point of explosion and is responsible for primary blast injuries, usually involving air-filled structures such as ears, lungs, and bowel.

9. **What are blast winds?**
   Following an explosion, the blast overpressure wave displaces environmental gases, causing high-speed blast winds away from the point of explosion. These winds can reach upward of 1000 mph and contribute to blast-related injuries.

10. **What are important scene safety concerns following an explosion?**
    - Responders must always consider the possibility of secondary devices placed in proximity to the scene and timed to detonate shortly after arrival of police, fire, and EMS personnel.
    - As responders approach the scene, consideration must be given to the possibility of an additive to the bomb such as a chemical agent or a radioactive material to create a "dirty" bomb.
    - After an explosion, the structural stability of any involved building must be evaluated for the potential for building collapse.
    - High particulate environments pose a risk of inhalation injury to unsuspecting responders who have failed to don appropriate personal protective equipment for the event.

11. **What are important scene legal concerns following an explosion?**
    The whole scene is a crime scene and should be managed as such. Care should be taken to preserve any evidence that may remain on the scene and when treating victims of the explosion.

12. **What is unique about primary blast injury with respect to the other form of blast injury?**
    In primary blast injury, the mechanism of injury is such that it often causes injuries that are not outwardly obvious to the prehospital provider, making them easy to overlook. As mentioned previously, these typically involve the lungs, tympanic membranes, and bowel.

13. **What are the mechanistic forces of primary blast injury?**
    - Shearing forces
    - Implosion–explosion forces
    - Spalling forces

14. **Describe shearing forces.**
    As the energy from a blast overpressure wave is transferred to tissue, it causes the tissue to move based on its density and internal fixation. Less-dense, less-fixed tissues will move to a greater extent than

higher density, more-fixed tissues. When these tissues juxtapose each other, structures that bridge or connect the tissues are damaged by the tethering structures.

15. **Which tissues are susceptible to shearing forces?**
    - Cerebral tissue—at the gray–white junction, resulting in diffuse axonal injury
    - Pulmonary tissues—where vascular, bronchial, and lung parenchymal structures are in close connection, resulting in bronchial vascular fistulas
    - Gastrointestinal tissues—where vascular, mesenteric, and enteric structures are at risk for tearing

16. **Describe implosion-explosion forces.**
    As the blast overpressure wave passes through an air-filled structure, the contained air becomes extremely compressed. Subsequently as the pressure wave passes by, the air expands significantly to occupy a much greater volume. This rapid (<10 msec) flux generates great stress on the walls of the air-filled cavity and may result in damage or perforation of the cavity's walls.

17. **Which structures are susceptible to implosion–explosion forces?**
    Mainly the gas-containing structures of the body, such as
    (a) Auditory structures—where the tympanic membranes (TM) can perforate as a result of the air-filled middle ear
    (b) Pulmonary—where the alveolar–capillary junction can be disrupted, resulting in pulmonary edema and parenchymal contusion
    (c) Gastrointestinal structures—where perforation and bowel wall injury can occur

18. **Describe spalling forces.**
    As the blast overpressure wave passes from a higher density media/tissue to a lower density tissue/media, the pressure wave reverberates at the interface causing fragmentation of the higher density media into the lower density media, resulting in tissue damage.

19. **Which structures are susceptible to spalling forces?**
    Anywhere varying tissue densities juxtapose, spalling forces can cause tearing of the tissue surfaces (central nervous system, pulmonary, gastrointestinal, etc.).

20. **At what peak blast overpressures above ambient air pressure (15 psi or 1 atm) is a body structure or victim at risk for primary blast injury?**
    - 2–5 psi: TM perforation
    - 10–15 psi: Pulmonary injury
    - 15–20 psi: Gastrointestinal injury
    - 50 psi–Lethal dose: LD_{50} (50% of victims die)
    - 99 psi – LD_{99} (99% of victims die)

21. **What factors are related to peak blast overpressure experienced by the victim?**
    - Explosive type—high-order explosives will create larger blast overpressures
    - Explosive size—a bigger explosive charge will create larger blast overpressures

- Distance from explosion—the closer a victim is to the explosion, the greater the blast overpressure experienced by the victim
- Conducting media of the pressure wave—underwater explosions generate higher pressures
- Reflecting surfaces in proximity to victim—a reflecting surface will increase the blast overpressure experienced by the victim up to a factor of nine times the original force
- Closed- vs. open-space explosions—contained explosions in a bus or room generate higher pressures within that space than do open-space explosions

22. Is a ruptured TM a marker of occult or impending pulmonary blast injury?

No. Although TMs rupture at a much lower psi, studies have demonstrated that this finding is not predictive of occult or impending pulmonary blast injury. Patients with evidence of blast lung may not have ruptured TMs and vice versa.

23. What percent of patients with blast injury have significant eye injuries?
- 10%

24. What are the clinical concerns of primary blast injury involving the lungs?
- Blast lung
- Vascular air embolism

25. What is blast lung?

Blast lung is a form of acute lung injury that results from the blast overpressure causing damage to the alveolar–capillary membrane and lung parenchyma. The end result is capillary leak with pulmonary edema and hemorrhage resulting in hypoxia and tissue damage.

26. What is the classic triad of clinical findings in blast lung?

1. Apnea
2. Bradycardia
3. Hypotension

27. Over what time frame does blast lung develop?

It often develops immediately following the blast injury, but may be delayed up to 48 hours from the explosion. As such, all patients exposed to a significant overpressure must be carefully screened for respiratory complaints and observed for at least 4-6 hours to assure that injury does not develop.

28. Discuss the significance of air emboli.

Air emboli result from bronchial–vascular fistulas. On a macroscopic level, air emboli can cause ischemia and dysfunction to almost any organ (brain, retina, cardiac, extremities, bowel) resulting in mental status or neurologic changes, visual disturbances, or vague cardiopulmonary and abdominal complaints. When air emboli are massive, they result in overt cerebrovascular, spinal, myocardial, or mesenteric ischemia syndromes.

29. How can the risk of air emboli be minimized in a person at risk for pulmonary blast injury?

When possible, avoid positive-pressure ventilation, which can worsen bronchial–vascular fistulas. If positive-pressure ventilation is required, it should be performed with 100% oxygen that is rapidly absorbed by surrounding tissues. Embolism of this gas is much less damaging than air, which contains 80% nitrogen or lower concentrations of oxygen. Delaying nonemergent surgeries for roughly 48 hours, when possible, may also help reduce the incidence of acute air emboli.

30. **What are unique concerns with respect to gastrointestinal injury from primary blast injury?**

    Gastrointestinal injury may present acutely due to the perforation of a hollow viscus but may also be delayed as much as 12–24 hours. In delayed cases, the perforations may be small and thus require time for inflammation to develop and generate symptoms. Alternatively, vascular injury, serosal hematomas, or mesenteric injury may result from focal bowel wall ischemia with delayed perforation.

31. **What time frame of observation is required to exclude gastrointestinal injury?**

    Patients with any complaints (abdominal cramping, nausea, or vomiting) must be evaluated for more severe injury. Patients with a significant blast pressure exposure must be closely observed for the development of delayed symptoms for 4–6 hours.

32. **What is the field treatment of a victim of blast injury?**

    Patients with obvious findings of blunt or penetrating injury should be treated as per standard trauma protocols. Patients with minimal or no signs of external injury are a greater challenge, as occult injuries and delayed onset of symptoms are not unusual. All such victims should be transported to the hospital for further evaluation and observation. Oxygen saturation should be maintained above 90% using supplemental oxygen as necessary. Patients must be closely observed for the early signs of blast lung including increasing tachypnea and decreasing oxygen saturation as well as for any signs of air embolism.

Pearls and Pitfalls

1. Prehospital scene safety is paramount following an explosion and should take priority.
2. Intact TMs following exposure to a significant blast overpressure wave do not exclude the possibility of pulmonary or gastrointestinal injury.
3. Primary blast injuries are often hidden injuries as external signs of trauma can be absent.
4. Secondary and tertiary blast injuries can usually be treated in a similar fashion to other blunt and penetrating injuries.
5. Following exposures to a significant blast overpressure wave, patients with no or trivial pulmonary or gastrointestinal complaints still must be observed for delayed presentations of primary blast injury.

References

1. Alfici R, Ashkenazi I, Kessel B. Management of victims in a mass casualty incident caused by a terrorist bombing: treatment algorithms for stable, unstable, and in extremis victims. Mil Med 171:1155–1162, 2006.
2. CDC. Explosions and blast injuries: A primer for clinicians. http://www.bt.cdc.gov/masscasualties/pdf/explosions-blast-injuries.pdf. Accessed 5/1/2011.
3. DePalma RG, Burris DG, Champion HR, et al. Blast injuries. N Engl J Med 352:1335–1342, 2005.

4. Gans L, Kennedy T. Management of unique clinical entities in disaster medicine. Emerg Med Clin North Am May;14(2):301–326, 1996.
5. Lavonis E, Pennardt A. Blast injuries. http://www.emedicine.com/emerg/topic63.htm. Accessed 5/1/2011.
6. Leibovici D, Gofrit ON, Shapira SC. Eardrum perforation in explosion survivors: Is it a marker of pulmonary blast injury? Ann Emerg Med 34:168–172, 1999.
7. Phillips YY. Primary blast injuries. Ann Emerg Med Dec; 106(15):1446–1450, 1986.
8. Wightman JM, Gladish SL. Explosions and blast injuries. Ann Emerg Med June; 37(6):664–678, 2001.
9. Wolf SJ, Bebarta VS, Bonnett CJ, et al. Blast injuries. Lancet 375:406–415, 2009.

Mass Gatherings

CHAPTER 26

Jedd Roe, MD, MBA, FACEP

1. **What is a mass gathering?**
   One dictionary defines a mass as a "large body of persons in a compact group" and a gathering as an "assembly or meeting." Those involved in the planning of prehospital care generally consider any event that involves at least 1000 persons to be a mass gathering.

2. **Why should medical care be provided at mass gatherings?**
   Most mass gatherings will involve substantially more than 1000 participants. For example, large sports stadiums generally hold at least 70,000 occupants. Thus, for several hours, the population of many small- to medium-sized cities can be found in a relatively small area. With a population base of this magnitude, a significant number of medical events are likely to occur. Most medical complaints involve only first aid, but it is important to be prepared to deal with the truly emergent problems that might occur, from cardiac arrests and childbirth to true mass casualty situations. In addition, if medical care is not provided on site, the local emergency medical services (EMS) system will be called for every medical complaint. This could easily overburden the EMS system and seriously impair its ability to meet its routine responsibilities.

3. **What is the framework for providing care at a mass gathering?**
   Essentially, one must create a microcosm of an EMS system. Each component of the system, including communications, personnel, medical equipment and supplies, onsite response, medical direction, and transport capability, will be required in order to provide care at a mass gathering.

4. **Do physicians need to be involved?**
   A strong case can be made for direct physician involvement on-site at mass gatherings. First, most of the published research on the medical care provided at mass gatherings has been done by physicians who have designed and implemented plans for such events. Although most of the medical care can and will be provided by paramedics or nurses, the emergency physician's greater medical expertise is occasionally required. Perhaps more importantly, the physician can accept the responsibility for treating and releasing patients who might otherwise require transport when common prehospital protocols are followed. Reducing the number of transported patients results in decreased costs of care and greater satisfaction for patients and event organizers.

5. **Where should planning begin?**
   Usually, the event organizer is contacted first to ascertain his or her expectations for the medical care that may be required. Those planning for the medical care should share the results of their prior experiences and those published in the literature for similar events to be sure that the expectations of the event organizers are reasonable. Financial issues regarding the cost of the medical care need to be addressed. Many for-profit events have funds budgeted for emergency care, and even if volunteer personnel are to be used, supplies may need to be purchased or donations solicited. Perhaps the most important issue to clarify is who will be in overall charge of all medical care. This is particularly important

for events that will use personnel from different agencies or volunteer groups. Many bands, sports teams, or speakers may have their own medical personnel with them. Determine the level of responsibility that you will assume for their care activities and how to meet other requirements they may have, such as transport.

6. **What other agencies or organizations are likely to be involved?**
For any large gathering, local police and possibly fire departments generally will be involved. Events may have their own security details or customer service representatives. Education of, and liaison with, each of these groups will enhance the ability of event participants to access medical care. Interagency communication may be facilitated by the use of a command post, usually containing a representative of each participating agency, for event coordination. In the case of events involving a head of state or other security concerns, agencies such as the U.S. Secret Service may be involved. Joint planning is especially important in such instances so that medical personnel receive appropriate clearances and care can be provided under the auspices of these special security concerns.

7. **How does the physical site of the mass gathering influence the planning for medical care?**
Planners must become familiar with the site in detail. Where will the concentrations of people be, and what are the points of access? This will aid in determining the required number and location of first aid stations. Plan for the ingress and egress of ambulances to the first aid room(s). What are the barriers to EMS response to event participants or access to first aid rooms? Determine where your responsibility for medical care ends and where those of the local EMS system begins. For instance, whose responsibility is the event participant who has collapsed in a distant parking lot? Arrange for public service announcements or signs that clearly identify the location of first aid rooms and how the public can access medical care.

8. **Is a first aid room necessary?**
Yes, at least one. First aid rooms serve as a central treatment facility and source of supplies and operations. They should be clearly identified and easily visible and accessible to the public. Cots or beds should be present so patients may lie down and, ideally, should allow for privacy from walk-in traffic. An EMS provider should always be in attendance at the first aid room—to be present for walk-in patients and prevent unauthorized use of supplies and equipment. If several first aid rooms are being used, it may be helpful to designate the largest room with best access to ambulance transport as the main first aid room where most of the supplies may be stored and seriously ill patients may be attended to while awaiting transport.

9. **Are outdoor events handled differently than indoor events?**
Yes. Outdoor events allow for exposure to the elements and may have additional special requirements. The largest environmental factor is usually temperature. Although hypothermia can be a concern for events held in cold temperatures, mass gatherings held in warm climates generally produce larger numbers of patients who experience dehydration and heat exhaustion. Sites near large bodies of water may require water rescue capabilities. Most indoor events are climate controlled and involve seated participants, thus decreasing the potential for medical problems.

10. **Are treat and release strategies effective?**
Yes, typically this policy is used where relatively simple medical problems are anticipated and very large attendances are anticipated. Because more minor cases are taken care of at the point of contact, event

resources at central treatment stations will then be kept available for more seriously ill or injured parties. This can involve the dispensing of simple pharmaceuticals such as acetaminophen or diphenhydramine using predetermined medical protocols. In times of need, other approaches can provide alternatives to traditional protocols such as for the rehydration of heat exhaustion victims at first aid stations. For instance, in the setting of typical heat exhaustion complaints and positive orthostatic vital signs, paramedic treatment teams can administer intravenous fluid and release those patients who respond appropriately.

11. **Can the estimated attendance at a mass gathering be used to help determine staffing levels?**
Generally, yes. While there have been a number of published recommendations, there is some consensus to provide one physician per 40,000–50,000 people and one emergency medical technician-paramedic or one nurse for every 10,000 people. Ideally, if a similar event has been held at a similar venue, one should have good data on which to base future planning. If this information is not available, other event characteristics become important in determining staffing levels.

12. **What other characteristics of a mass gathering are important?**
The type of event has been shown to influence the volume and categories of medical problems. For instance, one is likely to see more patients with sequelae of alcohol and drug use at rock concerts than at classical music concerts. The risk of violence or trauma varies greatly among events and rises dramatically at auto racing events or public demonstrations. Reported rates of medical encounters have varied from 16 per 10,000 people at the 1994 Los Angeles Summer Olympics to 185 per 10,000 people at the 1991 Super Bowl in Tampa, Florida.

The age of attendees may be an important factor. More significant medical problems could be anticipated from an older population. The environment and duration of an event can also be a potent factor. For instance, in sports and concert related events in Cleveland, Ohio, in 2003, critical diagnoses (e.g., cardiac arrest, chest pain, syncope, trauma, and dyspnea) occurred more frequently with football events than for baseball or arena venues. EMS transfer occurred most often for alcohol-related complaints at football games, whereas baseball transfers most often happened for injuries.

At one stadium, on a hot August day with a 12-hour rock concert, 10 times the number of patients were contacted than during an average 5-hour National Football League game at the same stadium. Severity of illness also increased, as evidenced by a similar rise in the number of patients requiring transport to a hospital. Rock concerts also can provide a wide diversity of medical problems that vary according to genre and scale. For instance, drug use among attendees can vary based on headliner, and concerts involving a physical form of dancing called "moshing" showed a traumatic injury rate 13 times higher than nonmosh events.

13. **How much medical capability is needed at a site?**
Although most medical problems will be minor, such as requests for first aid or acetaminophen, most authorities agree that preparations should be made for personnel and equipment to deal with life-threatening problems such as cardiac arrest, respiratory complaints, and traumatic injuries. At a minimum, if advanced life support is not available, automated external defibrillators and emergency medical technicians trained in their use should be present.

14. Are automated external defibrillators (AEDs) useful in these settings?

Yes. A large, prospective trial that used trained nonparamedic volunteers in high-risk areas such as shopping malls and apartment complexes demonstrated that trained laypeople can use AEDs in these settings. More importantly, those victims of out-of-hospital cardiac arrest in the cardiopulmonary resuscitation and AED group had a much higher rate of survival to hospital discharge. Motyka and colleagues describe a method for determining the number of AEDs in a stadium or arena setting that is based on translating predicted response times into distance and using those values to calculate the number of AEDs that a site requires (clearly, such a calculation is a starting point for an answer that will be influenced by the event factors already discussed).

15. Functionally, how would a medical response take place at a mass gathering?

First, preestablished lines of communication are paramount. An EMS representative in the command post might be notified of an incident by a security representative. Although it is helpful for the EMS representative to have radio contact with the local EMS system, medical operations should be conducted on a separate frequency or talk group (800 MHz). A paramedic is notified by radio and could respond by electric cart or on foot. Many systems have implemented responding by bicycle. In Denver, paramedics on mountain bicycles have achieved a 50% reduction in response time at many mass gatherings. Depending on severity of illness, a patient may be transported to the first aid room by wheelchair, stretcher, or electric cart for observation and therapy. Hospitals can be notified by radio of impending patient arrival, but telephone communication often improves the quality of communication.

16. Does every patient contact need to be documented?

Yes. For minor first aid and analgesic requests, one may elect to merely record demographic data (time, name, age), chief complaint, treatment, and disposition. Any complaint of greater severity requires the usual complete documentation required of an EMS response or emergency department visit. Compulsiveness in this area allows for greater medicolegal protection and data gathering for future planning and quality improvement.

17. Besides the typical events, do any other special situations warrant this sort of planning?

Most major airports should be considered in the same context as a mass gathering. They tend to be distant from major metropolitan areas, up to 23 million passengers may pass through annually, and as many as 15,000 employees may be on site. Yearly call volumes have ranged from 800 to 6000. Some airports staff on-site medical clinics with physicians and nurses, and others provide paramedic first response and first aid rooms. An independent system of providing on-site medical care should be established that conforms to Federal Aviation Administration regulations. Depending on the distance to a hospital, helicopter transport may be necessary for severely ill or injured patients.

18. What's the worst-case scenario?

Each mass gathering is a mass casualty event waiting to happen. The local EMS disaster plan can be initiated in such circumstances, but each mass gathering has a specific set of logistics that can be anticipated and analyzed beforehand. Fixed sites, such as stadiums, can have site-specific disaster plans, which can be tested by the use of tabletop and full-scale exercises.

Pearls and Pitfalls

1. For an average event, you will need one paramedic for every 10,000 of estimated attendance.
2. All events are not created equal; consider the type and anticipated age of attendees.
3. Create a disaster plan specific to each mass gathering site.
4. Plan for AEDs at mass gathering sites. Trained laypeople with AEDs can leverage traditional ALS coverage over a larger area.
5. Always take environmental conditions into account when planning for and covering a mass gathering.
6. You can easily be overwhelmed by patients with low-acuity illnesses or injuries.
7. Treat-and-release strategies are essential to avoid overwhelming local EMS with transports.

References

1. Cwinn AA, Dinerman N, Pons PT, et al. Prehospital care at a major international airport. Ann Emerg Med 17:1042–1048, 1988.
2. Erickson TB, Aks SE, Koenigsberg M, et al. Drug use patterns at major rock concert events. Ann Emerg Med 28:22–26, 1996.
3. Feldman MJ, Lukins JL, Verbeek PR, et al. Use of treat-and-release medical directives for paramedics at a mass gathering. Prehosp Emerg Care 9:213–217, 2005.
4. Grange JT, Green SM, Downs W. Concert medicine: Spectrum of medical problems encountered at 405 major concerts. Acad Emerg Med 6:202–207, 1999.
5. Hallstrom AL, Ornato JP, Weisfeldt M, et al. Public-access defibrillation and survival after out-of-hospital cardiac arrest. N Eng J Med 351:637–646, 2004.
6. Janchar T, Milzman D, Hill J, et al. Mosh-concert-related injuries vs standard concert seating (abstract). Ann Emerg Med 48:S76–S77, 2006.
7. Leonard RB. Medical support for mass gatherings. Emerg Med Clin North Am 14:383–397, 1996.
8. Motyka TM, Winslow JE, Newton K, et al. Method for determining automatic external defibrillator need at mass gatherings. Resuscitation 65:309–314, 2005.
9. Parrillo SJ. Medical care at mass gatherings: Considerations for physician involvement. Prehosp Disaster Med 10:273–275, 1995.
10. Paul HM. Mass casualty: Pope's Denver visit causes Mega MCI. J Emerg Med Serv 18(11):64–75, 1993.
11. Sanders AB, Criss E, Steckl P, et al. An analysis of medical care at mass gatherings. Ann Emerg Med 15:515–519, 1986.
12. Tallman TA, Peacock WF IV, Telban DJ, et al. Spectator risk at professional sporting events: An analysis of the Cleveland Clinic Event Medicine Program (abstract). Ann Emerg Med 46:S114, 2005.

Clinical Care

SECTION V

Chapter 27
Decision Making and Critical Interpretation of Vital Signs 193
Vince Markovchick, MD

Chapter 28
The Prehospital Patient Assessment 198
Arthur Hsieh, MA, NREMT-P

Chapter 29
Electrocardiogram Interpretation 203
Angel Burba, MS, NREMT-P, NCEC

Chapter 30
Cardiac Dysrhythmias 218
Paul Davidson, MD

Chapter 31
Cardiac Arrest 228
Jason Haukoos, MD, MSc

Chapter 32
Overview of Shock 234
Robert McNamara, MD, FAAEM

Chapter 33
Chest Pain 239
Christopher B. Colwell, MD, FACEP

Chapter 34
Acute Coronary Syndrome 245
Jeffrey J. Messerole, PS

Chapter 35
Altered Mental Status 257
Mike Stackpool, MD

Chapter 36
Acute Neurologic Emergencies 267
Julie Scadden, NREMT-P, PS

Chapter 37
Hypertensive Emergencies 273
James A. Temple, BA, NREMT-P, CCP and Christopher B. Colwell, MD, FACEP

Chapter 38
Seizures 278
Julie Scadden, NREMT-P, PS

Chapter 39
Fever 283
Cheryl Blazek, BS, EMT-P

Chapter 40
Abdominal Pain 287
Christina Johnson, MD, FACEP

Chapter 41
Gastrointestinal Hemorrhage 293
Mike Stackpool, MD

Chapter 42
Vomiting and Diarrhea 297
Cheryl Blazek, BS, EMT-P

Chapter 43
Dyspnea 300
Gregory J. Chapman, BS, RRT, REMT-P

Chapter 44
Extremity Pain and Trauma 304
Julie Scadden, NREMT-P, PS

Chapter 45
Overdose and Poisoning — 309
Kennon Heard, MD, and Vikhyat Bebarta, MD

Chapter 46
Hypothermia and Frostbite — 316
Daniel F. Danzl, MD

Chapter 47
Heat Illness — 322
Stephen V. Cantrill, MD

Chapter 48
Altitude Illness — 326
Ben Honigman, MD, and Kelly Bookman, MD

Chapter 49
Obstetric and Gynecologic Emergencies — 330
Cheryl Blazek, BS, EMT-P

Chapter 50
Allergy and Anaphylaxis — 335
Lance W. Jobe, MD, FACEP

Chapter 51
Diabetic Emergencies — 341
Jeffrey J. Messerole, PS

Chapter 52
Psychiatric and Behavioral Emergencies — 350
Eugene E. Kercher, MD, LFACEP, LFAPA, and Christopher E. Dong, MD

Chapter 53
Management of the Violent Patient — 361
James A. Temple, BA, NREMT-P, CCP

Chapter 54
General Trauma Principles — 367
Larry Mottley, MD

Chapter 55
Head Trauma — 373
Will Chapleau, EMT-P, RN, TNS

Chapter 56
Spinal Cord Injuries — 377
Will Chapleau, EMT-P, RN, TNS

Chapter 57
Neck Trauma — 382
Nicholas C. Johnson, MD

Chapter 58
Thoracic Trauma — 386
Jeffrey P. Salomone, MD, and Joseph A. Salomone, MD

Chapter 59
Abdominal Trauma — 390
Kelly Bookman, MD, and Lawrence Bookman, DO, FACEP

Chapter 60
Pelvic Trauma — 394
Jeffrey P. Salomone, MD, and Matthew Bitner, MD

Chapter 61
Interpersonal Violence — 397
Debra Houry, MD, MPH

Chapter 62
Thermal Burns — 402
Jeffrey S. Guy, MD, MSc, MMHC

Decision Making and Critical Interpretation of Vital Signs

CHAPTER 27

Vince Markovchick, MD

1. **Why is knowledge of vital signs important?**
   The accurate taking of, and critical interpretation of, vital signs is paramount in determining patient status and triage. If accurately taken and critically interpreted, they, when combined with a chief complaint, will help to identify the vast majority of life-threatened patients.

2. **What are vital signs?**
   Besides being the measurements of heart rate, blood pressure, respiratory rate, and temperature, vital signs are the patient's declaration of bodily function during or after insult or illness. Remember that *vital* means "contributing to, or essential for life." Vital signs alone can often determine the patient's clinical stability with or without a complete history, mechanism of injury, or the patient's own verbalization of a chief complaint.

3. **How is a patient's temperature taken in the field without a thermometer?**
   An accurate temperature cannot be determined without a thermometer. However, touching the patient will determine if they have a high fever or significant hypothermia.

4. **Why should mental status be discussed in a chapter on vital signs?**
   Mental status is a very sensitive indicator of cerebral perfusion and oxygenation. Mental status changes should serve as a red flag to the prehospital provider. Once any changes are noted, the provider should rapidly determine the cause of this alteration (see Chapter 35, Altered Mental Status).

5. **What are some of the mental status changes to look for?**
   Confusion, agitation, and decreased level of consciousness or unconsciousness.

6. **What factors affect "normal" vital signs?**
   Age—very young or elderly
   Physical conditioning
   Medications—sympathomimetics, beta blockers, calcium channel blockers, over-the-counter medicine
   Pregnancy

7. **How does age influence normal vital signs?**

Weight and Vital Signs by Age Group

Age	Weight	Respirations Breaths/min	Pulse Beats/min	Systolic Blood Pressure (mmHg)
Newborn	3–4 kg (6–9 lb)	30–50	120–160	60–80
6 mo–1yr	8–10 kg (16–22 lb)	30–40	120–140	70–80
2–4 yr	12–16 kg (24–34 lb)	20–30	100–110	80–95

(Continued)

Weight and Vital Signs by Age Group *(Continued)*

Age	Weight	Respirations Breaths/min	Pulse Beats/min	Systolic Blood Pressure (mmHg)
5–8 yr	18–26 kg (36–55 lb)	14–20	90–100	90–100
8–12 yr	26–50 kg (55–110 lb)	12–20	80–100	100–110
>12 yr	>50 kg (110)	12–20	60–90	100–120
Adult		12–20	60–100	120

8. **Are there any age-specific things I need to know about vital signs?**
   Yes. Children have a greater cardiac reserve than adults and are less likely to exhibit hypotension than adults with the same percentage of intravascular volume loss. On the other end of the age spectrum, the expected physiologic response manifested by abnormal vital signs such as tachycardia or fever may not occur. Therefore, "normal" vital signs in the elderly do not rule out an immediate life threat.

9. **What is the differential diagnosis of hypotension?**
   Shock—hypovolemia, cardiogenic, septic, neurogenic (spinal cord injury, anaphylaxis)
   Hypothermia

10. **Why is it important to touch the skin of a hypotensive patient?**
    Because feeling the skin of a hypotensive patient can help provide clues as to the type of shock the patient is experiencing. If the skin is cool and moist or diaphoretic, the patient is in cardiogenic or hypovolemic shock. Warm and dry skin is associated with neurogenic, septic, or anaphylactic shock.

11. **What is the differential diagnosis of hypertension?**
    Increased intracranial pressure
    Drug induced—cocaine or amphetamines
    Aortic dissection
    Eclampsia/preeclampsia
    Chronic essential hypertension

12. **What is the differential diagnosis of tachycardia?**
    Shock
    Hyperthermia—environmental or infection
    Cardiac—supraventricular tachycardia, ventricular tachycardia, or rapid atrial fibrillation
    Hyperthyroidism
    Pain
    Anxiety
    Medications/drugs of abuse—sympathomimetics, antihistamines, or anticholinergics

13. **What is the differential diagnosis of bradycardia?**
    Decompensated shock
    Heart block
    Hypothermia
    Cushing's reflex (increased intracranial pressure)
    Increased vagal tone

Medication overdose—beta blockers
Hypothyroidism
Excellent physical condition

14. What is the differential diagnosis of tachypnea?
Hypoxia
Metabolic acidosis
Hyperthermia
Hyperthyroidism
Drug overdose—cocaine or amphetamines
Pain
Anxiety

15. What is the differential diagnosis of bradypnea?
CNS depression—narcotics/sedative hypnotics/ethanol, increased intracranial pressure
Respiratory failure
Hypothermia

16. How do medications affect vital signs?
Many medications, such as antihypertensives, beta blockers, calcium channel blockers, and antidysrhythmics, may inhibit normal physiologic responses. For example, a patient in hypovolemic shock on beta blockers may not be able to manifest a compensatory tachycardia. It is important that the provider understands the mechanism of action of prescription medications and the potential effect they will have on the patient's vital signs.

17. What should I consider about nonprescription medications and recreational drugs in relation to vital signs?
Over-the-counter medications may blunt a fever (aspirin, ibuprofen and acetaminophen) or cause a tachycardia (antihistamines and pseudoephedrine). Sympathomimetics such as cocaine and amphetamines will cause tachycardia and hypertension.

18. What are "orthostatic" vital signs and how do I obtain them?
Orthostatic vital signs compare blood pressure and pulse in the supine position to the seated or standing position and are used to assess for the presence of hypovolemia. A blood pressure and pulse are measured with the patient in the supine position and a repeat blood pressure and pulse are again obtained immediately upon assuming the seated or standing position. If the patient develops symptoms of near syncope or has a decrease in systolic blood pressure >10 or more and an increase in pulse of >10, the orthostatic vital signs are usually considered positive.

19. When are orthostatic vital signs contraindicated?
Orthostatic vital signs should NOT be taken if the patient has a low blood pressure or elevated heart rate while supine or the patient complained of feeling dizzy or faint while standing, as these abnormalities are already telling you the patient is hypovolemic and in shock.

20. When should vital signs be performed in the physical exam?
As soon as possible after the status of the airway is assessed, as they are part of the breathing and overall condition assessment. However, vital sign acquisition should not take precedence over critical intervention skills such as airway management and O_2 administration.

Clinical Care

21. **What is the fifth vital sign and when should I obtain it?**
    Most, if not all, EMTs now have the capability to measure O_2 saturation via pulse oximetry. O_2 saturation should be determined in any patient who displays abnormal vital signs, appears seriously ill or injured, has respiratory complaints or appears dyspneic. Pulse oximetry should be obtained whenever intubation or active airway intervention is considered, as it is an invaluable aid in making this decision. It should be continuously monitored en route to the emergency department.

22. **How do I interpret O_2 sat readings?**
    The interpretation of "normal" must be adjusted for altitude. For example, at sea level a normal O_2 sat is 98–100%, at 5000 ft. O_2 sat is 95%, and at 8000 ft. O_2 sat is 87%.

23. **What can cause false pulse oximetry readings?**
    Carbon monoxide poisoning will cause a falsely elevated O_2 sat, whereas hypovolemic shock and vasoconstriction will result in a falsely decreased reading.

24. **What other considerations are important?**
    Vital signs are a matter of interpretation. If the findings are questionable, they should be repeated immediately; if they are abnormal, they should be repeated as soon as possible. Abnormal blood pressures should be confirmed by taking blood pressure in the opposite arm.

25. **When are "normal" vital signs abnormal?**
    When the patient is beyond the stage of compensation for his or her illness or injury, for example, a blunt trauma patient with intraabdominal hemorrhage who is no longer tachycardic or the acute asthmatic that no longer presents tachypneic and now has a "normal" respiratory rate. This period represents a time of imminent precipitous decompensation to the patient. The prehospital provider must recognize the patient at risk and intervene immediately and aggressively.

26. **What effect does improper sphygmomanometer cuff size have on blood pressure readings?**
    If the cuff is too small it will give a falsely elevated reading and if it is too large it will give a falsely low reading. Therefore, be sure to properly size the cuff used to measure blood pressure to the size of the patient.

27. **Are there any absolute "don'ts" concerning vital signs?**
    Don't ever estimate vital signs. The acquisition of vital signs is a simple act that requires little time. The importance of an accurate set of vital signs must not be underestimated. There are no excuses for not taking accurate and complete vital signs.

28. **What is the key question to ask when formulating a differential diagnosis?**
    What is the most serious possible cause of this patient's presenting signs and symptoms? If this question is not posed for every patient encounter, then potential life threats will be overlooked and proper measures to stabilize and treat the patient will not be carried out.

29. **How do I approach a patient with a chronic recurrent complaint?**
    Ask "is there anything different now about your complaint (e.g., headache, chest, back, or abdominal pain)?" Do not suggest new symptoms to the patient. For example, do not ask a question such as, "Is this the worst headache you've ever had?" Also, ask neutral, nonjudgmental questions.

Pearls and Pitfalls

1. Always count, never estimate, the respiratory rate.
2. Auscultate the blood pressure whenever possible.
3. Be aware when "normal" vital signs are really abnormal and identify an unstable life-threatened patient.
4. When formulating a differential diagnosis, always consider the most serious diagnosis first rather than the most likely.

References

1. Markovchick VJ, Pons PT, Wolfe RE, eds. Emergency Medicine Secrets, 5th ed. Philadelphia: Mosby, 2011.
2. Rosen P, et al., eds. Emergency Medicine: Concepts and Clinical Practice, 7th ed. Philadelphia: Mosby, 2010.

CHAPTER 28

The Prehospital Patient Assessment

Arthur Hsieh, MA, NREMT-P

1. **What is the purpose of the patient assessment?**
   The goal of doing a patient assessment is to rapidly **identify** and **treat** any potentially life-threatening illness or injury. The assessment then provides an objective database on which to establish treatment priorities. A good physical exam plus a well-taken history are the essential elements in making an initial diagnosis.

2. **What tools are needed to perform a patient assessment?**
   In today's modern world of medicine, there are many tools and devices that can provide valuable, objective information about the patient's condition. Examples include pulse oximeters, waveform capnography, electrocardiogram monitors, and blood glucometers. However, the main tools that a paramedic uses to assess any patient are his/her hands (palpation), eyes (inspection), and ears (auscultation) to elicit the key elements of the exam, and the brain, to organize the information and synthesize possible underlying causes for the presentation. In addition to these "tools," the paramedic should also have empathy, respect, and compassion to promote the trust necessary to elicit an accurate medical history.

3. **Patients seem so different from each other. Should I assess each of them differently?**
   No—in fact, a hallmark of a good practitioner is the consistency of approach to the patient assessment. There are always certain components of the patient assessment that must be conducted first, no matter how ill or well the patient presents. This is the primary assessment.

4. **Is the patient assessment just about the patient?**
   No. Because EMS providers work in the field, there are certain details that must be looked at, even before assessing the patient directly. Scene safety is paramount, for you and any one else on the rescue crew. Determine the number of patients involved and whether specific additional resources are needed. Observe scene clues to ascertain whether the patient's chief complaint is based in trauma, medical, or both.

5. **What are the components of a patient assessment?**
   After the scene size up, patient assessment can be broken down into three broad areas: The primary assessment, the secondary assessment (history and physical exam), and reassessment (or ongoing assessment). In addition, there are some differences between the assessment of a trauma patient and a medical patient. There are four general categories: trauma patients with major or minor mechanisms of injury and medical patients who are conscious or experiencing altered mental status.

6. **What are the components of the primary assessment?**
   Every primary assessment begins with an overall general impression of the patient's condition. This may be quite simple—the patient looks at you as you approach, shakes your hand when you extend it, and answers your questions appropriately and easily. Although the patient may still be ill, his or her basic body mechanisms are working well enough to perfuse the primary target end organ, the brain. On the other hand, a patient may present altered, unresponsive, or in cardiopulmonary distress or arrest. In these

critical situations, you must complete the following assessment and treatment steps before continuing with the assessment:

- **Airway**—establish and maintain a patent airway to ensure the passage and exchange of oxygen and carbon dioxide. Simultaneously, manually control the cervical spine if injury to the area is suspected. If the airway is not patent, perform manual airway maneuvers such as a head tilt, chin lift, or modified jaw thrust and insert an oral or nasal airway to control the tongue. Consider padding the shoulders to assist in lifting the head to correct airway positioning. Advanced procedures such as intubation or cricothyrotomy may be needed if basic procedures fail.
- **Breathing**—establish that the patient is able to ventilate and is receiving enough oxygen to sustain metabolic processes. Immediately correct any inadequate situation—begin manual ventilations with a bag mask device for a hypoventilating condition and provide supplemental oxygen if hypoxia is suspected. Specific procedures such as needle decompression and sealing a sucking chest wound may be needed to preserve breathing ability.
- **Circulation**—establish that the patient has a pulse and appropriate skin signs to indicate that there is adequate perfusion to the body. Control massive bleeding immediately and correct hypoperfusing conditions through body positioning and temperature control. Pharmacologic support and crystalloid volume infusion may be needed if basic procedures fail to correct the condition.
- **Disability**—identify if the patient is **A**wake, responsive to **V**erbal or **P**ainful stimulus, or is **U**nresponsive. This is the **AVPU** scale, a simple method of establishing the patient's level of consciousness.
- **Expose**—remove the patient's clothing as appropriate to visualize the entire body for signs of injury or illness. Maintain modesty and cover the patient with a blanket or sheet afterward to help maintain body temperature.

7. **When do I move to the secondary assessment?**

   Sometimes never. If the patient is experiencing a life-threatening condition you must intercede immediately. For example, you may need to expend all of your energy and attention to relieving a patient's fully obstructed airway and may never get finding out about the patient's past medical history.

   The general rule of thumb is, you should begin the secondary assessment only after you are satisfied that you have at least temporarily managed the problems found in the primary assessment.

8. **What are the components of the secondary assessment and how do I organize them?**

   There are two general components of the secondary assessment. History taking elicits both the subjective description of the patient's presentation (OPQRST: onset, provocation or palliation, quality of pain, severity, time (history), as well any past pertinent medical history, medications, medical allergies, oral intake history, and events leading to the current condition (AMPLE: allergies, medications, past medical history, last eaten, events leading). (See Chapter 6 for descriptions of OPQRST and AMPLE.)

   A physical examination searches the body for additional objective clues to the underlying cause of the patient's condition. The physical exam may be focused on one or more parts of the body that may be related to the patient's condition or it may be a detailed and thorough survey of the entire body.

   See Figure 28.1 for help in organizing the sequence of the secondary assessment components. For a trauma patient, conduct a physical exam of the patient's "potential kill zones" of the head, neck, thorax, and pelvis to find anything missed during the primary assessment. In a conscious medical patient, eliciting

Clinical Care

Major Trauma Patient	Minor Trauma Patient	Conscious Medical Patient	Altered Medical Patient
Begin transport	Problem-focused physical exam	OPQRST	Physical exam
Physical exam (kill zone)	Vital signs	Vital signs	Vital signs
Vital signs	OPQRST	SAMPLE	OPQRST (bystanders)
OPQRST	SAMPLE	Physical exam	SAMPLE (bystanders)
SAMPLE	Head-to-toe physical exam (as necessary)		
Head-to-toe physical exam			

FIGURE 28.1 Secondary assessment organization.

SAMPLE = Symptoms, allergies, medications, prior history, last meal eaten (events leading up to injury/illness).

the patient's history first may provide you more information related to possible conditions; following it with a physical examination may provide you the clues necessary to formulate a treatment plan.

9. **When do I perform a head-to-toe physical exam?**
   Once all major life threats are managed, and major secondary findings are determined, a thorough detailed physical exam may be performed to ensure that nothing else of substance is missed. In a critically ill or injured patient, this exam may never occur.

10. **How do vital signs fit into the patient assessment?**
    The patient's pulse rate, blood pressure, respiratory rate, and oxygen saturation are essential objective findings in evaluating the patient's breathing and perfusion status. These actions must be taken early, often, and accurately to spot trends in the patient's condition. The first full set of vital signs is usually taken after the completion of the primary assessment and every few minutes thereafter. Paramedics will often take one last set of vital signs just prior to arrival to the hospital.

11. **When should I reassess the patient?**
    This is a bit of a trick question. The answer is "always," as in the fact that the reassessment is constantly happening. While the patient is in your care, you are responsible for that person's airway, breath, and circulatory abilities. So, it makes sense that you are constantly performing a primary assessment. You will need to reassess the patient's vital signs and monitor for signs of improvement after each intervention.

12. **What other information is important to know when assessing the trauma patient?**
    As part of the scene size up, take into consideration the mechanism of injury that the patient sustained during the event. Determining whether blunt or penetrating forces were involved can help you predict the injury pattern that the patient may have received.
    If you suspect a real or potential critical injury, *do not delay transport.* Package the patient during the primary assessment. Begin transport as soon as possible.

13. What about the medical patient?
Unlike the immediacy of the events surrounding a trauma patient, the nature of the illness that may be causing the patient's complaints may have taken days, weeks, or even years to develop. Your ability to be a detective in sleuthing out the subtle details of the patient's OPQRST and AMPLE history will be paramount in establishing a list of possible causes for the patient's condition. For the unconscious or altered medical patient, this becomes even more crucial. You will need to gather as much information from scene clues and bystander accounts to come up with possible causes.

Similar to trauma, there are specific circumstances that warrant immediate transport. Patients with evolving myocardial infarctions and strokes will benefit greatly from a rapid transport to an appropriate receiving hospital.

14. Is making a diagnosis that important?
Absolutely not. A diagnosis is nice, but the most important principles are that a thorough history and physical examination are performed, life-threatening problems are identified, and that appropriate patient intervention is accomplished. If the diagnosis is not obvious, presupposition of the patient's condition should not be conveyed to the receiving facility. This information could mislead triage or delay making a definitive diagnosis.

15. Why shouldn't I be able to make a diagnosis?
Sometimes you will, and it would be wonderful if that were always the case, but it is not. A patient assessment is an exercise in subtlety. The signs and symptoms that a patient might have for a specific disease may not be *exactly* the same as the next patient with the same disease. Often, what you read and learn about disease states are the so-called classic signs and symptoms that the majority of patients tend to exhibit. Clearly, it is not all patients. Don't be fooled by the patient who does not present as a so-called textbook case.

16. What is psychosclerosis?
Psychosclerosis is a term used to describe the "hardening of categories." Others call it tunnel vision. Call it jumping to conclusions. Regardless of which term you use, the results are the same; if you rapidly come to the conclusion that a particular disease is causing the patient's signs and symptoms, you may do yourself (and the patient) an injustice. Many patients will experience a wide variety of signs and symptoms associated with a specific illness. In addition, many patients will have more than one underlying cause for the complaint they are experiencing. Locking yourself into one diagnosis will lead you astray and cause you to lose sight of the actual cause(s).

Pearls and Pitfalls

1. Remember your manners. Be empathetic, courteous, polite, and honest when assessing your patients.
2. First things first. Complete the primary assessment before moving on to the secondary assessment.
3. When in doubt go back to the beginning. If you find yourself getting confused or lost while managing the patient, stop and go back to the primary assessment.
4. Continuously monitor your patient. A disease or injury is an evolution of an event over time and frequent reassessment is mandatory.
5. Vital signs are vital; do not estimate any vital sign.
6. Patients do not read the book and do not always present with classic signs and systems.
7. Do not develop psychosclerosis or tunnel vision.

References

1. Bickley L. Bates' Guide to Physical Examination and History Taking, 9th ed. Philadelphia: Lippincott Williams & Wilkins, 2005.
2. Deakin CD, Low JL. Accuracy of the advanced trauma life support guidelines for predicting systolic blood pressure using carotid, femoral, and radial pulses: Observational study. Br Med J 321:673–674, 2000.
3. Edmonds ZV, Mower WR, Lovato LM, et al. The reliability of vital sign measurements. Ann Emerg Med 39:233–237, 2002.
4. Hooker EA, O'Brien DJ, Danzyl DF, et al. Respiratory rates in emergency department patients. J Emerg Med 7:129–132, 1989.
5. Lovett PB. The vexatious vital: neither clinical measurements by nurses nor an electronic monitor provides accurate measurements of respiratory rate in triage. Ann Emerg Med 45(1):68–76, 2005.
6. Markovchick VJ, Pons PT, Bakes KM. Emergency Medicine Secrets, 5th ed. St. Louis: Elsevier, 2011.
7. Marx JA, et al. (eds.): Rosen's Emergency Medicine: Concepts and Clinical Practice, 7th ed. Philadelphia: Mosby, 2010.
8. National Association of EMTs: Prehospital Trauma Life Support, 7th ed. St. Louis, MO: Mosby/JEMS, 2011.
9. Price S, Wilson L. Pathophysiology: Clinical Concepts of Diseases Processes, 4th ed., p. 587(t). St. Louis: Mosby Yearbook, 1992.
10. Thibodeau G, Patton K. The Human Body in Health and Human Disease, 4th ed., p. 512. St. Louis: Elsevier, 2005

Electrocardiogram Interpretation

Angel Burba, MS, NREMT-P, NCEC

CHAPTER 29

1. **What is an electrocardiogram?**
   An electrocardiogram (ECG) is a graphical recording of cardiac electrical activity.

2. **Is ECG interpretation best done in the emergency department?**
   Yes and no. The emergency department has the advantage of a controlled environment and ready access to 12-lead ECGs, but many abnormal heart rhythms cause serious symptoms, can be recognized on a cardiac monitor, and require immediate prehospital management. Many EMS systems have adopted 12-lead interpretation in the prehospital setting. The important point is to not get so wrapped up in analyzing the ECG that the patient's symptoms are ignored. Patient assessment remains the foundation on which rhythm management must be based.

3. **Electrical activity of the heart sounds complex—where do I start?**
   Most of the heart is comprised of muscle fibers, which, when stimulated by an electrical impulse in a process called depolarization, contract in an organized fashion. This electrical impulse comes from the second type of cardiac tissue, which is a specialized group of cells called pacemakers. These cells have two special properties. First, they initiate depolarization, and then they automatically begin recharging so that depolarization can be induced again. The electrical impulse generated by pacemaker cells is conducted through the heart by a specialized conduction system, and the integrity of this system is important for producing a coordinated contraction of the atria and ventricles (Figure 29.1).

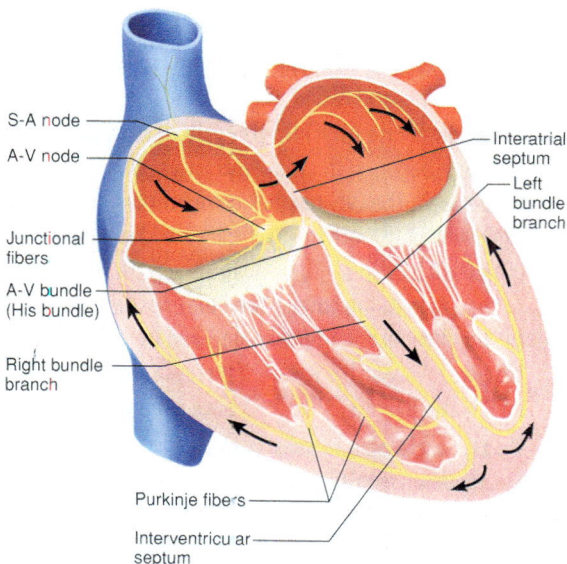

FIGURE 29.1 Anatomy and pathway of the electrical conducting system of the heart. (From Chapleau W et al. The Paramedic, McGraw-Hill, 2009. Reproduced with permission of The McGraw-Hill Companies.)

4. Where does electrical activity begin?

A normal cardiac impulse originates at the sinoatrial (SA) node located in the right atrium. The SA node usually discharges at a rate of 60–100 times per minute, and the impulse is conducted down a series of internodal pathways to the atrioventricular (AV) node, which lies near the junction of the atria with the ventricles. Here, the impulse is delayed to allow the atria to contract and augment ventricular filling with some extra blood. The impulse continues to the bundle of His, which divides into right and left bundle branches that conduct the impulse rapidly to the muscle fibers of the ventricles by a series of Purkinje fibers embedded within the ventricular walls. The result of the electrical wave moving through the ventricle is a muscular response in the form of a ventricular contraction. The normal ventricular contraction should yield a palpable pulse beat, which can typically be felt at any of the arterial pulse points.

5. Is the SA node the only pacemaker site?

No. The SA node is the usual pacemaker because it has the fastest discharge rate at 60–100 beats per minute (bpm) and thus discharges before the other pacemaker sites. Other sites, which take over when the SA node fails, include ectopic atrial sites (distinct from the SA node), AV node (junctional) pacemaker, and ventricular sites. The sympathetic and parasympathetic (through the vagus nerve) nervous systems may act on the SA and AV nodes to accelerate and slow down cardiac rate, respectively. Drugs and some disease processes also may alter a pacemaker's rate.

6. What are the inherent rates of firing for each pacemaker site?

When operating on their normal inherent rates, without the influence of the sympathetic or parasympathetic nervous system, the SA node fires at 60–100 bpm, the AV node fires at approximately 40–60 bpm, and the ventricles/Purkinje fibers fire at 20–40 bpm.

7. What does an ECG do?

The ECG is a tracing on a monitor or graph paper that shows cardiac electrical voltage (y axis) versus time (x axis). The graph paper is comprised of 1-mm squares. As the paper travels through the machine at 25 mm/sec, each square represents 0.04 sec. Voltage is measured in millimeters and is represented as the height of the waves. Each portion of the tracing corresponds to physiologic electrical activity of the heart.

8. What does one physiologic cycle of cardiac activity look like?

The cycle begins with atrial contraction, which is represented by the P wave of the ECG cycle (see Figure 29.2). The QRS complex occurs with ventricular depolarization, and the T wave follows as an expression of the recharging of the ventricles (repolarization). The QRS is typically the largest (tallest) complex. It is defined relative to the isoelectric (base) line. The Q wave is the first negative (downward) deflection from the baseline and may not be present in all tracings. The R wave is the first positive (upward) deflection from baseline, and the S wave is defined as the first negative deflection below baseline following the R wave. If there is a second positive deflection after the R wave, it is described as an R' wave (R prime). Like the Q wave, the S wave may not be noted in all cases.

9. Do the atria also repolarize?

Yes. However, repolarization of the atria occurs during ventricular depolarization, and the tracing of atrial repolarization is usually obscured by the higher ventricular depolarization voltages so no specific atrial depolarization wave is identifiable on the ECG tracing.

Electrocardiogram Interpretation

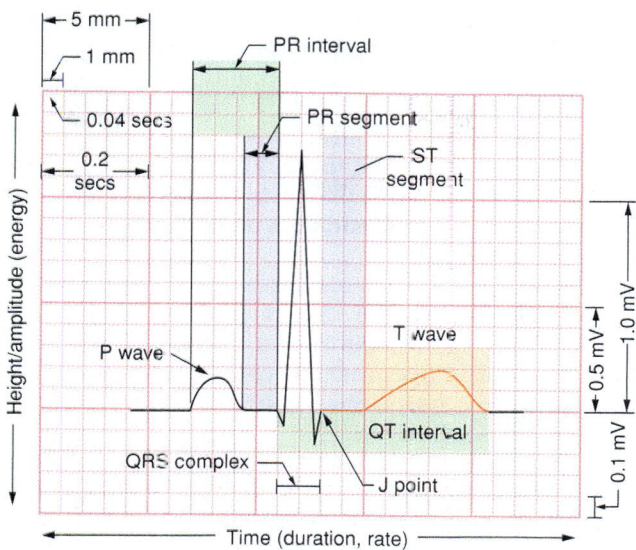

FIGURE 29.2 The cardiac cycle for one beat. (From Chapleau W et al. The Paramedic, McGraw-Hill, 2009. Reproduced with permission of The McGraw-Hill Companies.)

10. **What other portions of the ECG cycle are important?**

    The P–R interval (PRI) is defined as the time from the onset of the P wave to the beginning of the QRS complex (see Figure 29.2). This interval describes the time delay between atrial and ventricular contraction, and if conduction is slowed by disease or drugs, the P–R interval will be prolonged beyond the normal value of 0.20 sec. The QRS interval is measured from the first deflection from baseline (a Q wave or R wave) to the end of the S wave (or R' wave). A normal QRS complex is less than 0.12 sec long, and when conduction is pathologically delayed by disease of the septal conducting system, the QRS complex widens beyond 0.12 sec. The last important interval is the ST segment, which is the segment between the end of the QRS complex and the beginning of the T wave. Elevation of the ST segment above the baseline or isoelectric line is a crucial sign in diagnosing such entities as myocardial infarction or pericarditis. Depression of the ST segment can be seen with ischemia of myocardial muscle, drugs (e.g., digoxin), and thickening of the ventricular wall, which commonly results from chronic hypertension.

11. **What does the term "normal" mean when interpreting an ECG?**

    Normal refers to waves and segments that occur when the impulses are traveling through the electrical conduction system following the SA-AV-Purkinje pathways and the rhythm and origin of the impulses. In lead II, "normal" atrial activity is seen as an upright, round, and regular P wave, with a PRI of less than 0.2 sec long, followed by a narrow (less than 0.12 sec) QRS wave. Normal also indicates that there are no ectopic beats present.

12. **How do I obtain an ECG from the patient?**

    First, attach electrodes to the skin. These patches or metal pads function as receivers transmitting electrical data from the patient to the cardiac monitor through attached cables. The standard monitoring leads are I, II, and III, and electrodes are attached to the right arm, left arm, and left leg (with perhaps an additional cable attached to the right leg). As a wave of positive charges (depolarization) approaches a positive electrode, an upward deflection is recorded, and a downward deflection results as the electrical activity moves away from a positive electrode. The standard leads are represented as follows:

Lead	Positive Electrode	Negative Electrode
I	Left arm	Right arm
II	Left leg	Right arm
III	Left leg	Left arm

Because of the different electrode positions, each lead gives a view of the heart's electrical activity from a different perspective. In addition, 12-lead ECGs use the limb leads as a common negative electrode and place positive electrodes at six sites across the anterior chest. These precordial leads are numbered V1–V6, and enable closer examination of the septum and left ventricle.

13. **Can I use a standard field monitor to get information similar to that from the precordial leads of a 12-lead ECG?**
Yes. The addition of modified chest leads (MCLs) to the standard leads offers useful analogs to the precordial leads for the prehospital environment. MCL1 is one of the most commonly used, and in this case the positive electrode is placed in the fourth intercostal space (level of the male nipple), just to the right of the sternum, and the left arm acts as the negative electrode. This lead may be particularly useful for identifying P waves and determining whether a rhythm is of ventricular or supraventricular origin.

14. **What is meant by axis?**
Axis is a term that describes the direction in which depolarization spreads through heart muscle (see Figure 29.3). For reference purposes, the direction of electrical current in lead I is labeled 0°, whereas in lead II the direction is 45°, and in lead aVf 90°. Patterns noted in these leads demonstrate the alteration of axis in certain disease states:
   1. Normal axis. The QRS complexes are seen to be positive in leads I, II, and III.
   2. Left axis deviation. The QRS complex is positive in lead I and negative in leads II and III. This pattern is sometimes seen in the setting of myocardial ischemia or enlargement of the ventricular wall due to chronic hypertension.
   3. Right axis deviation. This pattern generates a negative QRS complex in lead I, whereas the QRS complex of lead III is positive. Right axis deviation is seen in some patients with chronic lung disease and enlargement of the right ventricle.

15. **What is the most important part of ECG interpretation?**
Stay organized. Choose a format for ECG analysis, and use it in exactly the same way for every tracing that you examine. Do not take shortcuts or fall into "pattern recognition" where you simply glance at a tracing and jump to a conclusion without performing an organized analysis. You should also get in the habit of printing a static strip in addition to looking at the rhythm in dynamic mode.

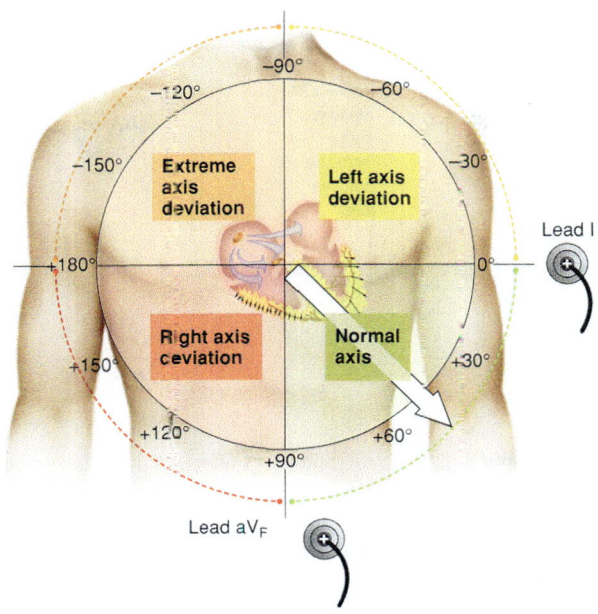

FIGURE 29.3 The electrical axis of the heart. (From Chapleau W et al. The Paramedic, McGraw-Hill, 2009. Reproduced with permission of The McGraw-Hill Companies.)

16. Is there an easy way to organize ECG interpretation?

Ask yourself questions in the following five areas:

1. Rate: what is the rate?
2. Regularity: is the rhythm regular or irregular? If it is irregular, is a pattern present? Is there any ectopy present?
3. P wave assessment: do you see P waves, and are they related to the QRS complexes? Is the relationship 1:1 (one P wave for every QRS complex?) Are there any QRS waves without Ps? Are there any Ps without QRS waves?
4. PRI assessment: is there a PR Interval? Is it consistent? If it varies, is there a detectable pattern?
5. QRS assessment: is the QRS complex wide (> 0.12 sec) or narrow (< 0.12, which is normal)?

Answering these questions usually allows you to diagnose the abnormal heart rhythms (dysrhythmias) that require prehospital management.

17. How do I calculate rate?

(a) Determine if the rhythm is regular or irregular as this will impact which counting method is appropriate.

(b) Always verify the heart rate displayed on the monitor with a comparison of the actual pulse rate. Remember, the ECG shows electrical activity only—it does not provide any information regarding mechanical response (i.e., it does not indicate if the heart is actually circulating blood via mechanical pumping).

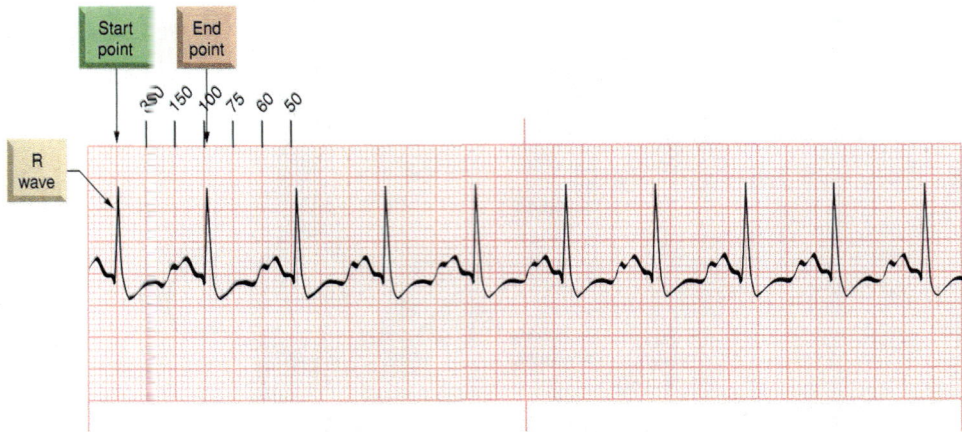

FIGURE 29.4 Counting method for calculating heart rate. (From Chapleau W et al. The Paramedic, McGraw-Hill, 2009. Reproduced with permission of The McGraw-Hill Companies.)

Counting methods: an inexact method is to find an apex of a QRS complex aligned with a solid line on the graph paper and count the big (5 mm) boxes before the identical point of the following QRS. The rate is obtained by dividing the number of boxes into 300. A second counting method is to count the number of small boxes between two QRS complexes and dividing that number into 1500. Both of these methods are the most accurate with a regular rhythm (see Figure 29.4).

Six-second strip method: most ECG paper has marks on the top or bottom of the paper every 3 sec. Therefore, the rate can be approximated by counting the number of QRS complexes in a 6-sec period and multiplying by 10. This method works best with a regular rhythm (see Figure 29.5).

Rate meter method: use a commercial rate meter and calipers to determine the rate. Although this provides a high level of precision, the individual is somewhat dependent upon having the correct tools when needed, so alternative methods should be available.

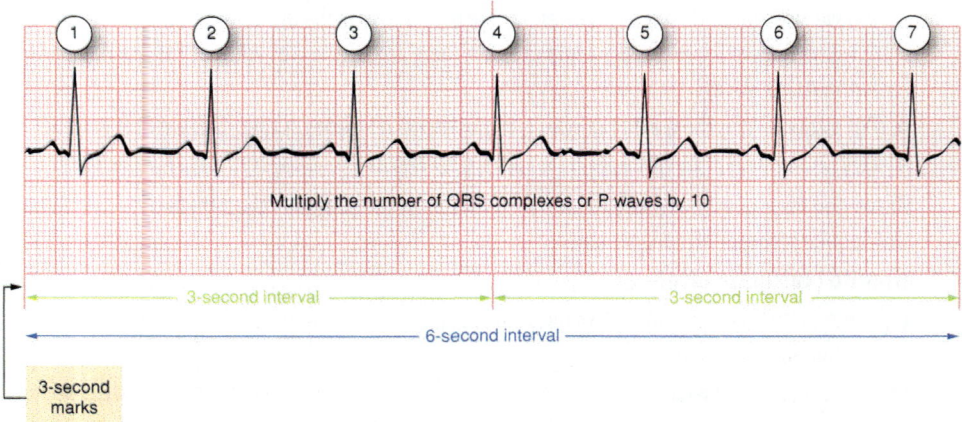

FIGURE 29.5 Six second strip method for calculating heart rate. (From Chapleau W et al. The Paramedic, McGraw-Hill, 2009. Reproduced with permission of The McGraw-Hill Companies.)

18. How do I determine whether a rhythm is regular?

First, the pulse corresponds exactly to each QRS complex, and the time between impulses is the same. Rhythm is easiest to measure by comparing the distance between neighboring R waves (R–R interval) at multiple different points of the ECG recording. One also may analyze the distance between P waves. Regular rhythms may originate from all pacemaker sites. When a normal P wave is associated with each QRS complex, the rhythm originates at the SA node and is called a normal sinus rhythm.

19. What if I see an irregular rhythm?

Try to determine whether there is any pattern to the irregularity. Some heart blocks may show irregular patterns that repeat predictably. This is termed "regularly irregular." Premature beats are the most common cause of irregular rhythms. They may arise from ectopic foci in the atria, junction (AV node), or ventricles. Premature atrial contractions (PACs) show a P wave with a slightly or obviously different shape from the normal P wave originating from the SA node. The remainder of the conduction proceeds as usual, giving a normal QRS complex. A premature junctional complex (PJC) originates near the AV node, and conduction moves in two directions, down to the ventricles and up the atria. Because conduction normally goes down the septum and ventricles, the QRS complex is normal, but conduction is reversed through the atria, showing an inverted P wave. The inverted P wave may occur immediately before the QRS (within 0.2 sec) during the QRS (as a buried wave) or immediately after the QRS. Ectopic beats originating from the ventricles are called "premature ventricular contractions" or PVCs. A widened, slurred QRS complex is seen, which may vary in shape and axis depending on whether the focus is high or low in the ventricle. Typically, a long compensatory pause follows a PVC, as the regular atrial impulse finds the ventricles in an absolute refractory period and conduction stops. The next atrial impulse generally proceeds as usual.

20. What is the significance of the QRS width?

When the normal conducting pathway from the AV node through the bundle of His to the bundle branches and Purkinje fibers of the right and left ventricles is followed, ventricular contraction follows in an organized fashion and produces a normal QRS (duration <0.12 sec). Impulses may arise in the ventricles below this conducting system. Thus, electrical activity flows more slowly from one working muscle fiber to another. The result is a widened QRS complex (duration >0.12 sec). This type of QRS morphology also may be seen with sinus or atrial pacemakers when conduction down the bundle of His or individual ventricular conduction bundles is delayed. For example, the typical finding of a right bundle-branch block (RBBB) is a P wave associated with a widened QRS complex showing an RSR' morphology in lead MCL1, whereas a left bundle-branch block (LBBB) shows an upright widened QRS complex in MCL6.

21. Are all P waves the same?

No. We have already noted that differently shaped P waves may occur with PACs. P waves from the SA node are positive when viewed in leads I, II, and III, whereas P waves originating close to the AV node are inverted and seen immediately before or after the QRS complex (e.g., PJCs). Atrial flutter shows sawtooth-shaped P waves with a fast rate of up to 300 waves per minute. Usually a variable number of P waves precedes each QRS complex, because some are blocked from proceeding; the result is an irregular rhythm. A close relative to atrial flutter is atrial fibrillation, and the pattern can often switch from one to the other. With atrial fibrillation, no organized atrial activity is seen—only a chaotic, disorganized pattern of electrical activity along the baseline between QRS complexes. Ventricular complexes are generated in an irregular fashion because of the chaotic activity in the atria.

22. **Are all P waves followed by QRS complexes?**
Under normal circumstances, yes. Each QRS is preceded by a P wave, and the P–R interval is constant (< 0.20 sec). In pathologic settings, these characteristics do not hold. A fixed relationship between the QRS and P wave may coexist with a prolonged P–R interval (>0.20 sec), as seen with first-degree atrioventricular (AV) block. Fortunately, this condition is usually benign, and no specific care is indicated. In other settings, one may see more P waves than QRS complexes. These P waves may be blocked in a regular fashion (e.g., three P waves:one QRS), an irregular manner (ratio varies), or completely blocked, with P waves occurring independently of ventricular depolarization.

23. **What dysrhythmias are important in terms of prehospital management?**
The easiest dysrhythmia to recognize is asystole, which occurs when no electrical activity is present. The patient is pulseless and unresponsive. One must take care to ensure that the monitor, cable, and electrodes are properly applied as well as verifying the presence of asystole in a second lead. Ventricular fibrillation, pulseless ventricular tachycardia, and pulseless electrical activity (PEA) are all lethal dysrhythmias. Also, to maintain adequate perfusion, the heart rate needs to be within a normal range, so extreme bradycardia and tachycardia can compromise blood pressure and perfusion, which can also be dangerous.

24. **What is ventricular fibrillation?**
Ventricular fibrillation is defined as chaotic, uncoordinated electrical activity of ventricular muscle fibers (Figure 29.6). There is no cardiac output, and the patient becomes pulseless and unresponsive. A tracing of ventricular fibrillation demonstrates irregular, chaotic ventricular waves of varying amplitudes. Initially the amplitude changes are coarser or greater in magnitude, but with time the changes become finer as the rhythm progresses to asystole. Care must be taken not to confuse this rhythm with an artifact seen with patient movement, loose connections, or defective electrodes.

25. **What bradycardic rhythms are concerning?**
Almost any bradycardic rhythm should be examined closely. Sinus bradycardia shows a regular pattern with positive P waves in lead II associated with each ventricular complex. Although this rhythm may be normal in athletes and younger people at rest, treatment should be considered when accompanied by symptoms suggesting decreased perfusion.

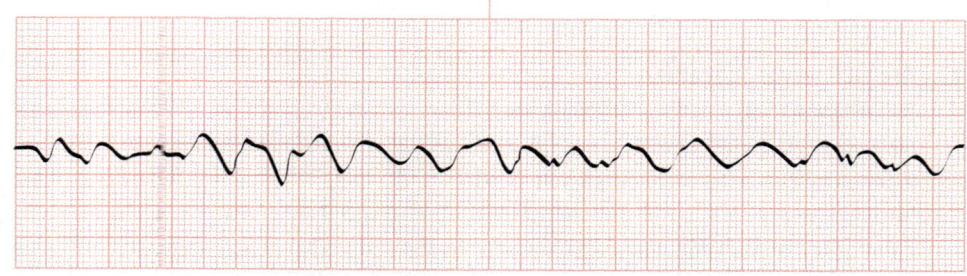

FIGURE 29.6 Ventricular fibrillation. (From Chapleau W et al. The Paramedic, McGraw-Hill, 2009. Reproduced with permission of The McGraw-Hill Companies.)

Electrocardiogram Interpretation

26. Can bradycardias arise from other sites?

Yes. If the SA node fails as a pacemaker, automaticity at other (escape) pacemaker sites will begin. After a pause in the rhythm that no longer inhibits the secondary pacemaker, the escape pacemaker will generate an impulse as a protective mechanism against cardiac arrest. If the AV node is the pacemaker site, junctional bradycardia may be seen. This rhythm is generally regular with a normal QRS complex; if P waves are seen, they are inverted in lead II and appear immediately before or after the QRS complex. Another escape rhythm is bradycardia of ventricular origin, also referred to as an idioventricular or agonal rhythm. The rhythm is usually regular with a widened QRS complex (>0.12 sec). Usually, P waves are not present, and hemodynamic compromise frequently results.

27. What are heart blocks?

Cardiac disease may slow conduction through the AV node. The consequence of partially or completely blocking these impulses is called heart block or, more accurately, atrioventricular (AV) block. AV block is classified into three types. First-degree AV block, which is more of a "delay" than a block because all impulses are eventually conducted, is a sinus rhythm with a prolonged P–R interval (>0.20 sec) (Figure 29.7).

In the two types of second-degree AV block, conduction of a P-wave impulse does not occur consistently. The first type of second-degree AV block is a variable block (also known as Wenckebach or Mobitz type I) in which the P–R interval progressively increases until conduction of the P wave is completely blocked, and a P wave is seen without a following QRS complex (Figure 29.8). Because the site of blockade

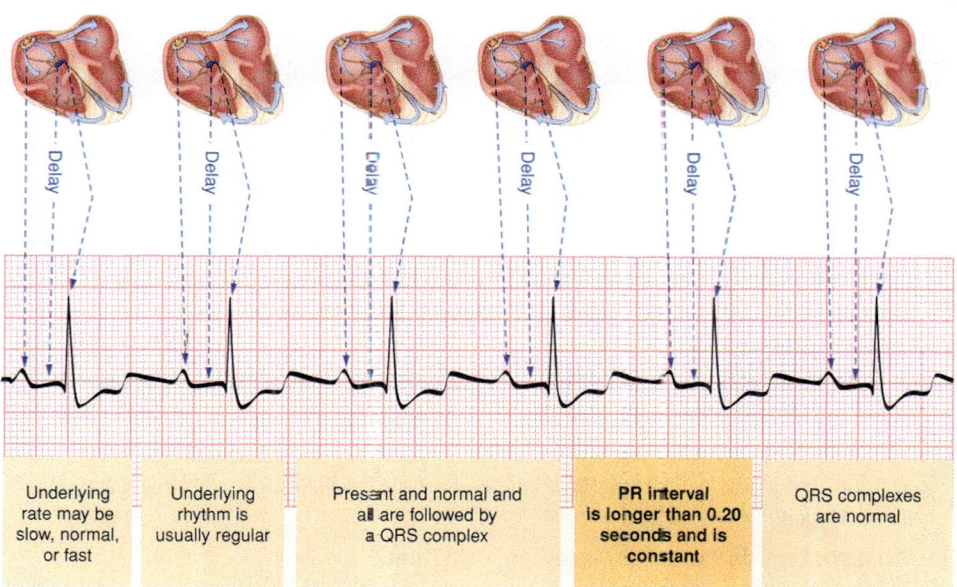

FIGURE 29.7 First degree atrioventricular (AV) block. (From Chapleau W et al. The Paramedic, McGraw-Hill, 2009. Reproduced with permission of The McGraw-Hill Companies.)

Clinical Care

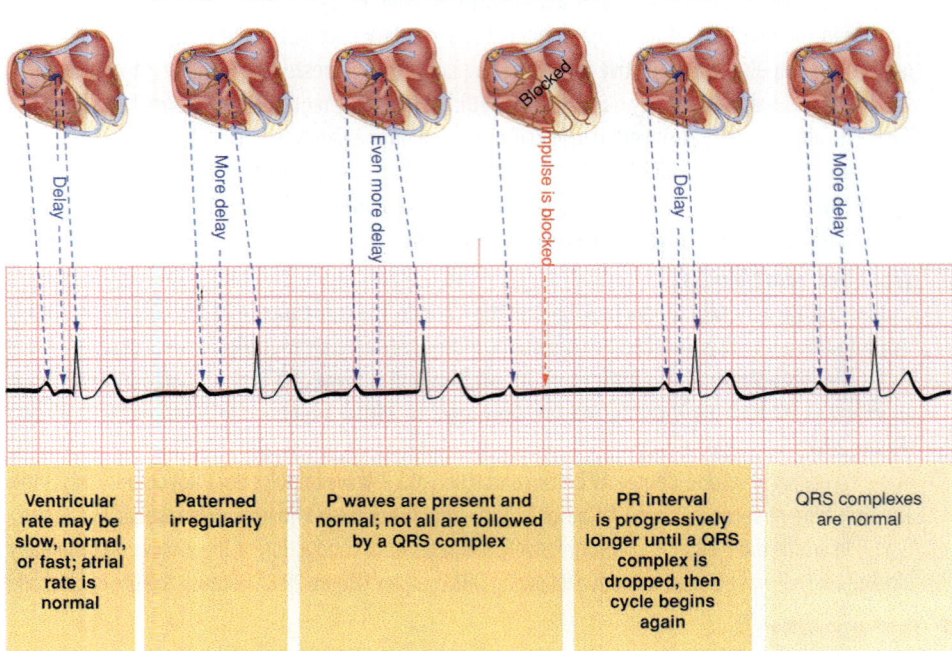

FIGURE 29.8 Second degree AV block, Mobitz type 1 (Wenckebach). (From Chapleau W et al. The Paramedic, McGraw-Hill, 2009. Reproduced with permission of The McGraw-Hill Companies.)

is at the AV node, normal width QRS complexes are seen, and there is little risk of progression to complete AV block.

In contrast, the second type of second-degree AV block, also known as fixed AV block, Classic, or Mobitz type II, presents with a constant PR interval, but occasional nonconducted beats (Figure 29.9). With 3:1 conduction, for example, two P waves are conducted through the AV node but the third is blocked. The site of block may be anywhere in the AV node, junction, or septum. The higher up the block occurs in the conduction pathway, the narrower the QRS complex. Blocks lower in the conducting system are associated with a widened QRS complex and a higher risk that the block will progress to complete AV block or asystole.

Third-degree AV block or complete AV block shows atrioventricular dissociation. In other words, both P waves and QRS complexes are present but show no relationship to one another and P–R interval measurements vary in a random nature (Figure 29.10). The atria are contracting independent of the ventricles. This situation often is unstable because the patient is bradycardic and often shows signs of hypoperfusion.

28. What strategy do you use for tachycardic rhythms?

The biggest danger with tachycardic rhythms is the potential compromise to blood pressure and perfusion because of inadequate time for ventricular filling.

Two important questions influence future management of the rhythm:

Electrocardiogram Interpretation

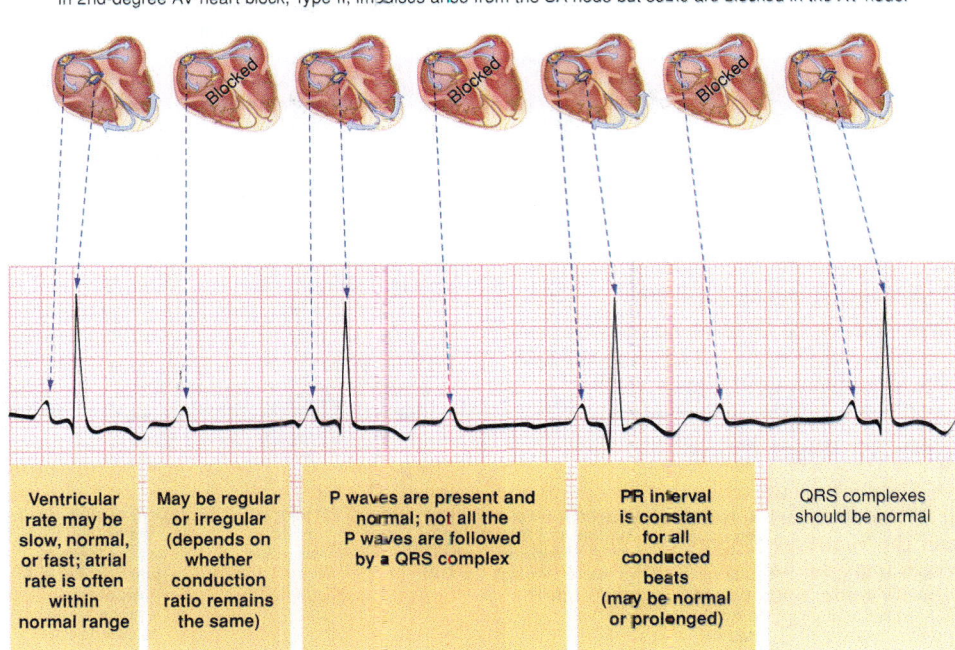

FIGURE 29.9 Second degree AV block. Mobitz type II. (From Chapleau W et al. The Paramedic, McGraw-Hill, 2009. Reproduced with permission of The McGraw-Hill Companies.)

(a) Is the rhythm regular or irregular?
(b) Is the QRS complex wide or narrow?

Irregular tachycardias should make one look for patterns suggestive of atrial fibrillation or flutter, ectopic beats, or tachycardias arising from ectopic foci. Regular tachycardias may arise from the same pacemakers as bradycardic rhythms and have the same characteristics as the slower rhythms from these sites. For example, sinus tachycardia shows the same P wave morphology (shape) as sinus bradycardia and a consistent relationship of the P wave to the QRS complex but has a rate over 100 bpm (but usually <150 bpm). The same is true for tachycardias from junctional or ventricular pacemakers.

29. I see a regular narrow complex tachycardia. What does that tell me?
Because the QRS complex is narrow, the impulse originates from a pacemaker at the AV node or higher in the conduction system (supraventricular). Because the rate is fast, usually over 160 bpm, the P waves of atrial depolarization are obscured by the QRS complexes. Vagal maneuvers may slow the rate so that underlying P-wave morphology (sinus, flutter waves, no P waves) may be appreciated.

30. Does a regular, wide complex tachycardia mean that the impulse originates below the AV node?
Yes, no, maybe. Tachycardia arising from a pacemaker below the AV node can produce regular tachycardia with a QRS complex greater than 0.12-sec duration. The problem is that a wide complex tachycardia also may arise from a pacemaker above the AV node if a conduction abnormality exists. Most commonly,

Clinical Care

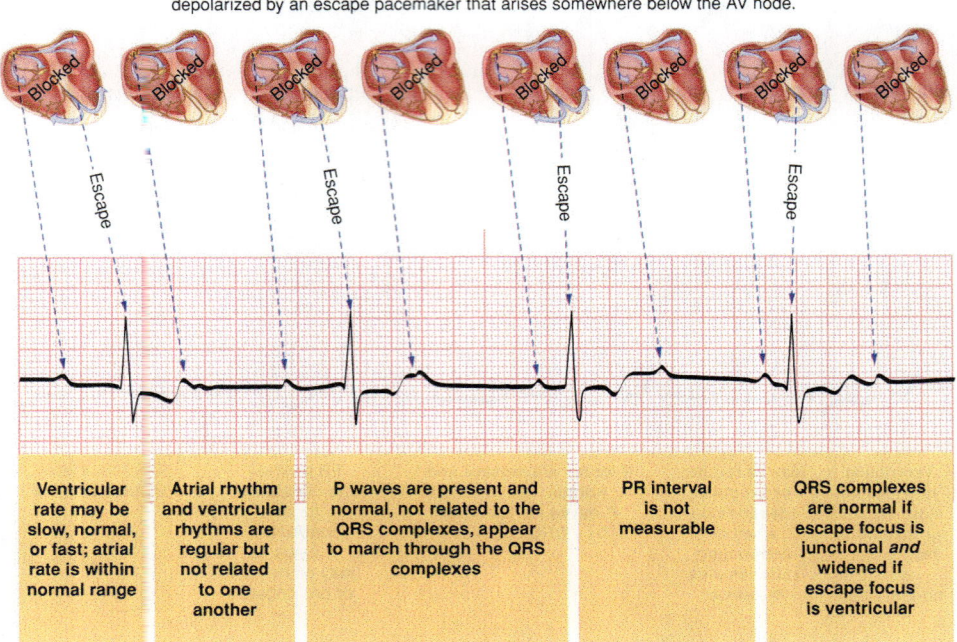

FIGURE 29.10 Third degree or complete A-V block. (From Chapleau W et al. The Paramedic, McGraw-Hill, 2009. Reproduced with permission of The McGraw-Hill Companies.)

such conduction abnormalities involve a bundle–branch block or an accessory pathway. An accessory pathway is a conduction pathway between the atria and ventricles in addition to the normal conduction system. If block is present at the AV node, conduction may proceed earlier than expected back to the atria through the accessory pathway. This type of retrograde conduction is responsible for producing wide complex tachycardias of supraventricular origin.

31. How can differentiate between ventricular and supraventricular rhythms?

First, ventricular tachycardia is more common, particularly in people over the age of 50 and those with a history of cardiac disease. It is commonly thought that patients with ventricular tachycardia appear more ill (e.g., lower blood pressure or altered mentation), but this is not necessarily the case. ECG criteria that may be helpful in distinguishing ventricular tachycardia include a QRS complex greater than 0.12-sec duration and AV dissociation, in which P waves may be seen that bear no relationship to the QRS complex.

A fusion beat may be seen when an impulse from the atria arrives at the septal conduction system at the same time as a ventricular impulse, and the resulting QRS complex is a combination of the bizarre, wide ventricular QRS complex and the normal, narrow QRS complex (Figure 29.11).

Unfortunately, both of these ECG characteristics may not be present in every case. It may then be necessary to examine the QRS morphology in MCL1 and MCL6 from a 12-lead ECG tracing. If the QRS complex in MCL1 shows an R wave greater than 0.03-sec duration or a deep, slurred S wave, a ventricular

Electrocardiogram Interpretation

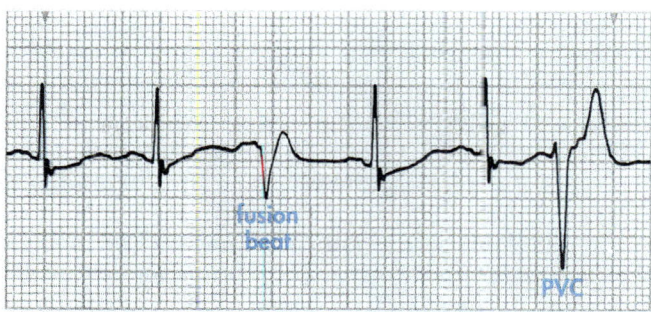

FIGURE 29.11 A fusion beat. (From Chapleau W et al. The Paramedic, McGraw-Hill, 2009. Reproduced with permission of The McGraw-Hill Companies.)

origin is suggested. In MCL6, a QR or QS complex is suggestive of a ventricular rhythm. In addition, if the axis points toward the right shoulder, as shown by negative QRS complexes in leads I, II, and III, chances are greater that the wide complex tachycardia is ventricular. If MCL6 is a primarily negative complex, chances are that the patient is in ventricular rather than supraventricular tachycardia.

In contrast, rhythms of supraventricular origin usually demonstrate QRS complexes with a duration of 0.12–0.14 sec and often show an RS complex in one of the MCL leads. The R–S interval is not over 0.10 sec in any MCL lead, and there is no evidence of AV dissociation. Morphology criteria suggestive of ventricular origin are absent.

32. **How come rhythms that arise from pacemaker sites other than the SA node (atria, junction, and ventricles) are not called "tachycardic" or if they fire faster than their inherent rates?**

    The terms "bradycardia" and "tachycardia" are tied to specific heart rate numbers. Bradycardia can apply for any heart rate less than 60 bpm and tachycardia applies for any heart rates greater than 100 bpm. Using this logic, rhythms arising from a site such as the AV node with a normal inherent rate of 40–60 bpm are labeled "bradycardic" because the rate is less than 60 bpms, even though the inherent (normal) firing rate is being met.

33. **Is it important to distinguish between supraventricular and ventricular tachycardia in the field?**

    Not necessarily. What is more important is to determine the perfusion status of the patient. It is more important to have an effective management strategy for all complex tachycardiac rhythms. Effective management should be based on the clinical status of the patient.

34. **What are artificial pacemakers?**

    An artificial pacemaker is usually implanted under the skin just below the clavicle. An easily palpable battery is connected to electrode wires that are passed through the subclavian vein to be embedded in the right side of the heart. The pacemaker has a sensing device to detect whether the heart is producing an impulse. If no impulse is detected in the required time, the pacemaker fires, thus initiating a contraction in the right ventricle. On the ECG, the pacemaker impulse is detected as a spike ("pacer spike") that is immediately followed by a widened QRS complex because the impulse began in the right ventricle (Figure 29.12). Some patients have an atrioventricular pacemaker that demonstrates two pacer

Clinical Care

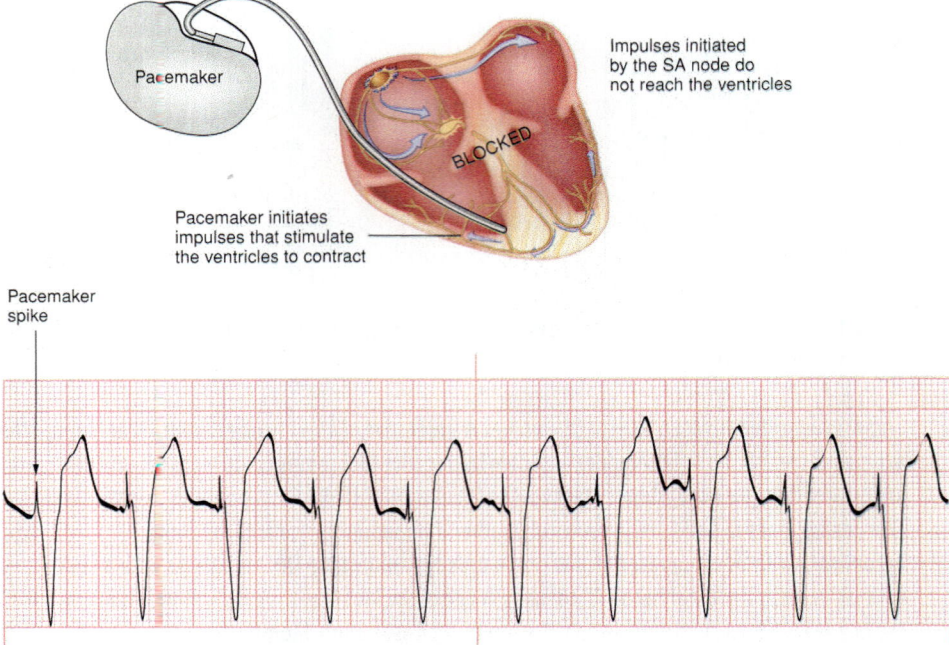

FIGURE 29.12 Paced cardiac rhythm. (From Chapleau W et al. The Paramedic, McGraw-Hill, 2009. Reproduced with permission of The McGraw-Hill Companies.)

spikes on the ECG. One corresponds to atrial contraction, and the other stimulates the ventricles.

35. Is a 12-lead ECG useful in the field?

Yes and no. Newer field monitors have the capability of producing a 12-lead ECG. The most useful application of a 12-lead ECG is in the diagnosis of myocardial infarction or ischemia. With the advent of thrombolytic and interventional therapy for myocardial infarction, many emergency medical service systems have implemented this management strategy for field use, and a 12-lead ECG is obtained to determine whether eligibility criteria for thrombolytics or angioplasty are met. One of the barriers to timely care in the emergency department is the time that it takes to obtain a 12-lead ECG. If the patient arrives at the emergency department with a 12-lead ECG, reperfusion therapy may be initiated more rapidly. In addition, many EMS systems are also completing check lists in the field to determine if thrombolytic therapy is appropriate. Serial, or repeat 12 leads can also provide valuable information on the evolution of ischemia and infarction and the EMS system can begin this process as well.

36. Can I diagnose myocardial infarction without a 12-lead ECG monitor?

The current standard is to obtain a 12 lead to evaluate for ST segment elevation and to obtain blood to look for the presence of cardiac enzymes. In addition, reciprocal changes in the form of ST depression are often seen in the side opposite the infarction. For example, with an inferior wall myocardial infarction, ST elevation will be seen in leads II and III, whereas ST depression will be noted on the anterior MCL leads.

Pearls and Pitfalls

1. The most important part of ECG interpretation is to be organized in your approach.
2. The approach to ECG interpretation requires answering six questions:
   (a) What is the rate?
   (b) Is the rhythm regular or irregular?
   (c) If it is irregular, is a pattern present?
   (d) Is the QRS narrow or wide?
   (e) Do you see P waves, and are they related to the QRS complexes (where the rhythm originates)?
   (f) Are the intervals and shape of the waves normal?
3. The biggest mistake is to treat the ECG and not the patient. The patient's clinical appearance should guide the need for intervention.
4. Wide complex tachycardia should be considered to be ventricular tachycardia until proven otherwise, particularly in patients with preexisting cardiac disease and those over the age of 50 years.
5. Twelve-lead ECGs performed in the field can save valuable time in the emergency department and expedite the care of the cardiac patient who requires reperfusion for a myocardial infarction.

References

1. Atkins JM. Basic rhythm interpretation. In Paramedic Field Care: A Complaint Based Approach, Pons P, Cason D, eds., pp. 181–209 St. Louis: Mosby, 1997.
2. Dubin D. Rapid Interpretation of EKGs, 3rd ed. Tampa, FL: Cover Publishing, 1983.
3. Yealy DM, Delbridge TR. Dysrhythmias. In Rosen's Emergency Medicine: Concepts and Clinical Practice, 5th ed., Marx J, et al., eds. pp 984–1024. St. Louis: Mosby, 2010.

Cardiac Dysrhythmias

Paul Davidson, MD

1. **What are the first questions to ask when approaching a patient with a cardiac dysrhythmia?**
   (a) Is the patient clinically and hemodynamically stable?
   (b) Is the rate fast or slow?
   (c) Are the complexes wide or narrow?
   (d) Is the rhythm regular or irregular?
2. **What is clinical instability?**
   Physical signs of poor cardiac output such as pulmonary edema, chest pain, obtundation, and diaphoresis.
3. **What is hemodynamic instability?**
   Definitions differ according to various authors, but certainly a systolic blood pressure <90 mmHg, a mean arterial pressure of <60 mmHg, or the absence of a radial pulse are concerning signs.
4. **Define a narrow complex tachycardia.**
   A rhythm that is narrow (<3 boxes wide) or 0.12 sec on an electrocardiogram (ECG) and fast (>100 bpm).
5. **Name the common causes of regular narrow complex tachycardia.**
   Sinus tachycardia, atrial flutter, junctional tachycardia, atrial tachycardias, and reciprocating tachycardias, such as atrioventricular (AV) node reentry tachycardia (Figure 30.1) and Wolff–Parkinson–White syndrome in orthodromic reciprocating tachycardia (Figure 30.2).

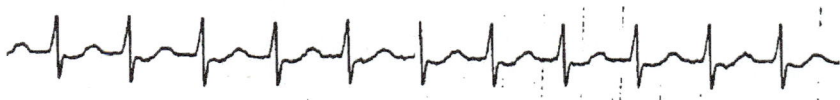

FIGURE 30.1   Atrioventricular node reentry tachycardia. Note the absent ("buried") P wave.

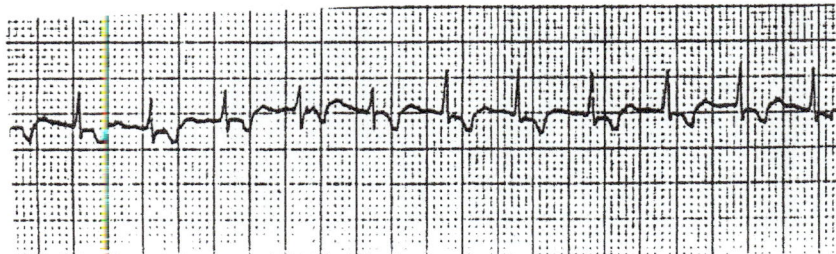

FIGURE 30.2   Wolff–Parkinson–White Syndrome, going "down the node and up the pathway." Note the inverted P waves after the QRS complex.

6. **Name the common causes of irregular narrow complex tachycardia.**
   Atrial fibrillation (Figure 30.3), atrial flutter with variable block (Figure 30.4), and multifocal atrial tachycardia (Figure 30.5).

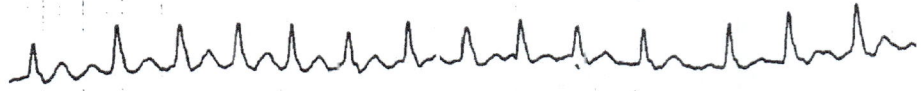

FIGURE 30.3   Atrial fibrillation. Note the irregularly irregular rhythm.

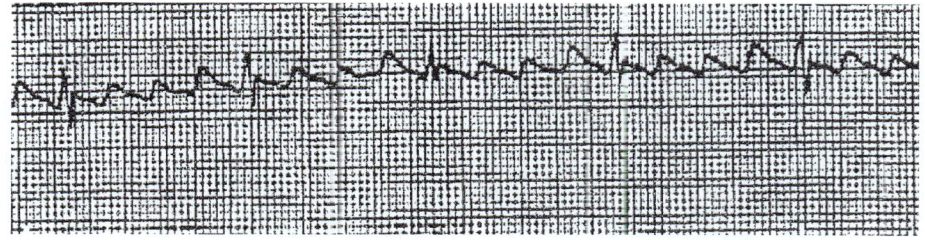

FIGURE 30.4   Atrial flutter with 4:1 conduction. Note the characteristic sawtooth pattern.

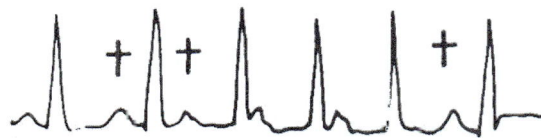

FIGURE 30.5   Multifocal atrial tachycardia. Note at least three different P wave morphologies.

7. **Why is it important to establish regularity vs. irregularity?**
   Because irregular rhythms (and some regular rhythms) are not treatable with adenosine. Patients with an irregular narrow complex rhythm who are stable should be transported. If patients are unstable, you should contact the base and prepare to cardiovert the patient.

8. **How do you make the diagnosis of atrial fibrillation with a rapid ventricular response?**
   Sometimes it is obvious from the rhythm strip, and at other times if the rhythm is fast and regular enough, the rhythm strip may look like a regular supraventricular tachycardia (SVT). The diagnosis is easy if you palpate a pulse and simultaneously look at the monitor or auscultate the heart. Atrial fibrillation is the only rhythm that results in an irregularly irregular pulse with varying intensity and a pulse deficit (fewer beats are palpated than are visible on the monitor or heard with the stethoscope).

9. **How should a stable narrow complex tachycardia be treated?**
   Assuming that you have ruled out sinus tachycardia, atrial flutter, and multifocal atrial tachycardia, use adenosine, 6 mg by rapid IV push, preferably in an antecubital or external jugular vein, followed by a 10-cc bolus of saline flush.

10. **What if adenosine, 6 mg IV, does not work?**
    Try adenosine, 12 mg by rapid IV push. The success rate of converting paroxysmal SVT is about 60% with 6 mg and over 90% with 12 mg.

11. How does adenosine work?

Adenosine puts the AV node in a "headlock" for about 6 sec and therefore terminates any dysrhythmia that uses the AV node as part of its circuit (i.e., AV node reentry tachycardia or Wolff–Parkinson–White in orthodromic reciprocating tachycardia. Figure 30.6). It will not convert sinus tachycardia, atrial flutter, or atrial fibrillation.

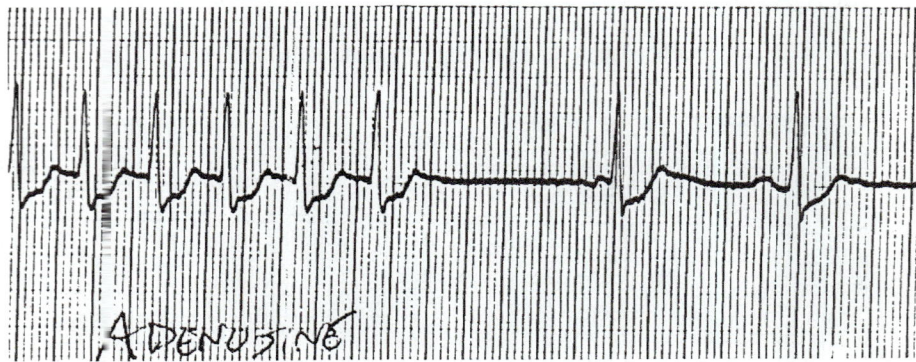

FIGURE 30.6 Atrioventricular node reentry tachycardia terminated with adenosine.

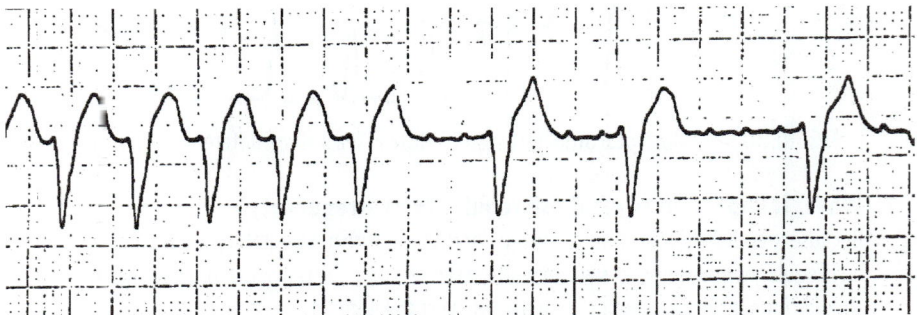

FIGURE 30.7 Adenosine uncovering atrial flutter as the cause of the tachycardia.

12. What are the three possible outcomes after you push adenosine?
1. Termination of the tachycardia
2. Unmasking of underlying atrial activity (such as atrial flutter. Figure 30.7)
3. No effect at all. The tachycardia actually "laughs" at you.

13. What prescription drugs interact with adenosine?
Dipyridamole (Persantine) and carbamazepine (Tegretol) enhance the effect of adenosine, whereas theophylline negates the effects of adenosine.

14. In what group of patients is adenosine relatively contraindicated?
Adenosine causes prolonged bronchospasm in asthmatic patients; in a few cases, it has precipitated respiratory arrest requiring intubation.

15. **What if adenosine does not work and the patient is still stable?**
    Initiate transport and consider IV verapamil (if available), 2.5–5 mg by IV push or IV diltiazem, 15–20 mg (0.25 mg/kg) given over 2 min.
16. **What is a wide complex tachycardia?**
    A rhythm that is wide (i.e., QRS >0.12 sec or 3 boxes on ECG) and fast (i.e., >100 bpm).
17. **What big decision must you make in patients with wide complex tachycardia?**
    Distinguishing between ventricular tachycardia and SVT with aberrancy.
18. **What does *aberrancy* mean?**
    Abnormal conduction of the electrical impulse from the atria to the ventricles. Examples of aberrancy include right bundle-branch block, left bundle-branch block, or conduction down an accessory pathway, as seen in Wolff–Parkinson–White syndrome.
19. **What should you generally assume that a wide complex tachycardia is?**
    Assume that it is ventricular tachycardia (VT), which is six times more common than SVT with aberrancy.
20. **With what must you *never* treat a wide complex tachycardia?**
    Verapamil or other calcium channel blockers because they cause cardiovascular collapse in patients with VT.
21. **Is the medical history of any value with wide complex tachycardia?**
    Yes—if the patient has had a myocardial infarction, there is a 98% chance that it is VT.
22. **Can you distinguish VT from SVT with aberrancy by vital signs?**
    No. Both may have stable or unstable vital signs, depending on the patient.
24. **Can the heart rate help to distinguish VT from SVT with aberrancy?**
    No. There is too much overlap between the two.
25. **How can you distinguish VT from SVT with aberrancy on a rhythm strip?**
    A few simple rules make the diagnosis of VT on a rhythm strip:
    (a) If the width of the complexes is greater than 3½ boxes, it is more likely to be VT.

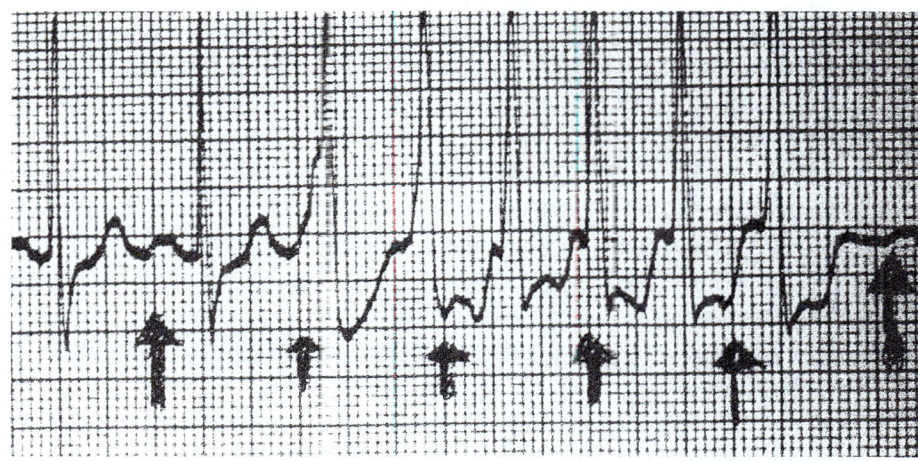

FIGURE 30.8 Ventricular tachycardia with visible P waves (evidence of atrioventricular dissociation).

(b) Atrioventricular dissociation, which is recognized by the P waves marching through the QRS complexes, is present with VT (Figure 30.8).
(c) A P wave may capture the ventricle at precisely the correct instant, leading to a "capture beat," which looks like a typical PQRST complex in the middle of the wide complex tachycardia.
(d) A fusion beat may be seen, which results when the ventricle is stimulated from itself and from the atrium at the same time. Its width is, therefore, less than a beat originating from the ventricle.

26. **Are all of the mental gyrations of attempting to distinguish VT from SVT with aberrancy worth the effort?**
No. Simply assume that it is VT and treat accordingly.

27. **What is the first drug to give a patient with stable wide complex tachycardia? Why?**
If the rhythm is VT or you are uncertain, give amiodarone 150 mg IV over 10 min. This is because VT is six times more common than SVT with aberrancy. Give repeat doses of amiodarone up to 2.2 g/24 hours, but beware of hypotension.

28. **What should you do if amiodarone does not work and the patient is still stable?**
If you are still certain that it is VT, repeat the amiodarone 150 mg IV over 10 min.

29. **What should you do if SVT with aberrant conduction is highly suspected?**
Attempt a vagal maneuver, but realize that it is about as useful as a screen door on a submarine most of the time. Give adenosine 6 mg rapid IV push, and if there is no conversion, try a 12-mg rapid IV push. Transport with continuous cardiac and patient monitoring.

30. **What if the patient becomes unstable en route?**
Synchronized cardioversion is the next step.

31. **Besides VT and SVT with aberrancy, what else can cause wide complex tachycardia?**
Hyperkalemia, torsades de pointes, and tricyclic antidepressant poisoning should be considered.

32. **A patient with stable VT suddenly loses pulses and becomes obtunded. What do you do?**
Start cardiopulmonary resuscitation (CPR) and immediately countershock the patient with 200 J monophasic or 120–200 J of biphasic depolarization as soon as the defibrillator is available. This is device specific. If the patient fails to convert, countershock with 360 J monophasic or a higher dose of biphasic depolarization. Again, know your defibrillator, as these energies are device specific. If the patient is still pulseless, start CPR, hyperventilate with 100% oxygen, intubate, and give IV epinephrine. (See advanced cardiac life support [ACLS] protocols for dosing.) Alternatively, 40 U IV vasopressin can be given to replace the first or second dose of epinephrine. If the patient is still pulseless, the ACLS algorithm recommends a third shock equivalent to 360 J monophasic and then amiodarone 300 mg IV or lidocaine 1–1.5 mg/kg.

33. **What is the rationale for this treatment approach?**
Most successful resuscitations depend on early CPR and defibrillation. Epinephrine restores coronary artery perfusion and increases the odds that countershock will restore spontaneous circulation.

34. **Is there any practical advantage to giving high-dose epinephrine to patients in cardiac arrest?**
No data prove that high-dose epinephrine improves survival or neurologic recovery compared with standard-dose epinephrine. Until such data become available, high-dose epinephrine should not be used routinely.

Cardiac Dysrhythmias

35. What is asystole? Under what circumstances is it reversible?
Asystole is most often a flat-line confirmation of death rather than a dysrhythmia to be treated (Figure 30.9). Rarely it results from heightened vagal tone or complete heart block and is potentially reversible.

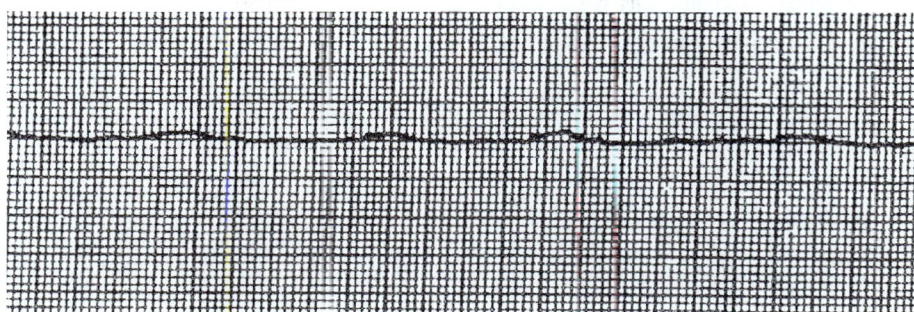

FIGURE 30.9 Asystole.

37. When is it necessary to confirm asystole in two leads?
The ACLS authors made this recommendation on the basis of one case report of a patient who was actually in ventricular fibrillation in two of the three leads, although the third lead showed asystole. The author of the case report surmised that ventricular fibrillation may have a vector (direction) and that all cases of asystole should be confirmed in two leads. Others say that this theory is hogwash and that the better reason to confirm asystole in two leads is to be sure that the monitoring equipment and leads are attached properly. You will find many more cases in which leads have fallen off than in which patients have ventricular fibrillation with a vector.

38. Should transcutaneous pacing be tried in all cases of asystole?
Absolutely not. Prehospital research has proved that the chance of reestablishing spontaneous circulation with pacing is very low if the period of asystole is more than 5 min. Save pacing for the rare patient with symptomatic bradycardia who does not respond to atropine administration.

39. What drugs are recommended for asystole?
After the patient is intubated and IV access is obtained, 1 mg epinephrine or 40 U vasopressin may be given to help restore circulation. If this is ineffective, epinephrine can be repeated every 3–5 min. Atropine is no longer recommended by the American Heart Association for treatment of asystole. If the patient remains asystolic after intubation, oxygenation, and ACLS drugs, seriously consider pronouncing the patient dead in the field, thus avoiding needless increased costs to the family.

40. Define absolute and relative bradycardia.
Absolute bradycardia is less than 60 bpm. Relative bradycardia refers to a heart rate above 60 in patients with low cardiac output who may benefit from an increased rate. Both absolute and relative bradycardia may need to be treated according to the ACLS algorithm.

41. When is a pulse of 40–59 bpm considered normal?
In a well-conditioned athlete, this is a normal resting pulse.

42. **Bradycardia should be treated under what three circumstances?**
    (a) Symptoms. The simple fact that a patient has a heart rate of 50 does not mean that you should bring out the atropine needle.
    (b) Mobitz 2 second-degree heart block (Figure 30.10).
    (c) Third-degree heart block (Figure 30.11).

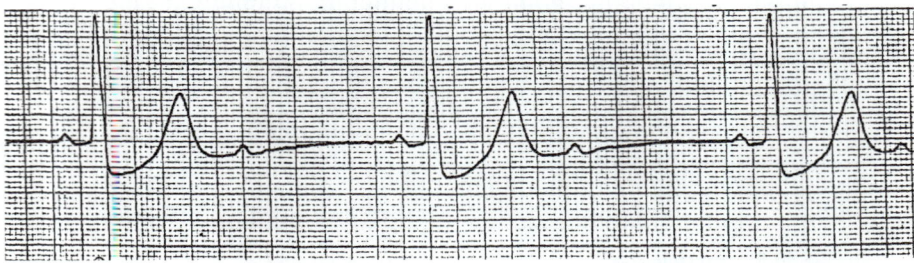

FIGURE 30.10 Mobitz type 2 atrioventricular block leading to bradycardia.

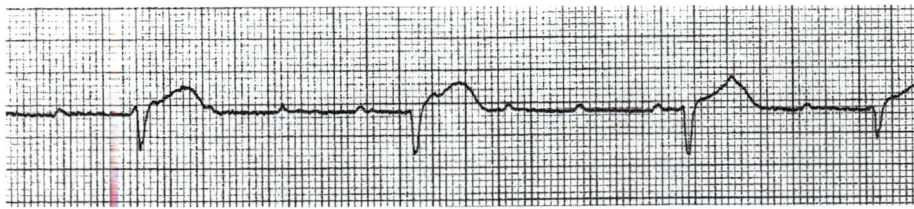

FIGURE 30.11 Complete (third-degree) heart block (in the setting of an acute inferior wall myocardial infarction).

43. **What is the first-line drug for bradycardia? How does it work?**
    Atropine exerts a strong anticholinergic effect on the AV node, thus blocking the bradycardic effect of the vagus nerve.
44. **When does atropine have no effect at all?**
    Atropine does not work in heart transplant patients, in whom the vagus nerve has been cut. Epinephrine is the drug of choice in transplant patients. Atropine may worsen bradycardias that result from heart block below the AV node, which seems paradoxical. However, atropine is still a first-line drug for bradycardia. If the ventricular rate decreases after a dose, be prepared to use epinephrine.
45. **What if additional rate increasing drugs are needed?**
    Dopamine 2–10 µg/kg/min is acceptable as is epinephrine infusion starting at 2–10 µg/min and titrating to response.
46. **A patient in third-degree heart block has a few premature ventricular contractions (PVCs). Should amiodarone or lidocaine be given?**
    No. Lidocaine and amiodarone suppress the ventricular pacemakers that are keeping the patient alive.

Cardiac Dysrhythmias

47. **What should I know about transcutaneous pacing?**
    Arrange the pads just to the left of the sternum in front and the spine in back. Most patients will capture with less than 70 mA. Capture may not occur in patients with big chests, chronic obstructive pulmonary disease, dilated cardiomyopathies, and pleural or pericardial effusions. It is proven therapy for bradycardia, as opposed to drugs that may have downsides, such as atropine. Benzodiazepines are often required concomitantly because the electric shocks can be painful.

48. **What is torsades de pointes?**
    It literally means "twisting of the points," which describes the spindle appearance of this unique type of polymorphic ventricular tachycardia (Figure 30.12).

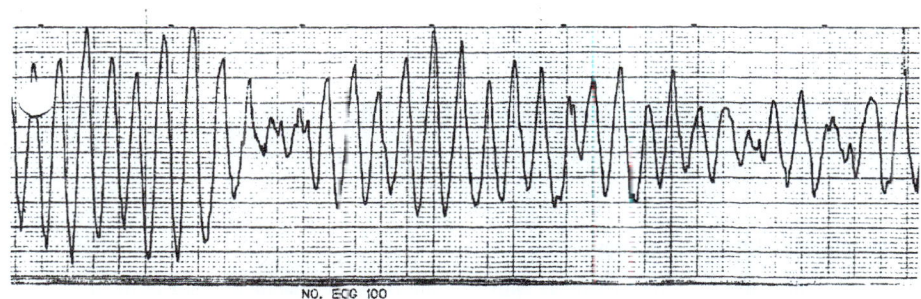

FIGURE 30.12   Torsades de pointes.

49. **What causes a patient to go into torsades?**
    Antidysrhythmic drugs (quinidine, procainamide, disopyramide, sotalol), antihistamines (benadryl, hismanal, seldane), electrolyte disturbances (hypokalemia, hypomagnesemia), and cardiac ischemia.

50. **How does torsades differ from garden variety monomorphic VT?**
    Torsades is often intermittent and fast (>300 bpm), and every beat looks different from the beat before it (i.e., polymorphic). It is associated with a long QT interval on the rhythm strip recorded before the patient develops torsades.

51. **How does treatment differ for torsades and monomorphic VT?**
    The primary treatment of stable patients with torsades involves removing the cause that lead to the prolonged QT interval, speeding the rhythm with dopamine, and/or overdrive pacing at the hospital with a transvenous pacer. By speeding the sinus rate, the QT interval therefore shortens and the propensity of the heart to go back into the torsades "spindle" is diminished. Magnesium sulfate, 2 g IV, is also an effective treatment for torsades and seems to work even in patients who are not hypomagnesemic. Lidocaine and amiodarone are ineffective, and IV procainamide and other class IA antiarrhythmics are absolutely contraindicated because they prolong the QT interval even further.

52. **What if a patient has a long spindle of torsades and becomes unstable?**
    Defibrillate the patient with 200 J. Multiple shocks may be required before the patient can be stabilized.

53. **What do you do about PVCs? Do they always require therapy?**
    No. They are common in adult medical patients (Figure 30.13).

Clinical Care

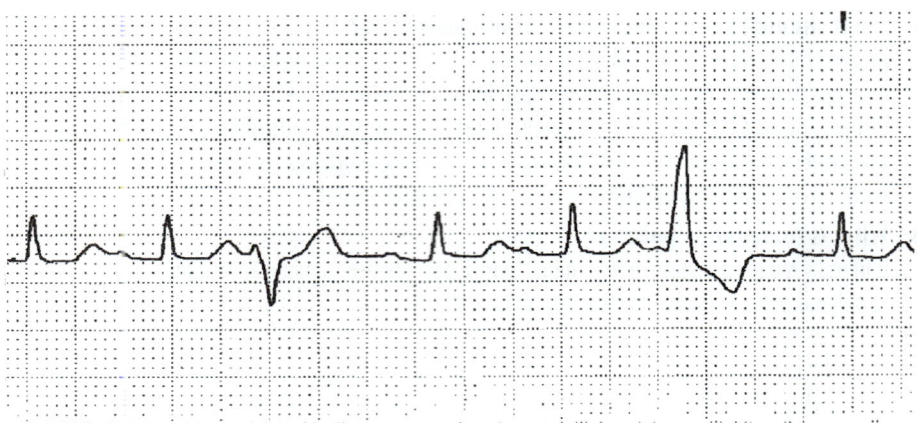

FIGURE 30.13   Multifocal premature ventricular contractions.

Pearls and Pitfalls

1. Treat the patient, not the monitor.
2. VT is six times more common than SVT with aberrancy. Assume a wide complex tachycardia is VT until proven otherwise. Look for the telltale signs of VT including a QRS complex greater than $3^{1}/_{2}$ boxes, capture beats, fusion beats, AV dissociation, and concordance (polarity on a 12 lead in leads V1–V6 is either all up or all down). Treating VT as SVT with aberrant conduction (i.e., giving verapamil to a VT case) can cause cardiovascular collapse.
3. Irregular narrow complex tachycardias including atrial fibrillation, atrial flutter with variable block, atrial tachycardia with variable block, and multifocal atrial tachycardia do not respond to adenosine.
4. Look before you leap. Take a few seconds to study the tracing before acting.
5. Waiting too long to administer life-saving therapies such as transvenous pacing, cardioversion, and antidysrhythmic drugs will decrease the potential for the desired response.
6. Prepare to deal with the potential downsides of therapies. For instance, amiodarone causes hypotension, dopamine and epinephrine can exacerbate ischemia and trigger ventricular dysrhythmias, atropine can exacerbate heart block, and transcutaneous pacing is painful and may require benzodiazepines.
7. Be careful to differentiate polymorphic torsades de pointes from monomorphic VT. It differs in its response to lidocaine and amiodarone, its treatment (magnesium, overdrive pacing, chronotropes), its propensity to recur, and the need for multiple countershocks until the QT interval can be shortened.

References

1. Field JM, Hazinski MF, Sayre MR, et al. 2010 American Heart Association Guidelines for Cardiopulmonary Resuscitation and Emergency Cardiac Care. Circulation 122; Supplement, Part 8: Adult Advanced Cardiovascular Life Support, pp. S729–S767
2. Harken AH. Cardiac dysrhythmias. Sci Am I(3):1–8, 1996.
3. Lowenstein SR, Halperin B, Reiter MJ. Paroxysmal supraventricular tachycardias. J Emerg Med 14:39–51, 1996.

4. Wagner GS. Marriot's Practical Electrocardiography, 9th ed. Baltimore: Lippincott Williams & Wilkins, 1994.
5. Wellens HJ, Bart FW, Lie KI. The value of the electrocardiogram in the differential diagnosis of a tachycardia with a widened QRS complex. Am J Med 64:27–33 1978.
6. Brugada P, Brugada J, Mont L, et al. A new approach to the differential diagnosis of a regular tachycardia with a wide QRS complex. Circulation 83:1649–1659, 1991.
7. Kao LW, Furbee RB. Drug induced Q–T prolongation. Med Clin N Am 89 1125–1144, 2005.
8. Gurevitz, OT, Ammash NM, Malouf JF, et al: Comparative efficacy of monophasic and biphasic waveforms for transthoracic cardioversion of atrial fibrillation and atrial flutter. Am Heart 149:316–321, 2005.
9. Raghavan AV, Decker WW, Meloy TD. Management of atrial fibrillation in the emergency department. Emerg Med Clin N Am 23:1127–1139, 2005.
10. Hood RE, Shorofsky SR. Management of arrhythmias in the emergency cepartment. Cardiol Clin 24:125–133, 2006.
11. Kudenchuk, PJ. Advanced cardiac life support antiarrhythmic drugs. Cardiol Clin N Am 20(1):79–87, 2002.

Cardiac Arrest

Jason Haukoos, MD, MSc

1. **How common is out-of-hospital cardiac arrest?**
   Approximately 350,000 people in the United States experience cardiac arrest each year.
2. **What percentage of all cardiac arrest patients survive to hospital discharge?**
   Approximately 5%.
3. **What are the most common causes of cardiopulmonary arrest?**
   The most common cause of cardiac arrest is acute coronary syndrome resulting from underlying coronary artery disease. This syndrome results in ventricular fibrillation (VF), the most commonly encountered initial rhythm in patients who experience cardiac arrest. Other etiologies of VF include drug toxicity, electrolyte disturbances (e.g., hyperkalemia), and prolonged hypoxia. If left untreated, VF will progress to asystole due to severe hypoxia and acidemia. Other causes of asystole include drug toxicity, electrolyte disturbances, and hypothermia. Pulseless electrical activity (PEA) also often results from prolonged, untreated VF. Other causes of PEA include hypovolemia, hypoxia, cardiac tamponade, massive pulmonary embolism, tension pneumothorax, profound acidosis, electrolyte disturbances, hypothermia, drug toxicity, or acute coronary syndrome.
4. **How should ventricular fibrillation be treated?**
   Standard treatment consists of immediate defibrillation. Recommended energy levels range from 120–200 J (biphasic). Stacked shocks are no longer recommended. Instead, providers should give one shock at a high energy level (e.g., 200 J biphasic), then resume chest compressions in an effort to minimize compression interruptions (Figure 31.1).
5. **How are chest compressions best performed, and why is it important to minimize chest compression interruptions?**
   In an adult, chest compressions should be performed at 100 per minute with a depth of approximately 2 in. (4–5 cm). The chest must be allowed to fully recoil after each compression, and compression–recoil times should be approximately equal. For best results, the patient should lie supine on a hard surface with the rescuer kneeling or standing at his or her side. If performed correctly, blood flow generated by chest compressions delivers a small but critical amount of oxygen and glucose to the brain and heart. It is important to minimize chest compression interruptions (e.g., to check for a pulse or evaluate the cardiac rhythm) because this results in a no-flow state and it becomes increasingly difficult to generate adequate blood flow after each interruption.
6. **What about chest compressions without ventilation?**
   The 2010 American Heart Association Guidelines for Cardiopulmonary Resuscitation (CPR) and Emergency Cardiac Care changed the basic life support sequence from "A-B-C" (Airway, Breathing, Chest Compressions) to "C-A-B" (Chest Compressions, Airway, Breathing). Although the best CPR method includes coordination of compressions with ventilations, rescuers should not delay initiation or interrupt the performance of chest compressions while providing ventilator support. It is thought that rescue breathing is not essential

Cardiac Arrest

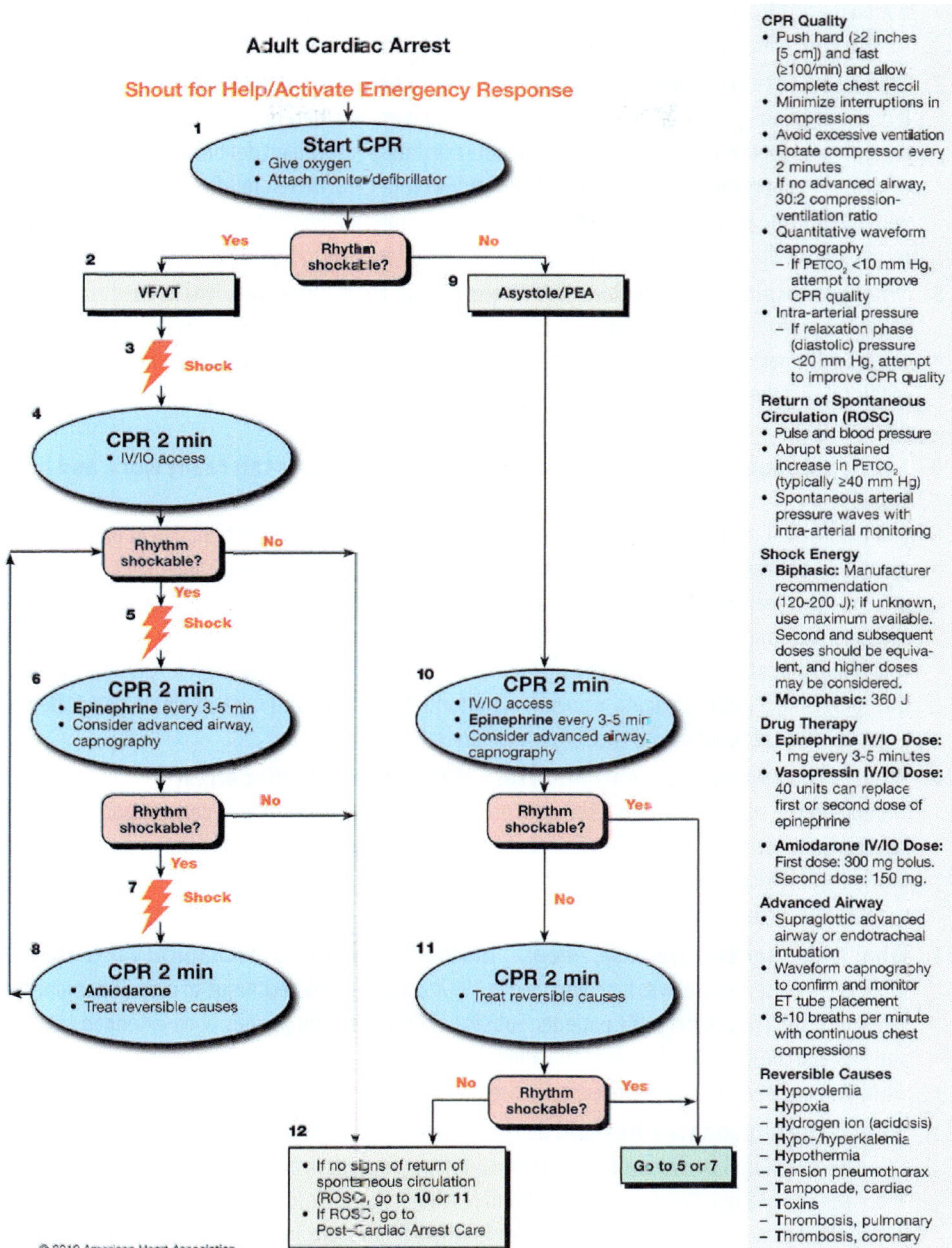

FIGURE 31.1 The ACLS pulseless arrest algorithm. Reprinted with permission. 2010 American Heart Association Guidelines for Cardiopulmonary Resuscitation and Emergency Cardiovascular Care, Part 8: Adult Advanced Cardiovascular Life Support Circulation.2010;122[suppl] 3]:S729-S767 ©2010 American Heart Association, Inc.

during the first 5 min of CPR. If the airway is open, occasional gasps and passive chest recoil likely provide some gas exchange.

7. **What percentage of patients with VF survive to hospital discharge?**
   It depends, but in general, if a patient develops VF and is immediately defibrillated, his or her survival percentage is approximately 80%. For every minute that transpires without defibrillation, this percentage decreases by approximately 10% (without CPR) or 5% (with CPR). Therefore, after approximately 8 min without CPR the patient's survival rate approaches 0%. This highlights the importance of immediate recognition of the onset of cardiac arrest, initiation of CPR, and performance of defibrillation.

8. **What prehospital interventions have been shown to improve survival in cardiac arrest?**
   Chest compressions and defibrillation. The most critical interventions during the first minutes of cardiac arrest are the performance of effective chest compressions followed by defibrillation. The only exception to this rule is if the patient arrests in front of the care provider who has the ability to perform immediate defibrillation.

9. **I've heard about "CPR before defibrillation." What is it, does this really work, and if so, how?**
   CPR before defibrillation refers to performing CPR for 2–3 min prior to defibrillation in patients with prolonged, untreated VF. This is based on the following evidence: (a) when you immediately defibrillate prolonged untreated VF, the resultant postshock rhythm is commonly PEA or asystole, two less treatable rhythms; and (b) performing CPR for a short duration prior to defibrillation increases the likelihood of converting the patient into a perfusing rhythm. CPR before defibrillation is thought to "prime the pump," thus providing a better circulatory environment for defibrillation, and it has been demonstrated to improve return of spontaneous circulation and survival.

10. **What is the appropriate ventilation rate of someone in cardiac arrest?**
    The appropriate ventilation rate is 12 breaths/min. Unfortunately, inadvertent hyperventilation in cardiac arrest is quite common. Two studies reported excessive ventilation during resuscitation by prehospital providers, and excessive ventilation has been demonstrated to be associated with decreased return of spontaneous circulation and survival.

11. **What is the "squeeze, release, release" method of providing mechanical ventilation?**
    "Squeeze, release, release" was first described in 1997 as a bag–mask technique to provide appropriate levels of ventilation to pediatric patients. Subsequently, this technique has been extended to adult patients, and consists of performing ventilation by squeezing the bag of a bag–valve at a rate consistent with someone saying, "squeeze, release, release."

12. **What is the impedance threshold device (ITD)?**
    This device is placed between the endotracheal tube or face mask and the bag–valve device and is about the size of a golf ball. It prevents influx of respiratory gases into the chest from chest wall recoil during chest compressions, thus lowering the intrathoracic pressure and improving blood return to the heart. It has been demonstrated in small studies to improve blood flow to the heart (i.e., coronary perfusion pressure) and subsequent return of spontaneous circulation. Definitive studies are currently being performed, and this simple device may serve to augment prehospital treatment of cardiac arrest in the future. However a recent study published in the New England Journal of Medicine failed to demonstrate a survival benefit to using the ITD.

Cardiac Arrest

13. **Does advanced cardiac life support (ACLS) work?**
    It depends. Only one study has systematically evaluated the addition of ACLS to an existing EMS system with basic life support and defibrillation capabilities. This study performed in Canada demonstrated no survival benefit for out-of-hospital cardiac arrest with the addition of ACLS services. This highlights the importance of the performance of good basic life support, including CPR and defibrillation.

14. **What are the adult doses of ACLS drugs?**
    Epinephrine: 1 mg IV push every 3–5 min.
    Atropine: 1 mg IV push every 3–5 min (maximum of 3 mg).
    Vasopressin: 40 U IV may replace the first or second dose of epinephrine.
    Amiodarone: 300 mg IV push (may be repeated at 150 mg IV push).
    Lidocaine: 1.0–1.5 mg/kg IV (may be repeated at 0.5–0.75 mg/kg IV every 5–10 min to a maximum of 3 mg/kg).
    Magnesium: 1–2 g IV push.

15. **How do pediatric advanced life support drug doses differ from adult doses?**
    Epinephrine: 0.01 mg/kg (0.1 mL/kg 1:10,000 IV push every 3–5 minutes.
    Atropine: 0.02 mg/kg IV push (minimum dose: 0.1 mg).
    Vasopressin: not indicated in pediatric arrest.
    Amiodarone: 5 mg/kg IV push (may repeat up to 15 mg/kg).
    Lidocaine: same as adult dosing.
    Glucose: 1 g/kg IV (D_{10}W: 5–10 mL/kg; D_{25}W: 2–4 mL/kg; D_{50}W: 1–2 mL/kg).

16. **How does defibrillation differ in pediatric arrest?**
    The lowest energy dose for effective defibrillation and the upper limit for safe defibrillation in infants and children are unknown. Biphasic energy dose is 2 J/kg.

17. **How do you determine the appropriate endotracheal size for a child?**
    (Age/4) + 4. For example, a 4-year-old child should require a 5.0 endotracheal tube: (4/4) + 4 = 1 + 4 = 5.

18. **What is an intraosseous (IO) line and what ACLS medications can be given through it?**
    Intraosseous needle placement provides a route for administering fluid, blood, and medications. An IO line is as efficient as an intravenous line and can be inserted quickly even in the most poorly perfused patients. The proximal tibia is the preferred site for an IO line. The needle should be inserted perpendicular to the bone with a screwing motion. It will release slightly when the marrow cavity is entered. Once in place and secured, the IO line should be flushed with 10 mL normal saline. All ACLS drugs can be given through an IO line.

19. **What is the most common cause of pediatric arrest?**
    Respiratory arrest is the most common cause of pediatric arrest. The first step in these situations, then, is to establish an airway and provide oxygenation and ventilation.

20. **What is "mild therapeutic hypothermia" and why is it used in cardiac arrest?**
    Mild therapeutic hypothermia describes the process of cooling a patient's core temperature to between 32 and 34°C for approximately 24 hours following return of spontaneous circulation. It is used in the

postresuscitation period to improve long-term neurological recovery and is generally well tolerated without significant complications.

21. **What benefit is expected when using mild therapeutic hypothermia?**
   The largest clinical trial to date demonstrated an improvement of 16% (55% good neurological recovery in the group of patients who received hypothermia versus 39% in the group who did not receive hypothermia) to 6 months postarrest. This translates to a number needed to treat for benefit to occur of only six patients.

22. **When should mild therapeutic hypothermia be initiated and is there a role for initiating it in the prehospital setting?**
   Although the major clinical study allowed for target core temperature to be achieved within 4 hours (and the median time to achieving target temperatures was 8 hours), most experts believe it should be started as soon as possible after return of spontaneous circulation. Unfortunately, little research has been done to best inform when to begin cooling, the optimal rate of cooling, or the duration of cooling. Some EMS agencies have begun initiating cooling prior to hospital arrival based on the assumption that beginning this process earlier has benefit. As yet, no evidence supports this approach.

23. **How does the management of traumatic arrest differ from that of nontraumatic cardiac arrest?**
   In traumatic arrest, closed-chest CPR is less effective. In trauma, the cause of the arrest may be cardiac tamponade, tension pneumothorax, or exsanguination from the thorax, abdomen, or extremities. Control of external hemorrhage, needle decompression for tension pneumothorax, and immediate transport to a trauma center are indicated.

24. **What is the most common injury found in those patients who survive traumatic arrest?**
   Pericardial tamponade.

25. **What other etiologies lead to cardiac arrest following trauma?**
   (a) Hypoxia due to respiratory arrest, airway obstruction, or tracheobronchial injury.
   (b) Severe head injury with secondary cardiovascular collapse.
   (c) Massive blood loss from thoracoabdominal trauma, leading to to hypovolemia.
   (d) Cardiopulmonary obstruction from tension pneumothorax, air embolism, or pericardial tamponade.

26. **How does treatment of cardiac arrest differ in a patient who is pregnant?**
   The best hope for fetal survival is maternal survival. The principal therapeutic differences in this setting include performing chest compressions higher on the sternum to account for the elevated diaphragm from the enlarged uterus and placing the patient in the left lateral position at approximately 15–30° from the horizontal plane. Tilting the patient shifts the gravid uterus to the left and away from the inferior vena cava and aorta, thus improving venous return to the heart and cardiac output, respectively.

27. **When may prehospital resuscitation efforts be terminated?**
   Prehospital resuscitation may be discontinued by EMS personnel when a valid no-CPR order is present or when the patient is deemed nonresuscitatable after an adequate trial of ACLS, including successful endotracheal intubation airway management, achievement of IV access and administration of indicated medications, determination of persistent asystole or an agonal rhythm, and when no reversible cause for the arrest is identified.

28. Where can I find more information about the management of cardiac arrest?
Visit the http://www.americanheart.org/ Web site.

Pearls and Pitfalls

1. CPR and defibrillation are the most important prehospital determinants of survival from out-of-hospital cardiac arrest.
2. Chest compression technique is critical to providing excellent treatment of patients in cardiac arrest. Do not overlook basic life support maneuvers.
3. Minimize chest compression interruptions during resuscitation. Each time CPR is interrupted, it becomes increasingly difficult to restore adequate cardiac output once CPR is resumed.
4. Do not hyperventilate patients in cardiac arrest. The appropriate ventilatory rate is 12 breaths/min, which equates to using the phrase "squeeze, release, release" as you use the bag-valve.
5. If intravenous access cannot be obtained, consider moving quickly to IO access. Administration of ACLS medications using an IO line is thought to be better than administering them through an endotracheal tube.
6. Remember, survival from out-of-hospital cardiac arrest is low, but prehospital medical care providers are the group most likely to impact this disease process. Diligence in resuscitation is important when approaching someone in cardiac arrest.

References

1. Aufderheide TP, Nichol G, Rea TD, et al. A trial of an impedance threshold device in out-of-hopsital cardiac arrest. N Engl J Med 2011;365:798-806.
2. 2010 American Heart Association Guidelines for Cardiopulmonary Resuscitation and Emergency Cardiovascular Care. Circulation;122:S640–S946, 2010.
3. Wik L, Hansen TB, Fylling F, et al. Delaying defibrillation to give basic cardiopulmonary resuscitation to patients with out-of-hospital ventricular fibrillation: A randomized trial. JAMA 289:1389–1395, 2003.
4. Aufderheide TP, Laure KG. Death by hyperventilation: A common and life-threatening problem during cardiopulmonary resuscitation. Crit Care Med 32:S345–S351, 2004.
5. Abella BS, Alvarado JP, Myklebust H, et a l. Quality of cardiopulmonary resuscitation during in-hospital cardiac arrest. JAMA 293:305–310, 2005.
6. Gausche M, Lewis RJ, Stratton SJ, et al. Effect of out-of-hospital pediatric endotracheal intubation on survival and neurologic outcome: a controlled clinical trial. JAMA 283:783–790, 2000.
7. Aufderheide TP, Pirrallo RG, Provo TA, et al. Clinical evaluation of an inspiratory impedance threshold device during standard cardiopulmonary resuscitation in patients with out-of-hospital cardiac arrest. Crit Care Med 33:734–740, 2005.
8. Stiell IG, Wells GA, Field B, et al. Advanced cardiac life support in out-of-hospital cardiac arrest. N Engl J Med 351:647–656, 2004.
9. Hopson LR, Hirsh E, Delgado J, et al. Guidelines for withholding or termination of resuscitation in prehospital traumatic cardiopulmonary arrest: A joint position paper from the National Association of EMS Physicians Standards and Clinical Practice Committee and the American College of Surgeons Committee on Trauma. Prehosp Emerg Care 7:141–146, 2003.
10. Bailey ED, Wydro GC, Cone DC for the National Association of EMS Physicians Standards and Clinical Practice Committee. Terminations of resuscitation in the prehospital setting for adult patients suffering nontraumatic cardiac arrest. Prehosp Emerg Care 4:190–195, 2000.

Overview of Shock

Robert McNamara, MD, FAAEM

1. **When does the body experience shock?**
   The body experiences shock when the oxygen demands of the tissues cannot be met by the circulatory system. When this happens, the tissues of the body are forced to revert to a much less effective form of energy production called anaerobic respiration. In most cases shock is caused by a problem with one or more of the components of the oxygen delivery system. In some cases, there is an increased demand for oxygen that cannot be met by the delivery system. This is called high output failure. For the purposes of this chapter we focus on shock secondary to damage of the oxygenation system.

2. **What are the components of the oxygen delivery system?**
   In order for oxygenation of the tissues to occur, there must be an intact oxygen delivery system with
   (a) An intact airway and respiratory system.
   (b) An adequate amount of normally functioning hemoglobin.
   (c) A closed circulatory system that has a normal volume and tone.
   (d) A normally functioning heart to pump.
   (f) Tissues that can properly offload and use the oxygen for energy production.

3. **What are the different types of shock?**
   (a) Hypovolemic: Due to a low circulatory volume. Causes a decrease in the pressure which perfuses tissues and therefore decreases the amount of blood and oxygen delivered.
   (b) Hemorrhagic: Causes both a decrease in volume and a decrease in oxygen-carrying capacity through loss of hemoglobin. (Some classify this as a subset of hypovolemic shock.)
   (c) Cardiogenic: Due to a poorly pumping heart. This can be intrinsic secondary to heart muscle damage or valvular disease. It can also be extrinsic due to compression of the heart from the outside by either the pericardium filling with blood or fluid and causing tamponade or due to pressure from a collapsed lung in the case of a tension pneumothorax. In both cases, the problem is decreased heart filling and therefore decreased output.
   (d) Neurogenic: Affects the vascular tone of the circulatory system by decreasing neurologic input to the smooth muscle of the vessels allowing them to relax and the blood vessels to dilate. This is generally only seen with a significant spinal cord injury.
   (e) Septic: In sepsis both the heart and the blood vessels can be affected by the toxins released by bacteria. The vessels lose tone and become leaky (low circulatory volume). Early on, the heart may be pumping vigorously and the picture is a high output failure, but eventually cardiac function also becomes depressed.

(f) Anaphylactic: In true anaphylaxis the vascular system both loses tone and becomes leaky resulting in shock from inadequate perfusion. Other signs of anaphylaxis are generally also present (dyspnea, wheezing, swelling, hives).

4. **What is anaerobic respiration?**
When the oxygen supply is able to keep up with demand, the cells make energy by aerobic respiration. This is a very efficient form of energy production that makes a lot of energy for cells to use to survive and function normally. When the demand for oxygen required by the cell cannot be supplied by the body, the cells are forced to produce energy by a much more inefficient means called anaerobic respiration. Anaerobic respiration produces a lot less energy and byproducts such as lactic acid that are toxic. It does not, however, require oxygen. Anaerobic respiration cannot meet the cells' energy need for very long and soon the cells will become damaged and die if they cannot make more energy by switching back to aerobic respiration. This process of cellular damage and death during anaerobic respiration is the basis of shock

5. **What are the stages of shock?**
Shock progresses through a series of stages as perfusion of the vital organs decreases and the body works to compensate. How quickly a patient passes through these stages depends on the degree of insult to the oxygen delivery system and the body's ability to compensate.
The outward signs of shock are the result of this battle between decreased perfusion and increasing compensation.

(a) Stage 1: This usually occurs when modest amounts of blood or volume are lost. The signs of this early stage are related to the effects of altered oxygen delivery on the brain, the most oxygen sensitive organ of the body. The patient may become anxious or agitated, not necessarily knowing what is wrong. The heart rate and blood pressure may be relatively normal.

(b) Stage 2: As further volume is lost, the body will begin to compensate by increasing the force with which the heart pumps. This causes a widening of the "pulse pressure". The systolic blood pressure goes up due to increased contractility and the diastolic drops due to decreased vascular volume or tone. There may also be the beginning of tachycardia. Respiratory rate will increase and mental status will become more confused. Late in this stage the skin may become cool as the body begins diverting blood from the less essential organs such as the skin to the more essential organs, including the brain and heart.

(c) Stage 3: The patient in this stage looks more like the typical picture one thinks of as shock. The mental status is abnormal. The patient is very tachycardic and pale as the body tries to maintain adequate oxygen delivery to essential organs. The blood pressure drops in this stage.

(d) Stage 4: The body decompensates. The patient becomes unresponsive; the respiratory rate is agonal. The heart may go from tachycardia to bradycardia as it also becomes hypoxic. The blood pressure drops as vascular tone can no longer be maintained and volume is very low. Death is imminent.

It is important to remember that the clinical presentation may not be typical in all patients. A normal blood pressure in the elderly may actually be relative hypotension and indicate hemodynamic instability. A normal heart rate in patients on beta blockers is not reassuring as the medication may mask a compensatory tachycardia.

6. What organs are affected by shock?
Every single organ system is affected by decreased perfusion. Some are more sensitive than others. The brain is generally the most sensitive organ to alterations in oxygen delivery and therefore a change in brain function is often the earliest and most subtle sign of decreased perfusion. Because the skin is the most resilient to shock and can last the longest with decreased perfusion, its blood supply is usually the first to be diverted. This shows up as diaphoresis, cool skin, and pallor. Bone, muscle, and then the gastrointestinal/genitourinary systems are generally affected next. This continues until the hypoperfusion is reversed or until death occurs.

7. What are the long-term effects of poor organ perfusion?
Each organ has its own threshold for irreversible injury. The brain is the most sensitive organ to hypoxia and even short-term hypoxia can lead to permanent anoxic brain injury. There can be liver failure and acute renal failure. Damage to lung tissue can lead to capillary leaking and acute respiratory distress syndrome, and body-wide tissue hypoxia can lead to cell damage triggering disseminated intravascular coagulation. The key is how long each kind of organ or cell has been deprived of adequate oxygenation.

8. What is the treatment of shock?
The two general strategies in shock treatment are (a) stop or at least lessen the cause for the shock and (b)) administer treatments directed at restoring the oxygen delivery system. Bleeding needs to be controlled by surgery if necessary. Problems with pump function need to be reversed. For example, if a tension pneumothorax is the cause of the problem, needle decompression will temporarily relieve the pressure causing decreased blood return to the heart. Other treatments, depending on the cause, include fluids, supplemental oxygen, assisted ventilation, agents to increase cardiac contractility and improve vascular tone, and proper antibiotic therapy.

9. Do fluids help in the treatment of shock?
There are some fairly clear indications for use of fluids in shock but some controversy exists over the use of fluids in hemorrhagic shock. Fluids are administered in most causes of shock. In the setting of cardiogenic shock fluids can potentially worsen pulmonary edema so providers need to be cautious if the patient has rales on lung examination. The biggest controversy relates to the use of IV fluids to treat shock from bleeding. Research has shown that the prehospital use of IV fluids may adversely affect trauma patients suffering from shock in two ways. The first is that the time taken in establishing an IV and starting fluids will delay transport and the definitive treatment needed to stop the bleeding. The second issue is that increasing blood volume using fluids dilutes clotting factors and disrupts clots by increasing vascular pressure. The research regarding this effect involved patients with penetrating trauma. It is useful to obtain and follow the recommendations of the local trauma centers. Regardless, the most important issue in hemorrhagic shock is to stop the cause of the bleeding as quickly as possible. Quoting a paramedic instructor, "The two most important drugs in the treatment of trauma are oxygen and gasoline and they both go in the carburetor."

10. What kind of fluids can I give my patient?
There are two kinds of fluids suitable for use in the prehospital setting: normal saline and lactated Ringers. Both crystalloids are isotonic (the same osmolarity as blood) and are considered safe. Other fluids such as hypertonic saline or colloids such as Dextran, Hespan, or albumin have been studied for use as resuscitation fluids but have not been widely adopted as the cost–benefit ratio is unclear.

Overview of Shock

11. **Should I get the IV started first then transport?**
    In patients suffering from traumatic injury, the most important factor in survival is rapid transport to a trauma center where definitive care can be provided. For this reason, time should not be spent on-scene in establishing IV lines. If transport is delayed due to other factors such as entrapment, IV fluids can be started. Otherwise, transport without delay and establish the IV fluids while transporting.

12. **We carry MAST on the rigs but do not use them any more. Why?**
    Military antishock trousers (MAST) were developed on the model of pressurized flight suits used by fighter pilots while doing very high G maneuvers. These suits would constrict and shunt blood to the brain preventing the pilot from passing out. MAST trousers were initially used in the hopes of also shunting or forcing blood from the less essential lower limbs to the more vital organs. Many different mechanisms were proposed for how they worked. It was hypothesized that they may have shunted blood from the lower extremities by directly forcing the blood out under pressure. This was called an autotransfusion from the extremities to the trunk. Another was that the trousers increased the peripheral vascular resistance of the limbs causing decreased extremity perfusion and keeping the blood in the trunk. However, studies never showed either of these facts to be true and MAST passed out of favor in the mid to late 1980s. Some pairs of MAST are still out there but there are few protocols left that include them. (See Chapter 83.)

13. **Why don't we give blood products on the ambulance?**
    There are two types of blood products. The first are the traditional blood products such as packed red blood cells (PRBCs) and plasma. Plasma and PRBCs are used in the hospital to treat hemorrhagic shock. The problem is that they must be kept refrigerated, and there are complications associated with their use such as transfusion reactions. For these reasons, and because of the limited supply of blood products, these are reserved for use in the hospital setting.
    Some research has been done in the area of synthetic oxygen-carrying hemoglobin substitutes. These substances have not yet shown any benefit for trauma patients in the prehospital setting and remain solely for use in research and clinical trials.

14. **How do I treat cardiogenic and neurogenic shock?**
    For the answer to this questions, see Chapter 34, Acute Coronary Syndrome and Chapter 56, Spine and Spinal Cord Trauma.

15. **How is diabetic shock different?**
    Diabetic shock is not shock in the traditional definition as there is no impairment of oxygen delivery to the tissues. However, the brain is dependent on glucose as an energy source and the effects of low blood sugar on the brain are essentially the same as inadequate oxygen delivery. The hypoglycemic patient will progress from restlessness and confusion to agitation (often violent) to poor responsiveness and coma just like the patient with a shock state. Thus the term diabetic shock will be with us for a long time.

Pearls and Pitfalls

1. The basic pathophysiology of shock is inadequate delivery of oxygen to tissues and cells.
2. "Compensated" shock is manifested by maintenance of systolic blood pressure but a widening of the pulse pressure and tachycardia.

3. Hypovolemic shock is manifested by hypotension, tachycardia, and increased systemic vascular resistance (cool, clammy skin).
4. Capacitance septic, neurogenic, or anaphylactic) shock presents with hypotension, tachycardia, and warm, dry skin.
5. The initial treatment of shock is administration of oxygen and an intravenous crystalloid bolus.
6. In trauma patients, who are actively hemorrhaging, starting an IV to administer fluids should not delay ambulance transport.

References

1. Bickell WH, Wall WJ, Pepe PE, et al. Immediate versus delayed fluid resuscitation for hypotensive patients with penetrating torso injuries. N Engl J Med 331:1105–1109, 1994.
2. Jones AE, Kline JA. Shock. In: Rosen's Emergency Medicine. Concepts and Clinical Practice, 7th ed., Marx JA et al., eds., pp 34-42. St. Louis: Mosby, 2010.
3. Mattox KL, Bickell W, Pepe PE, et al. Prospective MAST study in 911 patients. J Trauma 29:1104–1112, 1989.
4. Salomone JP, Pons PT, eds. PHTLS: Pre-hospital Trauma Life Support, 7th ed., pp 179–216. St. Louis: Mosby, 2011.
5. Haukoos JS: Shock. In Markovchick VJ, Pons PT, KM, eds. Emergency Medicine Secrets, 5th ed., pp. 28-34. St. Louis: Elsevier, 2011.
6. Sloan EP, Koenigsberg M, Gens D, et al. diaspirin cross-linked hemoglobin in the treatment of severe traumatic hemorrhagic shock: A randomized controlled efficacy trial. JAMA 282(19):1857–1864, 1999.

Chapter 33
Chest Pain

Christopher B. Colwell, MD, FACEP

1. **How big a problem is chest pain?**

   Very big! More than 5 million patients present to emergency departments each year with complaints of chest pain, representing almost 5% of all patients seen in emergency departments in the United States. More than 650,000 people die of coronary artery disease (CAD) each year, with almost two-thirds of these involving sudden cardiac death outside the hospital. Another 1.3 million people have nonfatal heart attacks each year, resulting in more than 1.5 million coronary care unit admissions per year. Pulmonary embolism is the third most common cause of death in the United States, at nearly 650,000 deaths per year. More importantly, studies have suggested that the diagnosis is missed almost 400,000 times per year. Finally, although not as common, untreated aortic dissection has a mortality of 25% at one day, 50% at one week, and 90% at one year. Chest pain obviously must be taken very seriously, and yet the large majority of patients who present with a chief complaint of chest pain do not have a significant pathologic process going on at that time. The complaint of chest pain takes up a large number of resources and time, and differentiating chest pain that represents serious pathology from that which does not can be very difficult.

2. **Does the location of the pain help in the diagnosis?**

   For the most part, no. There are two means by which the signals that communicate chest "pain" are transmitted. Somatic pain that arises from diseases affecting the chest wall is carried by very specific afferent nerves to the spinal cord and tends to be sharp, well-localized pain. This permits very specific mapping of the painful stimulus. On the other hand, visceral pain arises in the heart and lungs as well as the esophagus and stomach and tends to be dull, and achy. These organs are sparsely innervated, and signals enter the spinal cord at multiple levels, resulting in very poor specificity as to where the pain originated. As such, pain from unimportant causes can be identical to the pain from life-threatening causes, and both can present as pain virtually anywhere in the chest. Connections between somatic and visceral fibers can result in visceral pain being perceived as originating from or radiating to locations that are somatically inervated, such as the neck, jaw, or shoulder.

3. **What is the best initial approach to take with a patient complaining of chest pain?**

   There are two basic concepts to remember when evaluating a patient with chest pain. First, always focus on identifying life-threatening causes: ischemic heart disease or MI, pulmonary embolus, aortic dissection, pneumothorax, or esophageal rupture. Second, if there is any doubt, always treat the patient according to the worst possible scenario that the history and physical findings could represent. The most important tool for evaluating chest pain is a good history, followed by a physical exam and 12-lead electrocardiogram (ECG). Before diagnostic studies are undertaken, supplemental oxygen, intravenous access, and cardiac monitoring should be initiated in most patients.

Clinical Care

4. What are the important elements in the history of the patient's chest pain?

Certain key elements to be considered include location, onset, duration, character and quality, radiation, and associated symptoms (such as shortness of breath, nausea, sweating, or syncope). Precipitating factors such as exertion or inspiration can be helpful as well as any relieving factors such as rest, medications, or certain positions. Beyond a history of the current chest pain, a past medical history including risk factors for chest pain, medications, and pertinent family history can be useful.

5. What in a patient's history would suggest coronary artery disease?

Classically, the pain in CAD is described as dull or pressurelike and is retrosternal or felt in the left chest. In general, the pain crescendos, with a duration of 10 min or less for angina. Pain that radiates to the neck or arms is three to four times more likely to represent a MI as is pain that is associated with diaphoresis, nausea, or shortness of breath. Dyspnea is the sole complaint in approximately 15% of patients having an MI and is an associated symptom in 50%. Five key cardiac risk factors that should be assessed in every patient include a history of tobacco use, family history (MI in mother <age 55, father/brothers <age 45), diabetes mellitus, hypertension, and hypercholesterolemia, although the absence of risk factors should not, by itself, decrease the provider's concern for CAD. Without an ECG, it may be very difficult to differentiate unstable angina from an acute MI.

6. What about pain described as heartburn or "like gas pains"?

"Indigestion" is a very dangerous complaint, as it could represent a number of things, including cardiac ischemia, and yet the complaint itself may lead us to be less concerned. One study noted that of patients with "pressurelike" chest pain, 24% had infarctions and another 30% had anginal pain. They also noted that of patients describing "burning or indigestion," 23% had infarcts and 21% had unstable angina. There are numerous instances of patients with indigestion who have some relief after belching or a bowel movement but go on to be diagnosed with CAD. It has also been reported that 7–10% of patients with acute MI had complete relief of their pain with antacids alone.

7. What should be noted in the physical exam for CAD?

Probably the most important physical finding is what the general appearance of the patient is. A patient who is anxious and diaphoretic with a sense of impending doom may well have a significant problem. It is also very important to identify signs of cardiogenic shock (pale, cool, clammy, rales, hypotension, mental status change, jugular venous distention). Because the treatment for cardiogenic shock is the catheterization lab, these patients are best evaluated at a facility that can perform cardiac catheterization. Palpation may reveal localized tenderness, but remember that up to 10% of patients with acute coronary syndrome have reproducible pain on exam.

8. What about treatment?

All patients should receive oxygen as the basis of therapy. (Document whether it helps.) Unless they are allergic, all patients with nontraumatic chest pain should receive an aspirin (325 mg). The benefits of aspirin therapy in patients suffering from cardiac ischemia or infarction outway any risks associated with routine aspirin therapy. Sublingual nitroglycerin (either spray or tablet) acts as a direct coronary artery dilator and will often provide significant relief from the pain of angina but may show little effect with an MI.

9. When should I be concerned about pulmonary embolism?

More than 95% of cases of pulmonary embolism (PE) will present as one of three syndromes: (a) Pulmonary infarction with acute onset of pleuritic chest pain, dyspnea, and hemoptysis; (b) Acute cor pulmonale with acute dyspnea, cyanosis, right ventricular failure, and hypotension; (c) Unexplained dyspnea. These symptoms are very nonspecific and can be difficult to sort out, particularly if the patient has preexisting pulmonary disease. Only a few patients (approximately 20%) will present with the classic findings of pleuritic chest pain, dyspnea, and hemoptysis.

10. **What risk factors predispose one to development of PE?**
    Commonly described risk factors include a history of deep-vein thrombosis, injury or surgery to the lower extremities, immobility, obesity, cancer, tobacco and birth control pill use, history of coagulation disorders, and increasing age.

11. **What signs or symptoms suggest the existence of PE?**
    There are no signs or symptoms that are diagnostic of PE. A high index of suspicion for the disease is important. Common symptoms include dyspnea (84%), pleuritic chest pain (74%), apprehension (63%), and cough (50%). Syncope is more common with massive PE. The most frequent sign of PE is tachypnea (85%), whereas tachycardia, localized rales, and fever occur in about 50% of patients.

12. **Who is at risk for spontaneous (nontraumatic) aortic dissection?**
    Aortic dissection primarily occurs in individuals 50–70 years old. While aortic dissection is relatively rare before age 40, it does occur in select populations. Hypertension is the most common risk factor, occurring in 70–90% of patients with spontaneous dissection. The risk factors for patients younger than age 40 include connective tissue diseases (Marfan's and Ehlers–Danlos syndromes), congenital abnormalities (bicuspid aortic valve and aortic coarctation), chromosomal abnormalities (Turner's syndrome), and pregnancy (half of all female cases younger than age 40).

13. **How does the pain of dissection differ from CAD or PE?**
    The pain of aortic dissection is commonly described by the patient as "ripping" or "tearing." The pain often migrates, moving down the back as the dissection spreads. This occurs in up to 70% of patients. The pain is usually maximal in intensity right from the start rather than progressive, like ischemic pain. Only rarely (10%) does painless dissection occur. The pain is unlikely to improve with narcotic therapy. Providers should consider aortic dissection in any patient complaining of chest pain with any neurologic symptom since the dissection can interrupt the blood supply to the spinal cord and its nerve roots.

14. **What neurologic and other signs or symptoms are associated with aortic dissection?**
    Patients may have one of three patterns of neurologic findings: (a) stroke, (b) ischemic peripheral neuropathy (with an ischemic limb), or (c) paraparesis or paraplegia if the blood supply to the spinal cord is impaired. Patients may often appear "shocky" (clammy, cool, diaphoretic), although the blood pressure may be normal or elevated. Reduced peripheral pulses or unequal pulses when comparing limbs is very suggestive of dissection, but do not depend on this, as less than 50% of patients with aortic dissection will have decreased or unequal pulses. A blood pressure difference of more than 20 mmHg between the upper extremities should raise the concern for aortic dissection.

15. **What are the causes of a pneumothorax?**
    Trauma is the most common cause of a pneumothorax. Although more common in penetrating trauma, blunt trauma can cause a pneumothorax as well. Pneumothoraces can occur spontaneously, most commonly in males age 20–40 years who are taller than average. Other causes include asthma, tobacco use (emphysema), and barotrauma (diving accidents). Patients commonly describe chest pain (in 90%) that is pleuritic (sharp and worse on inspiration). Dyspnea also occurs in up to 80% of patients.

16. How should pneumothoraces be treated in the field?

If the patient is hemodynamically stable, high-flow oxygen should be administered via a nonrebreather mask. Only if patients are starting to show signs of tension pneumothorax (altered mentation, hypotension, absent breath sounds, and tachycardia) is a needle thoracostomy indicated. Remember that a deviated trachea is a late finding in a patient with a tension pneumothorax. Tension pneumothorax is rare in victims of blunt trauma.

17. How else can barotrauma occur?

One of the more common methods is coughing or forced exhalation against a closed glottis, such as when smoking crack or marijuana. This can result in either a pneumothorax or pneumomediastinum. Patients with pneumomediastinum often complain of sharp pleuritic substernal chest pain, similar to patients with a pneumothorax. They may have evidence of subcutaneous emphysema moving up into the neck. The classic physical finding is "Hamman's crunch," which is a crunchy sound heard in the substernal area over the heart.

18. Are there any other causes of pneumomediastinum?

Esophageal rupture can also result in pneumomediastinum. This is often referred to as Boerhaave's syndrome. It commonly occurs in male patients 50–70 years of age, often with a significant alcohol use history. A history of forceful emesis followed by severe chest pain, dyspnea, and subcutaneous emphysema is the classic presentation. Pleuritic chest pain and an acute abdomen are suggestive of esophageal rupture.

19. What type of chest pain is associated with cocaine use?

Chest pain is the most common cocaine-related medical problem, affecting about 64,000 patients per year. Cocaine can cause significant coronary artery vasospasm (potentiated by tobacco use), although this may not cause ischemia to the extent that was once suspected. Long-term cocaine use also causes accelerated atherosclerosis and should be considered a risk factor for CAD. True myocardial infarction occurs in less than 10% of cocaine chest pain. For the most part, cocaine chest pain is treated as you would treat any other ischemic chest pain. Those patients with significant anxiety, elevated blood pressure, or increased heart rate should be treated with benzodiazepines as a first-line agent. This reduces both the cardiac and central nervous system toxicity of cocaine. Do not forget aspirin when treating any patient with nontraumatic chest pain who is not allergic.

20. Beta blockers should never be used in patients that have used cocaine, correct?

Never say never. Although it is true that beta blockers should be used with caution in patients who have used cocaine and should be avoided in patients who are acutely cocaine toxic (tachycardic and hypertensive), patients may no longer be cocaine toxic when EMS is involved. In a patient with remote cocaine use and no signs of acute cocaine intoxication, beta blockers can safely be used when cardiac ischemia or infarction is suspected.

21. What about chest pain in patients with sickle cell disease?

The acute chest syndrome is a common complication of sickle cell disease. It is characterized by pleuritic chest pain, rales, and fever. It can be very difficult to distinguish from pneumonia, although cough may be more prominent in patients with pneumonia. Therapy includes aggressive oxygen therapy via nonrebreather mask as well as volume resuscitation with IV crystalloids.

22. How does the approach to chest pain differ with children?

Chest pain in children is not uncommon, with nearly 650,000 visits per year. Compared with adults, chest pain is more often chronic, with 30% of children having had it 6 months or more in one series. Fortunately, serious causes of chest pain are relatively rare, accounting for only about 5% of cases in most series.

23. How does the approach to chest pain differ with elderly patients?

Presenting symptoms are more likely to be atypical in elderly patients (as well as diabetics). Ischemic chest pain in the elderly may present as the sudden onset of shortness of breath, abdominal pain or fullness, weakness, dizziness, confusion, or syncope instead of chest pain. Although these symptoms can represent ischemia in any patient, they are more likely to be found in the elderly. Elderly patients (like those with diabetes) may have altered pain perception resulting in an atypical presentation.

24. What is the role of the 12-lead ECG in the prehospital environment?

Several studies have shown that paramedics are capable of obtaining prehospital ECGs of good quality, and that adding ECG data to the paramedic's clinical assessment, improves sensitivity for the detection of angina and MI (from 60% to 90%). It has also been shown that prehospital 12-lead ECGs correlate well with ECGs done at the emergency department (ED) and may speed the diagnosis of ischemic heart disease. At least one study has shown significant reductions in the time between arrival at the ED and receipt of thrombolytic therapy when prehospital ECGs are transmitted to the ED physicians. Recent studies have also suggested prehospital personnel with 12-lead ECG capabilities can reduce the time from arrival to the ED and delivery to the cardiac catheterization lab Repeat ECGs, particularly with a significant change in symptoms, can be very valuable.

Although it has been shown that prehospital personnel can obtain ECGs and that it increases their sensitivity for detecting ischemia, it has not yet been shown to improve patient care. Some studies suggest that prehospital personnel overcall ischemia. So much of the diagnosis of ischemia is dependent on history that a negative ECG in the field (or in the ED) cannot be used reliably to decide which patients do not have ischemic heart disease. Performing an ECG in the field may delay the patient's arrival at the ED. A number of EMS systems have instituted a program where prehospital personnel are activating the catheterization lab from the field based on the field 12-lead ECG. In such a system the added time to get a 12-lead in the field may be offset by reduced time to the lab in appropriate patients. More research is needed and already underway, but there have been significant advances in prehospital involvement in the activation of the cardiac catheterization lab which may impact door-to-balloon times more than any process changes that have been implemented after the patient's arrival to the ED. We may soon be looking at time of contact to balloon times more than door-to-balloon times.

25. Should thrombolytic therapy be initiated in the field?

Pro. Time is myocardium. It has been shown that the early administration of thrombolytic therapy leads to better outcomes and fewer complications. Several European studies have shown that giving thrombolytics in the field reduces the time to thrombolytic therapy by 40–50 min without significant complications.

Con. No study to date has shown improved outcome when thrombolytic therapy is given in the field by prehospital personnel. Although time to thrombolytic therapy is important, the major time delay comes from symptomatic patients not accessing emergency medical care, not from delays in receiving thrombolytic therapy. One U.S. study also showed that of patients classified as having an MI by virtue of their prehospital ECG, only 51% actually had one. Initiating thrombolytics in such patients exposes them to possible bleeding complications.

Pearl and Pitfalls

1. Always consider the life threats in every patient complaining of chest pain.
2. Think about pulmonary embolism and aortic dissection in addition to acute myocardial infarction in patients complaining of chest pain.
3. Treat chest pain associated with cocaine use like any other chest pain, but add benzodiazepines to your treatment regimen.
4. A simple pneumothorax does not require treatment in the field.
5. "Indigestion" is a very dangerous complaint.
6. Remember that anyone, in particular the elderly, women, and patients with diabetes, can have atypical symptoms and still be experiencing cardiac ischemia.
7. Repeat ECGs particularly with a significant change in symptoms, are very valuable.
8. Response to nitroglycerin or antacids does not make the diagnosis of, or rule out, cardiac ischemia.

References

1. McCaig, LF, Burt, CW. National Hospital Ambulatory Medical Care Survey: 2001 emergency department summary. Adv Data 335:1, 2003.
2. Brouwer MA, Martin JS, Maynard C. Influence of early prehospital thrombolytic therapy on mortality and event-free survival. Am J Cardiol 78:497–502, 1996.
3. Grijseels EW, Bouten MJ, Lenderink T. Pre-hospital thrombolytic therapy with alteplase or streptokinase. Practical applications, complications, and long term results. Eur Heart J 16:1833–1838, 1995.
4. Hollander JE. The management of cocaine-associated myocardial ischemia. N Engl J Med 333:1267–1272, 1995.
5. Pozner, CN, Levine, M, Zane, R. The cardiovascular effects of cocaine. J Emerg Med 29(2):493, 2005.
6. Levis, JT, Garmel, GM. Cocaine-associated chest pain. Emerg Med Clin North Am 23(4):1083, 2005.
7. Karagounis L, Ipsen SK, Jessop MR, et al. Impact of field-transmitted electrocardiography on time to in-hospital thrombolytic therapy in acute myocardial infarction. Am J Cardiol 66:786–791, 1990.
8. Goodacre, S, Locker, T, Morris, F, Campbell, S. How useful are clinical features in the diagnosis of acute, undifferentiated chest pain? Acad Emerg Med 9:203, 2002.
9. Kogan, A, Shapira, R, Silman-Stolar, Z, Rennert, G. Evaluation of chest pain in the ED: Factors affecting triage decisions. Am J Emerg Med 21(1):68, 2003
10. Goldman, L, Kirtane, AJ. Triage of patients with acute chest pain and possible cardiac ischemia: The elusive search for diagnostic perfection. Ann Intern Med 139(12):987, 2003.
11. Pope, JH, Aufderheide, TP, Ruthazer, R, et al. Missed diagnosis of acute cardiac ischemia in the emergency department. N Engl J Med 342(16):1163, 2000.
12. Manganelli E, Palla A, Donnamaria V. Clinical features of pulmonary embolism: Doubts and certainties. Chest 107:25s–32s 1995.
13. Lee, PY, Alexander, KP, Hammill, BG, et al. Representation of elderly persons and women in published randomized trials of acute coronary syndromes. JAMA 286:708, 2001.
14. Jones, ID, Slovis, CM. Emergency department evaluation for the chest pain patient. Emerg Med Clin North Am 19:269, 2001.

Acute Coronary Syndrome

Jeffrey J. Messerole, PS

1. **What is acute coronary syndrome?**
   As its name implies, an acute coronary syndrome (ACS) is a sudden onset of heart-related signs and symptoms that point to a particular disease, in this case, atherosclerosis. Atherosclerosis comes from the Greek words *athero* (meaning gruel or paste), and *sclerosis* (meaning hardness). In the body, this mixture is made up of calcium, lipids, fats, and is called plaque. As the plaque clings to the walls of the coronary arteries, it narrows the lumen of the artery, reducing the amount of blood and oxygen reaching the heart muscle. The plaque may harden or remain soft. When atherosclerosis is found within the coronary arteries it is referred to as coronary artery disease (CAD). Patients with CAD develop acute coronary syndromes (ACS). The two most common ACSs are angina pectoris and acute myocardial infarction (AMI). AMI can be further divided into ST-segment elevation myocardial infarction (STEMI), and non-ST-segment elevation myocardial infarction (NSTEMI).

2. **What is the difference between angina pectoris and AMI?**
   Angina pectoris literally means "chest pain" and is caused by an inadequate blood supply from a narrowed coronary artery partially occluded with plaque. Angina pain usually comes on with exercise or stress and lasts 3–5 min, sometimes up to 15 min. Rest and nitroglycerin relieve angina pain. Less common causes of angina include coronary artery spasm, arterial inflammation resulting from an infection, and extrinsic causes not related directly to the coronary artery such as hypoxia, hypotension, tachycardia, and anemia. Most patients who develop angina pain from these causes have a past medical history of CAD or angina. A rare form of an ACS may result from cocaine or methamphetamine use, as they increase myocardial oxygen demand and may cause coronary artery dissection.
   An AMI, on the other hand, is caused by a clot or thrombus that forms in a narrowed coronary artery where the plaque has ruptured, causing platelets to aggregate and a clot to form. If the coronary artery becomes completely obstructed, the cells in the heart muscle beyond the blockage will begin to die if circulation and enough oxygen-rich blood are not restored. This can cause permanent damage to the heart muscle and is commonly referred to as a heart attack.

3. **How will EMS become involved with cases of ACS?**
   EMS providers will get frequent calls for chest pain, the most common symptom associated with ACS. As effective treatment for ACS is time sensitive, it becomes important for the EMS provider to quickly recognize the potential presence of ACS and provide essential treatment within the first hours of onset to reduce the likelihood of sudden cardiac death.

4. **How prevalent is the CAD that causes ACS?**
   CAD is the most common type of heart disease, affecting an estimated 13 million Americans. It is the leading cause of death in the United States in both men and women. Approximately 1.2 million Americans

Clinical Care

suffered a heart attack as the result of CAD in 2007 and 452,000 of those died (320,000 out of hospital or in the emergency room). CAD is inevitable for many people as they age.

We can however reduce the rate at which CAD occurs, reducing our risk of developing ACS. By recognizing the presence of modifiable risk factors and taking steps to reduce them, CAD will be delayed and the chance of developing ACS is significantly reduced.

5. What risk factors are associated with CAD and the development of an ACS?

Several factors increase the risk of CAD and developing ACS. The more risk factors you have, the greater the chance of developing ACS. Some risk factors cannot be modified, but others can.

Risk factors we cannot modify include age, gender, and heredity. The older you get, the more likely your chance of having CAD. Men have CAD at an earlier age and are more likely to die from their ACS, but heart disease also remains the leading cause of death in women, particularly those who are postmenopausal. Estrogen in younger women has a cardioprotective effect; however, after menopause the incidence of ACS in men and women is similar. A family history of CAD increases the risk of developing ACS and may be directly linked to lifestyle. If your parents led a lifestyle of high risk for CAD, chances are you will as well. Those risk factors we can modify include hypertension, smoking, high cholesterol, diabetes, obesity, stress, and lack of physical activity. Hypertension as is defined by the American Heart Association (AHA) as a blood pressure greater than 140/90. It is easily diagnosed and can be successfully managed with diet, exercise, and medications. Hypertension causes the heart to work harder than it should and over time causes it to enlarge and weaken. Smoking increases your risk of developing ACS and is the single most preventable cause of death in the United States. Smokers' risk of heart attack is more than twice that of nonsmokers. Smokers who have ACS are more likely to die. The nicotine and carbon monoxide in tobacco smoke reduces the amount of oxygen in the blood, and damages blood vessel walls, causing plaque to build up. Tobacco smoke may trigger blood clots to form as well. Smoking promotes heart disease by reducing high-density lipoprotein (HDL) ("good") cholesterol. Quitting smoking reduces your risk of having ACS even if you have smoked for years. High cholesterol is another easily diagnosed problem that can be managed with diet, exercise, and medications. A heart-healthy diet high in fruits and vegetables and low in fats and carbohydrates reduces low-density lipoprotein (LDL) ("bad") cholesterol. Diabetes greatly increases the risk of heart disease. In fact, most people with diabetes die from some form of heart or blood vessel disease. Many people with diabetes also have high blood pressure, increasing their risk even more. Obesity, stress, and lack of exercise accelerate the atherosclerotic process increasing the chances of having ACS.

6. What consequences are associated with an ACS?

Angina is chest pain caused by an inadequate blood supply from a narrowed coronary artery that is often relieved by rest or nitroglycerin. In and of itself angina is a sign of serious heart disease and may lead to an AMI if it becomes unstable. Angina is considered unstable when it occurs with increasing frequency, at rest, or is more severe than the "normal" episodes of angina a patient experiences. If left untreated, unstable angina can lead to an AMI.

An AMI may lead to an irregular heart rhythm, a lethal heart rhythm such as ventricular fibrillation, or congestive heart failure (CHF), which may lead to the development of acute pulmonary edema or cardiogenic shock and death. Left ventricular infarction involving 40% or more of the heart muscle usually results in left heart failure, cardiogenic shock, and carries a high mortality rate. Right ventricular infarction or ischemia occurs in up to 50% of patients who present with an inferior wall AMI and may result in right heart failure or hypotension, especially if nitrates are administered for the complaint of chest pain.

Acute Coronary Syndrome

7. **What are the signs and symptoms of an ACS?**

   The classic signs and symptoms of ACS include a sudden onset of chest pain or pressure located in the center of the chest below the sternum. This pain or pressure may feel as if it is radiating to the neck, or jaw, and down the left arm. It is described as constant, usually lasting longer than 15 min. The patient may also complain of shortness of breath as if their chest is in a vise or an elephant is sitting on their chest making it difficult for them to breathe. Patients may also have the associated signs and symptoms of diaphoresis; pale, mottled, cool skin; weakness or lightheadedness; may complain of feeling nauseated; may vomit; and may have a feeling of impending doom. The presence of rales and rhonchi, with or without jugular vein distention, may be present with a large or a repeat AMI, indicating the presence of CHF. These classic signs and symptoms of ACS may all be present or only a few may be present. The elderly, those with diabetes, and postmenopausal women over 55 may present with no pain or discomfort but instead present as though they are having a sudden onset of flulike symptoms. Failure to consider flulike symptoms as ACS in elderly or diabetic patients, or postmenopausal women may lead to the development of serious and life-threatening consequences.

8. **How do I assess for an ACS?**

   Early recognition that a patient is having ACS is the primary goal of the assessment. Many patients will wait 2–3 hours before seeking medical help. This delay can result in lasting heart damage or worse, death. Because about 50% of all ACS patients may die before reaching the hospital, your assessment, as does the assessment of all medical patients, begins with the ABCs.

   The initial assessment begins with determining level of consciousness. Chapter 31, Cardiac Arrest, tells you what to do when a patient is unconscious and in cardiac arrest.

   If your patient is conscious and there are no serious life threats found when checking the ABCs, then a focused history and physical exam can begin. A SAMPLE history may be obtained and the patient's complaint of chest pain or pressure evaluated using the OPQRST mnemonic. Let us start first with the OPQRST.

   O, Onset—What was the patient doing when the chest pain or discomfort occurred? Remember you don't have to be working hard for an ACS to occur; in fact, most occur, at rest. If the pain occurred suddenly with activity or during a stressful situation, further assessment to determine a past medical history of angina is warranted. A gradual onset may suggest pericarditis, or an onset a day after heavy lifting or forceful coughing may suggest chest wall muscle involvement.

   P, Provocation—What makes the pain or discomfort better or worse? The pain from ACS is usually constant and it generally does not get worse with a deep breath, or when you palpate over the area where the pain is being felt. It is not made better by a particular position, or by splinting the chest with a pillow. If rest or nitroglycerin relieves the pain or pressure, then the ACS may be angina. If not, then the pain or discomfort could be the result of unstable angina or an AMI. If the pain increases with palpation or inspiration, then pneumonia, pneumothorax, or pulmonary embolism may be the reason for the pain or discomfort and further assessment for those signs and symptoms should occur.

   Q, Quality—Have the patient describe the pain or discomfort in their own words. Asking them if it is sharp or dull limits their response to those terms which may not accurately describe how they feel. Heart-related pain is often described as a feeling of pressure or squeezing. It can be described as indigestion in those patients denying the possibility of an AMI.

   R, Radiation—Does this pain or discomfort radiate or seem to go anywhere? Typically it will radiate to the neck, jaw, or down the arms, but it may also radiate to the back, into the abdomen or down the legs.

Clinical Care

It may radiate anywhere. Pain that is felt in the right shoulder may be referred from the heart or associated with gall bladder disease. The pain of an aortic dissection typically radiates straight through to the back and may settle in the flank or scrotum in males. Further assessments of those types of pain are warranted.

S, Severity—Have the patient rate their pain or discomfort on a 1–10 scale with 1 being the least amount and 10 the worst pain or discomfort they have ever felt. Giving the pain or discomfort a number informs you know where the pain is now. If the treatment you provide is effective, the number should go down. If the patient's pain or discomfort worsens the number should go up. Men typically will rate their pain a higher number than women. Often the treatment for chest pain in men is taken more seriously because of how they describe the intensity of their pain. Women may have little or no complaint of pain, but instead complain of a sudden onset of weakness with the associated signs and symptoms of AMI such as nausea, dizziness, and malaise.

T, Time—How long have they had this pain? Depending on how close the patient is to definitive therapy or a chest pain center capable of cardiac catheterization, the patient may need a fibrinolytic or "clot buster" medication or an angioplasty to help open the obstruction in the coronary artery if that is what is causing the ACS. There is a narrow window of opportunity in which the administration of a fibrinolytic will be beneficial. EMS providers should know what the capabilities are of the facilities they transport the patient to and which institutions have cardiac cath lab capability. Transport should never be delayed to obtain a complete history or physical exam.

After completion of the OPQRST you should have a good idea if your patient is likely experiencing ACS, and whether it is angina, unstable angina, or AMI. Chances are if they were shoveling heavy snow and suddenly developed chest pain that is substernal, constant, radiates to the neck, jaw, and down the left arm, making it hard for them to breathe, described as like an elephant sitting on their chest, and rated at 10+, and it has been going on for about an hour, and has not been relieved by rest or their own nitroglycerin, they are having an AMI. Although we have not completed a 12-Lead EKG or have the ability to look at cardiac markers, we can with some certainty develop the field impression of an AMI

9. What is the next step after I have obtained the history of the complaint?

If time permits, it is appropriate to get a little more information during transport by completing the SAMPLE history.

S, Signs and symptoms—look for those associated signs and symptoms of an ACS such as sudden onset of flu-like symptoms; weakness; dizziness; pale, cool, clammy skin, or the feeling of impending doom. Pertinent negatives such as the pain not being relieved by rest or after receiving nitroglycerin are important to note.

A, Allergies—Allergies to any medications are important, as this patient may be given aspirin along with other medications for their ACS.

M, Medications—Medications, including prescription, herbal, and over the counter, are important to determine and may indicate a past medical history of CAD, or that a patient has a previous heart history. Medications such as nitroglycerin, an aspirin a day, cholesterol-lowering medications, high blood pressure medications such as ACE inhibitors, beta blockers, or calcium channel blockers, and oral hypoglycemics indicating diabetes are all pertinent for the possibility of CAD. Note if the patient has taken any phosphodiesterase inhibitors (Viagra, Cialis, or Levitra) in the last 24–36 hours for erectile dysfunction. Nitrates should be avoided, as they may have a profound effect of lowering the blood pressure when combined with these medications.

P, Pertinent past medical history—Does a patient have a history of heart disease? Is there a family history of heart disease? Have they ever had an AMI, a coronary artery bypass graft, or a percutaneous transluminal coronary angioplasty with a stent to open a coronary vessel? Answering yes to these questions should make the EMS provider suspicious for likely ACS

L, Last oral intake—this may indicate the presence of a full stomach and an increased risk of vomiting should they become nauseated.

E, Events leading up to the call for 911—Was the patient engaged in physical activity, a high-stress situation, or did the patient wake up from a sleep with the pain or discomfort? Has there been any use of cocaine or methamphetamines?

10. **I have completed the history. Now what?**

    Now you can continue the physical assessment including a baseline set of vital signs and looking, listening and feeling those areas of the body associated with the chief complaints. The baseline vitals include recording:

    Respirations: Assess for rate, regularity, and depth. Respirations may be fast if the patient is anxious and believes they are having a heart attack, or if the patient is hypoxic. Normal respirations are 12-20 breaths per mintue effortlessly without pain and without noise. The patient should not be working hard to breathe or making noises while breathing. Noisy breathing is obstructed breathing and requires further assessment as to its cause. Consider left-heart failure with acute pulmonary edema in the patient with a positive history for ACS with rales and rhonchi.

    Pulse: Assess for rate, regularity, and strength. The normal pulse rate is 60–100 beats per minute and regular. A rapid, slow, or irregular pulse may indicate the presence of a dysrhythmia and a weak pulse may be an indication of inadequate blood pressure or an early sign of shock. A bounding pulse may be an indication for high blood pressure, or possible cocaine or methamphetamine use.

    Blood pressure: should be normal (120/80) unless the patient has a history of hypertension. It may be elevated as the result of anxiety, or it may be low indicating the presence of cardiogenic shock. It will also serve as an indicator of how well the patient is tolerating slow, rapid, or irregular heart rates.

    Temperature: Normal body temperature is 98.6°F or 37°C and is an important and often overlooked vital sign. An elevated temperature may indicate the presence of an infection, pericarditis, pulmonary embolism, aspirin overdose, or cocaine or methamphetamine use. Elevated temperatures increase myocardial oxygen demand by increasing the heart rate to the point of causing chest pain or discomfort. Also important to your assessment are the findings using the following diagnostics:

    Pulse oximetry should be monitored to assess for the presence or development of hypoxia as manifested by the complaint of shortness of breath, increased work of breathing, tachypnea, and oxygen saturations of less than 95% at sea level. Administering oxygen as soon as possible in ACS is a high priority and should not be delayed to get a pulse oximeter reading. Because what you see on a pulse oximeter is not real time, applying oxygen will not have an instantaneous effect on the number you see on your oximeter. Delaying oxygen administration in an obviously hypoxic patient in need of oxygen just to get the oximetry reading is strongly discouraged.

11. **Why is 12-lead ECG capability an important part of prehospital care?**

    A heart monitor with 12-lead ECG capabilities should be placed on all patients with ACS.

    Paramedics trained in the interpretation of acute changes on a 12-lead ECG and who notify the receiving facility in advance of arrival reduce door-to-drug or catheter lab times in patients who are candidates

Clinical Care

TABLE 34.1: Risk Stratification Based on a 12-Lead ECG

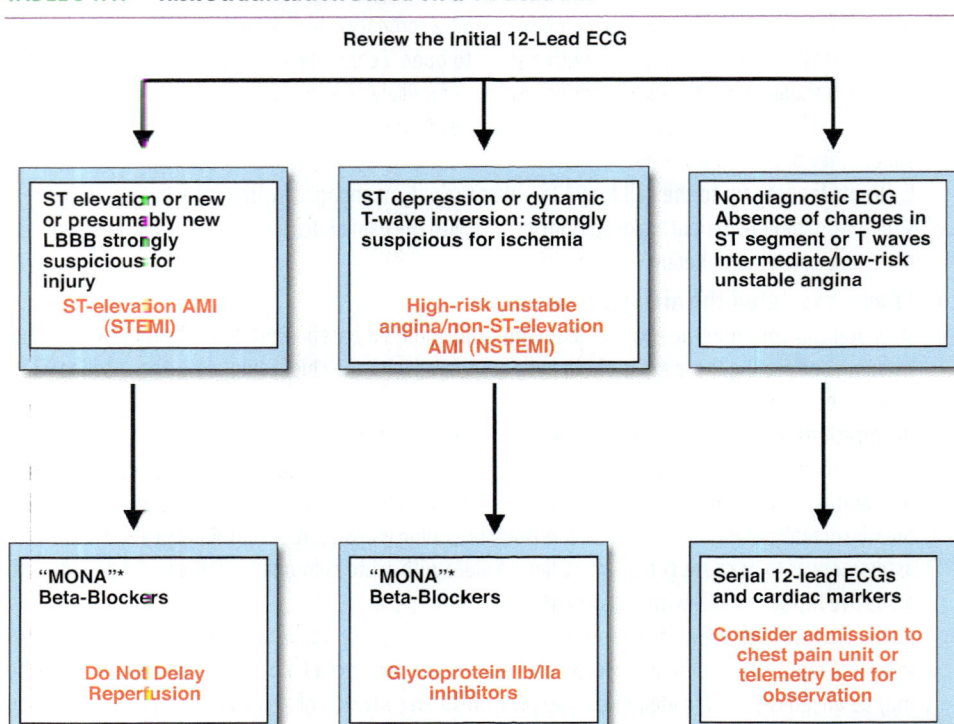

*MONA - morphine, oxygen, nitroglycerine, aspirin

for fibrinolysis or coronary angioplasty. Further classifying patients with ACS into one of three group subtypes based on 12-lead ECG findings guides the paramedic in treatment options as well as predicts the seriousness for potential complications (Table 34.1). Patients with STEMI or new left bundle-branch block (LBBB) are at the greatest risk of developing the serious complications associated with ACS and should be assessed for possible fibrinolytic administration. ST-segment depression defines the high-risk set of patients with unstable angina or NSTEMI who do not require reperfusion. Finally, those with normal 12-lead ECGs usually require serial ECGs and further assessment, as they may not yet be exhibiting the diagnostic signs, but their history is suspicious for ACS.

12. **Do I really need to know how to identify the location of an AMI on ECG?**
Yes. Knowing the location in the heart where the ischemia or injury is occurring and the expected complications associated with standard treatments will enhance the paramedic's ability to alter those standard treatments. (Table 34.2) For example, the paramedic should suspect right ventricular infarction in patients with inferior wall infarction as evident by elevated ST segments in leads II, III, and AVF. In patients with inferior wall infarction, the paramedic should obtain a right-sided ECG by moving the V leads on the left side of the chest to the right side of chest (Figure 34.1). ST-segment elevation greater than 1 mm in lead V4R is sensitive for right ventricular infarction. Patients with acute right ventricular

TABLE 34.2: ECG Lead Changes and Associated Complications

ECG Leads with Acute Changes	Related Artery	Area of Damage	Associated Complications
V1–V2	LCA:LAD–septal branch	Septum, His bundle, bundle branches	Infranodal blocks, Bundle branch blocks
V2–V3	LCA:LAD–diagonal branch	Anterior wall of left ventricle	LV dysfunction, CHF, BBBs, complete heart blocks, PVCs
I, aVL, V5–V6	LCA–circumflex branch	High lateral wall of left ventricle	LV dysfunction, AV nodal block
II, III, aVF	RCA–posterior descending branch	Inferior and posterior wall of left ventricle	Hypotension, sensitivity to nitrates and morphine
V_4R (II, III, aVF)	RCA–proximal branches	Right ventricle, inferior and posterior wall of the left ventricle	Hypotension, supranodal and AV-nodal blocks, A-fib/flutter, PACs
V1–V4 (marked ST depression)	Either LCA–circumflex, or RCA–posterior descending branch	Posterior wall left ventricle	Left ventricular function

LCA–left coronary artery, LAD–left anterior descending coronary artery, RCA–right coronary artery, LV–left ventricle, CHF–congestive heart failure, BBB–bundle branch block, PVC–premature ventricular contraction, AV–atrioventricular, PAC–premature atrial contraction, A-fib–atrial fibrillation.

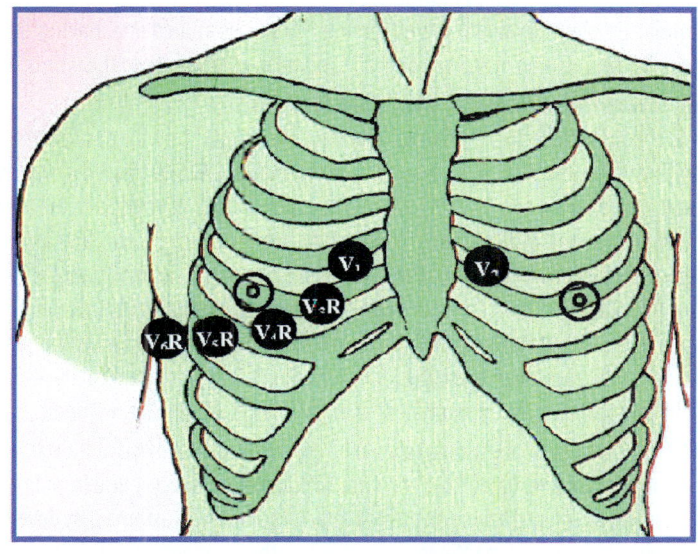

FIGURE 34.1 Lead placement for right 12-lead ECG.

Clinical Care

infarction are dependent on maintaining right ventricular "filling" pressure to maintain cardiac output. Any medications such as nitrates, diuretics, and other vasodilators (morphine, ACE inhibitors) that decrease preload should be avoided because they decrease right ventricular "filling" pressure and may cause severe hypotension. This hypotension may be corrected by an IV fluid bolus assuming you have the IV established before giving the nitroglycerin. Fluid administration of 1–2 L may be necessary and should be administered in aliquots of 250–500 mL as long as repeated examination shows that the lungs are clear and there is no evidence of acute pulmonary edema. Administering IV fluids in a patient with acute pulmonary edema will worsen the edema. Basic EMTs administering nitroglycerin not knowing the right ventricle is involved may cause hypotension, which reinforces the need for an advanced life support tier capable of 12-lead ECG interpretation whenever possible.

13. **Having completed the OPQRST, SAMPLE history, obtained baseline vital signs, and applied diagnostic equipment, what do I do now?**

The EMS providers' assessment should turn to completing the physical exam, focusing on the area of the body associated with the chief complaints. Lung sounds should be auscultated for the presence of rales or rhonchi. Wet lungs may be the result of left heart failure and acute pulmonary edema (APE) indicating cardiogenic shock. The presence of a cough with frothy pink sputum may also be evidence of APE. If the patient has a cough, do they normally have a cough? If so, why? Do they have a past medical history of chronic obstructive pulmonary disease (COPD)? If they normally cough, is it productive? Is what they are coughing up of normal amounts and color? A patient with COPD or pneumonia may have a productive cough. Noting if this is different may help you determine if what you are hearing is edema froth or normal productive sputum. Jugular vein distention and pedal edema may be present if right heart failure has occurred secondary to left heart failure. Examining the chest for previous scars indicating the presence of a pacemaker, or past heart surgery, would be beneficial to know as well and would support your field impression of ACS. Listen carefully to the heart and evaluate the rhythm as well as the presence of abnormal sounds such as murmurs. Examine the abdomen, as many abdominal processes can mimic cardiac problems. Evaluate the extremities for pulses and edema. Having completed your assessment, the field impression of ACS can be made and treatment specific to the type of ACS instituted.

14. **What field treatment options are available for ACSs?**

The EMT Basic should be able to provide the following prehospital care for a suspected ACS. Initially, until risk stratification occurs with 12-lead ECG interpretation, ACS is treated similarly. MONA is a mnemonic that is often used as a memory aid for the interventions needed once the field impression of ACS has been determined. MONA stands for morphine, oxygen, nitroglycerin, and aspirin. It does not suggest a particular order of administering the medications, or a particular importance of one medication over the other. Although EMT Basics are not permitted to administer narcotics (morphine), they all can provide oxygen and many states permit the administration of aspirin and assisting patients to take nitroglycerin if it has already been prescribed for them. Check with your medical director and scope of practice within your state for the appropriateness of EMT Basics administering medications.

- Aspirin 162–325 mg (2–4 baby aspirin) should be chewed and swallowed at the earliest sign of ACS. Providers should first assure that the patient is not allergic to acetylsalicylic acid (aspirin), has no history of recent bleeding ulcers, or is having an asthma attack. Patients with asthma may develop a condition known as aspirin-induced asthma. When given aspirin, asthma patients may develop an asthma attack

Acute Coronary Syndrome

that occurs gradually but is more intense and difficult to break. Early administration of aspirin in patients with ACS has been associated with decreased mortality rates in several clinical trials. Therefore aspirin should be given as soon as possible. The AHA advocates that prearrival instructions to take aspirin be given by dispatchers whenever possible. Aspirin suppositories (300 mg) are safe and can be considered for patients with severe nausea, vomiting, or disorders of the upper gastrointestinal tract.

- Oxygen, initially at 4 L/min via nasal cannula, is appropriate as administering oxygen increases the supply of oxygen available to the ischemic heart muscle tissue. If there are signs of hypoxia, oxygen should be administered at 10–15 L/min via nonrebreather mask. If shortness of breath is severe or acute pulmonary edema secondary to left heart failure is noted, then oxygen should be administered with continuous positive airway pressure (CPAP), or at least using a bag valve mask to provide positive pressure. Check with your medical director and scope of practice within your state for the appropriateness of EMT Basics administering CPAP.

- Nitroglycerin may be administered sublingually as a 0.4-mg tablet or metered dose spray. It may be repeated every 3–5 minutes three times as long as the patient's systolic blood pressure remains above 90 mmHg. Administering nitroglycerin more than three times may be appropriate after consultation with medical direction as long as the blood pressure remains above 90 mmHg. Nitroglycerin decreases the pain of ischemia by decreasing preload and cardiac oxygen consumption, and it dilates coronary arteries increasing cardiac collateral flow. Nitroglycerin should be given in patients with ACS, ST-segment elevation or depression, and for the consequences associated with AMI to include left ventricular failure (acute pulmonary edema or CHF). Use with extreme caution in right ventricular infarct because these patients require adequate preload. Nitroglycerin should not be given to patients with hypotension, extreme bradycardias, or tachycardias. Do not administer nitroglycerin to patients who have taken a phosphodiesterase inhibitor (Viagra, Cialis, Levitra) for erectile dysfunction within the last 24–36 hours. Nitroglycerin may further lower the blood pressure (BP) in a patient whose vascular system is already dilated. Watch for headache, a drop in BP, syncope, and tachycardia when nitroglycerin is given. The patient should sit or lie down during administration.

15. OK, those are the steps that all prehospital care providers should perform in patients with ACS; are there specific treatments advanced providers should consider?

Advanced EMS providers with their knowledge of rhythms and 12-lead ECG interpretation may:

- Establish an IV of normal saline as a route for administration of medications and fluid. If hypotension occurs following administration of nitroglycerin, judicious amounts of fluid should be infused quickly to increase right ventricular filling pressures. Some protocols call for 1–2 L in 500-mL boluses, checking blood pressure and lung sounds after each bolus. Fluids should be avoided in the presence of acute pulmonary edema secondary to left heart failure. Medications such as norepinephrine or dopamine may be infused to improve the pumping function of the heart.

- Some paramedic services will initiate an IV infusion of nitroglycerin for chest pain not relieved by rest, oxygen, sublingual nitroglycerin, or morphine. The infusion is often started at 10 µg/min and titrated until relief of pain, systolic pressure drops below 90 mmHg, or the blood pressure drops 30% from baseline, or 30 mmHg in the hypertensive patients.

- Administer morphine 2–4 mg IV titrated for pain relief. Be alert for a drop in blood pressure, especially in patients with volume depletion, or right ventricular infarction. Respiratory depression may occur and

Clinical Care

naloxone (Narcan™) should be available to reverse that complication. If the patient is allergic to morphine other analgesics may be an option. They may include fentanyl, Toradol™, or dilaudid. Check with your medical director and the scope of practice within your state regarding their use for these patients.

- In patients with ACS and hypotension or acute pulmonary edema, some services may consider infusing norepinephrine, dopamine, or dobutamine to improve BP and relieve pulmonary congestion. Strict adherence to protocol and ideally the use of infusion pumps for administering these medications are required. Local protocol, physician medical director involvement, and scope of practice within your state will determine if this is appropriate for your service.
- Furosemide (Lasix™) may also be administered in addition to nitroglycerin and morphine to relieve pulmonary edema in patients with systolic pressures greater then 90 mmHg. Generally 0.5–1 mg/kg IV push over 1–2 min is acceptable. Be cautious if the patient is volume depleted or dehydrated, as hypotension may result. If the patient is normovolemic he or she will make large amounts of urine in a short period of time.

Determining the presence of acute changes indicating ischemia or injury on the 12-lead ECG may support the need for further treatment including the following:

- Heparin bolus when used as adjunctive therapy with fibrin specific lytics in STEMI. Although most ground services are not infusing heparin drips, some are giving a bolus in STEMI confirmed by history and 12-lead ECG.
- IV beta-blocker administration reduces the size of the infarct, and mortality in patients who do not receive fibrinolytic therapy. They also reduce the incidence of ventricular ectopy and fibrillation. IV beta blockers decrease postinfarction ischemia and nonfatal AMI in patients who do receive fibrinolytic agents. IV beta blockers may also be beneficial for NSTEMI ACS. Because of this, IV beta blockers should be given to all patients without contraindications. Contraindications to beta blockers are moderate to severe left ventricular failure and pulmonary edema, bradycardia, hypotension, signs of poor peripheral perfusion, second-degree or third-degree heart block, and asthma. Metoprolol, atenolol, propranolol, esmolol, and labetalol are acceptable and paramedics should follow their local protocol. Vitals signs should be taken between doses to ensure that heart rate and blood pressure remain adequate.
- Out-of-hospital administration of fibrinolytics to patients with STEMI who have no contraindications is safe, feasible, and reasonable for patients with symptom duration up to 6 hours. Services offering out-of hospital fibrinolytics require a strict adherence to protocols, 12-lead ECG acquisition and interpretation, experience in ACLS, the ability to communicate with the receiving institution, and a medical director with experience in management of STEMI. A quality improvement process to evaluate all calls where fibrinolytics were used is required. Most EMS services have short enough transport times that they focus on early diagnosis with 12-lead ECG, completing a fibrinolytic checklist Table 34.3), administering first-line medications, and advance notification of the receiving facility. Selecting the proper fibrinolytic requires a thorough understanding of their properties and complications. Not being able to obtain a chest X-ray to determine the presence of a widened mediastinum, indicating an aneurysm, is another reason for not considering prehospital fibrinolytics.

16. What is the "chain of survival"?

The AHA advocates a chain of survival, with four links in that chain, each representing actions that if followed increase a patient's chance of survival should cardiac arrest occur. The four links are "early

TABLE 34.3: Fibrinolytic Checklist

This checklist is used to screen for ACS and to assist in field triage of those patients for whom fibrinolytic therapy or percutaneous coronary intervention (PCI) may be indicated.

I. Fibrinolysis **inclusion** criteria: In order for a patient to be a candidate for fibrinolysis or PCI, it generally requires that the first three items below are checked "Yes" AND that a 12-lead ECG indicates S–T elevations in at least two contiguous leads, and/or that there is a presumably new left bundle-branch block (LBBB).

	Yes	No
■ 12-lead ECG performed		
■ Ongoing nonpleuritic chest discomfort (>20 min and <12 hours)		
■ Patient is oriented and can cooperate		

II. Fibrinolysis **exclusion** criteria: In order to be considered an immediate candidate for fibrinolysis, all the following answers generally should be checked "No":

	Yes	No
■ BP >180/110 mmHg		
■ History of stroke or TIA		
■ Known bleeding disorder		
■ Active internal bleeding in past 4 weeks		
■ Surgery or significant trauma in past 4 weeks		
■ Terminal illness		
■ Jaundice, hepatitis, or kidney failure		
■ Use of anticoagulants		
■ CPR greater than 10 min		
■ Pregnancy		

TIA—transient ischemic attack.
Systolic/Diastolic Blood Pressure: _____ / _____ mmHg

access," "early CPR," "early defibrillation," and "early advanced care." EMS providers continue to play an important role in the reduction of death from ACS in all four of the links in the chain of survival by rapidly identifying the ACS and providing treatment to include, defibrillation, 12-Lead ECG interpretation, and medication administration. Patients with STEMI require prompt reperfusion. The shorter the time interval from symptom onset to reperfusion, the greater the benefit. Time is muscle, and the EMS provider can play a major role in salvaging that muscle. Patients with angina, NSTEMI, or nonspecific ECGs require risk stratification and appropriate treatment similar to STEMI before reaching the hospital. Efforts should also focus on early recognition of ACS by patients and family members as well. Many patients die before reaching the hospital because patients, their family members, and the general public may fail to recognize the signs of ACS and further fail to activate the EMS system. Only when we strengthen all the links in the chain of survival will we truly be doing all we can for patients with ACS.

Pearls and Pitfalls

1. Any complaint of chest pain should be taken seriously in all patients, as failure to recognize a patient's complaint of chest pain as ACS could lead to serious complications for the patient and significant medicolegal risk for the provider.
2. The elderly, people with diabetes, and postmenopausal women over 55 may present with atypical symptoms of ACS such as no pain or discomfort but instead complain of sudden onset of shortness of breath or flu like symptoms.
3. Although the pain of ACS is typically substernal and radiates to the left arm, the pain can be anywhere in the chest or upper abdomen and radiate to either side.
4. Nitrates should be avoided in patients taking medication for erectile dysfunction as they may have a profound effect of lowering blood pressure.
5. Early notification to the receiving hospital of the impending transport of a patient with suspected ACS will allow for activation of the cardiac interventional team and decrease the time from arrival to the hospital until reperfusion of the involved coronary artery.

References

1. Dalton A, Limmer D, Mistovich J, Werman H. Advanced Medical Life Support, 3rd ed., pp. 207–217. Upper Saddle River, NJ: Pearson Prentice Hall, 2007.
2. Aghababian R. Essentials of Emergency Medicine, pp. 97–116. Sudbury, MA: Jones and Bartlett, 2006.
3. Bledsoe B, Porter R, Cherry R. Essentials of Paramedic Care, 2nd ed.; pp. 1211–1224. Upper Saddle River, NJ: Pearson Prentice Hall, 2007.
4. Field J. Advanced Cardiac Life Support Provider Manual, pp. 65–78. Dallas, TX: American Heart Association, 2006.
5. American Heart Association. 2010 AHA guidelines for CPR and ECC. Circulation:122:S639–S946, 2010.
6. Field J, Hazinski M, Gilmore D. Handbook of ECC for Healthcare Providers, pp. 22–42. Dallas, TX: American Heart Association, 2006.
7. http://www.medpagetoday.com/Cardiology/AcuteCoronarySyndrome/tb/3723. Accessed June 3, 2011.
8. http://www.emedicine.com/EMERG/topic31.htm. Accessed June 3, 2011.
9. http://www.americanheart.org/presenter.jhtmL?identifier=4440. Accessed June 3, 2011.
10. http://www.clevelandclinicmeded.com/medicalpubs/diseasemanagement/cardiology/coronary-artery-disease/. Accessed June 3, 2011.
11. http://www.nhlbi.nih.gov/health/dci/Diseases/HeartAttack/HeartAttack_Treatments.html. Accessed June 3, 2011.

Altered Mental Status

Mike Stackpool, MD

CHAPTER 35

1. **What does "altered mental status" mean?**
   Confusion exists about how to describe confused patients. "Altered mental status" goes by many names. It may be called "delirium," "acute confusional state," "organic brain syndrome," "obtunded," "clouded consciousness," "stuporous," "acute brain syndrome," "toxic encephalopathy," or "metabolic encephalopathy." No matter how these are individually defined, there is overlap between groups.
   Altered mental status almost always combines a generalized reduction or alteration in the content of consciousness (a cortical function) with at least some reduction in total arousal (a brainstem function). This usually involves a defect in attention. The patient may not think clearly or quickly and can be easily distracted. Orientation, memory, and the ability to interpret stimuli may be faulty.
   Here we will use the term "delirium" as it is defined in the 2000 version of the *Diagnostic and Statistical Manual of Mental Disorders* (DSM IV–TR). This is a subset of acutely altered mental states. We will not discuss chronic changes in mentation such as comatose states, dementias, amnesias, or developmental delays.

2. **What is delirium?**
   Delirium is fundamentally a disturbance of *consciousness*: one's awareness of the environment and the ability to focus, sustain, or shift attention; and *cognition*: memory, orientation, and language. Frequently there are associated disturbances of perception (illusions, misinterpretations, visual hallucinations). Delirium is an acute process: it develops over a short period of time (usually hours to days) and tends to fluctuate during the course of a day. Frequently there are changes in the sleep–wake cycle. Finally, delirium is caused by an underlying medical condition.
   The terms "organic" and "functional" were once used to separate general medical disorders (organic) from psychiatric (functional). With the growing understanding that many psychiatric disorders have a basis in organic disease, this distinction is less helpful. Delirium is a medical condition presenting with psychiatric or behavioral manifestations.

3. **Are all patients with delirium the same?**
   No. There are three subtypes of delirium based on psychomotor activity. A patient's level of arousal may be hyperactive, hypoactive, or mixed. About 25% of patients are hyperactive. They may be very agitated, disoriented, and/or delusional. Patients with hypoactive delirium, another 25% of cases, are quietly confused. They tend to be disoriented and apathetic. The mixed subtype, 35% of cases, fluctuates between hyper- and hypoactive states. In about 15% of cases, psychomotor activity is normal. All may experience hallucinations, typically visual.

4. **How can I tell if the confusion is primarily medical or psychiatric?**
   It can be very difficult. Mental confusion associated with disorientation to person, place, and time and impaired language and memory may imply an underlying organic disorder. Hyperactive delirium can

mimic an acute manic phase or schizophrenic decompensation, whereas hypoactive delirium can be confused with profound depression. Preexisting illness and time course are key elements in discerning medical from psychiatric. Both bipolar and schizophrenic diseases are usually associated with a history of previous episodes. It is uncommon to develop severe psychiatric illness after age 40. Psychiatric symptoms tend to repeat themselves. New or unusual symptoms should suggest a nonpsychiatric cause. Delirium tends to develop more quickly and to fluctuate with periods of relative clarity, whereas psychiatric disorders are more stable. The onset of psychiatric disorders is nearly always subacute. Psychiatric disorders are more likely to manifest auditory hallucinations. Visual hallucinations tend to be medical or toxicological based. Vital signs tend to be stable in the psychiatric patient, whereas there can be marked autonomic instability in the delirious.

5. How prevalent is delirium?
Approximately 2.3 million patients each year are diagnosed with delirium, resulting in total annual health care costs of more than $4 billion. These figures are probably low, as it is well established that delirium is frequently missed.

Delirium accounts for 10–20% of admissions to acute care hospitals. Ten to 20% of patients 70 years or older admitted to the hospital are delirious at admission and another 10–20% become delirious during their stay. The incidence of postoperative delirium is also quite high. Nearly one in four patients experience delirium after elective procedures and twice that many do so after emergency surgical intervention. Cancer patients share the same incidence as elective surgery patients. Thirty to 40% of hospitalized HIV patients are delirious. Up to 60% of elderly nursing home residents may have delirium at any time. With earlier disposition from acute care settings to rehabilitation centers, nursing homes, and home care, the incidence of delirium in the community is likely to be increasing. In one recent study, 38% of patients who met criteria for delirium were discharged from the emergency department.

6. Who is at risk?
The hospitalized and the elderly are the largest at-risk groups. In addition to the aforementioned surgical, oncologic, and immune-compromised patients, patients with underlying central nervous system (CNS) disorders such as cardiovascular accidents, dementia, or Parkinson's disease, are taking more than three medicines, may have multiple medical conditions, chronic disease states, or any end-stage organ disease, may have terminal illness, may have sensory loss or deprivation (diminished hearing, macular degeneration, severe cataract disease), or are using drugs and alcohol or who suddenly stop can become delirious. In short, any significant underlying illness can predispose to delirium.

Physical illness is more commonly the cause in the very young and those older than 60 years. Delirium due to substance abuse is more common during the third and fourth decades of life.

7. Does delirium fully resolve?
Delirium is considered potentially reversible, but frequently there are long-term consequences. It doubles the mortality in the severely ill. Often there is long-term and irreversible functional decline. Delirium may persist for 12 months or longer. In one long-term follow-up study, only one-third of patients who had experienced delirium still lived independently in the community after two years. The impact is greater on patients who have delirium when they are hospitalized than in those who develop delirium during hospitalization.

8. **How do I know if someone is delirious?**

    Delirium is often missed. In some reports, this happens in more than 70% of cases. Knowing a patient's baseline mental status is difficult and yet it is an indispensable piece of information. Formal mental status testing need not be done prehospital. Patients are often unable to participate in their own history gathering so it is important to interview family members, friends, and facility staff. Ask about the patient's previous level of functioning. The hallmark features of delirium are deficits in attention, memory, and orientation. Their confusion fluctuates. Ask for examples. Simple observations and a few questions can rapidly assess a patient's level of confusion. Observe the patient's home and living arrangements. Is the appearance typical or unusual? Does the patient need instructions repeated or forget questions asked? Are they distracted? Attention can be tested by spelling WORLD backward or naming the days of the week backward. Always ask basic orientation questions. Patients may have difficulty with language and speech. Can they name simple objects (pencil, flashlight, hat)? Is their speech clear or gibberish? Is mumbled speech disorganized or simply poorly pronounced? One of the most sensitive tests is to name three objects and then repeat them a few minutes later.

    Children are considered at greater risk for delirium from ingestions and fever regardless of the source of the fever. Assessing cognition and attentiveness is difficult in the very young. Always ask the parents. Parents are far more attuned to subtle changes in behavior and attention. A child fussing on exam but consoling with parents, showing awareness of the surroundings, and making normal eye contact can be assumed to have normal alertness. Adolescents may have difficulty in clearly describing their symptoms.

9. **What other history questions should I ask?**

    What medications does the patient take, including any over-the-counter medicines and herbal supplements? What other medications are in the house? Could any have been borrowed or inadvertently accessed? Have there been any recent changes in the patient's drug regimen? Look specifically for street drugs, alcohol, and medication abuse. Ask about recent illness, surgery, or hospitalization. Ask about chronic medical and psychiatric conditions. Is there a preexisting endocrine disorder (diabetes or thyroid)? Has there been any recent exposure to toxins or environmental injury? Are there any previous episodes of confusion? It is useful to determine how long the patient has had mental status changes and whether the change was abrupt or gradual. In patients with chronic dementia or organic brain syndromes it is important to determine how their current mental status differs from their baseline mental status.

10. **What causes delirium?**

    Virtually any medical condition can precipitate delirium in a susceptible person. The conditions most commonly associated with delirium include underlying CNS disease (stroke, seizures), fluid and electrolyte disturbances (dehydration, hyponatremia, and hypernatremia), infections (meningitis, encephalitis, urinary tract, respiratory tract, skin, and soft tissue), drug or alcohol toxicity, withdrawal from alcohol or drugs, withdrawal or toxicity from psychoactive medications (SSRIs, neuroleptic medications, TCAs); metabolic disorders (uremia, hepatic failure), endocrine disorders (diabetes, thyroid), temperature extremes (hypo- and hyperthermia), low perfusion states (shock, heart failure), postoperative states, and toxidromes (sympathomimetic, narcotic, cholinergic, anticholinergic, aspirin, serotonin syndrome). In about 10–20% of patients, no cause is identified.

The exact pathophysiology of delirium is poorly understood. With so many disparate etiologies it's likely there are several mechanisms that share a common final pathway leading to global cognitive dysfunction.

11. Is there an easier way to remember this?

There are several well-known mnemonic devices for remembering the more common causes of delirium and triggering intervention. Try this one—DELIRIOUS EMT-Ps:

Drug abuse and drug withdrawal, particularly alcohol
Electrolyte (sodium, calcium) and **E**ndocrine disorders (diabetes, thyroid, parathyroid)
Liver disease (hepatic encephalopathy)
Infection (meningitis, kidney, lung, skin) and **I**schemia (cardiac and bowel)
Reduced sensory (diminished hearing and vision) and **R**eversal agents (naloxone and D-50)
Intracranial lesion (stroke, tumor)
Oxygen (hypoxic states and supplemental oxygen)
Uremia
Surgery and **S**eizure
Environment (hypothermia, hyperthermia, altitude)
Medications (more than three and recent changes) and **M**emory impairment
Toxidromes and **T**rauma
Perfusion
Scene safety

12. What exam findings should I look for?

The physical exam can be challenging in the agitated patient. Although there are few exam findings that will clearly reveal an underlying cause for delirium, there several typical stigmata of disease states.

In addition to the aroma of alcohol, the patients may have other odd odors. The ketoacidosis of diabetes has a fruity smell, whereas fetor hepaticus, associated with hepatic encephalopathy, is memorably foul. The hypoxic patient may appear dusky. Jaundice may reveal liver failure. Carbon monoxide poisoning can present as cherry-red lips. Are needle tracks or shooters' abscesses apparent? A bitten tongue or loss of bladder control may suggest a recent seizure and consequent concern for status epilepticus. Rebound abdominal tenderness or nuchal rigidity may localize a source of infection. Anticholinergic toxicity (red as a beet, dry as a bone, blind as a bat, mad as a hatter, and hot as a hare) can cause delirium in both the elderly taking multiple medications as well as a young patient abusing cough preparations.

Ascertaining focal neurologic signs may be confounded by the patient's inattention and altered consciousness. As best as possible, it is important to note pupillary responses and extraocular movements. Tremor and asterixis may be present in the awake patient. In severely obtunded subjects, decorticate and decerebrate posturing can occur.

Vital signs are often altered, as autonomic instability is characteristic of delirium. Consider preeclampsia in pregnant patients with hypertension.

13. What should I look for in a patient who has ingested alcohol?

Alcohol is the most common cause of abnormal mental status encountered by EMTs in the field. It initially may be manifested as stimulation or agitation. This may be followed by a depressant effect on the central nervous system, including a blunting of motor coordination and reflexes. Further elevation in blood alcohol can lead to coma and respiratory arrest.

It is of utmost importance, however to determine if the patient has other causes of altered mental status, including head injury or the ingestion of other toxins or poisons. It should be assumed that a patient has altered mental status from alcohol alone only after other treatable causes such as hypoglycemia or narcotic overdose have been ruled out.

In children it is important to consider the possibility of hypoglycemia caused by alcohol. In the naive drinker, particularly those with a thin body habitus, glycogen stores may be rapidly depleted during alcohol intoxication with a subsequent sudden drop in serum glucose. These patients are at particular risk for irreversible brain damage secondary to prolonged hypoglycemia if not recognized and treated.

14. How is a seizure patient with altered mental status evaluated?

Patients with a known seizure disorder who have abnormal mentation may be in a postictal state as a result of a recent seizure. These patients will typically be confused and combative. The postictal period is variable and can last briefly to as long as several days. Patients may require physical restraining during this period. Other physical findings that may support the diagnosis of a recent seizure should be sought, including tongue or lip biting or incontinence of bowel or bladder. One should observe for medical alert tags. Patients with a seizure disorder have a higher incidence of intracranial hemorrhage.

During seizure activity there is a switch from aerobic to anaerobic metabolism as a result of increased muscle activity and decreased or absent ventilation. Therefore, seizure activity will result in a metabolic acidosis reflected as a depression in serum CO_2. This can be measured from venous blood (red top) but will correct fairly rapidly after the seizure activity has stopped. It is important, therefore, to draw blood at the time an intravenous line is established.

15. How are diabetic patients evaluated?

Patients who are insulin dependent or take oral medications for diabetes are predisposed to two problems: hypoglycemia and hyperglycemia. Overmedication or intentional overdose of glucose-lowering drugs may result in hypoglycemia, which generally is manifested by a fairly sudden change in mentation associated with tachycardia and diaphoresis. These are sympathetic responses to sudden hypoglycemia. Neurologic manifestations may include paresthesias, cranial nerve palsy, transient hemiplegia, clonus, diplopia, and decerebrate posturing. Patients with hypoglycemia and fever should always be evaluated for a possible source of infection. Hypoglycemia may occur in chronic alcoholics with liver disease, acute alcohol intoxication in inexperienced drinkers, and in patients with insulin-producing pancreatic tumors.

Hyperglycemia results from a relative or absolute insulin deficiency and manifests in one of two disease states: diabetic ketoacidosis (DKA) (type I or insulin-dependent diabetes) or hyperosmolar nonketotic hyperglycemia (type II or adult-onset diabetes). Diabetic ketoacidosis is associated with Kussmaul respirations, dehydration, and a fruity (ketotic) odor to the breath. Nonketotic hyperosmolar states are associated with dehydration and hyperosmolality without ketoacidosis and are more likely than DKA to cause significant mental status changes primarily as decreased level of consciousness.

16. If opiate ingestion is suspected, how should the patient be treated?

The opiate syndrome is classically associated with depressed mentation, a blunted affect, and pinpoint pupils. Respiratory depression and respiratory arrest can be associated with opiate use. There is an additive central nervous system depressant effect with opiates and drugs such as alcohol, barbiturates, and benzodiazepines. Many opiate preparations are available for use as analgesics, cough suppressants, and antidiarrheals. It is important for the prehospital provider to recognize these medications.

Commonly Prescribed Opiate Preparations

Generic name	Trade name
Codeine	Tylenol #3
Meperidine	Demerol
Hydrocodone	Vicodin, Lorcet, Lortab
Oxycodone	Percodan, Percocet, Tylox
Hydromorphone	Dilaudid
Diphenoxylate	Lomotil

Opiates are popular street drugs that come in a variety of preparations containing heroin, methadone, morphine, opium, and codeine. They may come in a variety of strengths and purity. It is not unusual for an emergency department to experience a sudden increase in the number of opiate overdoses based on the arrival of a particularly potent batch of drugs. The effects of opiates are rapidly reversed with the use of naloxone (Narcan™), which should be administered for suspected opiate overdoses in 2-mg intravenous increments. Some opiates, particularly diphenoxylate, may require higher doses for satisfactory reversal. If there is an effect from naloxone administration and the patient's condition suddenly deteriorates, more naloxone should be administered. Absence of a response to naloxone may imply that there is a concomitant overdose with other central nervous system depressants that are not reversed by naloxone, such as barbiturates or benzodiazepines.

17. How can one determine if someone has altered mentation because of uremia or liver failure?
The alteration in mentation in a uremic patient occurs because of the increasing blood urea nitrogen and the subsequent changes in serum osmolality. Advanced uremic patients may develop a condition called uremic frost in which a high concentration of urea in sweat yields a "frosty" appearance to the skin as the sweat dries. The skin of a uremic patient may also get a sallow, yellow color resulting from an accumulation of carotenelike pigments.
Patients with advanced liver disease may develop a flapping tremor or asterixis, a precoma condition that results in a nonrhythmic lapse in a voluntary sustained posture of the extremities, head, and trunk. The patient also may be jaundiced and may have a distended abdomen secondary to ascites or liver enlargement.
Uremia or liver failure generally will be suspected because of the past medical history or findings suggesting the underlying illness, such as a renal dialysis shunt in the forearm or jaundice.

18. What should the examination include if the patient has a head injury?
In addition to all of the usual signs and symptoms of a head injury, every examination must include an evaluation of (a) the patient's mental status, (b) pupillary response to light stimulation, and (c) the best motor and verbal response in order to calculate the Glasgow Coma Score. One must always keep in mind

the potential for cervical spine injury in patients who have sustained a head injury. Mental status changes from head injury can vary from agitation and combativeness to vacillating levels of consciousness and ultimately to coma.

19. **How can temperature extremes change mentation?**
    The exact mechanism of cerebral dysfunction associated with temperature extremes is unknown; some well-recognized patterns exist. As core body temperature decreases, cerebral blood flow decreases and mental status changes occur that resemble alcohol intoxication: slurred speech, motor incoordination, mental confusion, and lethargy. These changes can occur at body temperatures below 32°C (90°F). As body temperatures drop below 30°C (86°F), coma, dilated nonreactive pupils, and cardiac dysrhythmias may occur.
    Elevation in body temperature can result in several distinct syndromes. Mental status changes are not usually associated with heat cramps or heat exhaustion. Heatstroke, however, is a true medical emergency associated with widespread organ (including neurologic) dysfunction and may occur at a body temperature of 41.1°C (106°F) or greater. The neurologic changes in heatstroke may include hallucinations, irritable or bizarre behavior, combativeness, pupillary abnormalities, posturing, hemi- or quadriplegia, status epilepticus, or coma. Sweating may or may not be present.
    Children with moderate to high fevers may exhibit altered mentation that may take the form of acute confusion, hallucination, and nightmares. These symptoms are temperature dependent and do not necessarily imply serious disease. Febrile seizures can be a cause of altered mentation and may require a special evaluation to exclude serious underlying pathology.

20. **What infectious processes can result in altered mentation?**
    Meningitis, encephalitis, as well as other conditions. Meningitis is a viral or bacterial infection of the meninges that initially will manifest as headache with fever and signs of meningeal irritation (stiff neck). The mental status may be normal but, as the disease progresses, the patient may have a progressive decrease in level of consciousness.
    Encephalitis is an infection that involves the brain parenchyma; it usually affects the temporal lobe but can involve other areas of the brain. With encephalitis comes a rather abrupt onset of an acute confusional state associated with agitation and disorientation that may progress to lethargy, ataxia, seizures, and coma. Patients with encephalitis may occasionally appear to be acutely psychotic. They may require physical and/or chemical restraints. Such patients can be a difficult diagnostic dilemma, but the presence of a fever will usually lead the clinician to the correct diagnosis.
    Brain abscesses may also result in confusion and are generally associated with headache and fever. Other symptoms may include focal neurologic deficits and seizures

21. **How does one approach the patient with a suspected poisoning?**
    The astute prehospital provider will have the standard toxic syndromes committed to memory. These toxidromes include sympathomimetic, narcotic, cholinergic, anticholinergic, and other syndromes. All patients with a suspected poisoning should first be detoxified. The attendant should be cautioned against potential self-contamination during the initial evaluation and treatment phase. Careful attention should be paid to the airway, breathing, and circulation (ABC) as well as initial treatment, including establishing an IV and administering oxygen. The patient should be placed on a cardiac monitor and transported expediently to the nearest treatment facility.

22. Can a stroke result in altered mentation?

Yes but not always. Stroke is a broad general term that refers to an intracranial vascular event, which may include an ischemic event such as a transient ischemic attack (TIA) or an actual infarction of brain tissue. It generally is due to an embolus or a thrombus blocking one of the cerebral blood vessels. Stroke also may refer to a hemorrhagic event in which there is bleeding into the parenchyma of the brain. A stroke can be associated with normal mentation but abnormal motor function, which may render the patient with slurred speech or an inability to express thoughts or enunciate words clearly. Such a state may appear to be mental confusion even when the patient has normal mentation.

23. Can shock result in altered mentation?

Yes.

24. How low does blood pressure need to be before mental status changes occur?

Physiologic mechanisms help to maintain cerebral blood flow when the systolic blood pressure (BP) drops. There is a critical point, however, beyond which the cerebral blood flow starts to decrease. This is usually heralded by generalized signs of poor perfusion, which may include decreased level of consciousness, poor capillary refill, and cool clammy skin. The signs are usually associated with other physiologic changes, including increased heart and respiratory rates, diminished peripheral pulses, and decreased urine output.

The exact BP at which cerebral blood flow decreases and altered mental status changes occur can vary. The point at which this happens may depend on underlying disease states such as atherosclerotic peripheral vascular disease and other factors. It is generally felt that a systolic BP less than 80–90 mmHg will result in altered mental status.

25. What treatment should be initiated?

First and foremost, ensure the safety of the patient and yourself. Only a small minority of patients will present aggressive and agitated. The agitated elderly may be inadvertently injured by well-meaning medics. Conversely, medics may be injured by the younger substance-abusing population.

As part of scene and personnel safety, any patient with a suspected environmental poisoning (i.e., pesticide) should first be decontaminated.

Once scene safety is established, follow the ABCs. Measure O_2 saturation and administer supplemental oxygen. Cardiac monitoring and IV line insertion are expected. Most agencies can now perform a full 12-lead electrocardiogram. Treat threats to life and consider empiric naloxone administration. Blood glucose measurement should be performed on all patients with altered mental status followed by D-50 administration if low.

Manage the airway when it is at risk or when the patient is comatose and has no response to naloxone or has a poor gag reflex.

There is no medication for treating agitation that is both fast acting and universally safe. Haloperidol has been studied most often in the symptomatic management of delirium but carries the risk of extrapyramidal side effects, QTc prolongation, and torsades de pointes. There is also a risk of oversedation, but in the extremely agitated patient this is an acceptable, if not desirable, outcome. Risperidone and olanzapine are relatively new atypical antipsychotics and may have better safety profiles, although they are not commonly used or available in the prehospital setting. Immediate sedation will not occur, as the onset of action for these drugs can be 30 min or more. Benzodiazepines have a more rapid onset of action than the antipsychotics, but they commonly worsen confusion and sedation. Benzodiazepines are the drugs of choice only in cases of sedative drug and alcohol withdrawal or cocaine and amphetamine agitated delirium. Use physical restraints as needed.

Sensory deprivation worsens delirium; remember to bring the patient's eyeglasses and hearing aids.

26. **What if the patient does not want to go to the hospital?**

    It is important to determine if a patient who is refusing care has normal decision-making capacity. This is unlikely in the setting of acute mental status changes or fluctuating confusion.

    The patient must have normal thought processes, orientation, and be able to make decisions that a "prudent layperson" would make with regard to their health care. The patient must understand their underlying condition and what the consequences of not treating the medical condition may be. When treating someone with altered mental status, implied consent laws should prevail. It is always best to act in the best interest of the patient regardless of the patient's expressed wishes. This may involve soliciting help from family or even law enforcement and physically or chemically restraining the patient. The medical record should fully reflect the patient's impaired capacity and why the patient does not have normal decision-making capacity.

27. **What about tasers and excited delirium?**

    There is much controversy on this subject. Electroconvulsive devices (ECD) are clearly here to stay. There is no question they are less lethal and safer than handguns or brute force. Nevertheless, some patients have died in police custody after an ECD has been used. Some of these deaths are associated with a prone or "hog-tied" restraint. Nearly all of these are associated with an agitated delirium. If called to a scene where an ECD has been used to subdue a suspect, treat the underlying agitated delirium and with the patient in a supine position, restrain them as necessary, either physically or chemically.

Pearls and Pitfalls

1. First, not suspecting it; delirium is underdiagnosed.
2. Assuming an altered state is psychiatric and thus overlooking a serious underlying medical condition.
3. Being distracted by threatening or combative behavior.
4. Missing the acute change in a chronic condition.
5. Failing to treat the reversible causes of delirium, especially hypoglycemia.

References

1. Francis J. Prevention and treatment of delirium and confusional states. UpToDate. January 10, 2007.
2. Francis, J, Young G. Diagnosis of delirium and confusional states. UpToDate. April 28, 2006.
3. Myer, E. Acute toxic-metabolic encephalopathy in children. UpToDate. July 4, 2006.
4. Diagnostic and Statistical Manual of Mental Disorders: DSM-IV-TR, p. 143. Washington, DC: American Psychiatric Association, 2000.
5. Strote J. Taser use in restraint-related deaths. Prehospital Emergency Care, Volume 10, Issue 4 December 2006, pages 447–450
6. Gerstein PS. Delirium, dementia, and amnesia...http://emedicine.medscape.com/article/793247-overview. Accessed June 3, 2011.

7. Vilke, G, Johnson WD, Castillo EM. Evaluation of in-custody deaths proximal to use of conductive energy devices: 75. Ann Emerg Med 48(4), Supplement:S23–S24, 2006.
8. Strote, J. The role of tasers in police restraint-related deaths: 301. Ann Emerg Med 46(3), Supplement:S85, 2005.
9. O'Halloran, R. Asphyxial death during prone restraint revisited: A report of 21 cases. Am J Forensic Med Pathol 21(1):39–52, 2000.
10. Pollanen, M. Unexpected death related to restraint for excited delirium: A retrospective study of deaths in police custody and in the community. CMAJ 158(12):1603–1607, 1998.
11. Chalela J, Kasner S. Acute toxic-metabolic encephalopathy in adults. UpToDate December 2006.
12. Hustey FM, Meldon SW. The prevalence and documentation of impaired mental status in elderly emergency department patients. Ann Emerg Med 39:248–253, 2002.
13. Flynn O'Brien F, Kifuji K, Summergrad P. Medical conditions with psychiatric manifestations. Adolesc Med Clin 17(1), 49–77, 2006.
14. Martini, D. Delirium in the pediatric emergency department. Clin Pediatr Emerg Med 5(3):173–180, 2004.

Acute Neurologic Emergencies

CHAPTER 36

Julie Scadden, NREMT-P, PS

1. **What causes a headache?**
   A headache results from activation of peripheral pain receptors within the cranium and other structures. Pain may originate from multiple sources, such as contraction of extracranial muscles of the neck and scalp or dilation and distention of intracranial vessels. It may also be caused by inflammation of the peripheral vessels and nerves of the head, neck, or meninges covering the brain, as well as traction on intracranial structures from meningeal irritation and increased intracranial pressure (ICP).

2. **Are there different types of headaches?**
   Four types of headache are commonly recognized: vascular, muscle contraction (tension), traction, and inflammatory.

3. **How does one differentiate the various types of headaches?**
   Migraine headaches, the most common type of vascular headache, are commonly characterized by severe pain on one or both sides of the head, accompanied by nausea and sometimes blurred vision.
   There are a number of different types of migraine headaches including some forms that can present with neurologic symptoms that could be mistaken for a stroke.
   Tension headaches are the most common type of headache overall. They are generally characterized as mild to moderate in severity and usually are not well localized.
   Traction headaches result when intracranial structures are pulled, displaced, or stretched as a result of some other disease process, for example, a brain tumor.
   Finally, inflammatory headaches occur as a result of infectious processes such as acute meningitis or from irritation occurring with entities such as sub-arachnoid hemorrhage.

4. **What is a "cluster headache"?**
   A cluster headache is a type of vascular headache that causes repeated "attacks" or episodes of severe pain, occurring in cyclical patterns or "clusters." Cluster "periods," or bouts of frequent attacks, may last from weeks to months, although each individual headache generally lasts only 1–2 hours.. They may then be followed by periods when attacks go into remission (stop completely), and no headache occurs for months or sometimes years. Although cluster headache attacks are extremely painful, they are not life threatening.

5. **What is ultimately important to understand about headache complaints?**
   Headache pain in and of itself usually isn't life threatening. Headache is most often not the result of underlying disease; however, it *can* indicate the need for further investigation if it is acute in origin or becomes chronic. Headaches that manifest abruptly and are severe, sometimes described as feeling like a "thunderclap," may be serious as they can represent a subarachnoid hemorrhage. Other types of headache, when accompanied by fever, stiff neck, rash, mental confusion, seizures, double vision, weakness, numbness, or speech difficulties can indicate a number of serious problems including, meningitis, encephalitis, brain tumor, and stroke.

Clinical Care

6. **Who seeks medical care for headaches?**
   People who seek medical advice or intervention for headache usually do so because they have never experienced a headache before, are having a change in the typical characteristics of their recurring headaches, or have chronic headaches that need additional pain management.

7. **What is a stroke?**
   A cerebral vascular accident (CVA), more commonly known as stroke, occurs when the blood supply to an area of the brain is disrupted, either through occlusion or from rupture of a blood vessel. This results in a loss of oxygen and other nutrients causing cellular damage to that part of the brain beyond the point of occlusion or at the point of rupture. A stroke can affect any part of the brain.

8. **What is a transient ischemic attack?**
   A transient ischemic attack (TIA) is a transient (temporary) stroke that lasts from a few minutes to a few hours (less than 24 hours). TIAs are caused by a temporary thrombotic or embolic occlusion in a blood vessel of the brain with subsequent restoration of the blood flow to the afflicted area. Although there is no lasting injury to the brain when a TIA is over, it is sometimes referred to as a "ministroke." TIAs can be an important predictor of a major stroke event to follow. More than one-third of people who experience one or more TIAs will later have a stroke.

9. **What are the symptoms of a TIA?**
   The symptoms of a TIA include the following:
   - Sudden numbness or weakness of the face, arm, or leg, usually on one side of the body
   - Sudden confusion, trouble speaking or understanding
   - Trouble seeing out of one or both eyes
   - Problems walking, dizziness, loss of balance, or coordination
   - Sudden, severe headache with no known cause

10. **You have been called to evaluate an elderly female whose family describes a complaint of headache, slurred speech, and weakness in her right hand. Observing the patient, there is no sign of dysphasia or weakness and she complains of only a mild headache that she states is "normal" for her. If her vital signs are within normal parameters, does she still need to go to the emergency department (ED)?**
    Yes, the patient's medical history alone dictates the need for transport. Physician-level evaluation of the patient within 60 min following a possible TIA is recommended. Identification of the source, or cause, of the TIA will help determine appropriate therapy, including drug therapy or surgery, to reduce the risk of further events or a full-blown stroke, or cardiovascular accident (CVA).

11. **Can a CVA and TIA be differentiated in the prehospital setting?**
    If the patient is still having neurologic symptoms at the time of your assessment, then the answer is no, you cannot differentiate between a TIA and CVA. Only if the symptoms have completely resolved in less than 24 hours can the episode be called a TIA.

12. **Are there different kinds of stroke?**
    Stroke is classified in one of two ways: occlusive or hemorrhagic.
    An occlusive stroke occurs when a cerebral artery becomes blocked, severely decreasing or obstructing blood flow. This deprives the distal cells of oxygen and nutrients, as well as blocking waste removal, causing ischemic brain cells to infarct, with no hope of recovery if perfusion is not quickly restored.

Hemorrhagic stroke occurs following the rupture of a cerebral artery. Without the flow of oxygenated, arterial blood, brain cells become ischemic and eventually infarct, just as it happens in occlusive stroke. Additionally, however, in hemorrhagic stroke, blood from the ruptured artery forms an intracranial hematoma, which can quickly expand, compressing and herniating brain tissue.

13. Is there more than one type of occlusive stroke?

Yes, thrombotic and embolic. Thrombotic stroke occurs after deposits of atherosclerotic plaque narrow the lumen of a cerebral artery, gradually decreasing the flow of arterial blood. When an artery is significantly narrowed, platelets adhere to the rough surface of the vessel walls, creating a thrombus that completely occludes the artery.

Embolic stroke, like the thrombotic stroke, occurs from the occlusion of a cerebral artery. The difference is that the occlusion results when an embolus (plaque) breaks free from a proximal site such as the heart or carotid artery and lodges in a more distal vessel such as a cerebral artery.

14. What are the "7 Ds of Stroke Care"?

A system for the treatment of stroke, the 7 Ds of stroke care are detection, dispatch, delivery, door (arrival and urgent triage in the ED), data, decision, and drug administration. This system provides a means for increased efficiency and effectiveness of stroke care and highlights the major steps in diagnosis and treatment, as well as the key points at which delays in treatment can occur.

15. Is it important to determine an occlusive stroke vs. a hemorrhagic stroke in the prehospital setting?

No, it is nearly impossible to definitively determine the "type" of stroke without a computed tomography scan, but it does not really matter as prehospital management goals are the same regardless of type of stroke. The goal in prehospital management is to treat the presenting signs and symptoms and effect rapid transport to the nearest, most appropriate facility to minimize brain injury and maximize patient recovery.

16. What tools can EMS providers use to identify stroke patients?

The signs and symptoms of stroke can be subtle and the need to identify potential stroke victims is a time-sensitive priority for best patient outcomes. Using out-of-hospital tools such as the Cincinnati Prehospital Stroke Scale (CPSS) or the Los Angeles Prehospital Stroke Screen (LAPSS) can help emergency medical service (EMS) providers to identify stroke patients with reasonable accuracy.

17. What is the CPSS?

The CPSS is based on physical examination only. Health care providers check for three findings: facial droop, arm weakness, and speech abnormalities.

First, check for facial droop by having the person smile or show his or her teeth. A normal response is that both sides of the face move equally. An abnormal response is that one side of the face does not move as well as the other (or at all). Next, check for arm drift. Have the patient close their eyes and hold their arms straight out in front for about 10 sec. If one arm does not move, or one arm drifts down more than the other, that is abnormal. Finally, check the patient's speech by having them say, "You can't teach an old dog new tricks," or some other simple, familiar saying. If the person slurs the words, gets some words wrong, or is unable to speak, that is an abnormal response. An abnormal finding on any of these three components could represent a stroke.

If any one of these signs is abnormal the statistical probability of stroke is 72%.

Clinical Care

18. What is the LAPSS?

LAPSS first requires health care providers to determine if the patient is over age 45, does not have a history of prior seizures, whether the neurologic complaints started within the past 24 hours, was able to ambulate before the onset of the new symptoms, and has a blood glucose level between 60 and 400 mg/dL. Then the responder must evaluate for abnormalities in any of three physical examination categories: facial smile or grimace, grip, and arm strength. If the answer to the all of the items in first part of the screening tool is yes and there is a physical abnormality, then there is strong likelihood of a stroke.

19. Why is determining time of symptoms onset so important when suspecting the diagnosis of stroke?

Studies have found that many stroke patients who received fibrinolytic ("clot-busting") drug therapy within 3 hours of the start of stroke symptoms were at least 30% more likely to recover with limited or no permanent disability after 3 months.

The current window for thrombolytic therapy has been increased from 3 to 4.5 hours for some patients. Rapid identification of the clinical signs of possible stroke, as well as community and professional education, is essential to successfully increasing the proportion of stroke victims that can be treated successfully with fibrinolytic therapy.

20. What are important factors for treatment and transport of stroke patients?

EMS determination or high suspicion of stroke includes establishing the last time (time "zero") the patient was observed to be normal. Initiation of rapid transport to a medical facility that is capable of providing definitive care for stroke management and pre-arrival notification to the receiving facility is paramount to best patient outcome.

While en route to the facility, support cardiopulmonary function, monitor neurologic status, and check for blood glucose (if authorized by protocol) as a part of your prehospital management. Oxygen should be administered to hypoxemic patients (oxygen saturation less than 95% at sea level). Additionally, monitor the patient for respiratory compromise from aspiration, upper airway obstruction, hypoventilation, and (although rare) neurogenic pulmonary edema.

Hospitals should predefine their capability for treating stroke patients, communicating this status to EMS and surrounding communities, to ensure stroke patients are being transported to the most appropriate facility for definitive stroke management.

21. List the steps and "time goals" generally accepted for prehospital stroke management.

The time goals of the National Institute of Neurological Disorders and Stroke describe the time-sensitive nature of management of acute ischemic stroke:

1. Identify signs of possible stroke.
2. Check critical EMS assessments and actions:
   - Support ABCs.
   - Administer O_2 as needed.
   - Perform prehospital stroke assessment.
   - Establish time of last-known normal presentation of patient.
   - Transport to a center with definitive stroke care if appropriate (bring witness if possible to confirm onset of symptoms).

- Alert the hospital.
- Check glucose if possible.

TIME GOAL: 10 min to ED arrival

22. Can children have strokes?

Yes. The effects of stroke in children are generally the same as seen in adults and can include hemiparesis, aphasia, decreased field of vision, and trouble with visual perception. Children may also experience loss of emotional control and mood changes, problems with memory, judgment, and/or problem solving, as well as behavioral and personality changes, or improper language or actions.

23. What causes stroke in children?

Identifying the cause of stroke in children is vital to providing the right treatment as well as the prevention of additional injury. The most common cause of ischemic stroke in children is a blood clot, often due to congenital heart defects or infection that forms in the heart and travels to the brain. In sickle cell disease, sickled blood cells cannot carry oxygen to the brain and blood vessels may have narrowed or closed. About 10% of children with sickle cell disease suffer one or more strokes. The risk of such events can be reduced with blood transfusions. Hemorrhagic strokes in children are most often caused by arteriovenous malformations or can be the result of physical abuse.

24. How well do children recover from stroke?

Stroke recovery for a child, as with an adult, is different for each child. Children often recover the use of their arms and legs, as well as their ability to speak after a stroke. In general, younger people will recover more of their abilities than older people following a stroke. Prompt recognition by EMS, rapid transport to appropriate medical treatment, and rehabilitation can improve recovery significantly.

25. What is the "stroke chain of survival"?

The stroke chain of survival describes links, or definitive actions, that should be taken by patients, family, and health care providers to maximize recovery from stroke including

- Rapid recognition and reaction to stroke warning signs
- Rapid EMS dispatch
- Rapid EMS system transport and hospital prenotification
- Rapid diagnosis and treatment in the hospital

Even high-risk patients fail to recognize the signs of a stroke, or they deny or rationalize it, making continuing efforts at educating patients, communities, and health care providers essential in management and outcomes of cerebral vascular accidents.

Pearls and Pitfalls

1. Headaches are a common, sometimes everyday occurrence; however, assuming they do not warrant further consideration is potentially extremely dangerous.
2. Like other types of pain, headaches can be a signal of a more serious illness.
3. A CVA is sometimes called a "brain attack" due to the progression from ischemia to infarction.
4. TIA and stroke are the same disease, but TIA is a mild, temporary manifestation, whereas stroke is severe and can cause permanent disability.

Clinical Care

5. Checking for bruits prior to carotid massage may prevent the caregiver from precipitating a stroke.
6. Transport bystander witnesses, family members, or caregivers (if possible) with the patient to verify time of symptoms onset.
7. Remaining on scene to complete an in-depth assessment and treatment delays the time until definitive care and should be avoided.

References

1. Jauch EC, Cucchiava B, et al. Part II adult stroke 2010 American Heart Association guidelines for cardiopulmonary resuscitation and emergency cardiovascular care. Circulation 122:S818–S928, 2010.
2. National Institute of Neurological Disorders and Stroke: NINDS headache information, http://www.ninds.nih.gov/disorders/headache/headache.htm Accessed Jun 4, 2011.
3. Mayo Clinic Staff. Cluster headache: Introduction/when to seek medical advice. http://www.mayoclinic.com/health/cluster-headache/DS00487 Accessed Jun 4, 2011.
4. Mayo Clinic Staff. Concussion: Signs and symptoms. http://www.mayoclinic.com/health/concussion/DS00320 Accessed Jun 4, 2011.
5. American Heart Association. Transient ischemic attack (TIA), http://www.americanheart.org/presenter.jhtml?identifier=478 Accessed Jun 4, 2011.
6. National Institute of Neurological Disorders and Stroke. NINDS transient ischemic attack information, http://www.ninds.nih.gov/disorders/tia/tia.htm Accessed Jun 4, 2011.
7. Huff, JS. Cerebellar hemorrhage: eMedicine., http://www.emedicine.com/neuro/topic51.htm Accessed Jun 4, 2011.
8. National Institute of Neurological Disorders and Strokes. Know stroke. Know the signs, act in time. NIIH Publication No. 02-4872, http://www.ninds.nih.gov/disorders/stroke/knowstroke.htm Accessed Jun 4, 2011.
9. American Stroke Association. Pediatric stroke, http://www.strokeassociation.org/presenter.jhtml?identifier=3030392 Accessed Jun 4, 2011.

Hypertensive Emergencies

James A. Temple, BA, NREMT-P, CCP and Christopher B. Colwell, MD, FACEP

1. What is hypertension?
The answer to this question varies, as hypertension has been defined in a variety of ways. Most practitioners agree that hypertension (HTN) is a systolic reading over 140 mmHg and a diastolic reading of over 90 mmHg. However, current medical literature breaks down hypertension according to the following criteria:
- Normal blood pressure: systolic BP (SBP) less than 120 and diastolic BP (DBP) less than 80 mmHg
- Prehypertension: SBP 120–139 or DBP 80–90
- Stage 1 HTN: SBP 140–159 or DPB 90–99
- Stage 2 HTN: SBP >160 or DBP >100

2. Can I make the diagnosis of HTN in the field?
A patient may have an elevated BP reading during a prehospital care encounter for a variety of reasons, including pain or anxiety, which may not indicate underlying HTN. Although markedly elevated BP readings in the field might be a good indication for primary care follow-up, prehospital care providers should be careful about labeling any patient as having underlying HTN until the diagnosis has been made in the primary care setting. A patient should have at least three elevated BP readings at three separate outpatient office visits before being diagnosed with HTN.

3. How common is HTN?
Very common, and it has been described as endemic. One quarter of all Americans have HTN. Exact numbers are not known, as up to 25% of those with HTN are unaware that they have it.

4. What is the most common cause of HTN?
The most common cause of HTN is essential HTN. In other words, the actual cause of HTN in the majority of patients is not known. Factors such as age, heredity, race, obesity, and amount of dietary sodium may play a role. Although essential HTN is the most common form of HTN, specific causes do exist including renal disease, arterial disease, steroid therapy, thyroid and parathyroid disease, and ingestion of foods containing large amounts of tyramine (such as aged cheeses or wine), particularly in patients taking monoamine oxidase inhibitors.

5. When does a hypertensive emergency exist?
Patients who exhibit acute impairment of an organ system (target organ damage, TOD) along with the finding of HTN are experiencing a hypertensive emergency. These hypertensive emergencies occur in about 1% of all hypertensive patients.

It is important to remember that the presence of a hypertensive emergency depends on the presence of acute TOD, not on the absolute value of the BP reading. In other words, always treat the patient, not the number.

6. What is TOD?
TOD is organ dysfunction that can be seen in the cardiovascular system, central nervous system, renal system, and even during pregnancy. Examples include hypertensive encephalopathy, acute myocardial infarction (MI), congestive heart failure, and preeclampsia/eclampsia. Contrary to what some might think, a headache alone in the setting of severe HTN is not a hypertensive emergency unless altered mental status is involved.

7. Can hypertensive emergencies be recognized in the field?
Yes, by recognizing evidence of end-organ damage (such as altered mental status or pulmonary edema) in the setting of severe HTN.

8. How is HTN treated in the field?
It usually is not. HTN is generally not treated in the field because of the risk of lowering BP too quickly with most of the medications used in the field, and the fact that acutely lowering BP is rarely needed. Exceptions include patients with chest pain that is concerning for acute coronary syndrome/MI or patients with pulmonary edema who are hypertensive. These patients may be treated in many cases with nitroglycerin to manage their symptoms, which will often lower their BP. Another exception to the not treated in the field guideline is the patient exhibiting signs of severe preeclampsia or eclampsia.

9. What should I do for a patient with severe HTN and evidence of pulmonary edema on exam?
Treat the pulmonary edema and you will also be treating the HTN. Sublingual nitroglycerin will help in treating the pulmonary edema by reducing the preload (and afterload to some degree), and lower the BP as well. Furosemide (Lasix™) can also be used but will be effective only after preload reduction is accomplished.

10. What are the central nervous system (CNS) consequences of HTN?
One major manifestation of hypertension involving the CNS is a higher risk of CVA, both hemorrhagic and ischemic. Another serious complication is hypertensive encephalopathy. This is usually seen as a sharp and sudden rise in BP, above the 200/130 mmHg level. Common signs and symptoms of hypertensive encephalopathy include severe headache, nausea, vomiting, seizures, altered mental status, aphasia, blindness, and other strokelike symptoms.

11. What is the best way to manage a patient with severe HTN and acute neurologic deficits in the field?
As a general rule, do not treat BP in the field. Although up to 85% of strokes are ischemic, and 15% hemorrhagic, it will be difficult to distinguish between these two in the field. Because HTN in patients with ischemic strokes is often close to the patient's baseline BP, and patients with hemorrhagic strokes may have very labile BPs, it is often quite difficult to safely manage BP in these patients. Lowering BP too quickly, or even bringing BP down to what the health care provider feels is a "normal" BP can be quite dangerous. HTN in the setting of a stroke should not be treated in the field. Prehospital management should concentrate on supportive care and rapid transport.

12. Why shouldn't I treat BP in the field in patients with altered mental status?
Cerebral autoregulation is the process by which cerebral blood flow is maintained at a constant rate despite an elevated peripheral BP. When autoregulation has occurred in response to chronically elevated BP, your patient may not be able to maintain adequate cerebral perfusion at what we might think of as

Hypertensive Emergencies

"normal" BP. Bringing BP down below the level to which the patient has autoregulated can result in cerebral hypoperfusion and worsen the brain injury. It will be impossible to know to what extent autoregulation has occurred in your patient, so you need to be very careful when lowering BP so as not to induce cerebral hypoperfusion.

13. **Does HTN lead to any other complications?**

    Absolutely. Over the course of time, the constant pounding of ejected blood from the left ventricle against the wall of the aorta may weaken the proximal aorta, increasing the risk for aneurysm. The damage leads to a tear in the wall of the vessel producing a dual lumen in the aorta; one is the true lumen and the other is referred to as a false lumen. With each contraction, blood is forced in between the damaged layers of the aorta as well as through the normal lumen. This dissection will eventually compromise blood flow to distal organs or rupture, and death quickly follows.

    In addition to thoracic aortic dissection, HTN may lead to an abdominal aortic aneurysm (AAA). This again can be a life-threatening situation brought about by weakening of the abdominal aortic wall. Patients may have these aneurysms and be completely asymptomatic until the expanding aneurysm puts pressure on adjacent structures or becomes so large that the weakened wall finally ruptures and the patient bleeds acutely into their abdomen.

14. **What are the typical complaints and findings of an aortic dissection?**

    Some of the findings you may expect to see are as follows:

    - Chest pain, or a "ripping, tearing" sensation, often between the shoulder blades. The patient may state it is the worst pain they have ever experienced.
    - Usually there are no other "precursory" symptoms. Pain is 10 on a 10-point scale and has a very sudden onset, with no warnings.
    - Poor or absent circulation to one extremity (arm or leg). Take a blood pressure reading in both arms; a difference of 10 mmHg or more suggests the presence of dissection.

    It is always a good idea to take BPs in both arms on any patient with chest pain or any other cardiovascular situation or complaint to help evaluate for a dissection.

    The patient with an aortic aneurysm has a few basic needs: rapid transport, oxygen, pain relief, and rapid transport. Patients need immediate evaluation in the ED and potentially a cardiovascular surgeon to repair the abnormality.

15. **What will I see in a patient with an AAA?**

    One of the hallmark findings with an AAA is a pulsating mass in the abdomen. Upon careful inspection and palpation, this can be identified, and should serve as a red flag indicating the need for rapid transport. In the event of rupture you will see the development of the classical AAA symptoms: low back pain, pain around the umbilicus with radiation down to the groin or scrotum in males and even into the thigh, an urgent need to defecate, syncope, tachycardia, and profound hypotension.

    Like the patient with aortic dissection, the patient with AAA requires rapid transport for definitive surgical care.

16. **What about HTN in the pregnant patient?**

    HTN is seen in up to 8% of pregnancies. The pregnant patient will typically have a BP that is lower than usual, so a BP of greater than 140/80 in the pregnant patient is cause for concern. This can typically occur anywhere between 20 weeks gestation and 2 weeks postpartum. The risk of pregnancy-induced

HTN is highest in women who are younger than 20, those in their first pregnancy (primigravida), and those with twin or molar pregnancies.

A molar pregnancy is also referred to as a hydatidiform mole. This results from fertilization of an egg that does not have a nucleus. No viable fetus develops; instead, abnormal tissue secretes HCG (human chorionic gonadotropin) which results in an increased incidence of hyperemesis gravidarum and early preeclampsia.

17. **When do I need to be worried about BP and preeclampsia in pregnant women?**
    Preeclampsia is defined as "an increase in SBP of 30 mmHg and/or an increase in DBP of 15 mmHg on two occasions that are at least 6 hours apart in association with peripheral edema and protein in the urine (which is not tested for in the field)." Keep in mind that in pregnancy, maternal BP usually drops, so what may be a "normal" reading of 124/80 may actually be hypertensive for a given patient. This depends on the baseline BP. If a woman's blood pressure was 90/70 early in her pregnancy, your current 124/80 is of obvious concern.

18. **What is severe preeclampsia?**
    Severe preeclampsia is marked BP elevation (generally greater than 160/110) associated with epigastric or liver tenderness, visual disturbances, or a severe headache. Severe preeclampsia should be managed in the same way as eclampsia.

19. **What is eclampsia?**
    Eclampsia is the occurrence of seizures in a patient with preeclampsia (or presumed preeclampsia). Progression from preeclampsia to eclampsia is unpredictable and can occur very rapidly. Eclampsia should be considered in any visibly pregnant woman who has experienced trauma (such as a motor vehicle crash or a fall) without an obvious cause.

20. **How is eclampsia treated?**
    In the United States, eclampsia and severe preeclampsia are treated with magnesium sulfate. The dose is 6 g IV, followed by 2 g IV per hour as needed. Beware of hypoventilation from respiratory depression or paralysis in patients receiving such large doses of magnesium. Valium can also be used for seizure control if magnesium is not available or does not stop the seizure activity. Ultimately, the field treatment of eclampsia is rapid transport of the patient for delivery of the fetus in the hospital in any patient not already in the postpartum period.

Pearls and Pitfalls

1. Hypertension rarely needs to be treated in the field.
2. The presence or absence of acute target organ damage determines whether a hypertensive emergency exists.
3. Patients without evidence of acute end-organ damage will rarely require urgent reduction of their blood pressure, either in the field or at the hospital.
4. Lowering BP too quickly, particularly in patients with symptoms of a stroke, can be dangerous.
5. As tempting as it may be, never treat a number, always treat the patient.

References

1. National Heart Lung and Blood Institute. Seventh report of the joint national committee of prevention, detection, evaluation, and treatment of high blood pressure (JNC 7):42, 2003.
2. eMedicine. Hypertensive emergencies: http://emedicine.medscape.com/article/1952052 Accessed 6/04/2011.
3. eMedicine. Hypertension: http://emedcine.medscape.com/article/241381 Accessed 6/04/2011.
4. Bledsoe BE, Porter RS, Cherry RA. Essentials of Paramedic Care, 2nd ed., update. Upper Saddle River, NJ: Pearson Education Inc., 2011.
5. Bledsoe BE, Benner RW. Critical Care Paramedic. Upper Saddle River, NJ: Pearson Education Inc., 2006.
6. Caroline NL, AAOS. Nancy Caroline's Emergency Care in the Streets, 6th ed. Sudbury, MA: Jones and Bartlett, 2008.
7. Pesola, GR, Pesola HR, Lin M, et al. The normal differences in bilateral indirect blood pressure recordings in hypertensive individuals. Acad Emerg Med 9(4):342–345.
8. Nguyen TT, Rohrback SM, Lenamond C. Distinguishing and managing hypertensive emergencies and urgencies. Emerg Med Pract 7(7):1, 2005.
9. Jones DW, Hall JE. Seventh report of the Joint National Committee on Prevention, Detection, Evaluation, and Treatment of High Blood Pressure and evidence from new hypertensive trials. Hypertension 43:1, 2004.
10. Sibai BM. Diagnosis and management of gestational hypertension and preeclampsia. Obstet Gynecol 188:1615, 2003.

Seizures

Julie Scadden, NREMT-P, PS

1. **What is a seizure and why should I know about them?**
   A seizure results from excessive and disorderly neuronal discharges in the cerebral cortex. An estimated 300,000 people will experience a first seizure each year with approximately 2.7 million Americans of all ages affected by seizures, making them among the most common prehospital chief complaints. You will definitely treat patients with seizures.

2. **Do the terms "seizure" and "epilepsy" mean the same thing?**
   A seizure results from paroxysmal and excessive electrical neuronal discharges in the cerebral cortex. Epilepsy is a group of related disorders characterized by the tendency for recurrent seizures. Seizures are a symptom of epilepsy.

3. **Are there different types of seizures?**
   Yes, seizures can be generalized (involving the whole body) or partial (focal or involving just a part of the body). Generalized tonic–clonic, or *grand mal*, seizures are caused by abnormal electrical activity that spreads throughout the entire brain, resulting in loss of consciousness and generalized tonic-clonic muscle activity. Absence, or *petit mal*, seizures usually involve only a brief, sudden loss or "absence" of conscious activity, usually lasting only a few seconds or minutes, but many episodes may occur in a single day. Simple partial or focal, seizures begin in a localized area of the brain and remain focal. Patients who experience a focal seizure also remain conscious.

4. **What is an "ictus"?**
   An ictus is the period when the seizure occurs. Thus, preictal describes the period before a seizure, and postictal is the period after the seizure. Patients who have seizures may have a preictal forewarning, or an aura, that the seizure is about to begin.

5. **What is a Jacksonian march?**
   As a focal seizure spreads across the cerebral cortex, you may see what started out as focal tonic–clonic activity spread to other parts of the body. For example, tonic–clonic activity may begin in a patient's arm and then spread to the face, other arm, and legs. This is known as a "Jacksonian march."

6. **What is a febrile seizure?**
   Febrile seizures are seizures usually associated with fever that occur in infancy or childhood, generally between the ages of 3 months and 5 years of age in children with no underlying neurological abnormalities. A febrile seizure usually is of brief duration (less than 5 min) and is isolated.

7. **Can anyone have a seizure?**
   Yes, any individual may have a seizure when placed under the right stressors, such as hypoxia, fever, hypoglycemia, toxins (cocaine or amphetamines), or an intracranial injury.

8. **Define the term "seizure threshold."**
    The concept of "seizure threshold" suggests that everyone has a certain balance, which is probably genetically determined, between excitatory and inhibitory forces in the brain. One may have a higher or lower threshold than others yet never have a seizure or have seizures for no obvious reason. This conceptual theory asserts that a low seizure threshold makes it easier for epilepsy to develop and/or easier for a person to experience a seizure.

9. **What are cryptogenic seizures?**
    Cryptogenic seizures, also known as idiopathic or primary seizures, are of undetermined etiology. They most commonly occur in childhood and may be associated with a genetic or physiological disposition. Often times, there is a family history of epilepsy; however, in all cases of cryptogenic seizures, the exact cause cannot be identified.

10. **What is the differential diagnosis of seizures?**
    Seizures may be confused with a number of conditions, including panic attack, syncope, migraine, vertigo, decerebrate posturing, hyperventilation, and movement disorders. Breath-holding attacks are commonly mistaken for seizures. Such events usually occur in children under the age of 6 years who are frustrated or angry. The children will present as crying, with uncontrollable shaking followed by cessation of breathing, then cyanosis. They may even progress to lethargy, limpness, and unresponsiveness. Proper differential diagnosis should be ascertained from the history of precipitating factors, along with appropriate diagnostic examinations if needed.

11. **What is "status epilepticus"?**
    Status epilepticus is traditionally defined as more than 5 min of continuous seizure activity or a series of seizures without full return of consciousness in between.

12. **What are some of the metabolic causes of seizure?**
    Hypoglycemia or hyperglycemia, hypernatremia or hyponatremia, hypocalcemia, hypomagnesemia, uremia, metabolic acidosis, and fever are causes.

13. **What are the the common antiseizure medications?**
    Phenytoin (Dilantin™)
    Carbamazepine (Tegretol™)
    Felbamate (Felbatol™)
    Tiagabine (Gabitril™)
    Levetiracetam (Keppra™)
    Lamotrigine (Lamictal™)
    Pregabalin (Lyrica™)
    Gabapentin (Neurontin™)
    Divalproex sodium (Depakote™)
    Valproic acid (Depakene™)
    Ethosuximide (Zarontin™)
    Phenobarbital

14. **You are called to the scene of a person down. Your patient is unresponsive but appears awake when you arrive. His friends tell you the patient has a history of seizures. What are the kinds of questions you should ask regarding what they saw?**

    What was the patient doing before the event?

    Did the patient lose consciousness?

    Did he fall?

    Did he get injured when he fell?

    How long did the seizure last?

    What did the event look like?

    Is there any history of recent head trauma or fevers?

    What was the patient's appearance immediately after the seizure activity stopped (postictal state)?

    Remember, all patients with grand mal seizures will have a loss of consciousness or may injure themselves as they fall. They are also commonly confused after the event. Generalized seizures may be manifested as generalized tonic, clonic, or tonic–clonic activity. Focal seizures rarely result in a loss of consciousness and normally involve only one limb or the face but may then spread under certain circumstances.

15. **Why is a syncopal event sometimes confused with a seizure?**

    People experiencing vasovagal syncope (a simple fainting spell) may have clonic activity (muscle twitching) believed to be caused by a temporary, but extremely low blood pressure during the synopal episode. This is often mistaken for seizure activity by witnesses. However, the patient's mental status is normal immediately after the event in contrast to the postictal state of a patient with a loss of consciousness secondary to a true seizure. Tongue biting, incontinence, and postevent confusion or amnesia are not normally associated with syncopal events as they are with seizure.

16. **How do I distinguish "pseudoseizures" (psychogenic seizures) from true seizures?**

    Pseudoseizures often last longer than true seizures and rarely have a postictal period. Patients are awake during these episodes and often remember events that occurred during the event. Some characteristics of motor activity that are associated with pseudoseizures include side-to-side shaking of the head, pelvic thrusting, asynchronous extremity movement (bicycling), weeping, stuttering, and arching of the back. Patients with pseudoseizures have no alterations on their electroencephalograph tracing during the "seizure" and have no transient anion gap acidosis immediately following.

17. **What findings are common on physical exam of a patient who has experienced a generalized tonic–clonic seizure?**

    Altered mental status (postictal confusion), intraoral trauma or tongue lacerations, lethargy, focal weakness or sensory loss, and incontinence are some common findings. Perform a complete exam to try to determine the underlying cause of the seizure. Check carefully for signs of general or head trauma, as well as evidence of alcohol or drug use. Finally, be sure to perform a neurologic exam.

18. **In addition to metabolic derangements, what other conditions can cause seizures?**

    Seizures may result from brain tumor, trauma, subdural hematoma, subarachnoid hemorrhage, stroke, and intracranial bleeding. Infections, including meningitis and encephalitis, can also cause seizure. Overdose or use of various substances such as tricyclic antidepressants, cocaine, amphetamines, antihistamines, theophylline, and isoniazid are other causes. Alcohol withdrawal is a common cause of seizures. One of the most common causes of a seizure is subtheraputic levels of antiseizure medication.

19. **In a patient who is 36 weeks pregnant and seizing, what is the most serious cause?**
   A generalized seizure in any third trimester pregnant woman must be assumed to be secondary to eclampsia. Eclampsia also includes hypertension, hyperreflexia, and proteinuria. Treatment is administration of 4–6 g of magnesium sulfate IV followed by emergent delivery of the fetus and placenta at the hospital.

20. **Are spinal precautions necessary in all seizure patients?**
   Cervical spine immobilization should be used for all seizure patients who have experienced a fall, even from standing. C-spine immobilization is not necessary in patients with a seizure that has not been associated with head trauma or a fall.

21. **How do I manage the actively seizing patient?**
   Protect the patient from injury secondary to tonic–clonic activity. Do not attempt to insert anything into the patient's mouth during the seizure. Administer oxygen, start an IV, and determine blood glucose level.

22. **What medications should be administered to treat seizure in the prehospital setting?**
   Most seizures are brief, self limited, and will have stopped spontaneously before or shortly after your arrival. If the patient is still seizing, or has a recurrent seizure, benzodiazepines are the drug of choice for use in the prehospital arena. Diazepam (Valium™) has traditionally been used in recommended doses of is 5–10 mg IV push for an adult (0.1 mg/kg in a child); Midazolam (Versed™), thiopental, or pentobarbital are also effective in controlling seizures. Additionally, a blood glucose determination should be performed in all patients with a history of seizure and diabetes. If the patient has low blood sugar, administer 25 g of $D_{50}W$ slow IV push.

23. **Your patient begins to have a seizure and you are unable to establish an IV. What do you do?**
   Diastat®, a gel form of diazepam, may be administered rectally with a recommended dose of 0.2–0.5 mg/kg. Midazolam (Versed), 0.2 mg/kg, can be administered intranasally, or via the buccal route, when IV access is not possible, especially in children.

24. **Do all seizure patients need to be transported to an emergency department?**
   New onset, or traumatic seizure, patients should be transported. Patients with a known seizure disorder, especially those experiencing a short postictal period and a return to normal mental status, may refuse transport; however, if they are not transported, you should clearly instruct them to not drive an automobile until cleared after follow-up with their primary care physician.

25. **Why is it important to obtain a blood tube in the field for serum electrolytes?**
   A transient (less than 30 min) metabolic acidosis occurs after a grand mal seizure. If the diagnosis of seizure is in question, normal electrolytes on field bloods drawn immediately after the seizure will prevent expensive diagnostic tests and labeling the patient with a diagnosis of epilepsy.

Clinical Care

Pearls and Pitfalls

1. Observe carefully and document the exact type of movements during the event in order to help determine what type of seizure the patient had.
2. Obtain a careful history about the circumstances of the "seizure."
3. Observe and document any postictal state.
4. Administer benzodiazepines for prolonged or recurrent grand mal seizures.
5. Assume the presence of eclampsia in a third-trimester pregnant patient with a seizure.
6. Remember the prehospital treatable causes of seizures are hypoxia and hypoglycemia.
7. Consider spinal precautions in any patient who has had a fall associated with the seizure.

Reference

1. Nair, DR: Epilepsy, The Cleveland Clinic: http://www.clevelandclinicmeded.com/medicalpubs/diseasemanagement/neurology/epileptic-syndrome/Accessed June 4, 2011.
2. Epilepsy Foundation: http://www.epilepsyfoundation.org/about/index.cfm Accessed June 4, 2011.
3. Simple partial seizures. http://emedicine.medscape.com/article/1184384-overview Accessed June 4, 2011.
4. Seizures in children. http://www.emedicinehealth.com/seizures_in_children/article_em.htm Accessed June 4, 2011.
5. National Institute of Neurological Disorderes and Stroke. Febrile seizures: http://www.ninds.nih.gov/disorders/febrile_seizures/febrile_seizures.htm Accessed June 4, 2011.
6. American Academy of Pediatrics. Pediatric Eduation for Prehospital Professionals Provider Manual, 2nd ed., pp. 106–112. Elk Grove Village, IL: Jones and Bartlett, 2006.
7. Bledsoe BE, Porter RS, Cherry R. Esssentials in Paramedic Care, 2nd ed., update, pp. 1264–1267. Upper Saddle River, NJ: Pearson Education, Inc., 2011.
8. McIntyre J, Robertson S, Norris E, et al. Safety and efficacy of buccal midazolam versus rectal diazepam for emergency treatment of seizures in children: A randomized controlled trial. Lancet 366(9481):205–210, 2005.
9. Wolfe, TR, Macfarlane, TC. Intranasal midazolam therapy for pediatric status epilepticus. Am J Emerg Med 23(3):343–346. http://www.sciencedirect.come/science Viewed: 3/25/2007.

Fever

Cheryl Blazek, BS, EMT-P

CHAPTER 39

1. **A patient with a temperature of 104°F has a fever. True or false?**
   Maybe. A fever in medical terms is defined as an elevation of body temperature that occurs because the body's internal thermostat has been "reset" at a higher level. This is most commonly caused by infections. Elevations of body temperature that are not caused by resetting the thermostat occur when the body's heat production exceeds heat loss. This is not defined as a fever; instead, the medical term for this condition is hyperthermia.

2. **How does the body regulate temperature?**
   The brain's hypothalamus regulates heat production (by increasing metabolism and shivering) and heat loss (by varying the blood flow to the skin and by sweating). It measures the blood temperature directly and has an intrinsic set point of about 98.6°F (37°C).

3. **What is the main source of heat production in the body?**
   The primary source of heat production is metabolism of food into energy. The basal metabolic rate can be increased or decreased depending on the body's needs. Heat is also produced during physical exercise.

4. **Explain the four ways that the body loses heat.**
   As a child, did an adult ever tell you to put a hat on when it's cold outside? That's because most body heat is lost through *radiation* of heat from exposed skin. *Evaporation* of sweat also allows for heat loss; the effectiveness of this method depends on the humidity of the ambient air. *Convection* is a third process of heat loss; wind blowing across exposed skin will "pull" heat from the body. Heat loss through convection is increased when the skin or clothing is damp. Heat loss may also occur through *conduction*—a direct transfer of heat from one's body to another object or substance. Conduction is responsible for a significant percent of heat loss when a person is immersed in water.

5. **Why is it important to know the anatomic site where the temperature was measured?**
   Rectal and tympanic membrane temperatures reflect the temperature in the body's core. In general, a rectal temperature is about 1°F (0.6°C) higher than oral temperature. Thus, a normal rectal temperature is 99.6°F (37.6°C). Conversely, temperatures taken in a patient's axilla will be about 1°F (0.5°C) lower than oral temperatures. An axillary temperature of 98.6°F is equivalent to an oral temperature of about 99.6°F. Axillary temperatures may take 5–7 min to obtain and are quite variable, and therefore are not completely reliable.
   A temperature should always be reported as the actual reading in the manner it was taken. For example, a rectal temperature should be reported as "102 degrees rectally." Do not report the temperature as "101 degrees" to adjust for the 1 degree elevation of a rectal temperature. Axillary and oral temperature readings should be reported in the same manner.

6. **How does an infection cause a fever?**
   Infectious agents (viruses, bacteria, or fungi) cause the release of chemicals known as pyrogens. Pyrogens result in an elevation of the hypothalamic set point above the usual set point of 98.6°F. It is thought a fever helps to fight off infection in the body. Some infections may be sensitive to a rise in body temperature. Fevers, however, may cause serious damage to the body. The common treatment approach is to lower the fever to a safe body temperature.

7. **What other conditions (besides infection) result in an elevation of temperature?**
   Strokes and tumors can affect the hypothalamus directly, resulting in dysfunction of the temperature regulatory system. Sympathomimetic drugs such as amphetamines or cocaine can result in increased heat production, as can the adrenergic state associated with drug or alcohol withdrawal. If the body is unable to lose this heat, an elevated temperature results. High environmental temperatures, high humidity, or extreme physical activity on a hot day can overwhelm the body's ability to lose excess heat.

8. **In a patient with a history of fever, what questions should be asked?**
   How old is the patient? When did the fever start? How high is the fever? Any recent travel? Are there any associated symptoms such as pain, vomiting, diarrhea or seizures? Are there any chronic medical conditions, particularly any that compromise the immune system? Has the patient recently been exposed to any illnesses? Is anyone else in the household ill? If the patient is a child, is he or she up to date on krecommended childhood immunizations? What antifever or antipyretic medications have been taken? When? What dose? What results were seen, if any, from the medication?

9. **What patients are at special risk from a fever?**
   Fever in infants and children should always prompt concern. Any fever in a child younger than 3 months old is abnormal and may indicate a life-threatening emergency such as meningitis. All of these children should be evaluated by a physician. Elderly patients may develop serious infections without a fever; the presence of a fever in this population requires a full medical evaluation. Fever in immunocompromised hosts, including patients with diabetes, AIDS, or cancer, may be the harbinger of serious illness.

10. **Explain the effect that elevated temperature may have on the other vital signs.**
    A patient's heart rate will increase approximately 10 beats per minute (bpm) for every 1°C (1.8°F) rise in temperature. In an effort to blow off excess body heat, the respiratory rate also increases as the temperature increases. Hypotension in the setting of a fever is an ominous sign and generally indicates a serious infectious process or sepsis.

11. **What is the most important exam finding to assess in febrile patients?**
    The most important observation to make is how well the patient is tolerating the fever. Does he or she look toxic? What is the mental status? In children, note whether they are playful, smiling, alert, and interactive with you and their caregivers, or if they are lethargic and not as alert as normal.

12. **What are purpura, and what is their importance?**
    Purpura are purple or maroon blotches on the skin that do not blanch with pressure. Purpura are often associated with meningitis. Other serious infections may result in a variety of rashes. Always perform a careful skin exam when evaluating a febrile patient.

13. **Define sepsis and bacteremia.**
    Bacteremia occurs when bacteria invade the bloodstream. These bacteria may release toxins that cause vasodilatation, hypotension, and shock. Sepsis refers to the life-threatening shock that may

result from bacteremia. All septic patients are bacteremic, but not all bacteremic patients are septic.

14. **You are treating a 62-year-old diabetic female who has a heart rate of 112, blood pressure of 88/64, and a respiratory rate of 28. She is slightly confused, and her skin feels warm and dry to the touch. What would be the appropriate field treatment?**
   Given the patient's age and past medical history of diabetes, she is at risk of developing a serious bacterial infection and all its consequences. Hypotension and altered mentation should be of concern; presume she is septic until proven otherwise. Field treatment will include application of high-flow oxygen, checking a blood glucose level and administering glucose if warranted. IV fluid administration to treat hypotension and dehydration is appropriate. A cardiac monitor can be applied to monitor any cardiac changes or abnormalities that may result from the patient's elevated body temperature.

15. **What is a febrile seizure? What are its characteristics? Who is at risk?**
   A febrile seizure is a generalized tonic–clonic seizure that may occur in children (usually between 6 months and 5 years old) when they have a rapidly rising temperature. Children who have had one febrile seizure are at increased risk of having a second seizure, either during the current infectious state or during a future febrile illness. Febrile seizures usually are brief, single seizures with short postictal periods. Children who present in status epilepticus who and are afebrile upon evaluation should have other causes considered. Children should be managed pharmacologically as directed by medical direction or standing order.
   A febrile seizure should be treated similar to any other seizure with regards to priority treatment given to airway, breathing, and circulation and protecting the patient from injury.

16. **List appropriate field treatments for elevated temperature.**
   Patients with elevated temperature are often dehydrated, and intravenous administration of fluids is critical. Oxygen should be given to all tachypneic patients as well as to those in respiratory distress, and cardiac monitoring should be considered. Field measures to lower temperature should be begun for patients with a temperature of more than 104°F.

17. **Describe appropriate methods to lower a patient's temperature.**
   Undress the patient as much as possible and place him or her in a cool environment. Sponging with tepid lukewarm water is very effective. Avoid ice-water baths; if the patient's skin is cooled too quickly, shivering will result and will lead to increased heat production.

Pearls and Pitfalls

1. A fever involves resetting the body's thermostat to a higher temperature.
2. Hyperthermia is when heat accumulation exceeds heat loss.
3. The heart rate goes up approximately 10 bpm for each degree Celsius rise in temperature.
4. Overly aggressive cooling measures will cause the patient to shiver and increase heat production.

References

1. Bledsoe BE. Environmental emergencies. In Paramedic Emergency Care, 2nd ed., Bledsoe BE, Porter RS, Shade B, eds. Englewood Cliffs, NJ, Prentice-Hall, 1994.

2. Dierking BH, Everidge JM, Ramenofsky ML. Initial prehospital assessment of the pediatric patient. JEMS: J Emerg Med Serv 13:59, 1988.
3. Goodykoontz C. Fever. In Prehospital Field Care: A Complaint-Based Approach, Pons PT ed. St. Louis: Mosby, 1997.
4. Thomas H, Folstad S. Fever. In The Clinical Practice of Emergency Medicine, 2nd ed., Harwood-Nuss A, ed. Philadelphia: Lippincott-Raven, 1996.
5. Zukin DD, Grisham JE. The febrile child. In Emergency Medicine: Concepts and Clinical Practice, 3rd ed., Rosen P, et al., eds. St. Louis: Mosby, 1992.

Abdominal Pain

Christina Johnson, MD, FACEP

CHAPTER 40

1. **Define the term "acute abdomen."**
   This is a term used by surgeons and emergency physicians to describe abdominal conditions that require surgical exploration. Examples of such conditions include a perforated appendix, perforated gastric or duodenal ulcer, strangulated bowel, ruptured intraperitoneal abscess, ruptured spleen or liver, and ruptured ectopic pregnancy. A patient with an acute abdomen typically has a rigid abdominal wall or rebound tenderness upon examination and prefers to lie still; he or she may complain about bumps in the road during the ambulance ride to the hospital.

2. **What are key pieces of information to elicit from the patient's history?**
   The patient's description of the abdominal pain is an important piece of the pain assessment. Pain that begins suddenly and is severe usually implicates a serious cause. The distribution and quality of the pain can narrow the differential diagnosis. For instance, pain that begins in the periumbilical region and progresses to the right lower quadrant is typical of appendicitis. In contrast, pain that is periumbilical and radiates to the back is more likely to be due to pancreatitis. Pain that is increased by deep inspiration can be due to irritation of the diaphragm, as in cholecystitis (or pulmonary embolus or pneumonia, which can mimic abdominal conditions). Acute onset of unilateral flank pain that radiates to the abdomen and groin on the same side suggests a diagnosis of renal colic.
   Precipitating and alleviating factors also provide clues to the possible diagnosis. For example, right upper abdominal pain that occurs after ingestion of a fatty meal is a clue to the diagnosis of cholelithiasis. Associated symptoms also can be important to the diagnosis. Fever and chills are present in cases of infection, whereas nausea, vomiting, and anorexia are nonspecific symptoms. Vomiting that follows the onset of abdominal pain may indicate intestinal obstruction, pancreatitis, appendicitis, or cholecystitis. The presence of intestinal bleeding is an important factor to consider in the diagnosis of abdominal pain. Menstrual history, history of alcohol use, presence of dysuria or hematuria, reports of weight gain or loss, and abnormal pattern of bowel movements also should be elicited. Finally, a history of previous similar pain and previous abdominal surgeries may help in diagnosing and managing the patient's abdominal pain.

3. **Name some cardiovascular causes of abdominal pain.**
   Weakening of the wall of the abdominal aorta leads to formation of an aneurysm. Aneurysms may enlarge, leak, or rupture, leading to significant abdominal and back pain. Arterial insufficiency in the abdomen (due to atherosclerosis, thromboembolism, or hypotension) can lead to intestinal ischemia and/or infarction of the bowel. Some patients with myocardial ischemia or infarction, pericarditis, or myocarditis experience pain that localizes or radiates to the epigastrium.

4. **How would a patient with an abdominal aortic aneurysm present?**

   Classically, a patient with a symptomatic abdominal aortic aneurysm (AAA) describes the acute onset of pain in the abdomen radiating to the back. The pain may be described as tearing and severe. A pulsatile abdominal mass may be noted on exam and one might find absent pedal pulses. Hypotension, often associated with syncope, is an ominous sign in a patient with an AAA because it suggests rupture of the aneurysm with bleeding into the abdominal cavity. The mortality of ruptured AAA is extremely high. Unfortunately, most patients who present with ruptured AAA have not been diagnosed with AAA in the past.

5. **What are examples of gastrointestinal causes of abdominal pain?**

Cause of Pain	Description
Gastritis	Inflammation of the stomach lining associated with excess gastric acid production and gastric irritants such as nonsteroidal anti-inflammatory drugs (NSAIDS) and alcohol
Gastric or duodenal ulcer	Erosion of the mucosal lining of the stomach or, more commonly, the duodenum. Often due to NSAIDs or *Helicobacter pylori*
Cholelithiasis	Formation of gallstones that may become obstructed and cause pain
Cholecystitis	Infection within the gallbladder
Bowel obstruction	Usually caused by adhesions from prior surgery or hernias
Appendicitis	Infection of the appendix, an appendage of the large intestine
Diverticulitis	Inflammation of diverticuli (small out-pouches) of the large bowel, seen in older patients
Inflammatory bowel	Ulcerative colitis and Crohn's disease may cause pain, bleeding, obstruction, and abscess disease
Pancreatitis	Inflammation of the pancreas, may be caused by obstruction by biliary gallstones, medications, or alcohol
Hepatitis	Inflammation of the liver caused by viral infection, alcohol, or medications
Gastroenteritis	Viral or food-borne infection associated with vomiting, diarrhea, and dehydration

6. **What are some examples of common genitourinary causes of abdominal pain?**

Cause of Pain	Description
Nephrolithiasis	Renal stones, particularly if they obstruct the lumen of the ureter, can cause pain that is referred to the abdomen, back, or groin
Pelvic inflammatory disease	Sexually transmitted diseases that are untreated may progress to infect the uterus, ovaries, or fallopian tubes, and can lead to a tubo-ovarian abscess
Ovarian torsion	Twisting of the ovary with resultant ischemia and unilateral pain

Ectopic pregnancy	A pregnancy located anywhere except its usual location within the uterus; frequently associated with intraabdominal and vaginal bleeding
Ruptured ovarian cyst	Leads to symptoms of peritonitis as the cyst fluid irritates the peritoneum diffusely
Cystitis	Infection of the bladder; usually with associated symptoms of dysuria and urinary frequency and urgency
Testicular torsion	Twisting of the testicle, causes severe pain in the scrotum that may radiate to the abdomen
Epididymitis	Infection of the epididymis that causes pain that may radiate to the abdomen

7. **Some diseases of organs that do not reside within the abdomen can cause abdominal pain. What are some examples of such diseases?**
Acute myocardial infarction can be associated with pain in the epigastrium. Lower-lobe pneumonia, pneumothorax, pulmonary embolus, or pleural effusion can cause inflammation of the diaphragm and lead to pleuritic upper abdominal pain. Patients with streptococcal pharyngitis, hypercalcemia, or diabetic ketoacidosis frequently complain of abdominal pain. Herpes zoster is another condition that may cause abdominal pain.

8. **What are key points of the prehospital physical examination in a patient with abdominal pain?**
One must start with a general assessment of the patient. How sick appearing is the patient? Is the patient diaphoretic and writhing in pain, or is the patient calmly conversing about the nature of his or her pain? Next comes assessment of the patient's vital signs. Is the patient tachycardic, as are most patients with an acute abdomen? Is the patient hypotensive? Causes of hypotension include gastrointestinal or vascular hemorrhage, sepsis, ruptured ectopic pregnancy, pancreatitis, and a vagal response to pain. Does the patient have a tactile fever? How intense is the pain on a scale of 1–10 (the so-called "fifth vital sign")? Is the patient pale, diaphoretic, or jaundiced? Further examination includes auscultation of the heart and lungs and visual inspection, auscultation and palpation of the abdomen. Is the abdomen distended? Are bowel sounds present? Is the abdomen soft or rigid? Always palpate away from the region of greatest abdominal pain first to obtain a reliable exam. Are pedal pulses present?

9. **How does the patient with colicky pain present?**
Patients with obstructing gallstones or renal stones may present with colicky pain. They have acute onset of abdominal pain and tend to writhe about, appearing restless in their attempts to find comfortable positions.

10. **What are some peritoneal signs?**
Peritoneal signs, or signs of peritoneal inflammation, include rebound tenderness (pain that is severe with releasing pressure from the patient's abdomen), pain with coughing, movement of the patient's stretcher or tapping the patient's heel, and pain that causes abdominal wall rigidity when palpated.

11. **What are the priorities for prehospital management of the patient with abdominal pain?**
The patient should be placed in a position of comfort. In the case of a hypotensive patient, that position should be supine. A patient who is nauseated should be placed in the left lateral decubitus position and

an emesis basin placed nearby. Antiemetics may be indicated. Given that bleeding or infarction of vital structures are possible in a patient with abdominal pain, oxygen should be provided. Intravenous fluid administration is appropriate in the prehospital phase, with the amount to be given dependent on the degree of abnormality in the patient's vital signs. Any patient older than 40 years may need a cardiac monitor en route to the hospital. Patients with abdominal pain should be prohibited from taking anything by mouth prior to their arrival in the emergency department (ED).

12. **Is it appropriate to give patients medication to relieve their abdominal pain en route to the hospital?**
Traditionally, opiates have been withheld until a patient with abdominal pain was examined by a surgeon because of concern that the administration of pain medication would mask physical findings and delay definitive diagnosis. Multiple studies have demonstrated that the administration of opiates such as morphine causes a reduction in abdominal pain without impairing or delaying the ability to diagnose the cause of the pain. In some cases localization and diagnosis of the pain are easier because of improved patient comfort after analgesia is administered. Currently, it is recommended that patients with significant abdominal pain be given narcotic analgesia. Hypotension is an important contraindication to administration of narcotic analgesia.

13. **What should the prehospital provider do if a patient with abdominal pain refuses to be transported to the hospital?**
Because it is difficult to diagnose the cause of a patient's abdominal pain in the field, it is equally difficult to reassure the patient about the nature of his or her abdominal pain. All patients with abdominal pain should be transported to the hospital for further evaluation and treatment as indicated. If the patient is competent and understands the risks of refusing further care, including potential catastrophic complications, a case can be made for allowing him or her to refuse care *against medical advice* and in consultation with the base station physician.

14. **If the patient is transported to the hospital for further evaluation of abdominal pain, what sort of procedures can he or she expect?**
In addition to a complete physical examination, including a rectal examination and in women a pelvic examination, the patient may have blood drawn for a complete blood count, pregnancy test (if indicated), and liver function tests or electrolytes depending upon the nature of the pain. Urinalysis is often performed. Ultrasonography, abdominal plain film radiographs, or computed tomograms may be ordered. Any patient with an acute abdomen will require surgical consultation. Despite such thorough workups, the most common ED diagnosis of abdominal pain is "abdominal pain of unknown cause." In such cases the patients are observed in the hospital or scheduled for close outpatient follow-up.

15. **In what ways might an elderly patient with abdominal pain differ from a younger patient?**
In general, the elderly patient poses a higher risk for serious conditions. Frequently, older patients have significant comorbidities such as cardiovascular or renal disease. They are more likely to delay seeking medical attention for their pain and when they do present their conditions may have deteriorated. Some conditions such as ruptured abdominal aortic aneurysm, acute mesenteric ischemia, diverticulitis and cancer are more common in patients over the age of 65. Although elderly patients

are often sicker, elderly patients also tend to have more subtle and less classic presentations of abdominal conditions. For example, they are less likely to be febrile or tachycardic with infection, are more likely to present with altered mentation with underlying abdominal pathology, and are less likely to manifest peritoneal signs. For all of these reasons, their rate of morbidity and mortality due to abdominal pain is increased.

16. **What are the most common diagnoses of abdominal pain in children?**
   In decreasing frequency: abdominal pain of unknown cause, gastroenteritis, appendicitis, constipation, urinary tract infection, viral illness, streptococcal pharyngitis, pneumonia, and otitis. Unusual but serious causes of pain in children include pyloric stenosis (typically seen in newborns and associated with projectile vomiting), intussusception (invagination of the bowel associated with colicky abdominal pain, vomiting and bloody stools), volvulus (malrotation of the bowel leading to obstruction), incarcerated inguinal hernia, and testicular torsion.

17. **How do the symptoms and signs of abdominal pain differ in pregnant patients?**
   Almost all pregnant patients experience some degree of abdominal pain during pregnancy. Symptoms such as nausea and vomiting may be due to pregnancy alone or to some other cause. Urinary frequency and urgency are common and may be the result of compression of the bladder by the uterus or urinary tract infection. As the uterus enlarges it displaces the abdominal contents and may distort the classic presentation of a surgical abdomen. For example, a pregnant patient with appendicitis may complain of right upper-quadrant pain because the appendix is displaced superiorly. Pregnant patients have heart rates that are faster than baseline, making interpretation of the severity of alterations in vital signs difficult. One must remain observant for any symptoms or signs of ectopic pregnancy because of the potential for rapid decompensation in a patient with a ruptured ectopic pregnancy.

18. **Why is it important to know if a patient is immunosuppressed?**
   Patients who are immunosuppressed because of cancer chemotherapy, human immunodeficiency virus, rheumatologic conditions, or other immune disorders may have abdominal pain due to any of the aforementioned conditions or a host of other unique etiologies of abdominal pain. For example, patients with intra-abdominal tumors may be more likely to have bowel obstruction, or because of cancer chemotherapy may be more susceptible to intra-abdominal sepsis. Patients with AIDS may have enterocolitis with severe diarrhea and dehydration or pancreatitis caused by retroviral medications. A patient with rheumatoid arthritis treated with immunosuppressive medication such as prednisone may not manifest a fever with significant infection or may be hypotensive because of adrenal suppression in the setting of intra-abdominal pathology.

Pearls and Pitfalls

1. Acute onset of abdominal and back pain in association with hypotension in a patient over the age of 50 years is a ruptured aortic aneurysm until proven otherwise.
2. Acute onset of abdominal pain and hypotension in a female of child-bearing age is a ruptured ectopic pregnancy until proven otherwise.
3. Epigastric pain can result from abdominal or cardiac causes.
4. Withholding analgesics until the patient is evaluated by a surgeon is an outdated concept.

References

1. American College of Emergency Physicians. Clinical policy: Critical issues for the initial evaluation and management of patients presenting with a chief complaint of nontraumatic acute abdominal pain. Ann Emerg Med 36(4): 406–413, 2000.
2. D'Agostino J. Common abdominal emergencies in children. Emerg Med Clin N Am 20(1):139–153, 2002.
3. Flasar MH, Cross R, Goldberg E. Acute abdominal pain. Prim Care 33(3):659–684, 2006.
4. Gallagher EJ, Esses D, Lee C, et al. Randomized clinical trial of morphine in acute abdominal pain. Ann Emerg Med 48(2):150–160, 2006.
5. Goldman RD, Crum D, Bromberg R, et al. Analgesia Administration for Acute Abdominal Pain in the Pediatric Emergency Department. Ped Emerg Care 22(1):18–21, 2006.
6. Kamin RA, Nowicki TA, Courtney DS, et al. Pearls and Pitfalls in the Emergency Department Evaluation of Abdominal Pain. Emerg Med Clin N Am 21(1):61–72, 2003.
7. Lyon C, Clark DC. Diagnosis of Acute Abdominal Pain in Older Patients. Am Fam Phys 74(9):1537–1544, 2006.
8. Martinez JP, Mattu A. Abdominal Pain in the Elderly. Emerg Med Clin N Am 24(2):371–388, 2006.
9. McCormick D. His and hers abdominal pain: Gender-specific factors. Emerg Med Serv 34(5):83–85, 2005.
10. Miller SK, Alpert PT. Assessment and differential diagnosis of abdominal pain. Nurs Pract 31(7):38–47, 2006.
11. Pointer JE, Harlan K. Impact of liberalization of protocols for the use of morphine sulfate in an urban emergency medical services system. Prehosp Emerg Care 9(4):377–381, 2005.
12. Ranji SR, Goodman LE, Simel DL, et al. Do opiates affect the clinical evaluation of patients with acute abdominal pain? JAMA 296(14):1764–1774, 2006.
13. Thomas SH, Silen W, Cheema F, et al. Effects of morphine analgesia on diagnostic accuracy in emergency department patients with abdominal pain: A prospective, randomized trial. J Am Coll Surg 196(1):18–31, 2003.
14. Trott AT, Lucas RH. Acute abdominal pain. In Emergency Medicine: Concepts and Clinical Practice, 4th ed., Rosen P, Barkin RM, eds., pp. 1888–1903. St. Louis: Mosby, 1998,

Gastrointestinal Hemorrhage

Mike Stackpool, MD

1. **How serious a problem is gastrointestinal (GI) bleeding?**
   The overall mortality of GI bleeding is 8–10% and has remained constant for more than a generation. Two percent of hospital admissions and 5% of emergency department admissions are for gastrointestinal bleeding. Ten percent of patients require intervention to control the hemorrhage and the bleeding resolves spontaneously in the remaining 90%. Upper gastrointestinal bleeding (UGIB) occurs in 100–200 cases per 100,000 population, whereas lower gastrointestinal bleeding (LGIB) occurs in 20–27 cases per 100,000 population. LGIB carries a mortality rate of 2–4%, much lower than UGIB. Bleeding that occurs while a person is an inpatient carries a much higher mortality

2. **How does GI hemorrhage present?**
   Upper GI bleeding commonly presents with hematemesis and/or melena. Lower GI bleeding usually presents with hematochezia or bright red blood per rectum.

3. **Upper? Lower? What is the difference?**
   In 1857 an Austrian physician and anatomist named Wenzel Treitz (1819–1872) described the suspensory ligament of the duodenum, the tissue that connects the duodenum of the small intestines to the diaphragm. The ligament consists of skeletal muscle from the diaphragm and smooth muscle from the third and fourth parts of the duodenum. This slip of tissue now bears his name. The ligament of Treitz is more than a convenient anatomical landmark. The upper GI tract is proximal to the ligament of Treitz, whereas the lower GI tract is beyond the ligament. Bleeding distal to the ligament of Treitz rarely refluxes back into the proximal duodenum and stomach.

4. **What is the difference between melena and hematochezia?**
   Melena is thick, black, foul-smelling or tarry-looking stool and typically indicates a source of bleeding from the upper GI tract. Occasionally melena will result from a right-sided colonic bleed. Melena may also present as a black liquid and has a very characteristic odor. It is blood that is partially degraded by digestion. At least 100 mL of blood is needed to form melena.
   Hematochezia is bright red or maroon-colored blood with or without fresh clots passing per rectum. Typically it indicates bleeding from the colon, although up to 11% of patients will have upper GI bleeding. A massive UGIB will present with hematochezia. There should be concomitant signs of volume depletion and hemorrhagic shock.
   Hematemesis is the vomiting of blood or coffee-ground-appearing emesis. Partially digested blood takes on a black appearance. This usually results from bleeding proximal to the ligament of Treitz. Vomiting coffee-ground emesis typically indicates a nonactive bleed. Bright red emesis, on the other hand, indicates a source of active bleeding. Swallowed blood can also appear to be hematemesis, so obtaining a careful history is important.
   Despite these typical distinctions, one cannot reliably attribute a source of GI bleeding based solely on stool color.

5. **What else can color stool?**
   Several foods and medicines may give stool a bloody or black appearance.
   Iron, bismuth (i.e., Pepto-Bismol™), and charcoal can turn stool black, and phenolphthalein and tetracyclines in syrup can turn it red.
   Diet will influence the color of stool. Cherries, Oreo™ cookies, and high-meat diets may color stool black. Beets and red Jello™ (or similar dyed foods) may turn stool red.
   Stool left standing will darken with time.

6. **How much red Jello™ do I have to eat to turn my stool red?**
   That is very difficult to say, perhaps very little. Cats that were fed 0.5 mL of baker's paste, a food dye, or $1/8$ teaspoon of glitter a day had distinctly colorful stools.

7. **What questions should be asked in the history?**
   It is important to know when the bleeding started, how often and how long it lasted, where it is from (i.e., emesis or bloody stools) and the color of the blood. Ask if the bleeding is painful or painless. Ask about the color and consistency of any associated stool. Any prior episodes of bleeding, past procedures (endoscopy, colonoscopy, or surgery), and the need for blood transfusions are also important pieces of information.
   Clinical history is crucial. Ask if the patient has any predisposing diseases such as peptic ulcers, diverticulosis, cancer, or inflammatory bowel disease. Include questions about underlying liver disease (easy bruising, jaundice, and changes in stool color), coagulation disorders (hemophilia, deep-vein thromboses), abdominal surgeries (abdominal aortic aneurysms or vascular grafts), hypertension, and cardiovascular disease. In infants, ask about feeding habits, weight loss, and irritability.
   Many medicines can erode the walls of the stomach and intestine and lead to GI hemorrhage. Particularly troublesome are the nonsteroidal anti-inflammatory drugs (NSAIDs) and aspirin, but be sure to ask about Coumadin or "blood thinners" and steroid use.
   A drug history should specifically ask about beta blockers (which may mask tachycardia), proton pump inhibitors or H-2 blockers (indicating underlying ulcerative disease), and anticoagulation agents.
   Alcohol may be the most pervasive and erosive GI irritant and is commonly associated with severe and repeated GI bleeds.
   Finally, always ask about associated symptoms. The stress of significant blood loss can overly tax a weak heart and may result in myocardial infarction.

8. **What causes GI bleeding?**
   In adults, most UGIB is from peptic ulcer disease and erosions, esophagogastric varices, arteriovenous malformations, Mallory–Weiss tears, tumors, and Dieulafoy's lesion (a congenital abnormality of submucosal arteries). Over the last couple decades the incidence of peptic ulcer disease has fallen. Gastric mucosal irritants such as alcohol, aspirin, or ibuprofen are also causes of UGIB.
   LGIB arises most commonly from diverticulosis; angiodysplasia (dilated tortuous submucosal vessels); colitis (inflammatory bowel disease, ischemia, and infections), cancer, proctitis, and hemorrhoids.
   Although most patients have minor bleeding, diverticulosis accounts for 30–50% of cases of massive LGIB. Bleeding is painless and there are no signs of diverticulitis (inflammation/infection of the diverticulae).

9. Are there age differences in gastrointestinal hemorrhage?

Hematochezia may be more likely in children than in adults (particularly in neonates and infants) due to shortened intestinal transit time.

The causes of GI bleeding in children vary with the child's age. Across all ages, the common UGIB causes are gastric and duodenal ulcers, esophagitis, gastritis, varices, and exposure to NSAIDS, whereas common causes of LGIB are infectious or allergic colitis and anorectal fissures.

The older the child, the more similar the causes of bleeding are to an adult.

Newborns: Age-specific causes of GI bleeding include cow's milk allergy, congenital malformations, and swallowed maternal blood.

Necrotizing enterocolitis is a severe cause of bleeding in this age group. Although most infants with NEC are born prematurely, one in 6 cases occur in term infants. These infants usually appear ill and toxic. Term infants are likely to have an underlying illness or congenital defect.

Infants and toddlers: In this age group, consideration must be given to the possibility of foreign body ingestion, including pill esophagitis and caustic ingestion.

This is the age group to consider ileocolic intussusception and Meckel's diverticulum. Intussusception, where one portion of the bowel invaginates into the adjacent section of bowel, typically occurs in infants between 3 months and 3 years of age, with most cases occurring before age 2. Patients may be awakened from sleep with severe and *cyclic* abdominal pain. Classically, they are irritable, draw up their legs, vomit, and pass a "currant jelly" (bloody and mucoid) stool. Meckel's diverticulum is a congenital outpouching malformation of the small bowel. Meckel's diverticulae follow the "rule of twos." It occurs in 2% of the population, has a male-to-female ratio of 2:1, is found within 2 feet of the ileocecal valve, and is 2 inches long; 2% percent of the population develop a complication. Bleeding is usually painless.

At the other end of the age spectrum, neoplasm is responsible for approximately 10% of cases of rectal bleeding in patients over age 50 years. Damage to GI mucosa from radiation treatments may also lead to hemorrhage. Elderly patients are also susceptible to ischemic colitis and concomitant bleeding. Aortoenteric fistulas are a rare cause of acute UGIB. Fistulas are a direct communication between the aorta and the GI tract and typically form from atherosclerotic aortic aneurysms or previous surgery with placement of a prosthetic aortic graft. Patients may present with an initial herald bleed or intermittent bleeding that is manifested by hematemesis and/or hematochezia. Other physical findings may include pain, fever, a toxic appearance, an abdominal bruit, or a palpable abdominal mass. An untreated aortoenteric fistula will result in the patient's death.

Under the age of 50 years, hemorrhoids are the most common cause of rectal bleeding.

10. What should I do to treat a patient with GI bleeding?

Whether the source of bleeding is the upper or lower GI tract, field treatment is similar. The administration of supplemental oxygen is always appropriate, as these patients will have diminished oxygen-carrying capacity secondary to their blood loss. Immediate transport should be initiated for patients with obvious signs of shock, as needed blood replacement can only occur at the receiving hospital and urgent transport considered for all other patients with GI hemorrhage, as the bleeding is not visible and these patients may deteriorate rapidly. Intravenous access and volume administration should be accomplished as per local protocol. Rarely, upper GI bleeding may be massive and compromise a patient's airway, necessitating active airway intervention such as endotracheal intubation.

Pearls and Pitfalls

1. Gastointestinal hemorrhage is a life-threatening problem with a mortality rate of approximately 10%.
2. The dividing line for upper versus lower GI bleeding is the ligament of Treitz in the duodenum.
3. The airway must be protected from aspiration of blood or stomach contents. If the patient is obtunded or in shock, emergent airway management is indicated.
4. Always consider GI bleeding to be an underlying etiology in patients with syncope, cardiac syndromes or arrest, confusion, hypotension, and cardiovascular accidents.
5. Treatment for GI hemorrhage, including transfusion and endoscopy, can only be accomplished at the receiving hospital; therefore, transport should be considered early in the prehospital course.
6. Because most GI hemorrhage is not visible externally, patients may appear stable and then suddenly deteriorate.

References

1. AGA guideline: Evaluation and management of occult and obscure gastrointestinal bleeding. Gastroenterology 2000; 118:197.
2. AGA technical review: Evaluation and management of occult and obscure gastrointestinal bleeding. Gastroenterology 2000; 118:201.
3. Ramsook C, Endom EE. Approach to lower gastrointestinal bleeding in children. UpToDate, December 13, 2006.
4. Villa X. Approach to upper gastrointestinal bleeding in children. UpToDate, June 23, 2006.
5. Wolfson AB, Hendey GW, Henry, PL, et al., eds. Harwood-Nuss' Clinical Practice of Emergency Medicine, 4th ed., Philadelphia: Lippincott Williams & Wilkins, 2005.
6. Schanler RJ. Clinical features and diagnosis of necrotizing enterocolitis in newborns. UpToDate, July 25, 2006.
7. Saab S, Jutabha R. Approach to the adult patient with lower gastrointestinal bleeding. UpToDate, November 14, 2005.
8. Jutabha R, Jensen DM. Approach to the adult patient with upper gastrointestinal bleeding. UpToDate, December 4, 2006.
9. Saab S, Jutabha R. Etiology of lower gastrointestinal bleeding in adults. UpToDate October 2, 2006.
10. Jutabha R, Jensen DM. Major causes of upper gastrointestinal bleeding in adults. UpToDate, October 4, 2006.
11. Jutabha R, Jensen DM. Uncommon causes of upper gastrointestinal bleeding. UpToDate, September 14, 2006.
12. Wallach J. Interpretation of Diagnostic Tests, 7th ed. Philadelphia: Lippincott Williams & Wilkins, 2000.
13. Marx JA, Hockberger RS, Walls RM. Rosen's Emergency Medicine: Concepts and Practice, 6th ed. Phildelphia: Mosby-Elsevier, 2006.
14. Guelrud M. Mallory-Weiss syndrome. UpToDate August 31, 2006.
15. Chawla S, Seth D, Mahajan P, et al. Upper gastrointestinal bleeding in children. Clin Pediatr 46(1):16–21, 2007.
16. Griffin B. The use of fecal markers to facilitate sample collection in group-housed cats. Contemp Top Lab Anim Sci 41(2):51–56, 2002.
17. Hoedema R. The management of lower gastrointestinal hemorrhage. Dis Colon Rectum 48(11):2010–2024, 2005.
18. Arvola T. Rectal bleeding in infancy: Clinical, allergological and microbiological examination. Pediatrics 117(4):e760–e768, 2006.

Vomiting and Diarrhea

Cheryl Blazek, BS, EMT-P

1. What should I note in the history for a patient with vomiting?

Emesis (vomiting) is seen in a variety of medical conditions, including gastrointestinal (GI) problems. Thus, it is important to start with very general questions. Inquire about abdominal pain, diarrhea, and fever. Note exactly how the emesis appears. Is it bloody, or does it look like coffee grounds? Bilious vomiting (yellow bile-stained fluid) in children must be differentiated from the normal regurgitation of milk or formula associated with burping. In a distal small-bowel or large-bowel obstruction, the patient will eventually vomit feculent material. Always ask about trauma, because a head injury can cause vomiting. Other neurologic complaints such as headache or seizures may indicate the possibility of a neurologic cause. Always ask for a medication list; this can suggest a toxic ingestion (e.g., aminophylline) or metabolic problems (e.g., diabetic ketoacidosis). Never forget that myocardial ischemia can present with nausea and vomiting, with or without chest pain. This is frequently seen in inferior-wall myocardial infarction. Ask and note the frequency of episodes and when the vomiting started. Ask if the patient has been able to keep food or liquids down in order to assess for the likelihood of dehydration. Ask about the patient's medical history and if the patient is on any regular medications. Patients who have health conditions regulated by medication can have serious acute medical repercussions if they are not able to keep their medications down long enough for them to work.

2. What is important in the physical exam?

Carefully evaluate the vital signs. A fever may indicate an infectious cause. Orthostatic changes in blood pressure and pulse are indicative of extensive fluid loss and dehydration. A careful inspection of the abdomen may reveal surgical scars. Previous abdominal surgery is a risk factor for bowel obstruction. Note tenderness, guarding, and rigidity of the abdomen. A rigid abdomen may be caused by an intra-abdominal catastrophe requiring surgical intervention. Observe the emesis for the presence of bile, blood, or fecal odor. Note the appearance of skin and mucosal areas for signs of dehydration.

3. What are the complications of vomiting?

In addition to dehydration, the patient is at risk for electrolyte abnormalities and esophageal or gastric tears leading to perforation or bleeding usually after prolonged forceful vomiting. A tear in the esophagus after vomiting is referred to as a Mallory–Weiss tear, and complete rupture of the esophagus is called Boerhaave's syndrome.

4. What about the airway?

Don't forget airway, breathing, and circulation just because the patient primarily has a GI complaint. It is imperative to evaluate the airway of any patient with vomiting because he or she is at risk for aspiration and subsequent pneumonia. If a patient is intoxicated or has an altered mental status, aspiration is more likely. It is particularly important to be aware of possible aspiration in any patient immobilized in a supine position on a backboard in a cervical collar. These patients will aspirate if they do not have a gag reflex and may require advanced airway maneuvers such as intubation.

5. **Shouldn't a patient who is intoxicated and vomits be intubated to protect his or her airway?**
   No. Intoxication and vomiting by themselves are not good indications for intubating a patient unless the patient cannot be positioned on the left side with the head down (e.g., after trauma), the patient does not have a gag reflex, or the patient is clearly hypoventilating (i.e., has a respiratory rate less than 10 breaths per minute that does not increase with stimulation).

6. **What drug ingestions can cause vomiting?**
   Many different medications can cause vomiting. Some common overdoses that cause nausea and vomiting include acetaminophen and iron (particularly common in children), digoxin, and theophylline.

7. **What does it mean when a patient vomits "coffee grounds"?**
   This is a common description of the emesis in a patient who has previously bled into the stomach. The stomach acid changes the color and appearance of the blood. Treatment is the same as for any patient who vomits bright red blood. Two large-bore peripheral IV lines should be quickly inserted and a bolus of IV fluids (20 mL/kg of normal saline or lactated Ringer's) given if the patient is hypotensive or tachycardic.

8. **What are the symptoms of food poisoning?**
   Different types of food poisoning will cause different syndromes. Many bacterial etiologies of food poisoning cause either primarily vomiting or primarily diarrhea. Onset of symptoms after ingestion of the offending agent may begin shortly after the meal (only 1–2 hours), or it may take days for symptoms to appear, depending on the exact cause. It can be difficult to make a diagnosis of food poisoning unless multiple patients report symptoms after ingestion of a common meal.

9. **What is important about the medical history in diarrhea?**
   Always ask about the frequency and amount of diarrhea because the severity of symptoms may suggest associated dehydration. It is important to note whether the diarrhea is bloody because this may indicate infection, inflammatory bowel disease, or gut ischemia. A history of black, tarry, foul-smelling stool suggests melena, which is the result of upper GI bleeding (usually from the stomach or proximal duodenum). The blood darkens with exposure to stomach acid; it acts as a cathartic and travels rapidly through the bowel. Recent travel to another country is often associated with infectious diarrhea.

10. **Is there anything different about kids with vomiting and diarrhea?**
    Children with multiple episodes of vomiting or diarrhea are more likely to become dehydrated and to appear ill or lethargic because they have a smaller volume of body fluids than adults and are unable to tolerate fluid losses. True projectile vomiting in an infant requires medical evaluation for pyloric stenosis, a congenital defect requiring surgical repair. Bilious emesis is never normal in infants and should always be evaluated in an emergency facility for the possible presence of an obstructive intestinal lesion. Children with violent coughing spells may vomit after they stop coughing, as in pertussis (whooping cough) or asthma.

11. **What about geriatric patients with prolonged or multiple episodes of vomiting or diarrhea?**
    Like children, elderly adults often have fewer physiologic reserves than younger adults and are more prone to dehydration. Severely dehydrated patients may appear confused or even comatose.

12. When should I administer an antiemetic in the field?
There is no need for the routine administration of an antiemetic unless the patient has intractable, persistent, severe retching. Such episodes of vomiting may cause rupture of the esophagus (Boerhaave's syndrome).

13. What antiemetic should I administer?
Metoclopramide (Reglan), 5 mg intravenously or intramuscularly or prochlorperazine (Compazine) are effective antiemetics if there are no contraindications such as pregnancy, neuroleptic malignant syndrome, or Parkinson's disease.

Pearls and Pitfalls

1. Most adult patients with vomiting or diarrhea do not become dehydrated.
2. Dehydration is common in children with vomiting and diarrhea.
3. Antiemetics are usually not needed unless the vomiting is persistent.
4. Failure to position the patient properly to protect the airway can lead to aspiration.

References

1. Marx JA, Hockberger RS, Walls RA, et al., eds. Rosen's Emergency Medicine: Concepts and Clinical Practice, 7th ed. St. Louis: Mosby, 2010.
2. Strange G, Ahrens W, Lelyveld S, et al., eds. Pediatric Emergency Medicine: A Comprehensive Study Guide, 2nd ed. New York: McGraw-Hill, 2002.

Dyspnea

Gregory J. Chapman, BS, RRT, REMT-P

1. **What is dyspnea?**
   Dyspnea is the subjective perception of shortness of breath.

2. **How do I assess a patient who is dyspneic?**
   Visually determine the mental status, skin color, obvious signs of respiratory distress including the presence of nasal alar flaring, use of accessory muscles, and respiratory rate, and assess the A and B of the ABCs (airway, breathing, circulation). Is there any evidence of upper-airway obstruction? Is the patient tachypneic? Are breath sounds present and equal? Are there any abnormal sounds (i.e., wheezing, rales, and rhonchi)? What is the oxygen saturation on room air (if a pulse oximeter is available)? Ominous findings revealing that the patient is becoming tired include an altered mental status, two- to three-word dyspnea, or combativeness (from hypoxia) often manifested by pulling off the oxygen mask or refusing the nebulizer.

3. **What should be done concomitantly with this assessment?**
   Stop and stabilize when an abnormality is determined. Examples include placing all patients with dyspnea on oxygen. Suctioning of secretions, placement of a nasopharyngeal airway, and intubation for upper airway obstruction may be needed. Administration of bronchodilators such as albuterol via nebulizer is indicated for wheezing.

4. **Why should I place all dyspneic patients on oxygen?**
   All such patients should be presumed to be hypoxic, and supplemental oxygen may improve this. In addition, if a patient should deteriorate and sustain a respiratory arrest, preoxygenation will provide more time in which to establish an airway or intubate the patient prior to the patient's O_2 saturation falling to a dangerously low level.

5. **What conditions cause dyspnea and pleuritic chest pain?**
   Pulmonary embolus, pneumothorax, pneumonia, and pleurisy.

6. **What conditions cause dyspnea and diffuse wheezing?**
   Bronchiolitis (in children younger than 2 years), acute bronchial asthma, anaphylaxis, chronic obstructive pulmonary disease (COPD) such as emphysema or chronic bronchitis, congestive heart failure (CHF), and bronchitis.

7. **How do I distinguish between COPD and CHF?**
   Do a chest X-ray. Unless you have this available in your ambulance, it is often impossible to make this determination with certainty in the field. Having said that, a careful history will often be helpful, as many patients will know what their underlying pulmonary disease is and if the current symptoms are typical of their prior episodes.

8. **Why is morphine contraindicated in a patient with COPD?**
   Morphine may suppress the respiratory drive and may cause hypoventilation, carbon dioxide retention, and respiratory failure.

Dyspnea

9. **If I can't use morphine to treat a patient whose wheezing may be due to CHF, what should I use?**
   Sublingual nitroglycerin will reduce afterload without suppressing the respiratory drive. Administration of albuterol may improve bronchial constriction secondary to concomitant COPD, asthma, or bronchitis.

10. **Is there anything else I can do to support the patient with acute pulmonary edema?**
    Yes. Continuous positive airway pressure (CPAP) is being used in many EMS systems with great success. By increasing the pressure remaining in the airways at the end of expiration, the alveolus is held open against the pressure of the pulmonary edema fluid, thus increasing oxygen exchange. It often may avert the need for endotracheal intubation when used proactively. Some EMS systems are now using BiPAP which is a bilevel positive pressure device that utilizes a higher pressure during inspiration and a lower pressure during expiration to make exhalation easier.

11. **Are there any contraindications to CPAP?**
    Yes. Adding pressure to the thoracic cavity decreases preload. While this may be beneficial in acute pulmonary edema when the patient has an increased blood pressure, if the patient is in cardiogenic shock, decreasing the preload will lower blood pressure further.

10. **Define asthma.**
    Asthma is bronchiolar constriction caused by intrinsic or extrinsic factors, manifested by dyspnea and diffuse wheezing.

11. **How should I treat asthma?**
    Oxygen (100%) and the administration of inhaled $beta_2$-agonists such as albuterol. They may be given continuously or in line to intubated patients. There is some evidence that intravenous magnesium administration may offer some benefit in severe asthma cases; however its use remains controversial and no studies have been done to document using it in the prehospital setting.

12. **When is a normal vital sign very abnormal in an asthmatic?**
    A "normal" respiratory rate of 12–18 is an ominous sign in a patient with diffuse wheezing and indicates respiratory failure and impending respiratory arrest. A respiratory rate of more than 24 indicates that the patient still has the capacity to perform the work of breathing necessary to maintain adequate oxygenation.

13. **What is hyperventilation syndrome?**
    Decreased levels of CO_2 in the blood caused by very deep and rapid respirations secondary to acute anxiety and emotional upset.

14. **What are the symptoms of hyperventilation syndrome, and why do they occur?**
    The patient will have a rapid respiratory rate associated with numbness and tingling, first apparent around the mouth and lips, which is followed by carpopedal spasm or tetany. This occurs because hyperventilation dramatically decreases the pCO_2 in the blood, which causes respiratory alkalosis and hypocalcemia.

15. **I've heard that patients who are hyperventilating can be treated with rebreathing into a bag or mask.**
    Absolutely not, as patients who are hypoxic or severely acidotic from other causes will also present with tachypnea and sometimes deep breathing or increased tidal volume. If this is treated with rebreathing techniques, it may further decrease the O_2 level in the blood and lead to disastrous consequences.

16. If rebreathing into a paper bag is dangerous, how do I manage a patient who appears to have hyperventilation syndrome?

First, you must rule out other causes of dyspnea and hyperventilation. A calm and reassuring approach and an attempt to "talk them down" to decrease the depth and rate of breathing are most often successful and always safe. Other causes of hyperventilation such as diabetic ketoacidosis or hypoxia will not improve all these patients should be treated with O_2 by mask or nasal cannula.

17. How do I suspect the diagnosis of pneumonia?

The presenting signs and symptoms of pneumonia, which is pus in the alveoli of the lungs, include productive cough with green–yellow sputum, dyspnea, tachypnea, fever, chills, pleuritic chest pain, localized rales, and flaring of the nasal alae with inspiration. All such patients should be treated with high-flow O_2.

18. What is a pulmonary embolus?

A pulmonary embolus (PE) is a blood clot that originates in the veins of the lower extremities or pelvis, breaks off, and is carried into and through the right ventricle and on to the lungs via the pulmonary artery.

19. How do I make the diagnosis of PE?

The diagnosis cannot be made in the field; it is a difficult diagnosis to make even with the aid of sophisticated diagnostic imaging techniques. It should be suspected in any patient with sudden onset of pleuritic chest pain, dyspnea, tachypnea, and tachycardia.

20. What patients are at highest risk for development of PE?

The elderly (i.e., older than age 70), postpartum women, women taking birth control pills, anyone who has prolonged immobility (e.g., bed rest or long leg cast), and patients with cancer or hypercoagulable states (e.g., proteins C or S deficiency).

21. What is the treatment?

High-flow O_2 via a nonrebreather mask, cardiac monitoring, transport to the emergency department (ED) for evaluation, and treatment with heparin and possibly thrombolytics.

22. What is HAPE?

High Altitude Pulmonary Edema, which occurs in susceptible individuals who travel to locations above 8000 feet elevation. It may become life threatening if not treated and resolves with administration of O_2 and rapid descent (often of as little as 1000 feet) to a lower altitude.

23. Which vital sign taken in the field is most likely to be inaccurate and why?

The respiratory rate is often estimated rather than counted over 20–30 seconds, as most prehospital providers (and, for that matter, most hospital providers) are action oriented and sometimes do not take the time necessary to determine the respiratory rate accurately in patients who do not complain of dyspnea or who look dyspneic.

24. Why is estimating the respiratory rate a dangerous practice?

Some very sick patients may be overlooked, particularly those with metabolic acidosis secondary to sepsis or toxic ingestions, as many of these patients have no complaints of dyspnea and do not appear to be in respiratory distress.

25. What's the message of this chapter?

Count the respiratory rate and administer O_2 to every dyspneic patient.

26. What technology is there to help me monitor my patient?
Pulse oximetry is currently available on most ambulances, both basic life support and advanced life support. Pulse oximetry should be used to augment good patient assessment skills. Although many experienced providers can easily determine if a patient is hypoxic without the use of a pulse oximeter, the pulse oximeter is a great tool to trend changes in the patient's oxygenation status.

27. Will the pulse oximeter tell me about the patient's ventilations?
No. However, end tidal CO_2 ($EtCO_2$) capnography will. $EtCO_2$ capnography monitors are available as either a stand alone unit or built into cardiac monitors. The $EtCO_2$ monitor can be attached to patients who are spontaneously breathing by using a device similar to a nasal cannula or can be attached to an endotracheal tube, laryngeal airway, or dual-lumen airway.

28. Does $EtCO_2$ correlate directly to $PaCO_2$ in an arterial blood gas?
There is good correlation between $EtCO_2$ and arterial PCO_2 in patients with good cardiac output. Studies have shown that $EtCO_2$ is about 4 mmHg lower than the arterial PCO_2.

29. When should I use $EtCO_2$ capnography?
As a matter of practice, continuous monitoring of $EtCO_2$ in patients with good cardiac output with waveform capnography is recommended on all intubated patients. Consensus documents from the National Association of EMS Physicians point to many studies that show that the use of capnography both for confirmation of endotracheal tube placement and as detection of a dislodged tube produce better rates of prehospital intubation success upon arrival at the ED.

Pearls and Pitfalls

1. All dyspneic patients should have an O_2 saturation measurement and be placed on oxygen.
2. Wheezing should be treated with inhaled bronchodilators.
3. Narcotics should be avoided in dyspneic patients since they may suppress the respiratory drive.
4. Continuously monitor all dyspneic patients with an O_2 saturation monitor.
5. CPAP is a useful adjunct for the treatment of pulmonary edema, COPD, and asthma.
6. Severe metabolic acidosis (e.g., diabetic ketoacidosis) may be manifested as dyspnea and hyperventilation.

References

1. Asthma and chronic obstructive pulmonary disease. In Markovchick V, Pons PT, Bakes KM., eds. Emergency Medicine Secrets, 5th Edition. Elsevier Mosby, St. Louis, 2011, pp 174–187.
2. Breathing and ventilation. In Markovchick V, Pons PT, Bakes KM., eds. Emergency Medicine Secrets. 5th Edition. Elsevier Mosby, St. Louis, 2011, pp 169–173.
3. Wolf SJ. Venous thromboembolism. Markovchick V, Pons P, Bakes KM, eds., Emergency Medicine Secrets, 5th Edition. Elsevier Mosby, St. Louis, 2011, pp. 188–194.
4. Barton CW, Wang ES Correlation of end-tidal CO2 measurements to arterial $PaCO_2$ in nonintubated patients. Ann Emerg Med. 23(3):560–563, 1994.
5. Grmec S, Mally S. Prehospital determination of tracheal tube placement in severe head injury. Emerg Med J 21(4):518–520, 2004.
6. Workgroup on EMS Management of Asthma Exacerbations. A model protocol for emergency medical services management of asthma exacerbations. Prehosp Emerg Care 10(4):418–429, 2006. PMID: 16997769
7. Hubble MW, Richards ME, Jarvis R, et al. Effectiveness of prehospital continuous positive airway pressure in the management of acute pulmonary edema. Prehosp Emerg Care Oct-Dec;10(4):430–439. 2006. PMID: 16997770

Extremity Pain and Trauma

Julie Scadden, NREMT-P, PS

1. **Who can develop painful extremity problems?**
   People of all ages can have extremity problems causing pain and discomfort. The age of the patient and the history obtained will help determine the likely cause of the patient's pain. Pediatric patients often fall onto an outstretched hand (sometimes referred to as FOOSH). This type of fall can result in a fracture of the radius and ulna or, more proximally, the distal humerus. Older patients also will often fall leading to fracture of the hip or shoulder, many times even when falling only a few feet (such as trip/fall mechanism from a standing position) because they have fragile bones secondary to osteoporosis. In addition, a wide variety of nontraumatic problems can produce extremity and joint pain in patients of all ages.

2. **You are called to the home of an elderly female complaining of knee pain. What is the most important piece of history you should know about this complaint?**
   The most important piece of the patient's past pertinent history is whether there has been any trauma to the extremity. Did the patient fall on her hip or side? Did she land on or twist her knee? In addition to direct injury to the knee, injury of the hip may present with pain referred to the knee, and occasionally knee pain will be the only complaint.

3. **How can I tell if a hip is fractured?**
   The only way to tell for certain is by X-ray evaluation, but the clinical exam can be suggestive. Most elderly patients fracture the hip at the femoral neck, and the leg will usually appear shortened when compared to the other leg and externally rotated. Most patients will not be able to bear weight and can have severe pain; others may be able to ambulate. Always suspect a fracture in an elderly patient with hip or knee pain complaints.

4. **Why is determining the mechanism of injury important when dealing with extremity injury?**
   Determining the mechanism of injury can lead to the recognition of critical injuries. Energy transference in low-energy versus high-energy impact or a fall from a stationary object versus being thrown from a moving object produces differing injury patterns and severity. Knowledge of the typical patterns of injury associated with different types of energy transference will help guide your assessment of anticipated injuries.

5. **What is the "path of injury"?**
   The "path of injury" refers to how energy is transferred within the body after a trauma mechanism and the likely injuries it will produce. There are a number of examples to be aware of:
   (a) If a patient falls, landing on his or her feet first, you would suspect primary injury to occur to the inferior extremities and move superiorly through the skeleton and organs. The path of injury, therefore, would begin with possible fractures of the calcaneus (heel bone), tibia, fibula, femur, pelvis, and spine and could include hollow organ or aortic shear injuries. Additionally, there may be secondary

abdominal or head injuries resulting from any continued tumbling forward of the body. Finally, the type of surface impacted may affect the potential severity of injuries in this path.

(b) A child who runs into the street and sees an oncoming vehicle will typically freeze in place, facing the vehicle. Once the child is struck by the moving vehicle, typically the bumper will impact one or both thighs producing fracture of the femurs. The impacted child will then fall toward the vehicle striking his or her chest causing thoracic injuries, and then the head will hit producing head trauma and finally be thrown, resulting in additional injuries.

(c) In contrast, an adult who sees an oncoming vehicle will typically turn to one side trying to avoid the collision, resulting in the bumper striking and fracturing the tibia and fibula. The adult will then fall toward the hood striking the lower chest and lateral abdomen followed by the head hitting the windshield and finally being thrown off.

6. **Why should you always check for pulses, movement, and sensation of the extremity before and after splinting?**
A pulseless extremity indicates either a vascular injury or a compartment syndrome. It is important to establish a baseline presence for pulses, movement, and sensation prior to splinting because a loss of any of these important clinical indicators could signal inadequate splinting and extremity management with the potential to cause addition injury to the limb.

7. **What is compartment syndrome?**
Compartment syndrome is a limb-threatening condition where increased pressure in the compartments of the extremity's muscles can compress the blood vessels within the compartment and compromise the blood supply to the extremity. The two most-common causes of compartment syndrome are hemorrhage from a fracture or vascular injury and third-space edema created when ischemic muscle tissue is reperfused following a period of diminished or absent blood flow, as when an extremity is crushed.

8. **When should I suspect compartment syndrome?**
The two earliest signs of a developing compartment syndrome are pain and paresthesias. When considering the mechanism of a fracture, crush injury, or compression of the extremity, the physical exam may reveal a tense and tight feeling in the muscles of the involved compartment of the extremity, coupled with pain on movement of the distal part of the extremity and tenderness on palpation. As the compartment syndrome progresses and ischemia develops, the patient will develop the "Five P's."

9. **What are the "Five P's"?**
The Five P's are pulselessness, pain, paresthesia, pallor, and paralysis.
You can check these five clinical signs to determine if there is evidence of limb ischemia. A palpable pulse would indicate acceptable perfusion; however, if the limb is cool and pale, it may not be perfused. Paresthesia (a tingling sensation) may reflect ischemia and nerve damage. Severe nerve ischemia over a prolonged period of time may result in paralysis of the muscle. All or some of these signs may be evident in compartment syndrome. Assessment and recognition of these signs and urgent transport are important in mitigating further loss of function or loss of the extremity itself.

10. **What else can cause compromised arterial blood flow?**
Arterial occlusion of a limb will present as a pulseless extremity. Arterial occlusion can happen as a result of trauma (e.g., gunshot wound or tear of the inner lining of an artery), embolus from a blood clot in the heart or clotting of a partially occluded artery (similar to an acute myocardial infarction). As ischemic

time progresses, the limb will become pale, cool, and insensate. The limb may be salvaged if treated in time.

11. What can happen when a vein is occluded?
Occlusion of a deep vein in the leg or pelvis is a deep venous thrombosis (DVT). Occlusion of a deep vein leads to swelling and pain of the extremity; sometimes you may palpate a tender cord in the extremity that represents the involved vein. A clot can break off and travel to the heart and out into the pulmonary circulation, causing a pulmonary embolus. A patient presenting with signs and symptoms of DVT needs a formal medical evaluation, most often with ultrasound, to make this diagnosis. A DVT requires treatment with anticoagulants (i.e., heparin) to prevent the clot from propagating.

12. What about dislocations?
A dislocation is a disruption in the normal anatomic relationship of the bones that make up a joint. The patient may have a history of previous dislocations; in addition, dislocations may also be associated with a fracture. Anterior dislocation of the shoulder is the most common type and is usually caused by a fall onto the inside of an upper arm, which is then abducted and externally rotated. Always check for distal pulses and sensation during the assessment of a dislocation, then splint the affected area in the position found. Do not attempt to relocate the joint in the field; instead, transport the patient in their position of comfort and consider pain management enroute.

13. How should pain be managed in patients with extremity injuries?
Whether you are treating a fracture, dislocation, or even a sprain, basic interventions such as immobilization, ice packs, elevation, and good communication with the patient to decrease anxiety should be initially attempted when treating extremity injuries. Administration of analgesic medications such as morphine sulfate, fentanyl, meperidine, hydromorphone, nitrous oxide, or nonsteroidal anti-inflammatory drugs should also be considered in patients with isolated extremity trauma.

14. What is "nursemaid's elbow"?
This is a layman's term for subluxation of the radial head at the elbow joint in a small child. This occurs most often between the ages of 1 and 5 years. The injury usually results from the pulling, or yanking, of the extended and pronated arm, which can occur when lifting a child by the arm. The child often presents with crying and will not use the affected extremity. There is no obvious deformity and no neurovascular compromise. Field treatment is splinting, symptomatic pain relief measures, and transport for evaluation and relocation of the subluxed radial head in the emergency department (ED).

15. What is Buerger's disease?
Buerger's disease is an acute inflammation and thrombosis (clotting) of arteries and veins affecting the hands and feet, typically found in smokers, predominantly young males. Symptoms include pain in the feet and/or hands induced by insufficient blood flow during exercise or pain in these areas at rest. The pain may be very intense in the affected regions. Additional signs and symptoms can include numbness and/or tingling in the distal extremities, including the presence of Raynaud's phenomenon, a condition in which the skin of the distal extremities (fingers, toes, hands, and feet) turns white when exposed to cold. Skin ulcerations and gangrene of the fingers and toes are common.

16. Why do patients with sickle cell disease get bone pain?
Constant, severe bone pain may occur due to the presence of abnormal sickled red blood cells that occlude small, nutrient blood vessels to the bone, thus causing ischemia during a vaso-occlusive crisis.

In infants, dactylitis (hand–foot syndrome), caused by infarctions of the small bones and presenting as a painful symmetrical swelling of the hands and feet, may be the initial manifestation of sickle cell anemia.

17. How do you treat extremity pain in children experiencing a sickle cell crisis?
Prehospital treatment of sickle cell crisis is determined via thorough information gathering, including patient age, location and severity of the pain, and pain management protocols. Direct online medical control may be necessary in atypical cases. The therapy for vaso-occlusive crises is hydration and analgesia. Intravenous isotonic solution is administered at a rate of 1–1.5 times the maintenance rate if oral hydration cannot be sustained. The use of analgesia is based on the severity of symptoms and the response to at-home therapies prior to the patient's presentation in the ED. Mild pain can often be controlled by ibuprofen, acetaminophen, or ketorolac. Morphine sulfate, meperidine, hydromorphone, or oxycodone are also used for pain management and some pediatric patients have benefited from high-dose IV methylprednisolone

18. What causes a red and warm joint?
There are multiple possibilities, and specific causes are difficult to diagnose in the field setting. Most commonly seen is *gout*, a type of arthritis caused by uric acid crystals forming in the joint space. This often affects the big toe and may be so painful that even the weight of a bed sheet makes the patient cringe. It is difficult to tell gout from an infected joint by exam, and diagnosis requires aspirating fluid from the joint space.
A joint that has a bacterial infection can present in similar fashion and is quite serious because the infection can destroy tissue and cartilage, leaving a deformed, useless joint if untreated. Cellulitis is an inflammation of the soft tissue, often of an extremity, and can become quite serious. The presence of cellulitis generally indicates an acute, uncontrolled spreading infection of the dermis and subcutaneous tissues via the lymphatic or circulatory systems. Microorganisms, usually Gram-positive bacteria, can trigger an inflammatory response that results in pain, redness, warmth, and swelling when left untreated.

19. What is osteomyelitis?
Osteomyelitis is an acute or chronic bone infection usually caused either by bacteria that originate in another part of the body and spread to the bone through the blood or as a result of direct bone injury, most commonly after penetrating trauma or open fracture. Other factors known to increase the risk of osteomyelitis include diabetes, hemodialysis, sickle cell disease, splenectomy, and intravenous drug use. Symptoms include pain in the bone, local swelling, redness, and warmth to the extremity, as well as fever, nausea, and malaise. In cases of chronic osteomyelitis, drainage of pus through the skin may occur. The objective of treatment for osteomyelitis is to eliminate the infection and prevent its return through long-term antibiotic therapy. Prehospital treatment will be limited to management of the symptoms, primarily fever and pain management.

20. What are rheumatic disorders?
Rheumatic disorders are a nonspecific class of autoimmune disorders affecting the bones, joints, and skin, as well as the heart, kidneys, and lungs. The terms "arthritis" and "rheumatism" alone cover at least 200 different conditions. Some of the major rheumatic disorders you may encounter during prehospital assessment are bursitis/tendonitis, fibromyalgia, neck pain, osteoarthritis, rheumatic fever, rheumatic heart disease (a long-term complication of rheumatic fever), rheumatoid arthritis, and lupus. Rheumatic

disorders share two characteristics: they cause chronic (often intermittent) pain and they are quite common. Prehospital treatment for rheumatic disorders is generally position of comfort and pain management.

21. **What joint problems do hemophiliacs get?**
Hemophiliacs can bleed into both muscle and joint spaces after sustaining relatively minor trauma. The severity of the bleeding depends on the severity of the disease. Patients with a very low level of clotting factors will usually be diagnosed at a young age and have multiple episodes of bleeding leading to severely deformed joints.

Pearls and Pitfalls

1. Gross deformity of extremities can distract providers from the evaluation of potential life-threatening internal injuries.
2. Assuming that if a patient can walk on it, it isn't broken.
3. Checking the five clinical signs of limb ischemia should occur both before *and* after splinting the extremity, not before *or* after.
4. Dislocations often have associated fractures.
5. Knee pain can indicate injury to the hip and pelvis.
6. Analgesics manage pain; sedatives address anxiety.

References

1. National Association of Emergency Medical Technicians. PHTLS: Prehospital Trauma Life Support, 7th ed., pp. 333–353. St. Louis: Mosby JEMS Elsevier, 2011.
2. Arnold JL. Sickle Cell Anemia. http://emedicine.medscape.com/article/205926-overview Accessed Oct 28, 2011.
3. King RW. Osteomyelitis. http://emedicine.medscape.com/article/785020-overview Accessed Oct 29, 2011
4. Herchline TE. Cellulitis. http://emedicine.medscape.com/article/214222-overview Accessed Oct 28, 2011.
5. Parrillo SJ. Rheumatic Fever in Emergency Medicine. http://emedicine.medscape.com/article/808945-overview Accessed Oct 28, 2011.
6. Centers for Disease Control and Prevention. Arthritis Overview. http://www.cdc.gov/arthritis/Accessed Oct 28, 2011.
7. Patel K. Deep Venous Thrombosis. http://emedicine.medscape.com/article/1911303-overview Accessed Oct 28, 2011.
8. Rasul AT. Acute Compartment Syndrome. http://emedicine.medscape.com/article/307668-overview Accessed Oct 28, 2011.
9. Wolfram W. Pediatrics: Nursemaid Elbow. http://emedicine.medscape.com/article/803026-overview Accessed Oct 28, 2011.
10. The Johns Hopkins Vasculitis Center. Buerger's Disease, 1998–2006. http://www.hopkinsvasculitis.org/types-vasculitis/buergers-disease/ Accessed Oct 28, 2011.

Overdose and Poisoning

Kennon Heard, MD, and Vikhyat Bebarta, MD

1. **How big a problem is exposure to poisons?**
   The American Association of Poison Control Centers recorded 2,479,355 cases of human poison exposure in 2009. Approximately 90% of these occurred in the home, and approximately 85% were accidental. The vast majority of these cases resulted in no or only minor illness. More than half of all exposures involve children younger than 6 years old; however, only 2% of the 1261 reported deaths involved children younger than 6 years old. Although suicidal intent was present in only 8% of cases, suicidal exposures accounted for approximately half of the the deaths. The vast majority of calls to a poison center do not result in referral to a health care facility.

2. **What are the most common substances involved in exposures reported to poison centers?**
   The most common substances are analgesics, household products, plants, sedative/hypnotic/antipsychotic medications, and toys/foreign bodies/miscellaneous.

3. **What are the most dangerous substances?**
   The six categories with the largest number of fatalities are analgesics (including narcotics), sedative/hypnotic/antipsychotic medications, antidepressants, stimulants and street drugs, cardiovascular drugs, and alcohols.

4. **How are patients exposed to poisons?**
   Ingestion is the most common route of exposure, followed by dermal, inhalation, or ocular exposures; bites and stings; and parenteral (intravenous) or aspiration exposures. In an ingestion, the poison must be absorbed across the gastrointestinal (GI) mucosa before toxic symptoms occur. The stomach can serve as a reservoir of poison for the small intestine where most absorption occurs. Inhalation injuries from noxious fumes may be immediate or delayed. Hypoxia is the greatest threat to life and occurs from airway obstruction caused by edema, laryngospasm, or bronchospasm or to displacement of oxygen by the inhaled gases themselves. Absorption from skin contact is usually slow unless the skin barrier is disrupted from abrasions, lacerations, or burns. Dermal exposure to corrosives can be very painful and disfiguring, but with few exceptions, it is not a life threat. Despite a rapid blink reflex the eye is relatively unprotected from exposures. Ocular damage can be immediate and irreversible. Intravenous routes are obviously the fastest routes of exposure. These may occur in IV drug abusers or inadvertently in the setting of home IV therapy.

5. **What are the scene priorities for an unknown exposure?**
   The first priority, as always, is scene safety for the rescuers. Environmental dangers or hazardous materials may require special equipment or protective gear. However, as most exposures occur in a public or residential setting, extraordinary measures will generally be unnecessary. Obtain as much information as

possible from family and bystanders. The time, amount, and route of ingestion are crucial pieces of information. Long-acting or extended-release medications are concerns for delayed or prolonged poisonings. Make sure to ask about the patient's illegal and prescription drug use as well as any available drugs or medications on the scene. Try to determine if the ingestion was intentional or accidental. *Gather any empty bottles and transport them with the patient.* If there is more than one patient, ask about exposures common to all, such as food, work or industrial chemicals, smoke, or heat sources (carbon monoxide). Manage the airway, breathing, and circulation, as in any illness, but be aware that a precipitous decline may follow ingestion or exposure.

6. What kind of decontamination can be done in the field?

Remove the patient from the source of exposure. Evacuate the area of potentially inhaled poisons and remove contaminated clothing. Irrigate the skin and eyes with normal saline or plain water. Apply high-flow oxygen by mask. Nebulized inhaled water may help dilute nasopharyngeal irritants. Never try to "neutralize" a base with an acid or an acid with a base. This will only further contaminate the patient, and the reaction is likely to release large amounts of heat and add thermal burns to the initial chemical injury.

7. What about GI decontamination? Is there a role for the prehospital administration of activated charcoal?

Recently, several studies have evaluated prehospital administration of activated charcoal as a treatment for oral poison exposure. Although these studies have shown that this intervention shortens the time to charcoal administration, studies in the emergency department have found that activated charcoal is not useful for the management of routine ingestions. As the utility of charcoal as an intervention is unclear, there is no role for routine prehospital charcoal administration.

8. What are the dangers of drinking the different kinds of alcohol?

Anyone who works in the prehospital setting soon appreciates the damage that alcohol abuse can wreak. Ethanol is the alcohol found in beer, wine, and liquor. Other easily available alcohols are methanol (in windshield washer fluid), isopropanol (in rubbing alcohol), and ethylene glycol (in antifreeze). All alcohols are central nervous system (CNS) depressants and will exhibit the familiar signs of intoxication: ataxia, nystagmus, slurred speech, emotional lability, and decreased sensorium. Eventually, severe toxic ingestions progress to respiratory depression and coma. Methanol is metabolized to formic acid, which causes a severe metabolic acidosis followed by decreased vision and even blindness beginning 6–12 hours after ingestion. Isopropyl alcohol leaves an odor of acetone on the breath. It can cause coma at blood levels that would be only mildly intoxicating with ethanol. Ethylene glycol is sweet tasting and often visually attractive. This makes it appealing to children and animals. The metabolism of ethylene glycol produces a metabolic acidosis and renal failure over several hours after exposure.

9. Many people are taking medication for depression. Are there serious dangers with an overdose of these medicines? How is an overdose treated?

Absolutely. Between 10% and 20% of the general population will become depressed at some point during their lives. It is the most common psychological disturbance. There are several families of medication aimed at relieving the symptoms of depression. The tricyclic antidepressants (TCAs) cause the most concern, whereas the newer serotonin reuptake inhibitors have a wider safety margin. TCAs include imipramine, amitriptyline, desipramine, and doxepin, among others, and have a confusing array of brand names. Symptoms of overdose include delerium, coma, seizures, hypotension, cardiac dysrhythmias, and cardiovascular collapse. Symptoms can progress quickly and patients may progress from normal to severe toxicity within an hour. The treatment for delirium and coma is intubation for airway protection. Seizures are treated with benzodiazepines. Hypotension requires volume resuscitation and adrenergic vasopressors such as dopamine or epinephrine infusions. Wide complex tachycardia should be treated with hypertonic sodium bicarbonate (1–2 meq/kg).

Overdose of other antidepressants usually produces somnolence, but this may progress to coma mandating airway management. Seizures may occur and usually respond to benzodiazepines. Dysrhythmias are very uncommon but should be treated with sodium bicarbonate (1–2 meq/kg).

10. **Acetaminophen is found in many over-the-counter drugs, so it must be safe, right?**
    When taken as directed, it is safe and effective. In larger quantities, however, it can be fatal. One of the difficulties with an acetaminophen (APAP) overdose is recognition of the ingestion itself. First, there are numerous over-the-counter and prescription drugs that are combined with APAP. Most cold or sinus medicines and analgesic prescriptions contain APAP. Second, acetaminophen poisoning does not produce symptoms for up to 24 hours after exposure. Consequently, every ingestion is routinely screened for APAP. Twenty extra-strength tablets or 30 regular-strength pills are toxic in an average-sized adult. Because the primary site of damage is the liver, alcoholics or patients with preexisting liver damage are at an increased risk for injury. Initially, there may be little evidence of toxic effects; nevertheless, the optimal time for antidote therapy with acetylcysteine is within 8 hours of ingestion.

11. **Aspirin is also found in many prescription and over-the-counter remedies. Are there any characteristic findings in an overdose?**
    The chemical name for aspirin is acetylsalicylic acid. Salicylates are the family of compounds that include aspirin and its cousin preparations of bismuth subsalicylate (Pepto-Bismol™), magnesium salicylate (Doan's Pills), methyl salicylate (oil of wintergreen), and other prescription medicines for inflammatory bowel disease and pain control. In an overdose, these medications may form concretions called *bezoars* in the stomach, which may delay and prolong absorption. Thirty tablets of aspirin in an adult is the minimum acute toxic dose; twice that can result in severe intoxication. Initially, patients present with nausea, vomiting, abdominal pain, hyperventilation, and tinnitus, which is a ringing or buzzing in the ears. This can develop over 10–15 hours into evidence of worsening mental status, dehydration, and deafness. Symptoms of severe or late salicylism include seizures, respiratory depression, hyperthermia, hypotension, and coma. Treatment is generally supportive and may include advanced management of the airway, IV fluids, and diazepam for seizures. Infusion of sodium bicarbonate can increase the excretion of aspirin, but patients with severe salicylate poisoning require dialysis.

12. **How do patients who take too much of their heart medicine present?**
    Calcium channel blockers (CCB) are used for hypertension, angina, and heart failure. Several are currently available. The more common ones are diltiazem, verapamil, nifedipine, and amlodipine. These drugs act to slow atrioventricular (AV) node conduction, slow sinus node activity, and cause vasodilatation in both the coronary and peripheral circulations. Consequently, a patient with CCB overdose will present with hypotension and bradycardia.

    Beta blockers (BB) are another widely prescribed medication used not only for hypertension and heart disease but also for hyperthyroidism and occasionally for migraines. Again, hypotension and bradycardia are cardinal features of an overdose. Hypoglycemia or seizures may occur following a BB overdose.

Digoxin is used in the treatment of congestive heart failure and atrial fibrillation. Some degree of toxic symptoms is believed to occur in 5–20% of patients taking digoxin. Toxicity initially presents with GI disturbances. Nausea, vomiting, diarrhea, and abdominal distention are common complaints. In addition, the patient may complain of blurred or yellow-colored vision, lethargy, and confusion. Finally, cardiac conduction disturbances are the most life-threatening toxic effect. Paroxysmal atrial tachycardia with AV block is classic, but any combination of tachycardia and heart block is suspicious for digoxin overdose. Treatment is similar for all three ingestions. Initial treatment includes cardiac monitoring, IV fluids for hypotension, and atropine for bradycardia. Cardiac pacing may be required. Hypotension from CCB or BB poisoning may respond transiently to IV calcium. Adrenergic vasopressors (dopamine or epinephrine) are the next important therapy. Magnesium or lidocaine may be helpful in the treatment of digoxin-induced dysrhythmias.

13. **What are toxidromes and how can they help me identify poisonings?**
    Toxidromes are a distinctive constellation of symptoms that are caused by poisonings. Several common toxidromes, their symptoms, and common causes are shown in Table 45.1. Although toxidromes are useful when they are present, they are not universally present and may be altered by coingestion of another poison.

14. **Are there any toxic exposures common to the rural setting?**
    The most common insecticides (organophosphate and carbamates) are related to nerve gases and chemical warfare agents. These compounds inhibit acetylcholinesterase, which leaves the cholinergic nervous system effectively "locked on." The symptoms can be remembered by the SLUDGE acronym shown in Table 45.1. In severe cases, muscle fasciculations and seizures may occur. The initial

TABLE 45.1: Common Toxidromes: Their Symptoms and Causes

Toxidrome	Symptoms	Poisons
Cholinergic	Salivation, lacrimation, urination, diarrhea, GI cramping, emesis (SLUDGE)	Carbamate and organophosphate pesticides, nerve gas (such as sarin), some mushrooms
Anticholinergic	Flushed skin, dry mouth, decreased bowel motility, delirium, seizures, dilated pupils	Antihistamines, atropine, scopolamine, Jimson weed
Opioid	Respiratory depression, decreased mental status, small pupils	Heroin, morphine, codeine, and other opioids
Sympathomimetic	Tachycardia, diaphoresis, anxiety, dilated pupils, seizures	Cocaine, amphetamine, caffeine, methylphenidate

management is airway protection and patient decontamination followed by IV atropine. Large doses of atropine are often required. Pralidoxime (2-PAM) blocks the action of some organophosphates and will typically be given in the emergency department.

There are many other common pesticides used. Rat and mouse poisons usually contain warfarin or related anticoagulants. In general, a single ingestion in an otherwise healthy person does not cause significant bleeding; however repeated exposures may cause a coagulopathy 24–72 hours after the exposure. There are many other pesticides used; most are benign but some can contain strychnine, cyanide, or other potentially dangerous poisons. It is critical to ascertain the exact product.

15. What is the treatment for patients with anticholinergic poisoning?

Patients with anticholinergic poisoning usually require little more than supportive care. However, patients with agitation may require sedation with benzodiazepines. Benzodiazepines are also used to treat seizures. Patients with CNS depression may require intubation. Very rarely patients with antihistamine overdose will develop cardiac dysrhythmias that require treatment with sodium bicarbonate boluses (1–2 meq/kg).

16. What about street drugs?

Cocaine, amphetamines, and related sympathomimetics are commonly available illicitly, in over-the-counter diet medicines, and by prescription. The sympathomimetic toxidrome is described in Table 45.1. The life-threatening complications of these poisons are seizures, hyperthermia, and ventricular dysrhythmias. In some cases, psychosis will develop that is indistinguishable from schizophrenia or the manic phase of bipolar disorder. Myocardial infarction and stroke have occurred secondary to cocaine use. The treatment for these patients is rapid sedation with benzodiazepines.

Opioids are very commonly encountered. Patients may be exposed through medication overdose, injection or inhalation of heroin, or even from transdermal use or abuse of the fentanyl patch. The first step of treatment is to open the airway and initiate ventilation. After ventilation and oxygenation, respiratory depression can be reversed with naloxone. The initial dose, 2 mg IV, may be repeated in cases of suspected severe overdose. Naloxone should not be routinely adminstered to patients without respiratory depression. Naloxone commonly causes withdrawal symptoms in opioid-dependent patients.

17. Speaking of withdrawal, how dangerous is it?

That depends on what the patient has been taking. Onset of symptoms can vary from a few hours in the case of cocaine and alcohol overdose to one or two days for some opiates. Ethanol is associated with the most common withdrawal syndrome, which may be life threatening. It manifests as intense sympathetic nervous system stimulation. A blood alcohol level of zero is not required for withdrawal to occur. In chronic alcoholics, serum alcohol levels over the legal limit of 100 mg/dL may produce symptoms. Ethanol withdrawal has four stages beginning with tremulousness, tachycardia, hyperthermia, and hypertension. This is followed by a progression through seizures, hallucinations, and finally frank delirium. Diazepam or lorazepam is the treatment of choice for sedation and control of autonomic dysfunction.

Opiate withdrawal is much more benign, albeit very uncomfortable. The constellation of symptoms includes rhinorrhea, lacrimation, vomiting, diarrhea, agitation, and mild elevations in heart rate and blood pressure. Piloerection (hair standing on end) is common, whereas seizures, mental status changes, and hyperthermia are rare. Withdrawal may be precipitated by naloxone use. Naloxone has a short half-life, however, and symptoms should resolve in two or three hours.

Cocaine or amphetamine withdrawal typically ends with depression and lethargy. No specific treatment is indicated.

18. What are the important inhaled poisons?

Carbon monoxide is produced in a fire and also by gas heaters, engine exhaust, and coal burners. It binds to hemoglobin 200 times greater than oxygen. Hemoglobin bound by carbon monoxide cannot transport oxygen. The earliest symptom is headache followed by dyspnea, irritability and fatigue, tachycardia, confusion, coma, and seizures (with increasing toxicity). Treatment is high-flow oxygen and possibly hyperbaric oxygen.

Cyanide gases from burning plastics or industrial settings is easily absorbed. Patients rapidly decline and complain of headache, nausea, and anxiety. They appear confused, and initial hypertension and bradycardia can progress to hypotension and tachycardia and quickly to apnea. High-flow oxygen and inhaled amyl nitrite are the initial measures. Then sodium nitrite IV and thiosulfate are given. These are all contained in a prepackaged cyanide antidote kit. Recently, hydroxocobalamine was approved in the United States as an antidote for cyanide. It has become the preferred prehospital treatment for cyanide poisoning.

19. What about plant ingestions?

Although plant ingestions rank fourth overall in frequency, they are not in the top 15 causes of death from ingestion. In fact, plant ingestions are generally benign, with few exceptions. Plant preparations of steeped teas or powdered seeds can be dangerous. Treat the symptoms of the ingestion rather than the ingestion itself. Bring a sample of the plant or preparation to the ED if it is available. Mushrooms grow almost everywhere, and poisonous varieties tend to be GI irritants. The nondescript white *Amanita phalloides* mushroom is dangerous and can result in fatal hepatic necrosis. These are different from the colorful *Amanita muscaria* dancing in *Fantasia*. These mushrooms cause an anticholinergic syndrome.

20. What should be done for the unknown ingestion?

The first step should be standard resuscitation: Secure the airway, administer high flow oxygen, and ventilate the patient. Because many poisons cause a metabolic acidosis, overdose patients should generally be hyperventilated. Hypotension should be treated with isotonic fluid boluses followed by an adrenergic vasopressor if necessary. Give sodium bicarbonate for wide complex tachycardias. Treat agitation and seizures with high doses of benzodiazepines. Finally, remember to check the blood glucose in patients with altered mental status.

Pearls and Pitfalls

1. Presume wide complex tachycardia that occurs following an overdose is caused by a drug that blocks sodium channels. Administer sodium bicarbonate to these patients.
2. Most poisoned patients die from losing their airway—manage the airway early.
3. Although most poisoned patients require little more than supportive care, patients with symptoms caused by other causes (such as trauma or infection) require specific treatment. Never assume a poisoning diagnosis when other problems may account for the patient's symptoms.
4. Failure to bring labeled containers with the patient can lead to a missed diagnosis or inappropriate treatment.

References

1. Vanden Hoek TL, Morrison LJ, Shuster M, et al. Cardiac arrest in special situations. Part 12. 2010 AHA guidelines for CPR and ECC. Circulation 122:S829–S861, 2010.
2. Cooper GM, Le Couteur DG, Richardson D, Buckley NA. A randomized clinical trial of activated charcoal for the routine management of oral drug overdose. QJM 98(9):655–660, 2005.
3. DeWitt CR, Waksman JC. Pharmacology, pathophysiology and management of calcium channel blocker and beta-blocker toxicity. Toxicol Rev 23(4):223–238, 2004.
4. Heard K. Gastrointestinal decontamination. Med Clin North Am 89(6):1067–1078, 2005.
5. Hoffman RS. Cocaine. In Goldfrank's Toxicologic Emergencies, 9th ed., Nelson LS, Lewin NA, Howland MA, et al., eds., pp. 1091–1102 New York: McGraw-Hill, 2011.
6. Isbister GK; Dawson AH, Whyte IM. Feasibility of prehospital treatment with activated charcoal: Who could we treat, who should we treat? Emerg Med J 20(4) 375–378, 2003.
7. Kao LW, Nanagas KA. Carbon monoxide poisoning. Med Clin North Am 89(6):1161–1194, 2005.
8. Lai MW; Klein-Schwartz W, Rodgers, GC, et al. 2005 Annual Report of the American Association of Poison Control Centers' national poisoning and exposure database. Clin Toxicol (Phila) 44(6–7):803–932, 2006.
9. Liebelt EL. Cyclic Antidepressants. In. Goldfrank's Toxicologic Emergencies, 9th ed., Nelson LS, Lewin NA, Howland MA, et al., eds., pp. 1049–1059. New York: McGraw-Hill, 2011.
10. Mokhlesi B, Leiken JB, Murray P, Corbridge TC. Adult toxicology in critical care: Part I: General approach to the intoxicated patient. Chest 2003 Feb; 123(2):577–92.
11. Mokhlesi B; Leikin JB, Murray P, and Corbridge TC. Adult toxicology in critical care: Part II: specific poisonings. Chest 2003 Mar; 123(3):897–922.
12. Betz JM. Plants. In Goldfrank's Toxicologic Emergencies, 9th ed., Nelson LS, Lewin NA, Howland MA, et al., eds., pp. 1537–1560. New York: McGraw-Hill; 2011.
13. Wiener SW. Toxic Alcohols. In Goldfrank's Toxicologic Emergencies, 9th ed., Nelson LS, Lewin NA, Howland MA, et al., eds., pp. 1400–1410. New York: McGraw-Hill, 2011.
14. Stork CM. Serotonin reuptake inhibitors and atypical antidepressants. In Goldfrank's Toxicologic Emergencies, 9th ed., Nelson LS, Lewin NA, Howland MA, et al., eds., pp. 1037–1048. New York: McGraw Hill; 2011.
15. Wills B, Erickson T. Drug- and toxin-associated seizures. Med Clin North Am 89(6):1297–1321, 2005.
16. Yip L, Dart RC, Gabow PA. Concepts and controversies in salicylate toxicity. Emerg Med Clin North Am 1994 May; 12(2):351–364.

Hypothermia and Frostbite

Daniel F. Danz, MD

CHAPTER 46

1. **What is accidental hypothermia?**
   Hypothermia occurs when the core temperature of the body drops below 35°C (95°F). Hypothermia is categorized as mild (32.2–35°C, 90–95°F), moderate (27–32.2°C; 80–90°F), severe (<27°C, <80°F).

2. **Why do I need to know about hypothermia?**
   In the United States, hypothermia can occur anywhere. Additionally, the injured, the sick, the young, and the old are particularly susceptible to cold. Therefore, EMS providers must be familiar with the causes, prevention, and care of hypothermia.

3. **What causes hypothermia?**
   Hypothermia occurs whenever the body loses heat into its environment faster than it can produce it. Hypothermia may also result from impaired thermoregulation or decreased heat production.

4. **What are the mechanisms of heat loss?**
   Heat is lost by five mechanisms: conduction, convection, radiation, evaporation, and respiration, so certain environmental factors can increase loss.
   1. Conductive loss is enhanced by direct contact with cold objects (such as lying on concrete or snow or a metal surface) and moisture, as water conducts and removes heat much faster than air. For example conductive heat loss increases 25-fold with immersion in cold water.
   2. Convective loss is increased by air movement, so windy conditions remove much more heat than calm, thus the concept of wind chill.
   3. Radiation increases with removal of clothing and other insulating layers. Radiation may account for more than 50% of heat loss.
   4. Evaporative heat loss increases with windy conditions and low humidity.
   5. Respiration in cold environments loses heat.

5. **Who is prone to hypothermia?**
   Patient characteristics that increase heat loss or decrease heat production include increased surface area compared to volume (infants and children), decreased metabolism (elderly, shocky, intoxicated), increased fluid loss (sweating, diarrhea, burns), and being disrobed for evaluation and treatment of illness or injury.

6. **How do you diagnose it?**
   Reliable core temperatures are difficult to obtain in the field. Simplified clinical assessment is recommended, but be aware that many other conditions cause a similar clinical picture.

Mild	Poor judgment
	Slurred speech
	Normal blood pressure
	Strong shivering
Moderate	Little or no shivering
	Dysrhythmias
	Pupils dilate
	Stupor/poor perfusion
Severe	No reflex or response
	Significant hypotension
	Maximum risk of ventricular fibrillation
	No pupil response

7. When should hypothermia be suspected?
Subtle presentations are common in urban areas. Mental changes can mimic intoxication as well as any neurologic or psychiatric condition.

8. Besides insulation to prevent further heat loss, how is hypothermia treated in the field?
A succinct summary is rescue, examine, insulate, and transport. During mountain rescue, consider sleeping bags, body-to-body contact, chemical heat pads, and hot water bottles. The type of power in the transport vehicle is another determinant. If available, heated IV infusions should be administered. Most patients are volume depleted. Limit active rewarming to heated inhalation and truncal application of heat (Figure 46.1).

9. How should hypothermic patients be prepared for transport?
Always attempt to keep the patient horizontal. Do not allow exertion. Gently remove or preferably cut off wet clothing, and use dry insulation. Stabilize fractures and cover open wounds during packaging.

10. When should CPR be initiated on the severely hypothermic patient?
Cardiopulmonary resuscitation (CPR) should be started in all hypothermia patients except those with:
  DNR status
  Obviously lethal injuries
  A frozen chest wall that cannot be depressed
  Any signs of life (implies perfusion)
  When the rescuers will be endangered by evacuation delays or changing conditions
Do not withhold CPR only because continuous compressions cannot be assured. Intermittent flow may be preferable to none. A physician was successfully resuscitated from 13.7°C (56.7 F) after 165 minutes of CPR.

11. Can I mistake hypothermia for death?
You bet you can, and it has occurred many times. Profoundly hypothermic patients may appear to be dead due to the dramatically decreased metabolic rate (i.e., slow shallow respirations and bradycardia).

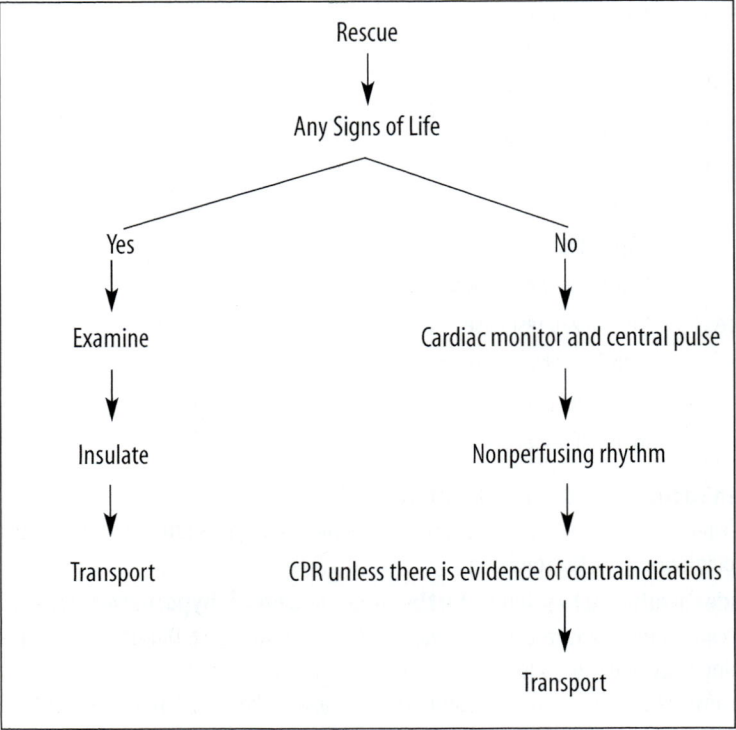

FIGURE 46.1   Algorithm for prehospital treatment of hypothermia.

12. What are the current ACLS guidelines in hypothermia?
The cold heart is less responsive to medications, electrical stimulation, and defibrillation. A single defibrillation attempt is indicated for ventricular fibrillation (VF) as well as a single round of advanced cardiac life support (ACLS) drugs. If no response is obtained, rewarm above 30°C (86°F) before attempting further.

13. Should the severely hypothermic patient be tracheally intubated?
Airway is always the first priority and should be secured in the hypothermic patient. The concern that endotracheal intubation can cause VF is overemphasized. In addition, preoxygenation with high-flow oxygen and bag–mask ventilation will help prevent this dysrhythmia from occurring. Endotracheal intubation will facilitate the use of humidified, heated oxygen systems as well as protecting the patient's airway.

14. What are some strategies to give fluids in the field?
Improvisation during transport can help. Plastic IV containers maybe be placed under the patient and insulated. Heat-producing packets can be taped to IV bags. A variety of commercial in-line heaters are available for both DC and AC power. Intraosseous infusions are another option in vasoconstricted dehydrated patients.

Hypothermia and Frostbite

15. What special consideration should be given to the hypothermic trauma patient?
The hypothermic trauma patient is a unique challenge. Research shows that because of the physiologic changes associated with hypothermia (impaired coagulation, altered platelet function, and disseminated intravascular coagulation), considerably increased blood loss can occur. The patient most at risk will have blunt or penetrating abdominal trauma as well as hypothermia. Aggressive efforts should be made to rewarm these patients or to minimize their heat loss. Avoid use of cold intravenous fluids, ventilation with cold oxygen, and exposing the patient for long periods of time.

16. Can I cause hypothermia?
Yes. Exposure of the very young and the very old by removal of clothing, even for relatively brief periods of time, will cause hypothermia. Also, the application of wet dressings to a body burn of greater than 10% of body surface area will cause hypothermia.

17. What is frostbite?
Frostbite occurs whenever the tissue temperature is below 0°C. Ice crystals will develop, damage cells, and cause microvascular thrombosis.

18. What are some risk factors?
Common ones include skin contact with good thermal conductors (metal, water, volatiles), wind chill exposure, and wet constrictive clothing or footwear.

19. What are the symptoms?
Initially various sensory deficits occur. Frostnip is simply transient tingling or numbness. Frostbite involves anesthesia of the affected part.

20. Should frozen tissues be thawed in the field?
Not in severely hypothermic patients. The cold extremity blood returning to the heart will further lower the heart temperature—this is termed core temperature afterdrop. Tissue refreezing is also disastrous. Ideally, rapid complete thawing by immersion in 40°C (77°F) circulating water is best in any setting. Never use dry heat, and do not rub or massage the tissue.

Pearls and Pitfalls

1. Accurate assessment of core temperature in the field is very difficult. Assume that unresponsive patients who are not shivering are severely hypothermic.
2. Computer software usually misdiagnoses J waves as injury current on 12-lead electrocardiograms (ECGs) (Figure 46.2). Prehospital thrombolytic therapy in hypothermia could exacerbate coagulopathies and be fatal.
3. Cold hearts fibrillate easily. Avoid rough handling such as rolling gurneys rapidly or "code 3 full lights and sirens" rapid transport. Consider aeromedical evacuation in rough terrain.
4. Remember that no prognostic neurologic scale, including the Glasgow Coma Scale, is valid during hypothermia. As an extreme example, many patients have recovered completely in the morgue.
5. Peripheral pulses are difficult to palpate in profoundly bradycardic vasoconstricted patients. Check the monitor for at least a minute before starting compressions, as iatrogenic ventricular fibrillation is a real hazard.

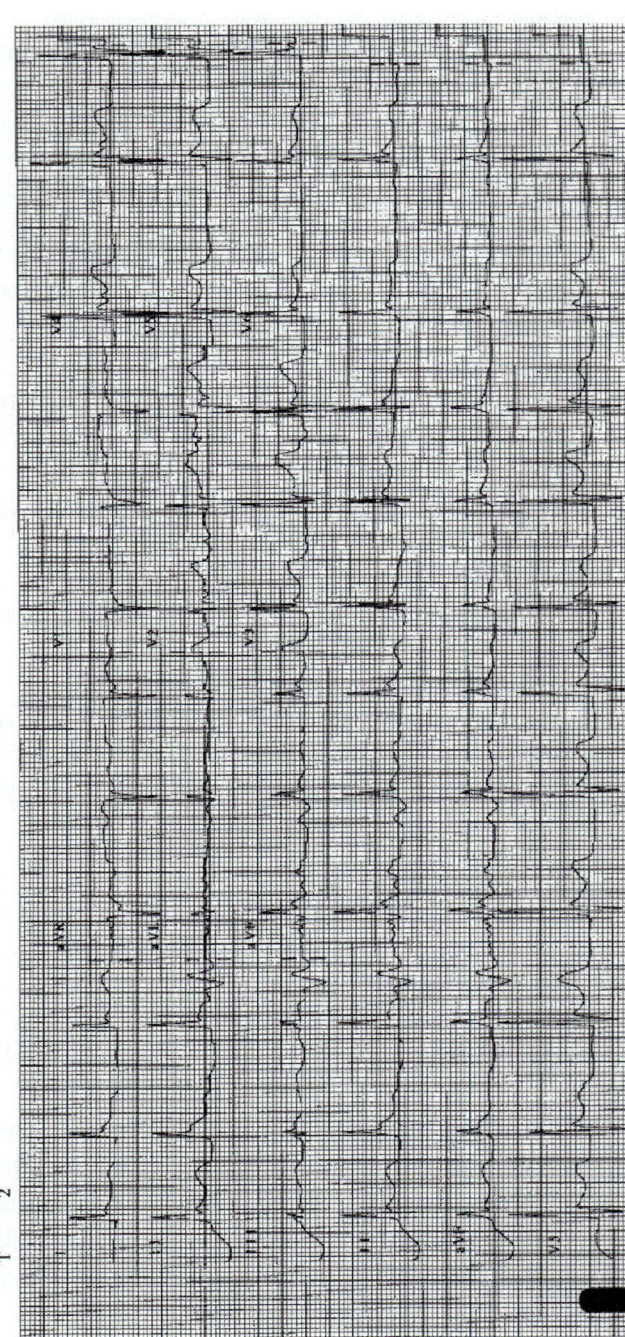

FIGURE 46.2 ECG showing classic J Waves associated with hypothermia.

6. Overinflation of an endotracheal tube cuff with frigid ambient air can kink the tube when the air in the cuff heats and expands.
7. If monitor leads do not stick to cold skin, try benzoin or use needle electrodes that can be made by simply puncturing the gel foam conventional monitor pad with a small-gauge needle and inserting the needles into the usual lead placement locations.
8. An extremely common error is overzealous assistance of ventilation. Carbon dioxide production is minimal, and hypocapneic ventricular irritability is dangerous.
9. For long transports, the ideal vehicle ambient temperature is unclear. The comfort of rescue personnel is important for performance, and an interior temperature around 25°C is unlikely to induce vasodilation and harm the patient.
10. Avoid prehospital thawing of frostbitten tissue if there is a possibility of refreezing—more tissue will be lost.

References

1. Centers for Disease Control and Prevention: Hypothermia-related deaths - United States, 1999-2002 and 2005. MMWR 55:282, 2006.
2. Delaney KA, Vassallo SU, Larkin GL, Goldfrank LR. Rewarming rates in urban patients with hypothermia: prediction of underlying infection. Acad Emerg Med 13:913, 2006.
3. Kempainen RR, Brunette DD. The evaluation and management of accidental hypothermia. Resp Care 49:192, 2004.
4. Headdon WG, Wilson PM, Dalton HR: The management of accidental hypothermia. BMJ 338:2085, 2009.
5. Gilbert M, Busund R, Skagseth A, et al. Resuscitation from accidental hypothermia of 13.7° C with circulatory arrest. Lancet 355:375, 2000.
6. Silfvast T, Pettilä, V. Outcome from severe accidental hypothermia in Southern Finland—A 10-year review. Resuscitation 59:285, 2003.
7. American Heart Association. 2010 Guidelines for cardiopulmonary resuscitation and emergency cardiovascular care, part 12.9: Cardiac arrest in hypothermia. Circulation 122-S845-S846, 2010.
8. Danzl DF. Hypothermia. Semin Respir Crit Care Med 23:57, 2002.
9. Hildebrand F, Giannoudis PV, van Griensven M, et al. Pathophysiologic changes and effects of hypothermia on outcome in elective surgery and trauma patients. Am J Surg 187:363, 2004.
10. Van der Ploeg G, et. al: Accidental hyopthermia: Rewarming treatments, complications and outcomes from one university medical centre. Resuscitation 81:1550, 2010.

Heat Illness

Stephen V. Cantrill, MD

CHAPTER 47

1. **What is heat illness?**
   Heat illness represents a spectrum of disease brought on due to exposure of the body to excessive heat and/or the inability of the body to rid itself of excess heat. Heat illness includes the entities of heat cramps, heat exhaustion, and the sometimes lethal heat stroke.

2. **Describe heat cramps.**
   Heat cramps occur in muscle groups that are fatigued by heavy work and are brought on by prolonged strenuous exercise, as in construction workers, sugar cane cutters, and miners. The onset occurs *after* finishing heavy work and during relaxation. They differ from the muscle cramps of athletes, which occur *during* exercise and resolve spontaneously. Heat cramps are the result of copious sweating during exertion with inadequate replacement of the salt lost in the sweat. Treatment of heat cramps consists of sodium chloride (NaCl) replacement, which can usually be accomplished orally or by the intravenous administration of normal saline. Body temperature is usually normal with heat cramps.

3. **What are the symptoms and signs of heat exhaustion?**
   The patient may complain of any combination of weakness, fatigue, frontal headache, vertigo, nausea and vomiting, thirst, decreased urine output, and cramps. This is felt to be due to volume depletion and electrolyte loss. The body temperature is normal or minimally elevated. Mental function remains normal. Tachycardia, orthostatic hypotension, and clinical dehydration may occur. The skin is pale, cool, and clammy and may be flushed. Sweating persists and may be profuse.

4. **What is the treatment for heat exhaustion?**
   Rest in a cool, shady spot. Fluid and electrolyte replacement is essential. Oral rehydration with solutions such as Gatorade™, Powerade™, or dilute sugar drinks with a half teaspoon of salt per liter can be very effective. If significant hypotension is present, intravenous fluids should be started. The patient should be monitored for further signs of progressive illness because heat exhaustion may progress to heat stroke.

5. **What is heat stroke?**
   Heat stroke is defined as having a rectal body temperature of 40.5°C (105°F) or greater after strenuous exercise and/or exposure to increased temperature and humidity with presence of an altered mental status or other neurologic dysfunction (ataxia, hallucinations, coma, seizures). Because most prehospital care providers do not have the ability to take a temperature in the field, the field diagnosis must be made based upon patient presentation and history. Note that sweating or its absence is *not* a criterion for heat stroke.

6. **Why is a rectal temperature of 40.5°C the cutoff?**
   Any temperature above this threshold indicates the failure of the body to dissipate excess heat and represents a failure of the body's thermoregulatory mechanism.

7. **What are the two types of heat stroke? How do they present?**

   Classic heat stroke is not associated with exercise but with exposure to high heat and humidity over time. This form of heat stroke has a slow onset, often developing over days. It is common in the elderly and the chronically ill, who may present with anorexia, nausea, vomiting, headache, dizziness, confusion, and hypotension. Anhidrosis (lack of sweating) is common.

   Exertional heat stroke usually affects young people in good health who are exercising in a hot, humid environment. It is rapid in onset. Nausea, dizziness, and confusion are common. Fatigue, ataxia, seizures, coma, and nuchal rigidity or posturing may also occur. These patients often are sweating at the time of presentation.

8. **Which populations are at increased risk for developing heat stroke?**
   - Extremes of age—due to relatively poor temperature regulation in the young and old
   - Chronically ill—especially those on drugs that predispose to heat illness
   - Military recruits—especially unacclimated northerners training in the South
   - Athletes—most commonly, football players and runners
   - Laborers—especially if water losses have not been replaced
   - Obese individuals—heat dissipation is compromised
   - Persons dressed inappropriately for their environment or activity level

9. **What is the "mean heat index" and how is it useful?**

   The "mean heat index" is a recently devised measure developed by the National Weather Service as a measure of how hot the environment actually feels to a person over the course of a day. This value is computed from a multiple regression equation based upon ambient temperature and humidity extremes encountered during a 24-hour period. Values of greater than 85°F (29.5°C) are felt to be dangerous to the population at large. The National Weather Service has developed methodology to create a forecast giving the probability of a locale exceeding a certain mean heat index for up to 7 days in the future. These forecasts can then be used by local health and emergency officials to prepare the public for times of increased risk from heat and heat stroke.

10. **What is the mortality rate of heat stroke?**

    Mortality rates vary from zero to 76% in different reports. This high variability is due to the differences in the populations studied. Young, healthy individuals with exertional heat stroke usually do quite well, whereas the elderly, chronically ill suffering classic heat stroke often fare quite poorly.

11. **What differential diagnoses should be considered in patients presenting with a rectal temperature greater than 40.5°C?**

Meningitis	Neuroleptic malignant syndrome
Typhus	Malignant hyperthermia
Falciparum malaria	Thyroid storm
Rocky Mountain spotted fever	Delirium tremens
Hypothalamic brain lesion	Anticholinergic drug overdose
Cocaine overdose	Amphetamine overdose

12. What is the most important aspect in the treatment of heat stroke?

Rapid cooling. Heat stroke is a true medical emergency where minutes count. Poor patient outcome is related more to the length of time the temperature remains elevated than to the absolute degree of hyperpyrexia. Field treatment should begin as soon as the diagnosis is suspected and should include removal of the patient from the hot environment, removal of constrictive clothing, and institution of rapid cooling.

13. What treatment modalities are effective for rapid cooling?

Immersion in ice water is effective, although many feel this must be accompanied by vigorous skin massage to counteract the cutaneous vasoconstriction that may actually impede heat loss. This modality may not be appropriate in the comatose or combative patient and is generally not practical in an ambulance. Aggressive evaporative cooling, consisting of treatment with water spray and a forced air stream from a fan (or transport in an ambulance with open windows), has proved successful and is preferred by many. Ice packs and massage may also be used. Cooling efforts should cease when the patient's temperature falls to 38.5°C (101.3°F) to avoid temperature undershoot and shivering.

14. How can heat illness be prevented?

- Keep well hydrated. This is essential to prevent heat illnesses.
- Avoid prolonged exposure to hot, humid environments and rest frequently during strenuous exercise.
- Wear well-ventilated, loosely woven, breathable clothing to keep cool, and wear a hat for protection from direct sun exposure.
- Avoid drugs that predispose to poor thermoregulation, such as amphetamines, diuretics, antihistamines, cocaine, and alcohol.
- Remember that heat illness is completely preventable.

Pearls and Pitfalls

1. The presence of sweating does not rule out the diagnosis of heat stroke.
2. The prehospital care rendered to patients with heat stroke may be life saving. Cooling should begin in the field as soon as the diagnosis is suspected.
3. Spraying the patient with tepid water, followed by fanning is a simple prehospital method to begin patient cooling.
4. Heat illness is completely preventable.

References

1. American College of Sports Medicine, Heat and cold illnesses during distance running. Med Sci Sports Exerc 28(12): i–x, 1996.
2. Bourchama A, Knochel J, Heat stroke. N Engl J Med 346:1978–1988, 2002.
3. Costrini A: Emergency treatment of exertional heatstroke and comparison of whole body cooling techniques. Med Sci Sports Exerc 22:15, 1990.
4. Horowitz BZ, The golden hour in heat stroke: Use of iced peritoneal lavage. Am J Emerg Med 7:616, 1989.
5. Hubbard RW, Matthew CB, Durkot MJ, et al. Novel approaches to the pathophysiology of heatstroke: The energy depletion model. Ann Emerg Med 16:1066–1075, 1987.

6. Hubbard RW. Heatstroke pathophysiology: The energy depletion model. Med Sci Sports Exerc 22:19, 1990.
7. Knochel JP. Environmental heat illness: An eclectic review. Arch Intern Med 133:841–864, 1974.
8. National Athletic Trainers Association. Inter-association task force on exertional heat illness consensus statement, 2003. Available at http://www.nata.org/sites/default/files/inter-association-task-force-exertional-heat-illness.pdf (Accessed June 4, 2011)
9. Shibolet S, Lancaster MC, Danon Y. Heat stroke: A review. Aviat Space Environ Med 47:280–301, 1976.
10. Vicario SJ, Okabajue R, Haltom T. Rapid cooling in classic heatstroke. Am J Emerg Med 4:394–398, 1986.
11. White JD, Riccobene E, Nucci R, et al. Evaporation versus iced gastric lavage treatment of heatstroke: Comparative efficacy in a canine model. Crit Care Med 15:748–750, 1987.
12. Yarbrough B, Vicario S: Heat illness. In Rosen's Emergency Medicine, Concepts and Clinical Practice, Marx J, et al. eds., pp. 1997–2009. St. Louis: Mosby, 2002.
13. Binkley HM, Beckett J, Casa DJ, Kleiner DM, Plummer PE. National Athletic Trainers' Association Position Statement. Exertional heat illnesses. J Athl Train 2002;37(3):329–343 Available at: http://www.nata.org/sites/default/files/ExternalHeatIllnesses.pdf (Accessed June 4, 2010)

CHAPTER 48

Altitude Illness

Ben Honigman, MD, and Kelly Bookman, MD

1. **How is altitude measured, and why are people affected by increases in elevation?**
   Altitude is measured in feet or meters above sea level. The partial pressure of oxygen (the amount of oxygen available in the air we take in with each breath) decreases with an increase in altitude. Therefore, the symptoms and signs associated with high altitude are directly and indirectly a result of hypoxia. Each individual has a different response to this hypoxia and, therefore, different susceptibilities to altitude illness. Within a few minutes at altitude, a decrease in blood oxygen saturation can be detected and ventilation is increased. This result is called the hypoxic ventilatory response. Altered fluid homeostasis also occurs, causing a redistribution of fluid from the intravascular space to the intra- and extracellular spaces that results in peripheral and, occasionally, pulmonary and cerebral edema.

2. **What are the most common syndromes caused by altitude illness?**
   Altitude illness is a continuum of symptoms and signs that can range from a mild loss of appetite and headache to cerebral and pulmonary edema, coma, and death. For the purposes of classification, these syndromes have been described as mild, moderate, and severe acute mountain sickness (AMS), with severe AMS also called high-altitude cerebral edema (HACE) or high-altitude pulmonary edema (HAPE).

3. **What are the symptoms, signs, and treatments for mild AMS?**
   Symptoms and signs: Headache relieved by rest and medication, nausea, fatigue, dizziness, anorexia, and insomnia. There are no characteristic physical exam findings.

   Treatment: It is important to keep well hydrated and continue adequate nutrition even in light of anorexia. Ibuprofen, aspirin, or acetaminophen can be beneficial for the treatment of headache. Most individuals can acclimatize within one to two days. Acetazolamide will help reduce symptoms. One should not continue to ascend until the symptoms have diminished.

4. **What are the symptoms, signs, and treatments for moderate AMS?**
   Symptoms and signs: Headache not relieved by rest or medication, anorexia, nausea with vomiting, fatigue and weakness at rest, and insomnia.

   Treatment: Descent of at least 1000 ft and sometimes 2000 ft or greater is necessary. Hydration and nutrition are essential. Oxygen will significantly improve symptoms because hypoxia is the underlying cause of AMS. Because the descent itself is the equivalent of providing additional oxygen, one should never delay descent to wait for supplemental oxygen. Pain medications for headache and, if persistent vomiting is present, an antiemetic such as prochlorperazine by suppository or odansetron orally disintegrating tablets (zofran) are recommended. Acetazolamide will also be helpful. It is important to closely monitor the patient for deterioration.

5. **What are the symptoms, signs, and treatments for severe AMS?**
   Symptoms and signs: All the above findings for moderate AMS plus ataxia, fatigue, and personal neglect. Neglect may progress to the point that the patient is not eating, drinking or dressing himself. There is dyspnea and tachycardia at rest. HACE and/or HAPE may develop. HAPE and HACE can be seen independently, but both are usually present to some degree.

   Treatment: Successful treatment depends on early recognition of the progression of AMS. Immediate descent of at least 1500–3000 ft is the treatment of choice. Oxygen is essential if available. Acetazolamide and dexamethasone can be used for HACE if descent is delayed. However, if medication does not work on its own—descent is mandatory.

6. **If descent is not an immediate alternative, is there anything else I can do?**
   The Gamow bag is a portable, inflatable neoprene bag that can be inflated to 2 psi to simulate a descent of 4000–6000 ft. This barometric change will usually improve the patient's symptoms. One to two people can fit in this device, which provides a temporizing measure until formal descent can be made.

7. **What is HAPE?**
   HAPE develops insidiously with fluid accumulation in the lungs, initially causing decreased endurance and a persistent dry cough. It usually strikes the second night at a new altitude and rarely happens after more than four days at a particular altitude. Scattered rales may be heard on lung auscultation. Late in the illness, a cough productive of blood-tinged frothy sputum may develop. Resting tachypnea and tachycardia, as well as hypoxia, progress. Fever may be present. Descent and/or oxygen are almost always successful in resolving symptoms. Mild to moderate HAPE can be treated with rest and supplemental oxygen without descent. Pulse oximetry can be used to guide treatment. If a patient does not improve to greater than 90% saturation after 5 min of high flow oxygen, descent is indicated. If HACE is also present, descent is mandatory. Medication is indicated if neither descent nor oxygen is available. Nifedipine can be used for treatment, as well as prevention, of HAPE. Inhaled beta-agonists have also been shown to be useful for treatment and prevention. Positive end expiratory pressure via mask can be used as a temporizing measure. Furosemide is not indicated because HAPE is noncardiogenic in origin. Sildenafil (Viagra) is currently under study as another treatment for HAPE and has shown initial success in preliminary studies and case reports.

8. **What is HACE?**
   HACE is the end-stage of AMS. It is manifested by a change in mental status that may include disorientation, somnolence, confusion, combativeness, stupor, and coma. The cause of death from HACE is brain herniation secondary to cerebral edema. Immediate descent is imperative. Dexamethasone is indicated for HACE.

9. **What are prevention measures for AMS?**
   The best prevention is gradual ascent. Once an individual is above an altitude of 10,000 ft, the sleeping altitude should not increase more than 2000 ft in 24 hours and an extra day should be spent acclimatizing

for every increase of 2000 ft. Acetazolamide is the preferred drug for prevention of AMS but dexamethasone works as well. Ginkgo biloba has not consistently been shown to be helpful. Prophylactic aspirin will reduce the headache associated with AMS. Keeping well hydrated is a must. Sedatives and alcohol should be avoided because they may cause hypoventilation, which can exacerbate AMS symptoms.

10. **Is there a difference between treating altitude illness at moderate altitude (8000–10,000 ft) versus higher altitude?**
    Yes. At moderate altitudes such as mountain resort communities, oxygen, acetazolamide, dexamethasone, and nifedipine may be used and allow the patient to remain at altitude. However, in the wilderness at higher altitudes, in addition to the above interventions, a Gamow bag or access to aeromedical evacuation should be available and descent becomes mandatory.

11. **What is acetazolamide, how does it work, and what are its indications for use?**
    Acetazolamide is a diuretic that indirectly causes enhanced ventilatory acclimatization and decreases cerebral spinal fluid production. It is the drug of choice for prophylaxis of AMS. It is also indicated for use during rapid ascent (i.e., for those partaking in a rescue effort), for persons with a past history of moderate AMS or HAPE, and for treatment for AMS that has already developed.

12. **Does acetazolamide have any side effects?**
    Yes. It is a sulfa-based drug and allergies may exist. Because acetazolamide is a diuretic, it causes polyuria and can lead to dehydration if adequate intake is not maintained. Peripheral paresthesias, myopia, and impotence can also occur. An unpleasant side effect is that it ruins the taste of carbonated beverages.

13. **What is dexamethasone, how does it work, and what are its indications for use?**
    Dexamethasone is a steroid that has anti-inflammatory effects. It is effective in treating AMS and HACE. However, symptoms can rebound once the medication is stopped. Therefore, its use as a prophylactic medication for AMS is limited to those with intolerable side effects from acetazolamide.

Pearls and Pitfalls

1. Mild acute mountain sickness (AMS) is manifested by headache, anorexia, insomnia, fatigue, and nausea.
2. Oral hydration, rest, and analgesics are the treatment for mild AMS.
3. Moderate AMS is treated by descent of at least 1000-2000 ft.
4. Severe AMS may be life threatening and must be treated by immediate descent or a Gamow bag.
5. A Gamow bag is a portable inflatable bag that can be pressurized to 2 psi, thus simulating a descent.
6. HACE is the most serious and life-threatening form of AMS.
7. Acetazolamide (Diamox) is used in prophylaxis of AMS.

References

1. Bartsch P, Bailey DM, Berger MM, et al. Acute mountain sickness: Controversies and advances. Review. High Alt Med Biol 5(2):110–124, 2004.

2. Chow T, Browne V, Heileson HL, et al. Ginkgo biloba and acetazolamide prophylaxis for acute mountain sickness: A randomized, placebo-controlled trial. Arch Intern Med 165(3):296–301, 2005.
3. Hackett PH, Roach RC. High-altitude illness. Review. N Engl J Med. 345(2):107–114, 2001.
4. Honigman B, Theis MK, Koziol-McLain J, et al. Acute mountain sickness in a general tourist population at moderate altitudes. Ann Intern Med 118(8):587–592, 1993.
5. Richalet JP, Gratadour P, Robach P, et al. Sildenafil inhibits altitude-induced hypoxemia and pulmonary hypertension. Am J Respir Crit Care Med 171(3):275–231, 2005.

Obstetric and Gynecologic Emergencies

Cheryl Blazek, BS, EMT-P

1. **How do women with obstetric or gynecologic emergencies present to EMS?**
   Generally, women with acute obstetric or gynecologic emergencies will call for EMS assistance because of complaints of abdominal pain, vaginal bleeding, or both.

2. **When should you consider that a woman with medical complaints may be pregnant?**
   Any female that is of the age of menses (generally 10–50 years of age) may be pregnant unless she's had a hysterectomy. The possibility of pregnancy must always be considered in the differential diagnosis, particularly when a woman presents with acute abdominal pain or vaginal bleeding. In addition, pregnancy must be a consideration even if the patient denies that she is pregnant. Cases abound where a female patient adamantly denied any possibility of pregnancy only to discover that the cause of the complaint was, in fact, pregnancy-related.

3. **In addition to complaints of pain or bleeding, what should I ask in the history?**
   Important information to obtain in the history includes the date of the last menstrual period: was it normal in terms of duration and amount of bleeding, birth control methods used, vaginal discharge, previous pregnancies and their outcome, and prior operations?

4. **What causes a miscarriage and how does it present?**
   Miscarriage, or spontaneous abortion, is relatively common, occurring in about 20% of women who are pregnant as confirmed by chemical tests. Of women who have vaginal bleeding in pregnancy, almost half have normal pregnancies and the other half miscarry. About 80% of miscarriages occur in the first 3 months, and most are caused by abnormal growth of the fetus, due either to chromosomal abnormalities or to abnormalities within the uterus. In the second trimester, after 14 weeks, miscarriage may be more complicated and associated with heavier bleeding. The common symptoms are lower abdominal cramping and vaginal bleeding. Before the uterus actually expels fetal tissue, the miscarriage is considered to be *threatened*. When the cervix opens, miscarriage is considered *inevitable* or *incomplete*. A *completed* miscarriage occurs after all pregnancy-related tissue has been expelled. To help in the assessment of the patient in the emergency department, it is mandatory to bring all the clots and tissue that the patient shows you. Pathologic analysis of this tissue can help to determine if miscarriage has occurred and if it is complete or not.

5. **What is an ectopic pregnancy and how does it present?**
   An ectopic pregnancy is a pregnancy that implants and grows outside of the uterus. The fertilized egg may implant in the fallopian tube (most common), in the ovary, or in the peritoneal cavity. It causes symptoms in the first 12 weeks of pregnancy, sometimes even before the patient misses a menstrual period. It is a problem because if the ectopic pregnancy ruptures, bleeding can be significant, hidden in the peritoneal cavity, and life threatening. Ectopic pregnancy should be considered in the prehospital assessment in any woman of childbearing age who presents with unilateral or bilateral lower abdominal pain.

Obstetric and Gynecologic Emergencies

6. **Name some physiologic changes that occur during pregnancy.**
   - Increased heart rate
   - Increased respiratory rate
   - Normal or low blood pressure
   - Decreased respiratory reserve
   - Increase venous pressure in legs
   - Supine hypotension
   - Loss of abdominal findings such as guarding

7. **How should a pregnant patient be transported?**
   After 20 weeks, supine positioning can cause hypotension, which occurs when the gravid uterus presses on the inferior vena cava, obstructing venous return to the heart. In 20% of pregnant women, this can result in decreased cardiac output, known as *supine hypotensive syndrome*. For this reason, after 20 weeks, the patient should be transported on her left side or, if immobilized on a backboard, with the backboard wedged and tilted 15° to the left.

8. **What are the main causes of bleeding in a woman who is more than 20 weeks pregnant?**
   The two primary causes of vaginal bleeding in the second half of pregnancy are placenta previa and abruptio placentae. *Placenta previa* is due to low implantation of the placenta on or near the cervix. As the uterus grows, small bridging vessels overlying the cervix can tear and cause bleeding, which is usually painless and bright red. A digital exam of the cervix can cause uncontrolled bleeding and therefore should never be performed in the prehospital arena. *Abruptio placentae* is premature separation of the placenta away from the wall of the uterus, which is usually painful and associated with uterine tenderness and contractions. Risk factors for abruptio placentae include trauma to the abdomen, cocaine use, hypertension, and eclampsia. Prehospital treatment of patients with placenta previa or abruption is focused on volume resuscitation and rapid transport to an appropriate hospital. Other causes of vaginal bleeding after 20 weeks include early labor and other local lesions of the cervix.

9. **What is preeclampsia, and how are preeclampsia and eclampsia differentiated?**
   Preeclampsia is a vasospastic condition unique to pregnancy in which the patient develops edema, protein in the urine, and hypertension.
   Eclampsia is the occurrence of seizures in a pregnant patient with preeclampsia. Eclampsia can occur up to a week postpartum. Vasospasm associated with eclampsia causes injury to multiple organs, including the liver, kidney, and brain. Warning signs for eclampsia include hyperreflexia, visual disturbances, right upper quadrant pain, and severe headache.

10. **How should eclamptic seizures be treated?**
    With diazepam 5–10 mg IV, as with seizures in nonpregnancy. The specific treatment of choice is magnesium sulfate, 4 g of 10% solution IV over 20 min in 250 mL of D_5W. During the infusion, reflexes should be monitored and respiratory depression should be treated with assisted ventilation.

11. **What else can cause seizures in pregnancy?**
    Patients can have increased frequency of epileptic seizures; thrombotic strokes, or intracranial bleeds and seizures due to toxins or overdoses. Never forget the possibility of hypoglycemia in the pregnant patient with seizures.

12. **How should paroxysmal superventricular tachycardia be treated in pregnancy?**
    Much the same as it is in nonpregnant women. The first priority should be to ascertain that the tachycardia is indeed primary and is not secondarily caused by hypovolemia, sepsis, fever, or another illness. Adenosine can be used safely in pregnancy, and cardioversion also is safe for the fetus.

13. **When do you consider the fetus separately when the mother is critically ill?**
    After 24–26 weeks, at which point the fetus is potentially viable outside the uterus. Rapid transport for consideration of emergent cesarean section should be done whenever the dome of the uterus is at or above a position halfway between the umbilicus and the xiphoid process.

14. **What may cause cardiac arrest in pregnancy?**
    Causes specific to the pregnancy need to be considered: hypovolemia due to uterine rupture or abruptio placenta, hepatic or splenic rupture, or ruptured ectopic pregnancy lead the list. In addition, pulmonary emboli, amniotic fluid embolus, and other complications can occur. Cardiopulmonary resuscitation is difficult in pregnancy due to the large size of the uterus. Up to 26 weeks, the goal should be maximal resuscitation of the mother. After 26 weeks, two patients exist: the fetus and the mother. Fluids should be administered; supplemental oxygen and early airway management are mandatory; the patient should be tilted at least 15° to the left side; and the usual advanced cardiac life support (ACLS) drugs and defibrillation should be used. Because cardiopulmonary resuscitation has such a dismal outcome, expeditious transport for possible cesarean section or thoracotomy is indicated.

15. **In a motor vehicle accident, what are the special risks in pregnancy?**
    One major concern is abruptio placentae. Also, common physical exam signs of blunt abdominal trauma are often more difficult to evaluate in the pregnant trauma victim, and the patient must be considered to have significant injury until proven otherwise. Therefore, when the visibly pregnant patient is in a motor vehicle accident, it is necessary to be aggressive with fluid resuscitation, avoid the supine position, and ventilate with high-flow oxygen. The hospital should be advised if the patient appears to be more than 26 weeks pregnant, as a two-patient resuscitation should be instituted in the emergency department.

16. **When do you stop the ambulance with a woman in labor and prepare to deliver?**
    Imminent delivery should be considered if the patient is bearing down, if there is crowning of the head, or if the patient is a multiparous woman who knows that she is about to deliver.

17. **What are the priorities for prehospital delivery of a pregnant woman?**
    The first priority is to control the speed of delivery and thus the trauma to the maternal perineum. This is done by having the patient pant and using your gloved hand to put some gentle counterpressure against the baby's head to maintain flexion and slow delivery. After the head has delivered, you must check around the baby's neck for the umbilical cord and, if present, disengage it or double clamp and cut the cord if you are unable to remove the cord from around the neck. After the head is delivered, suction the infant's airway and wait for the rest of the delivery. External rotation will occur so that the head will realign with the anterior and posterior shoulders. The anterior shoulder should be delivered first with gentle downward traction on the next contraction, and then upward traction is followed rapidly by delivery of the posterior shoulder and the rest of the baby. Do *not* pull on the baby's neck—gentle guidance is all that is required.

18. **Should you wait for the placenta to deliver?**
    The patient can be transported after delivery of the baby and cross-clamping of the cord. Manual traction on the placenta can cause tearing and incomplete separation of the placenta and uncontrolled bleeding. Therefore, it is best to leave delivery of the placenta to occur on its own or by hospital personnel.

19. **Summarize the treatment of critical illness in pregnancy.**
    - Early airway management
    - Aggressive fluid resuscitation
    - Position on left side/backboard 15° to left
    - ACLS—normal protocols
    - Rapid transport after 24 weeks of gestation for consideration of fetal rescue

20. **What prehospital considerations are important in the patient who is a victim of alleged sexual assault?**
    The paramedic is responsible for treating traumatic injuries and for preserving evidence. All clothes worn by the victim during the assault should be brought in with the patient, the police should be notified, and the emergency department should be alerted that a possible sexual assault victim is being transported. The patient needs to be as active a participant in her care as possible, as the trauma has involved powerlessness. Only the history that is necessary to perform a competent medical examination and treatment should be obtained by prehospital personnel. Sensitivity to the victim's emotional state should be demonstrated at all times.

21. **What are some of common causes of gynecologic-related abdominal pain in the nonpregnant female?**
    In addition to the nongynecologic causes of pain, such as appendicitis or gall bladder disease, the gynecologic considerations include such problems as ovarian cysts, ruptured ovarian cysts, torsion of the ovary, and pelvic infections such as acute salpingitis (infected fallopian tube) or tubo-ovarian abscess. A careful, detailed history will often help to narrow down the possibilities.

22. **What should I do to treat the patient who likely has a gynecologic cause for her abdominal pain and is probably not pregnant?**
    The field management is primarily supportive. Intravenous fluids are appropriate for any patient who appears volume depleted. Supplemental oxygen may be administered to patients who are tachycardic, hypotensive, or have signs of shock. Treatment of the patient's discomfort with analgesics is also appropriate.

Pearls and Pitfalls

1. The possibility of pregnancy must always be considered in all women of child-bearing age.
2. Sudden onset of abdominal pain and hypotension, with or without vaginal bleeding, in women of childbearing age is an ectopic pregnancy until proven otherwise.
3. The best care for the fetus is appropriate care of the mother.
4. Any clots or tissue passed vaginally by a pregnant woman should be transported to the hospital with the patient for evaluation.

Clinical Care

References

1. Abbott J. Complications related to pregnancy. In Emergency Medicine: Concepts and Clinical Practice, 4th ed., Rosen P, Barking RM, eds. St. Louis: Mosby, 1997.
2. Abbott JT, Emmans L, Lowenstein SR. Ectopic pregnancy: The common pitfalls in diagnosis. Am J Emerg Med 8:515, 1990.
3. Cunningham FG, MacDonald PC, Gant NF, et al. Williams' Obstetrics, 19th ed. Norwalk, CT: Appleton & Lange, 1993.
4. Goodwin TM, Breen MT. Pregnancy outcome and fetomaternal hemorrhage after noncatastrophic trauma. Am J Obstet Gyneco 162:665, 1990.
5. Lipsky A. Acute Pelvic Pain. in Marx JA, Hockberger RS, Walls RM, et al. (eds). Rosen's Emergency Medicine: Concepts and Clinical Practice. 7th Edition, pp. 193-198, Mosby Elsevier, St Louis, 2010.
6. Pearlman MD, Tintialli JE, Lorenz RP. Blunt trauma during pregnancy. N Engl J Med 323:1609–1613, 1990.
7. Tibbles CD. Selected Gynecologic Disorders. in Marx JA, Hockberger RS, Walls RM, et al. (eds). Rosen's Emergency Medicine: Concepts and Clinical Practice. 7th Edition, pp. 1325-1332, Mosby Elsevier, St Louis, 2010.
8. Houry DE, Salhi BA. Acute Complications of Pregnancy. in Marx JA, Hockberger RS, Walls RM, et al. (eds). Rosen's Emergency Medicine: Concepts and Clinical Practice. 7th Edition, pp. 2279-2297, Mosby Elsevier, St Louis, 2010.

Allergy and Anaphylaxis

Lance W. Jobe, MD, FACEP

CHAPTER 50

1. **What is anaphylaxis, and why does it occur?**
   Anaphylaxis is a serious, rapidly developing systemic reaction resulting from a cascade of immunologic factors that may result in death. It occurs as a result of the immune system recognizing and then reacting to a perceived foreign invader. Technically, anaphylaxis is an IgE (immunoglobulin E)-mediated response resulting in, among other effects, mast cell degranulation. A clinically indistinguishable event that is not IgE mediated is termed anaphylactoid reaction. However, from a clinical standpoint, these are treated the same and can be considered under the single term "anaphylaxis." In fact, the term anaphylactoid may be on its way out in favor of dividing anaphylaxis into immune-mediated (IgE) and non-immune-mediated (anaphylactoid). Until recently, there has been no agreed-upon definition of anaphylaxis. This has hampered diagnostic accuracy, research efforts, and comparisons of studies in the literature. In July 2005 the National Institute of Allergy and Infectious Disease and the Food Allergy and Anaphylaxis Network convened, in part, to work toward a universally accepted definition of anaphylaxis. This symposium proposed that the diagnosis could be made when there is an acute onset of illness with skin involvement (hives, itching, swollen lips-tongue-uvula) accompanied by either respiratory compromise or hypotension (including collapse, syncope, or incontinence). This definition has gained a foothold and is now the standard definition of anaphylaxis. There are some other criteria we will cover later, but these will capture the vast majority of cases.

2. **What are IgE and mast cells?**
   The human body's immune system is a mind-numbing array of cells and proteins designed to defend the castle from "foreign invaders." That's good for our bodies but not so good for trying to understand the mechanism. Immunoglobulins (Ig), also known as antibodies, are protein molecules that can be constructed with a zillion (actually estimated at 1×10^{15}) different combinations to recognize foreign invaders. There are five classes of Ig, of which IgE is one. Mast cells are individual cells located in connective tissue and concentrated, among other places, near mucosal surfaces, blood vessels, and in the skin. These cells contain preformed chemicals ready to be released into the surrounding tissue. When IgE located on the surface of the mast cells recognize and bind an antigen, the cells release their store of chemicals that cause the resulting signs and symptoms.

3. **What is an antigen?**
   Antigen is simply a name given to the bad guy, the foreign invader, that sets off the whole reaction. Antigens are also commonly referred to as allergens. For example, penicillin could be an antigen, as can the venom injected as a result of a bee sting. Some of the most common antigens are food sources, such as eggs, nuts, shellfish, and milk.

Clinical Care

4. **How do these chemical factors affect the body?**
   The most recognized chemical mediator released by mast cells is histamine, although several other mediators are also involved. Histamine causes vasodilatation and increased vascular permeability (think lots of little holes in your water pipes leaking water all over the house) that results in the most common clinical finding of allergic reactions: the cutaneous findings of hives, flushing, and/or itching. These vascular changes may also cause hypotension; in some cases profound and refractory hypotension. Histamine may also result in swelling (edema) of the face and mucous membranes, thereby narrowing or even closing off the upper airway. Histamine also causes smooth muscle spasm that may result in wheezing, abdominal cramping, and/or diarrhea. The bottom line is that airway, breathing, and circulation can all be profoundly and rapidly affected.

5. **What is the difference between an allergic reaction and anaphylaxis?**
   Allergies are immune disorders that encompass a broad spectrum of illnesses. On the one end is anaphylaxis, which we have defined already. Other less life-threatening allergic syndromes include contact dermatitis, atopic dermatitis (eczema), and acute urticaria, or hives. Hives may develop from an allergic reaction: however, without the associated respiratory or cardiovascular compromise, it would not be classified as an anaphylactic reaction.

6. **If I am giving a drug that a patient has never had before, could he or she have an anaphylactic reaction?**
   Yes and no. An IgE-mediated anaphylactic reaction requires that there was a previous exposure to induce "memory" of that particular antigen. So anaphylaxis, as defined previously, would not develop. However, non-immune anaphylactic reactions (anaphylactoid) may occur on first exposure. These reactions cause direct release of histamine without the need for binding with IgE. Systemic reactions to drugs such as NSAIDS (e.g., ibuprophen), opiates, and radiocontrast material are generally non-immune anaphylactic reactions. In addition, reactions to physical factors, such as heat, cold, and exercise fall in this category. These reactions run the continuum from simply hives and pruritis to life-threatening airway and vascular compromise.

7. **Can it be difficult to recognize anaphylaxis?**
   Generally not. Most patients will tell you that they think they are having an allergic reaction, and they are usually right. Furthermore, greater than 90% of patients will have cutaneous findings such as hives, flushing, pruritis, or angioedema. Angioedema, a delayed allergy that is most commonly associated with the drugs known as angiotensin-converting enzyme (ACE) inhibitors, often presents with isolated lip or tongue swelling, which can be so severe as to completely occlude the airway. Other potential airway emergencies, such as foreign body obstruction, epiglottitis, or retropharyngeal abscess, will generally show obvious clues from the history or secondary survey. Scromboid fish poisoning, caused by bacteria on the dark meat of fish such as tuna, mahi-mahi, or mackerel, presents with skin flushing and sometimes hives, which can be confused with an allergic reaction. When this type of fish is improperly handled, bacteria thrive and produce histamine-like toxins that, when ingested, result in flushing and hives. Patients often develop diarrhea, headache, palpitations, and abdominal cramps. Nausea and vomiting may occur as well. These toxins are heat stable and therefore not affected by cooking. The attack rate is very high,

Allergy and Anaphylaxis

and therefore other persons will likely be affected, which is a good clue that the symptoms are caused by scromboidosis rather than an allergic reaction.

8. **What about the patient who is hypotensive but has no rash or skin flushing?**
   There are occasional cases of anaphylaxis with hypotension, but no cutaneous, respiratory, or gastrointestinal findings. The symposium includes these patients in the definition of anaphylaxis if there was an exposure to a *known* allergen. An example might be a child at school with a known peanut allergy, who unknowingly eats a friend's cookie containing peanuts. He suddenly becomes ill and is found to be hypotensive but without the other clinical findings discussed above. In this patient, anaphylaxis must be considered in the differential of possible causes. However, it is important to emphasize that the provider must think of and look for other possible causes for hypotension. A third diagnostic criteria for anaphylaxis proposed by the symposium takes into account the patient exposed to a *likely* allergen with the rapid development of two of the following four criteria: mucocutaneous involvement, respiratory compromise, hypotension, or persistent gastrointestinal symptoms. Thus, the patient who recently ate shellfish and now presents with respiratory compromise or hypotension along with abdominal cramping would meet the criteria for anaphylaxis.

9. **How should I approach the patient with possible anaphylaxis?**
   As always, start with the ABCs and remember to reassess them periodically while you are with the patient, since things can change quickly. Oxygen should be immediately provided. If the patient is talking, he has a patent airway and will be helpful in telling you if he is having more difficulty breathing. Also, listen for stridor, hoarseness, and wheezing, and watch for any inability to handle secretions. A definitive airway may be needed in severe cases. Obtaining an accurate blood pressure and repeating it periodically is critical. If hypotensive, place the patient in the supine position with the legs elevated. This simple, but often forgotten, maneuver increases stroke volume and cardiac output in the patient in shock. The secondary survey should also assess for the presence of cutaneous findings. A brief history and assessment of the skin, in addition to airway, breathing and circulation (ABC), are all that is needed to assess whether a patient meets the criteria for anaphylaxis. If the criteria are met, then immediate administration of epinephrine is indicated. Intravenous access should be established, except in the most minor cases of hives without evidence of airway, breathing or vascular compromise.

10. **What should I do if the airway is compromised?**
    Immediate action is indicated. Besides preparing to intubate the patient, you should administer epinephrine 1:1000, 0.3–0.5 mg intramuscularly (IM) in the anterolateral thigh, which can be a life-saving action. Do not delay giving epinephrine in order to establish an IV or place the patient on a cardiac monitor. If the patient does not have an airway and cannot be ventilated with a bag mask, preparation for a surgical airway should occur simultaneously with the administration of epinephrine, as endotracheal intubation may be impossible. Epinephrine may be repeated every 5–15 min, or more frequently for the patient in extremis. Nebulized epinephrine may be considered in addition to the IM form in patients with primarily respiratory symptoms; however, there is limited evidence supporting the use of aerosolized epinephrine in anaphylaxis. If used, 2–3 mL of 1:1000 epinephrine combined with 3 mL normal saline is a reasonable dose.

Clinical Care

11. **If the patient is wheezing, should I administer albuterol?**
    Yes. In patients with bronchospasm (wheezing), nebulized albuterol may be beneficial. However, epinephrine remains the treatement of choice and should be administered first.

12. **What are the indications for intubation in the field?**
    If the airway is lost in anaphylaxis due to massive tissue edema, intubation can be extremely difficult, and failed attempts may convert a tenuous but usable airway into a completely obstructed airway. For the unresponsive patient in whom mechanical bag–mask ventilation attempts are unsuccessful, intubation, or even a surgical airway, may be necessary. If at all possible, however, patients in distress should be immediately treated and transported in a position of comfort to the closest facility. Communication with the receiving hospital should be clear regarding the potential need for a surgical airway.

13. **We have covered the airway and breathing, but what about circulation?**
    A blood pressure (BP) reading and IV access should be obtained in all patients with anaphylactic reactions. Hypotensive patients will need a bolus of normal saline or lactated ringers. Rapid infusion of a liter of fluid (20 mL/kg) and then reevaluation are the first steps. In elderly patients and those with possible cardiac disease, a 500-mL bolus followed by reassessment of the patient would be a more prudent approach. Any unstable patient should be placed on a cardiac monitor. Again, the primary drug treatment will be epinephrine 1:1000, 0.3–0.5 mg IM, prior to attempting to obtain IV access. Additional IV access and multiple liters of crystalloid may be required in the persistently hypotensive patient. In these rare cases, consider IV epinephrine. The safest mode of administration is to prepare an epinephrine infusion by diluting 1 mL of 1:1,000 epinephrine (1 mg; watch the dilution carefully) in 250 mL of dextrose 5% in water to yield a concentration of 4 µg/mL. This should be infused with a microdrop apparatus (60 drops/min = 1 mL/min = 60 mL/hr) starting with a rate of 1 µg/min (15 drops/min) and titrating slowly upward until an adequate blood pressure has been obtained. Epinephrine could also be given as a slow IV bolus by diluting 1 mL of 1:10,000 epinephrine (0.1 mg) in 10 mL normal saline and administering it slowly over 3–5 min.

14. **Why give epinephrine intramuscularly rather than subcutaneously (SC)?**
    Several studies in nonanaphylactic persons have shown more rapid absorption and higher plasma epinephrine levels when administered in the anterolateral thigh rather than subcutaneously. Furthermore, plasma epinephrine levels were higher and more quickly attained when given IM in the anterolateral thigh than when given IM in the upper arm (deltoid). Therefore, current recommendations are for the administration of epinephrine in the anterolateral thigh. However, it should be noted that no studies have been completed to show improved outcomes with this route of administration.

15. **Should I administer epinephrine to a patient who only has hives?**
    In general, diphenhydramine (Benadryl), 25–50 mg PO or IV, is all that is necessary for this non–life-threatening but uncomfortable condition. However, in the appropriate clinical setting, such as the patient with a history of life-threatening anaphylaxis to bee stings who was just stung by a bee and now has rapidly progressing hives or flushing, administering epinephrine may be appropriate. It should be noted that delayed administration of epinephrine in anaphylaxis has been associated with worse outcomes. Antihistamines, such as diphenhydramine, have little effect on blood pressure and have a

Allergy and Anaphylaxis

longer onset of action than epinephrine. Therefore, they are considered to be second-line therapy in anaphylaxis.

16. **What about pediatric patients?**
 The major difference is the dose of medication. The dose of IM epinephrine is 0.01 mg/kg of the 1:1000 solution (which will be 0.01 mL/kg; maximum dose 0.5 mg IM). Start an epinephrine drip at 0.1 μg/kg/min, increasing in increments of 0.1 μg/kg/min to a maximum of 1.5 μg/kg/min. The dose of diphenhydramine is 1 mg/kg (max 50 mg).

17. **What are the relative contraindications to epinephrine?**
 The key word here is "relative." In the patient with life-threatening anaphylaxis, there is no contraindication to the use of this life-saving treatment. It should however, be used with caution in the elderly, patients with significant hypertension, known coronary disease, or ischemic chest pain. Consider starting with smaller doses in these patients. There is very little evidence of adverse outcomes from IM or SC epinephrine. Most adverse events reported in the literature are related to the IV administration of epinephrine or to the failure to administer epinephrine when indicated.

18. **I've heard that glucagon is sometimes used in anaphylaxis. Why is that?**
 Glucagon can increase the strength of myocardial contractions (inotrope) as well as the heart rate (chronotrope) independent of the alpha and beta receptors in the heart. This can increase the stroke volume, which in turn increases cardiac output and blood pressure. The shock associated with anaphylaxis is largely due to both hypovolemic and distributive shock. However, in some cases there may also be a component of cardiogenic shock, especially in those patients on beta-blockers. Therefore, in refractory hypotension, glucagon 1 to 5 mg may be given IV at a rate of 1 mg/min in an effort to improve cardiac output and blood pressure.

19. **Should every patient with an allergic reaction be transported to a hospital for further evaluation?**
 If any treatment is implemented at the scene, the patient should be transported to the ED for further treatment and observation. The reason for this is twofold. First, the medications given in the field are relatively short acting, and the reaction could recur when the epinephrine wears off. Second, up to 20% of patients who experience an anaphylactic reaction will have a second reaction up to 72 hours later, though most occur within 6–8 hours. This is referred to as the biphasic reaction. Unfortunately, there is no way to reliably predict which patients are likely to have this reaction. Therefore, a period of observation in the emergency department or the hospital is generally recommended. Finally, most patients are additionally treated with corticosteroids. However, because of their slow onset of action, they are not useful in the primary management of anaphylaxis.

Pearls and Pitfalls

1. Even if a patient has never been exposed to a particular food or drug, they may still have an anaphylactic reaction.
2. Intramuscular epinephrine is the treatment of choice for anaphylaxis.
3. Most adverse reactions from epinephrine occur when administering it through the IV route. Watch the concentrations closely.

4. Errors of omission outnumber errors of commission when it comes to epinephrine administration in anaphylaxis.
5. Failed attempts at laryngoscopy will increase tissue swelling and could turn a tenable airway into a completely obstructed airway. Most of the patients can be oxygenated via bag–mask ventilation.
6. Most fatalities associated with anaphylaxis occur in patients with a prior history of reactive airway disease. Be extra vigilant with these patients.
7. Patients should be strongly discouraged from refusing transport even after experiencing marked improvement with treatment.

References

1. Tran TP, Muelleman RL. Allergy, hypersensitivity, and anaphylaxis. In Rosen's Emergency Medicine: Concepts and Clinical Practice, 7th ed., pp. 1511–1529, Marx J, Hockberger R, Walls R, eds., Philadelphia: Mosby, 2010.
2. Sampson HA, Munoz-Furlong A, Campbell RL, et al. Second symposium on the definition and management of anaphylaxis: Summary Report—Second National Institute of Allergy and Infectious Disease/Food Allergy and Anaphylaxis Network Symposium. Ann Emerg Med 47:373, 2006.
3. Lieberman P. Anaphylaxis. Med Clin North Am 90:77, 2006.
4. Lieberman P, Kemp SF, Oppenheimer J. The diagnosis and management of anaphylaxis: An update practice paramater. J Allergy Clin Immunol 115:Suppl 2:S483, 2005.
5. Anchor J, Settipane RA. Appropriate use of epinephrine in anaphylaxis. Am J Emerg Med 22:488, 2004.
6. Markovchick VJ, Markovchick NS. Anaphylaxis. In Emergency Medicine Secrets, 5th ed., Markovchick VJ, Pons PT, Bakes KM, eds., pp. 120–124. St. Louis: Elsevier, 2011.
7. Brown S: The pathophysiology of shock in anaphylaxis. Immunology and Allergy Clinics of North America 27: 309, 2007.
8. Tole J, Lieberman P: Biphasic Anaphylaxis: Review of Incidence, Clinical Predictors, and Observation Recommendations. Immunology and Allergy Clinics of North America 27: 165, 2007.

Diabetic Emergencies

Jeffrey J. Messerole, PS

1. **What is diabetes?**

   The word "diabetes" came from Greece in 200 AD and means to siphon or pass through. Diabetes described the constant urination of patients who had the disease. Centuries later, the Latin word "mellitus" was added and meant honey or sweet, as medical practitioners noticed the urine of diabetics contained sugar (although we will not ask how they figured that out). Little was known of the disease until two nineteenth-century discoveries shed a great deal of light on diabetes mellitus (DM). In 1869, while examining pancreatic tissue under a microscope, German medical student Paul Langerhans noticed groups of tiny cells like islands in the midst of a sea. He did not know it at the time, but these islets of Langerhans, as they are called today, contain the beta cells that produce insulin. In 1889, while exploring how the body metabolizes fat, European scientists Joseph von Mering and Oskar Minkowski found that when they removed the pancreas from a dog, the animal started to urinate uncontrollably. They tested the urine and found that it contained glucose. Recognizing that the dog had developed DM, the scientists concluded that the key to the illness resided in the pancreas and had something to do with beta cells, and what they produced. The discovery and isolation of insulin at the University of Toronto in 1921–1922 was one of the greatest events in the history of medicine. For the first time, medical practitioners knew that diabetes was caused by lack of insulin production leading to excess levels of glucose in the bloodstream and now had insulin therapy that would commute the death sentence associated with the diagnosis of insulin-dependent DM.

2. **How common is diabetes?**

   DM has been and still is the most common endocrine disorder and, unlike other diseases, is on an alarming rise, particularly in children. An estimated 20.8 million people in the United States—7% of the population—have diabetes, a serious, lifelong condition. Of those, 14.6 million have already been diagnosed, and 6.2 million have yet to be diagnosed. In 2005, about 1.5 million people ages 20 years or older were diagnosed with diabetes. The EMS system is called on frequently by patients, their families, or bystanders when a diabetic emergency occurs. It is important for prehospital providers to know the types of diabetic emergencies, what treatment options can be used, and to be aware of not only the problems directly associated with DM but also complications related to the disease.

3. **What is a normal glucose level and what are the effects of abnormal levels?**

   Normal glucose metabolism keeps blood sugars within the range of 70–110 mg/dL. Because diabetes is associated with abnormalities in glucose metabolism, blood glucose levels may be abnormally high or low, which affects many organs, and if left untreated will lead to multiple complications. Over time, having too much glucose in your blood can damage your eyes, kidneys, and nerves. Having too low a blood glucose level can lead to brain damage and death. Diabetes also increases the risk of heart disease, stroke, blindness, and peripheral vascular disease leading to limb amputation.

4. What is insulin, and what does it do?

Insulin is a hormone produced in the pancreas by the beta cells of the islets of Langerhans and is released into the blood stream in response to elevations in blood glucose levels. Insulin assists in glucose metabolism and uptake by the cells, allows excess glucose to be stored in the liver and muscle, and is used in fat synthesis. Lack of a sufficient amount of insulin or no insulin leads to an excess of glucose in the bloodstream as there is no insulin to facilitate glucose transport into the cells. Other cells in the body make different hormones that are also important in glucose metabolism. One of these is glucagon. When glucose is not getting into cells, because of either lack of food intake or lack of insulin production, the body perceives a fasting state and releases glucagon to attempt to increase the level of blood glucose. Glucagon causes the breakdown of stored sugars in the liver and then of stored body fat, which results in the production of ketones as a breakdown product. Ketones are acidic and lead to a lower blood pH (acidosis). It is this process of ketone and acid formation (ketoacidosis) that may lead to one of the serious complications seen in the diabetic. In the absence of glucagon, another counterregulatory hormone is released—epinephrine. Epinephrine assists in mobilizing glucose but usually not until the blood glucose levels are less than 50 mg/dL. The release of epinephrine is the cause of several of the signs and symptoms of low blood glucose level (hypoglycemia).

5. How does DM affect blood glucose levels?

DM is caused by inadequate amounts of insulin. Because insulin is required for glucose to be transported into cells, inadequate amounts or a lack of insulin lead to elevated blood glucose levels (hyperglycemia). Because the cells think they do not have enough glucose, compensatory mechanisms result in the release of glucagon, which converts stored glycogen into glucose. Glucagon further breaks down protein and fat to release glucose and ketones into the blood stream, but without insulin to transport the glucose into the cell, blood glucose levels rise.

6. What types of DM are there?

DM can be separated into two disease presentations. Type I, also referred to as insulin-dependent DM (IDDM) or juvenile-onset DM, usually develops prior to early adulthood but can occur at any age, so the term "juvenile onset" is not used unless it does develop early in life. Patients with Type I IDDM produce almost no insulin and consequently may develop markedly high glucose levels (hyperglycemia). Patients with IDDM are dependent on insulin therapy for survival and account for about 10% of the diabetic population.

Type II, also known as non–insulin-dependent DM (NIDDM), results from a combination of insulin resistance with relative insulin deficiency. NIDDMs are able to produce insulin but do so in decreased amounts, and what is produced is often not used properly by the body. Most Americans who are diagnosed with diabetes have Type II diabetes. Type II NIDDM is occurring at an alarming rate in children. A disease once seen in patients in their forties and older is now seen in patients in their twenties, with 45% of all-new Type II diabetes being seen in adolescents. Type II NIDDM accounts for 90% of the diabetic population. Patients with Type II NIDDM require diet control, oral medication, or, in some cases, additional insulin to control blood sugar levels. Ketoacidosis rarely occurs in patients with Type II diabetes because some insulin is produced. The differences between the two types of diabetes are listed in Table 51.1.

Gestational diabetes affects about 4% of all pregnant women, resulting in about 135,000 cases in the United States each year. The placenta supports the baby as it grows and hormones from the placenta help the baby develop. However, these hormones also block the action of the mother's insulin in her body.

TABLE 51.1: Types of DM

	Type I DM	**Type II DM**
Name	Insulin-dependent DM	Non–insulin-dependent DM
Pathology	No insulin production	Decrease production
Required treatment	Insulin	Diet control, oral agents, insulin
Ketoacidosis	Strong tendency	Rare tendency

This problem is called insulin resistance. Insulin resistance makes it hard for the mother's body to use insulin. She may need up to three times as much insulin. Gestational diabetes starts when the mother is not able to make and use all the insulin she needs for pregnancy. Many women who have gestational diabetes go on to develop Type II diabetes years later. There seems to be a link between the tendency to have gestational diabetes and Type II diabetes.

7. **Why do diabetic patients access the 911 system?**
Because of either too little or too much sugar (glucose) in the blood. Abnormally low blood sugar, referred to as hypoglycemia, may result when a patient with Type I diabetes takes their insulin but does not eat, eats later than intended, or eats the wrong type of food for the amount of insulin they have given themselves.
Patients with Type II diabetes who are not on insulin but who take oral hypoglycemic agents (Table 51.2) are also at risk for hypoglycemia up to 36 hours after taking these medications. Unrecognized hypoglycemia can lead to death. The cells of the body, especially the brain, are dependent on glucose to function. Permanent brain damage may occur in patients who survive hypoglycemic events because the cells of the brain do not have the ability to store or use other sources of energy as does the rest of the body. Hypoglycemia is a true medical emergency requiring immediate recognition and treatment to prevent permanent brain damage.
Abnormally high blood glucose levels, referred to as hyperglycemia, may result in a patient with undiagnosed diabetes, or when a patient with known diabetes does not take their hypoglycemic agent, or adhere to their diabetic diet. Insufficient amounts of insulin cause a lack of glucose transported into the cells, raising the blood sugar; in turn the liver releases stored glucose into the blood, causing further hyperglycemia. Once these stores have been depleted, body fats containing fatty acids are broken down to form more glucose. As blood glucose levels rise, the increasing osmotic pressure pulls water from the cells, dehydrating them and altering their ability to function. Once blood sugar reaches 185 mg/dL, the kidney's ability to retain glucose becomes overwhelmed, and glucose is lost into the urine. Glucose in the urine causes the kidneys to draw water and electrolytes out of the blood and into the urine as well. This causes increased urination secondary to the large amount of glucose in the urine, resulting in volume loss and dehydration. Volume loss in adult patients ranges from 4–10 L. In addition to the hyperglycemia, the resulting by-products of fatty acid breakdown are acidic ketones, which cause the blood pH to become acidic. Diabetic ketoacidosis (DKA) is the term given for this hyperglycemia with electrolyte imbalance and metabolic acidosis, and it is a dangerous complication of DM. The patient develops metabolic acidosis and also significant dehydration. The overall mortality is 5–15% per episode. It generally occurs in patients

TABLE 51.2 Hypoglycemic Oral Medications

Drug Class	Brand Name	Generic
Sulfonylureas	DiaBeta	Glyburide
	Micronase	Glyburide
	Glynase	Glyburide (micronized)
	Glucotrol	Glipizide
	Glucotrol XL	Glipizide
	Amaryl	Glimepiride
Meglitinides	Prandin	Repaglinide
	Starlix	Nateglinide
Biguanides	Glucophage	Metformin
	Glucophage XR	Metformin
Thiazolidinedione	Actos	Pioglitazone
	Avandia	Rosiglitazone
Alpha-glucosidase inhibitor	Precose	Acarbose
	Glyset	Miglitol
Combination	Glucovance	Glyburide/metformin

who are insulin dependent but has been reported to be the first manifestation of undiagnosed DM in 20% of all cases of DKA. In 70–80% of insulin-dependent diabetics with DKA, infection and medication noncompliance were common precipitating factors.

8. Does an elevated blood glucose level always lead to DKA?
No. Elevated blood glucose levels (hyperglycemia) can occur in some patients without the development of DKA. With Type II diabetes, following a meal the blood sugar rises and there is just enough insulin to allow for partial cell nourishment. The excess glucose not used remains in the blood, causing the blood glucose levels to rise. Normal acid–base status is maintained as the cells do receive some glucose so the need for fat metabolism is absent. Dehydration from excess blood glucose levels is the issue. This condition known as nonketotic hyperosmolar coma (NKHC), is more common in persons older than 60 years of age, and is characterized by central nervous system dysfunction associated with severe hyperglycemia and dehydration. Mortality may be as high as 50%. The predominant presentation is abnormal mental status, which may vary from lethargy to coma, and is caused by the dehydration and electrolyte imbalance. These symptoms resolve by treating the hyperosmolar state with insulin and aggressive fluid therapy.

9. What factors may cause problems in controlling DM?
Many diabetic patients administer insulin to themselves in the morning with a long-acting insulin to carry them through the day and then multiple injections throughout the day to cover what they have just eaten. Others use an insulin pump with a set basal rate and can increase the insulin amount or inject with a different type of insulin depending on diet and activity. (See Figure 51.1.) If food intake is

Diabetic Emergencies

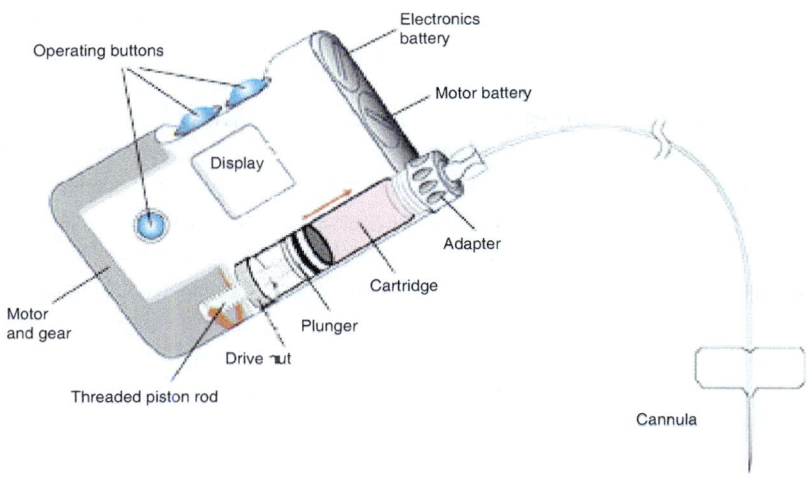

FIGURE 51.1 Insulin pump.

delayed, if diabetics miscalculate the dose or type of insulin, or if they exercise more than planned and use more glucose, then hypoglycemia ensues. The blood glucose level may also fall precipitously during exercise because metabolic requirements increase.

Common precipitating factors in the development of hyperglycemic states include infection, or an illness, medication noncompliance, or a malfunctioning insulin pump. Infection and illness cause a rise in blood sugar as the stress it puts on the body releases epinephrine and cortisol to help boost energy and fight the infection. The liver releases sugar stores and the blood glucose levels rise. Over a longer term, the patient who is ill may skip eating, reach for a quick fix (foods high in carbohydrates or simple sugars like chips, or candy), overeat, or may not feel like taking their medication. Improper diet, not taking their insulin, an insulin pump that malfunctions or is unknowingly disconnected, and the catecholamine release all lead to hyperglycemia.

10. **What is the goal of patient assessment?**
In assessing a diabetic patient who enters the EMS system, the prehospital provider is generally trying to differentiate hypoglycemia from hyperglycemia and the need for aggressive fluid therapy. These conditions, which must be recognized promptly and treated appropriately, are frequently identified by a focused history, physical exam, and rapid blood glucose determination. Because hypoglycemia may cause brain damage or death, and it is easily reversible, recognition of hypoglycemia is the primary goal of patient assessment, and management may precede completing your focused history and physical exam. A simple blood test will determine the presence of hypoglycemia and should be performed on all patients suspected or known to have diabetes as well as those with altered mental states.

11. **Can physical signs be helpful in distinguishing between hypoglycemia and hyperglycemia?**
Upon arrival at the scene, after ensuring scene safety and proper body substance isolation, look for environmental clues that the patient has diabetes. Are there insulin syringes or insulin vials visible?

Clinical Care

Is there a glucagon kit, or glucose paste or diabetic sugar tablets? Are there diabetic testing supplies such as a glucometer, lancets, or testing strips? Is there a prosthetic device indicating the loss of a limb? Is the patient wearing an insulin pump or have a MedicAlert tag indicating they have diabetes?

Typically, patients with hypoglycemia demonstrate pale, cool, clammy skin, with varying levels of diaphoresis. Hypoglycemic patients are usually well hydrated and will have normal skin turgor as well as moist skin and mucous membranes. Their heart rate is usually fast with a bounding pulse because of sympathetic nervous system activation and the release of epinephrine. Hypothermia can be a common presentation from evaporative heat loss and lack of glucose to produce heat. The respiratory rate is usually slowed or normal. Mental status changes occur rapidly, within minutes. Initially, patients may exhibit bizarre behavior, irritability, or combativeness prior to unresponsiveness. Seizures may occur secondary to hypoglycemia and usually resolve with administration of glucose and the correction of blood glucose levels to near normal levels. This presentation may easily be confused with that of an alcohol-intoxicated patient, and to assume the patient who smells or acts intoxicated has no other problem may lead to the hypoglycemia going undiagnosed and permanent brain damage or death may occur. A more prudent strategy is to assume the opposite—that hypoglycemia is present when alcohol is involved.

Typically patients with hyperglycemia present with signs of dehydration as they may experience 4–10 L of volume loss. Examine the skin for signs of dehydration to include dry, warm skin that tents when pinched, indicating poor turgor. Important facial features may include sunken eyes, a furrowed tongue, and dry mucous membranes. The patient may have gastrointestinal complaints such as nausea, vomiting, and abdominal cramping and pain. The heart rate is tachycardic from dehydration, and blood pressure may be decreased as well. A fruity odor on the patient's breath indicates the presence of ketones, suggesting the presence of DKA. A slight increase in respiratory rate is seen early with DKA as the patient attempts to blow off CO_2 in order to correct for the metabolic acids of fat metabolism. Kussmaul's respirations (deep, rapid, and intense respirations) may develop in more severe cases of DKA. Mental status changes are gradual in onset, usually occurring over several days and progress from restlessness and lethargy (an apathetic appearance) to unresponsiveness and are caused by dehydration, electrolyte imbalance, and acidosis. With hyperglycemia the brain cells get all the sugar they need. Instead, their dysfunction is related to the dehydration, electrolyte imbalance, and metabolic acidosis. The patient exhibits the "polys"—polydipsia (excessive thirst), polyuria (frequent urination), and polyphagia (desire to eat frequently), which are common presenting symptoms of new-onset or worsening diabetes and are also characteristics of the hyperosmolar state and dehydration seen with hyperglycemia.

The patient must have hyperglycemia, electrolyte imbalance, and metabolic acidosis to be in DKA. Although the blood glucose level can be measured in the field, electrolytes and pH cannot; therefore, we must rely on our ability to recognize the clinical signs and symptoms of DKA. Table 51.3 outlines the differences between hypoglycemia, hyperglycemia, and HHNC.

12. What management strategies are appropriate for diabetic patients?

Any patient with respiratory distress requires an assessment of the airway and administration of high-flow oxygen by mask. Pulse oximetry, skin color, and signs of respiratory distress need to be evaluated to determine if the tachypnea is respiratory in nature or related to metabolic acidosis associated with

TABLE 51.3: Signs and Symptoms of Diabetic Emergencies

Hypoglycemia	Hyperglycemia—DKA	HHNC*
Comes on within minutes	Comes on gradually over 3 days	Comes on gradually over 12 days
Type I IDDM	Type I IDDM	Type II NIDDM
Took insulin, did not eat	Did not take insulin	Not taking oral medications
Eating late or not the right food	Binge eating	Diet high in sugar and carbohydrates
Excessive exertion	Tired, illness	Tired, illness
Pale, cool, clammy	Dry, warm, tenting skin	Dry, warm, tenting skin
Tachycardia	Tachycardia	Tachycardia
Bounding pulse	Weak pulse	Weak pulse
Elevated blood pressure	Lower blood pressure	Lower blood pressure
Blood glucose <60	Blood glucose >180	Blood glucose > 600
Bizarre behavior, seizures, altered mental status from lethargy to coma	Altered mental status from lethargy to coma	Altered mental status, seizures, hemiplegia
	"Polys"—polyuria, polydipsia, polyphagia	"Polys"—polyuria, polydipsia, polyphagia
	Kussmaul's respirations	Ketosis does not occur, no Kussmaul's respirations
	Fruity odor on breath	No fruity odor on breath
	Nausea, vomiting, abdominal cramping	Nausea, vomiting, abdominal cramping

*Hyperosmolar hyperglycemic nonketotic coma.

DKA. Deep rapid breathing should not be written off as a patient who is just hyperventilating and the patient given a mask or brown paper bag to rebreathe their CO_2. Cardiac monitoring in any patient with a rapid pulse or altered mental state is appropriate. The need for a 12-lead electrocardiogram may also be necessary, as diabetics may have silent acute coronary syndromes. A diabetic having an acute coronary syndrome (ACS) may present with weakness or flulike symptoms and no crushing chest pain with radiation. Failure to recognize the difference in how a diabetic may present when having an ACS may lead to mistreatment and the potential for the syndrome to worsen. If available, the patient's temperature may be measured to check for hypothermia or elevated values suggesting an infectious process or illness. A rapid blood sugar determination is appropriate for all patients suspected or known to have diabetes and all patients with altered mental status, preferably prior to glucose administration. Any adult who is not awake and aware and any patient with a blood glucose reading of 70 or less should receive 50 mL (one amp) of 50% dextrose (D_{50}) intravenously through a free-flowing large-bore IV

Clinical Care

catheter. Extravasation of D_{50} will cause tissue necrosis, so ensuring that the IV is free flowing is important. Children should receive 2–4 mL/kg of 25% dextrose (D_{25}). This is achieved by mixing an equal amount of sterile water or normal saline (NS) with the D_{50}, thus diluting it to D_{25}. Awake patients with glucose levels of less than 70 may be given juice or other oral forms of glucose by mouth, so long as they are capable of drinking the liquid themselves without assistance. If an IV cannot be established, then the patient should receive 1 mg of glucagon intramuscularly. The glucagon will liberate any sugar stores left in the liver increasing the blood sugar. It may take up to 15 min for the peak onset of action of glucagon to occur. Hypotensive patients and other patients with signs of dehydration or hypoperfusion should be given IV fluids such as NS or lactated Ringer's solution to replenish the fluid volume. Children should be given 20 mL/kg of NS as an initial fluid bolus. This can be repeated twice if vital signs do not respond. Adults should be given fluid boluses of 500 mL of NS, which can be repeated to a total volume of 2 L. Fluid replacement is the mainstay of therapy for DKA and NKHC and should be administered aggressively to replace the huge amount of fluid volume already lost. The adminstration of insulin, correcting the electrolyte imbalance, and metabolic acidosis is a complex issue and accomplished after transport to the hospital.

13. **What if I cannot determine the blood sugar level in the field?**
    For unresponsive patients with an unknown blood glucose level, IV glucose should be administered. If the patient is hypoglycemic you will prevent possible brain damage or death. If the patient is hyperglycemic a single dose of 50% dextrose has not been shown to have a deleterious clinical effect. The only concern has been the administration of glucose to a patient who is having a stroke. Glucose can exacerbate the amount of damage ultimately produced. Therefore, if hypoglycemia is a real concern in a patient with a potential stroke, glucose determination is preferred prior to administration of sugar. If transport time is short and glucose measurement is not available in the prehospital setting, glucose infusion can be delayed until arrival at the hospital. Otherwise, glucose should be administered. Please refer to your protocols and medical director for input.

14. **Are there specific considerations for alcoholic or emaciated patients?**
    Yes. If there is a possibility that the patient is alcoholic or emaciated, D_{50} administration should be preceded by 50–100 mg of thiamine given intravenously if your protocol allows. Thiamine is used as a cofactor in the metabolism of glucose, and the alcoholic or emaciated patient generally has depleted most of their stored thiamine. Although controversy exists about this, some evidence suggests that Wernicke's encephalopathy may be precipitated by a large load of glucose, which then rapidly depletes the small amount of stored thiamine.

Pearls and Pitfalls

1. Hypoglycemia is a true medical emergency that can result in permanent brain damage if not recognized and corrected.
2. Hypoglycemia is easily identified in the field with a bedside glucometer.
3. A blood glucose level should always be checked in any patient who presents with altered mentation, even if the presumed cause is apparent.
4. Volume loss in cases of DKA or HHNC can lead to significant dehydration (4–10 L).

5. Diabetic patients having an acute myocardial infarction may present with atypical symptoms such as weakness or the "flu" and not complain of chest pain.
6. Extravasation of D_{50} may cause tissue necrosis, so be certain you have a patent IV line.

References

1. Dalton A, Limmer D, Mistovich J, Werman H. Advanced Medical Life Support, 3rd Edition, Chest Discomfort Or Pain 6:207–217; 2007, Pearson Prentice Hall, Upper Saddle River, New Jersey
2. Schneider SM. Disorders of glucose metabolism. In Essentials of Emergency Medicine, Aghababian R, ed., pp. 199–205, 2006. Sudbury, MA: Jones & Bartlett.
3. Bledsoe B, Porter R, Cherry R. Cardiology. In Essentials of Paramedic Care, 2nd ed., pp. 1211–1224, Upper Saddle River, NJ: Brady Pearson Prentice Hall, 2011.
4. Mistivich J, Karren K. Altered Mental Status and Diabetic Emergencies. In Prehospital Emergency Care, 8th ed., pp. 469–482., Upper Saddle River, NJ: Pearson Prentice Hall, 2008.
5. Pollack A. Endocrine emergencies. In Nancy Caroline's Emergency Care in the Streets, 6th ed., Caroline NL, ed., pp. 29.9–29.14. Sudbury, MA: Jones & Bartlett, 2008.

Web sites accessed May 2011:

http://www.answers.com/topic/diabetes-mellitus
http://www.nlm.nih.gov/medlineplus/diabetes.html
http://www.diabetes.org
http://www.cdc.gov/diabetes/statistics/index.htm#prevalence
http://www.ndep.nih.gov/
http://www.diabetes.niddk.nih.gov/dm/pubs/statistics/#7

Psychiatric and Behavioral Emergencies

CHAPTER 52

Eugene E. Kercher, MD, LFACEP, LFAPA, and Christopher B. Dong, MD

1. **What is a behavioral emergency?**
   It is a situation in which the patient presents with behaviors that are unusual, disordered, or socially inappropriate. Typically the onset of the behavior is relatively quick.

2. **What are the categories of behavioral emergencies?**
   The main categorization is based on the underlying cause of the behavioral emergency—organic versus functional. In patients with an organic cause, abnormal behavior is the result of a well-defined physiologic illness or toxin such as hypoglycemia, hypoxia, infection, metabolic disorder, endocrine disease, alcohol, or drugs. In patients with a functional cause, there is no definable physiologic cause for their behavior and it is thought to result from abnormal intrinsic brain function, true psychiatric illness, or a transient psychotic disorder brought on by an acute stress or crisis.

3. **Is it important to distinguish between these two broad categories in the prehospital setting?**
   It is extremely important to have an understanding of this concept because the treatment will ultimately be very different. It would be considered poor form to bring an out-of-control, delusional patient to the emergency department only to find out later that the patient had a blood glucose of 30 (and all that time was rapidly losing brain cells) or was hypoxic, both of which could have been easily treated in the field. Therefore, even if a distinction cannot be made in the field, gathering the data that may help make that distinction is very important.

4. **Why don't we just give them all dextrose and oxygen and let the physicians figure it out?**
   Simply because the information available from or obtained in the field may be the only solid clue to a diagnosis.

5. **What are examples of organic causes of behavioral disorders?**
   Meningitis, head trauma, hypoglycemia, hypothermia, hypoxia, hyponatremia, thyroid disease, liver failure, and dysrhythmias. The most common cause of disturbed behavior is alcohol or other drugs.

6. **What clues would help to differentiate organic causes from functional (psychiatric) causes?**
   Obviously, obtaining the history of the current illness as well as the past medical history will often provide initial clues. Encourage family members to come to the emergency department. If no family is available, try to obtain a phone number of a person who knows the patient.
   - Patients with organic disease often have:
     - altered level of consciousness
     - lethargy

- visual hallucinations
- abnormal vital signs (including pulse oximetry)
- changes in behavior that are acute occuring over hours to a couple of days
- evidence of drugs, alcohol, and medications on scene
- Patients with a functional disorder typically:
  - do not have an alteration of consciousness
  - are usually oriented and have no problems with recent memory
  - have a disordered thought process
  - manifest auditory hallucinations

Diagnosing a patient with a functional disorder who has no previous psychiatric history should be done carefully.

7. Is there a memory tool that can help me remember the factors that can be useful in differentiating organic from functional causes?

Yes, the mnemonic MADFOCS.

	Organic	**Functional**
Memory deficits	Recent impairment	Remote impairment
Activity	Psychomotor retardation	Repetitive activity
	Tremor	Posturing
	Ataxia	Rocking
Distortions	Visual hallucinations	Auditory hallucination
Feelings	Emotional lability	Flat affect
Orientation	Disoriented	Oriented
Cognition	Islands of lucidity	Continuous scattered thoughts
	Perceives occasionally	Unfiltered perceptions
	Attends occasionally	Unable to attend
	Focuses	
Some other findings	Age >40	Age <40
	Sudden onset	Gradual onset
	Physical examination often abnormal	Physical examination normal
	Vital signs may be abnormal	Vital signs usually normal
	Social immodesty	Social modesty
	Aphasia	Intelligible speech
	Consciousness impaired	Awake and alert

Modified from Frame DS, Kercher EE, Acute psychosis: Functional vs. organic. Emerg Med Clin North Am 9:123, 1991.

8. **What should I do if an organic cause is suspected?**
   Checking blood glucose level and pulse oximetry are two simple tests. If results are abnormally low, you should intervene immediately to correct the deficiency.

9. **Why do some patients with behavioral emergencies act so bizarrely?**
   Bizarre behavior and speech are manifestations of psychosis and are the result of a loss of touch with reality. Typical psychotic symptoms are categorized as delusions, hallucinations, and behavioral changes.
   - **Delusions** are erroneous beliefs that usually involve a misinterpretation of perceptions or experiences. These false beliefs have no foundation in fact or reality. Common delusions include:
     - persecution (people are out to get them, the government is monitoring them)
     - reference (people/media are talking about them)
     - control (the patient's thoughts or feelings are being controlled or inserted by others)
     - grandiosity (the patient has special powers, is famous, or is important)
   - **Hallucinations** are false perceptions of sensory stimuli that do not exist.
     - Auditory hallucinations, hearing voices, are the most common and are typically seen in patients with functional disorders.
     - Visual hallucinations are the next most common hallucination. They are more likely to be seen in patients with organic disease but are not rare in patients with functional disease.
     - Tactile, taste, and olfactory hallucinations are uncommon and suggest organic causes.
   - **Behavioral changes** are actions and responses that do not seem to be appropriate for the environment. They can be the result of patients responding to their hallucinations or acting in relation to their delusions or disordered thought process.

10. **Psychosis is typically associated with mental illness, schizophrenia in particular. Should I assume any patient with psychosis is schizophrenic until proven otherwise?**
    No. Psychosis can be seen in patients with mood disorders, such as depression, as well as in schizophrenia. One also needs to consider the possibility of an organic cause for the psychotic behavior. Many metabolic and toxicological disorders can have symptoms that mimic functional psychotic disorders. Two of the most common organic causes for psychotic like behavior are drug intoxication and drug withdrawal syndromes.

11. **How should I approach patients with behavioral emergencies?**
    Clearly identify yourself and explain your purpose. Speak in as calm a voice as possible. Establish rapport with the patient through active listening. Demonstrate that you are interested in him or her and their current situation. Although it is important to validate the patient's feelings, one should be careful to avoid validating delusions or irrational thoughts as this may make the psychosis worse. Try to be a calm and supportive force by attempting to reduce stress and avoid confrontation.

12. **Should I expect patients with behavioral emergencies to be violent or dangerous?**
    Most psychotic patients are not violent or imminently dangerous. However, they do have an increased potential for violent behavior because of a difficulty in impulse control and tendency to act on internal stimuli. Therefore, one should always be alert to the potential for danger and be prepared to respond.

Psychiatric and Behavioral Emergencies

13. **Because these patients may be violent or easily prone to violent behavior, how should they be approached?**
    - Clearly identify yourself and explain your purpose, speaking in as calm a voice as possible and avoiding threatening statements.
    - Respect the patient's personal space.
    - If the patient backs away, do not immediately try to approach them again; they are telling you to back off.
    - Do not touch the patient without asking for their permission first.
    - Approach with an open posture and try to ensure that your position and posture do not make the patient feel threatened or cornered.
    - Do not block their exit pathway, but be sure that you also have an exit.
    - Avoid crossed arms.
    - Do not have your hands behind your back or speak to others in a whispered voice. Patients may interpret these actions as you are trying to hide something or planning to do something to them.
    - As you approach the patient continuously assess the scene for the potential of violence.
    - Trust your gut instinct.

14. **Are there any clues as to which patients may become violent?**
    First, if you don't think of violence as a possibility, you will not be able to diffuse it before it starts. In general, if alcohol or drugs are involved, there is a greater potential for violence because of a loss of impulse control. Obviously, situations in which violence has already occurred are inherently dangerous. In assessing the potential for violence one should consider four areas: past history, posture, vocal activity, and physical activity.
    - A **past history** of hostile, aggressive, or violent behavior means there is a greater likelihood that the patient may become violent again.
    - **Posture**-related warning signs include sitting on the edge of a chair, standing, rigid musculature, clenched fists, and appearing visibly tense.
    - **Concerning vocal signs** include loud threatening speech, obscenities, and erratic speech.
    - **Physical activity** warning signals are pacing, psychomotor agitation, avoiding eye contact, startling easily, and being protective of physical boundaries.

15. **What should I do to maintain personal and scene safety?**
    - First and foremost, always be attentive and alert to the potential for violence.
    - Trust your gut instinct. If you feel you are in danger, act appropriately.
    - Remain a safe distance from the patient when direct patient contact is not required for physical assessment or treatment. Keep at least an arm and leg's length away from the patient to prevent you from easily getting punched or kicked by the patient or from invading the patient's personal space.
    - Always keep an unobstructed escape pathway between you and the exit. Do not allow the patient to get between you and the exit while being mindful not to make the patient feel trapped by blocking the patient's exit pathway yourself.

Clinical Care

- Assess the scene for objects that could be used as weapons. If present, then calmly work to deny the patient easy access to those objects.
- Avoid threatening statements and body language and confrontation.
- Follow the patient's lead. If he or she is backing away, then the patient is feeling threatened so give them their space. If the patient is becoming more agitated then give them more space and assess the scene for what may be agitating them.
- Try to reduce the amount and intensity of stimuli affecting the patient by excluding persons from the scene who may be agitating the patient or by removing the patient from a hostile environment. Friends or family may be used to help defuse the situation if they appear to be a calming force.
- If the patient is approaching you and you do not feel safe, move away from the patient until you are at a safe distance.
- Do not allow a single EMT or paramedic to be alone with the patient.

16. **Can I physically restrain a patient?**
When a patient is a danger to himself or to others, physical restraints may be necessary. It should be considered as a last option when verbal commands for the patient to cooperate and control himself or herself are not successful and there is a reasonable risk of violence. Obviously, this is not a black-and-white situation and judicious use of restraints is needed. If restraints are necessary, wait for assistance. (A minimum of five people is desirable, one for each extremity and one for the head.) Ideally, patients should be restrained by or with the assistance of law enforcement. When applying physical restraints, use the least amount of force necessary. If it is considered safe to do so before placing the patient in physical restraints, offer the patient a chance to cooperate with the applying of the restraints. After a show of force some patients will allow the restraints to be applied without resistance. If force is required to physically restrain a patient, apply the restraints as humanely as possible.

17. **After the patient has been placed in physical restraints, what else do I need to do?**
A physically restrained patient needs frequent monitoring of their respiratory, circulatory, and musculoskeletal status. One needs to make sure the patient's respiratory and circulatory systems are not being compromised by the physical restraints or the patient's positioning. One needs to be sure the restraints are not causing physical injury to or neurovascular compromise of the patient's extremities. If restraints need to be repositioned or loosened, it should be done one limb at a time with an adequate number of people present to safely control the patient. These patient reassessments and corrective actions, if any, should be documented in your report as well as the behaviors that necessitated the physical restraints. All patients should be restrained in the supine position, as restraining a patient in the prone position has been associated with sudden death.

18. **When are chemical restraints indicated?**
If patients are still violently thrashing despite physical restraints, they may still be in a position to hurt themselves or others. In addition, further medical evaluation and care may be impossible. In these situations, chemical restraints are needed.

19. **What drugs are used for chemical restraint?**
The drugs most often used are neuroleptics (i.e., droperidol or haloperidol) and benzodiazepines (i.e., lorazepam and midazolam). Neuroleptics and benzodiazepines have been effectively used alone or in

combination for rapid tranquilization of agitated or violent patients. The use of a neuroleptic and a benzodiazepine together has been shown to provide more effective sedation than either alone and is common practice in EDs. These medications can be administered intramuscularly (IM) or intravenously (IV). In the agitated/violent patient establishing an IV may be a risky proposition so the most likely route of medication administration will be intramuscular. Typical IM doses are droperidol 2.5 mg, haloperidol 5–10 mg, lorazepam 2 mg, and midazolam 5 mg. The onset of action for these medications is 10–20 minutes. The drug and dose that you use to chemically restrain patients will depend on your local treatment protocols.

20. What are the potential adverse effects of benzodiazepines and neuroleptics?
Benzodiazepines can cause excessive sedation or respiratory depression. Neuroleptics can cause hypotension, dystonia, akathisia, and the rare neuroleptic malignant syndrome. Dystonia is the involuntary continuous contraction of muscles of the face, neck, or back. Dystonic reactions can be treated with 25–50 mg of diphenhydramine. Akathisia is motor restlessness characterized by a physical need to be constantly moving. Patients do not want to be constantly moving but feel the need to do so. Although it is not a first-line treatment for akathisia, 25–50 mg of diphenhydramine can be used. Administration of neuroleptics is contraindicated in patients with a prolonged Q-T interval on their electrocardiogram.

21. What do I need to know about depression?
Prehospital personnel are often dispatched to situations in which depression is the underlying reason for the call. Diagnostic criteria are explicitly laid out by the American Psychiatric Association. They categorize the symptoms into areas of mood, psychomotor activity, cognition, and vegetative signs. These include feelings of hopelessness, loss of interest in pleasurable activities, reduced or slowed motor activity, decreased concentration and productivity, sleep and appetite disturbance, as well as recurrent thoughts of death. These symptoms need to be persistent and last for more than 2 weeks before a patient is diagnosed with major depression.

22. How can patients with depression present?
Displays of depression may be as overt as the person standing on a bridge threatening to jump or as subtle as the elderly individual, living alone, who calls because he or she is "not feeling well." Patients can also demonstrate psychotic symptoms. If delusional, they may state that they are already dead or their body is rotting. If hallucinating, they typically will describe hearing voices that are making negative statements about the patient or telling them to harm themselves. Suicide, of course, is the main life threat that must be addressed and is the eighth leading cause of death in the United States. If there is any concern about depression, the patient should be asked about thoughts of suicide and if they have made any attempts to harm themselves.

23. If I question a person about suicide, isn't there a risk that I'll be giving them the idea?
No. There is no evidence that asking about suicidal ideation causes people to attempt suicide. People who are depressed will be thinking about suicide, to some degree, long before you question them. Patients who are depressed and have thought about suicide often are willing to talk about it when asked but may be hesitant to bring it up on their own. Therefore, if you do not ask, they might not tell you and an opportunity to help them and possibly save their life will be missed.

24. What else should I know about potentially suicidal patients?
Suicidal thoughts or ideation are categorized as passive or active. Passive suicidal ideation means the patient has thought of suicide, but has not thought about how he or she would actually do it. Active suicidal ideation means the patient not only has suicidal thoughts but has also decided on a plan on how to commit suicide. A patient with active suicidal ideation is a much greater threat to himself or herself than one with passive suicidal ideation. It is important to recognize the signs and symptoms by which a patient at risk for suicide may present. In addition to overt acts or statements, be suspicious of nonverbalized suicidal ideation such as poorly explained or implausible accidents or injuries or statements by the patient that could be interpreted as demonstrating a lack of concern about his or her safety or well-being. If you have any concern or suspicion that the patient could have suicidal thoughts, ask the patient directly about it. Most people who have committed suicide provided some type of warning about their intent prior to their attempt.

25. What is the difference between a suicide attempt and a suicidal gesture?
In a suicide attempt patients cause harm to themselves with the realistic expectation that they will die. In a suicidal gesture, patients cause harm to themselves but do not expect that they will die from it. However, do not be fooled into thinking that because the patient made a suicidal gesture that they are not in danger of serious illness, injury, or death. Although their intent may not have been to put their life at significant risk, unbeknownst to them, what they did to make the gesture may in fact be potentially deadly.

26. Is there a way to identify patients at high risk for suicide?
Yes, the modified SAD PERSONS scale. Although this scale is useful for assessing suicide risk factors and trying to quantify risk for suicide, it should not be used in the pre-hospital arena to determine if a patient should be transported to a hospital or not. All patients actively voicing suicidal thoughts or in whom there are concerns about the patient being a danger to themselves need to be transported to the hospital. When used, a SAD PERSONS score of 6 or greater would put the patient at higher risk.

Factor	Points Assigned
Sex (male)	1
Age (<19 or >45)	1
Depression or hopelessness	2
Previous attempts or psychiatric care	1
Excessive alcohol or drug use	1
Rational thinking loss	2
Separated, divorced, or widowed	1
Organized or serious attempt	2
No social supports	1
Stated future intent	2

From Hockberger RS, Rothstein RJ, J Emerg Med 6:99, 1988.

27. What is bipolar disorder?

Bipolar disorder, or manic-depression, is a mood disorder, just as depression is a mood disorder. People afflicted with bipolar disorder will have episodes of severe depression; however, the depressive episodes are separated by periods of mania, or elevated mood. The mood cycles between mania, normal, and depression may occur over hours but typically take days, months, or up to two years. Signs and symptoms of mania include agitation, restlessness, constant movement, uncontrolled thinking, racing thoughts, rapid or pressured speech, and emotional outbursts. In more severe episodes of mania individuals can demonstrate psychotic symptoms. In the manic phase, people tend to lose self-control and impulse control and have a hyperinflated self-esteem or delusions of grandeur. They may be out in the street directing traffic or out spending money irrationally (e.g., they may spend all they own, including house and car, in a matter of days).

28. What do I need to know about schizophrenia?

Schizophrenia is a disorder of thought processes. This alteration in thought process can be seen as a loss of linear or rational thought processing that can affect their perception of self and their relationship to the real world.

- Thought content can be abnormal with delusions, ideas, or beliefs that have no factual basis and in general are obviously false. Common delusions include
  - persecution
  - possession of special abilities (can fly, can read minds, bodies are indestructible)
  - being on "special missions" for the government
  - hyperreligiosity
- Perception of sights and sounds can be altered; manifested as hallucinations, typically auditory, but can be visual, tactile, or olfactory.
- Impairment of perception and thought processing makes it difficult for individuals to differentiate between real-world stimuli and the internal stimuli (voices in their head or visual hallucinations) so they respond to their hallucinations as if they were real. This is one of the reasons for the characteristic apparently bizarre behaviors seen in people with schizophrenia.
- Disordered thought processing results in impaired judgement and puts their personal safety and those around them at risk because individuals may act on their delusions or hallucinations and harm those they perceive as a threat.
- Individuals are at high risk for suicide or accidentally injuring themselves due to their distorted perception of reality.
- Having schizophrenia does not eliminate the possibility of an organic cause for individuals' behavioral emergency.

Although people with schizophrenia typically demonstrate psychotic symptoms when they decompensate, a patient with psychosis is not necessarily a schizophrenic. That patient may have a mood disorder with psychotic features, a severe stress reaction, or an organic cause.

29. How should I manage patients with hyperventilation syndrome?

Although patients with hyperventilation syndrome may feel like they cannot breathe, are lightheaded, and are going to die, in reality this will not happen and it rarely causes any harm to the patient. In severe cases patients can develop circumoral and carpopedal paresthesias and spasms; however, these symptoms are reversible once the patients stop hyperventilating. The main treatment is reassuring the patient that they are breathing adequately and are not going to die and to have them slow down their breathing. Having a patient breathe into a paper bag has been described in the lay and some medical literature as a treatment for hyperventilation syndrome. It was believed that by rebreathing their exhaled air and carbon dioxide the patients would correct the low carbon-dioxide levels in their blood brought on by the hyperventilation and reverse the symptoms. However, studies have shown that breathing into a paper bag does not significantly raise carbon dioxide levels in the blood and can cause significant hypoxia, which could harm the patient. Having a patient breathe into a paper bag therefore cannot be recommended as a therapy for hyperventilation syndrome.

30. I have heard about mental health holds (MHHs). Who would qualify for an MHH?
Although there is some variation from state to state (and you should know what the law says in your state), an MHH can be placed on patients who are a risk to themselves (suicidal), a risk to others (homicidal), or gravely disabled (unable to provide food, shelter, and clothing for themselves) as a result of psychiatric illness. The MHH allows the patient to be held against their will for a specified amount of time (usually a maximum of 72 hours) in order to evaluate him or her psychiatrically. It is important to understand that MHHs are intended to be used for patients with functional psychiatric illness and not for patients with grave disability due to organic disease.

31. Who can place a patient on an MHH?
This also varies from state to state but generally includes health care workers and police officers who are certified to do so. Interestingly, in most, although not all, states, EMTs and paramedics are usually not included, even though they often contact patients who need to be placed on holds. Thus, they are required to involve the police in placing a hold in the field.

32. What about patients who refuse care?
Allowing patients with behavioral emergencies to refuse care and sign against medical advice is a high-risk proposition. Before that can even be considered, one needs to make a five-point assessment of the patient to determine if refusal of care is even a possible option.

- Patients must have decision-making capacity to refuse medical care by demonstrating that they have a clear understanding of the situation, what you want to do to care for them, the risks the patient may engender by refusing, have a rational line of reasoning for refusing, and comprehend the consequences of their decision.
- An organic etiology for their behavior has been reasonably ruled out.
- The patient is neither currently showing nor has shown in the past suicidal or aggressive behavior.
- The patient is known to have a psychiatric history with similar behavior and has not required evaluation, stabilization, or hospitalization.
- The patient has appropriate social support available and is willing to accept and use that support.

If a patient does not meet all those screening points to your satisfaction, he or she should not be allowed to refuse care. The policy and procedure under which the patient will be transported against their will depends on state mental health law and your local EMS system.

Psychiatric and Behavioral Emergencies

Pearls and Pitfalls

1. Keep at least an arm and a leg's length distance from your patient.
2. Keep an unobstructed pathway between you and the exit.
3. When patients require physical restraints, make a show of force, and offer them one last opportunity to cooperate and voluntarily allow the restraints to be applied.
4. Restrained patients need frequent monitoring of their respiratory and circulatory systems.
5. Never restrain a patient in the prone position.
6. The symptoms of psychosis and behavioral emergencies may be from an organic cause. Be sure to look for and correct reversible causes.
7. A patient with psychosis does not mean he or she has schizophrenia. Psychosis can be seen in mood disorders and with organic illness.
8. Patients with known psychiatric illness can also have organic causes for their abnormal behavior.
9. MADFOCS is a mnemonic that can be used to help differentiate between organic and functional causes of behavioral emergencies.
10. The SAD PERSONS scale is a useful tool to assess suicide risk.
11. Talking to a patient about suicidal thoughts does not increase their risk of suicide. In fact, it is often a relief to be asked and relate their thoughts.
12. Hyperventilating patients should not be made to breathe into a paper bag, as this can cause hypoxia.
13. Patients who you believe may be a danger to themselves or others, or are unable to care for themselves, should not be allowed to refuse care and transportation to a hospital.
14. MHHs are intended to be used for patients with functional, not organic, disorders.

References

1. Amin M. Acute psychosis. In Emergency Medicine Secrets, 5th ed., Markovchick VJ, Pons PT, Bakes KM, eds., pp. 557–663. St. Louis: Elsevier, 2011.
2. Rund DA, Saveanu RV. Depression and Suicide. Emergency Medicine Secrets, 5th ed., pp. 663–670. St. Louis: Elsevier, 2011.
3. American Psychiatric Association. Diagnostic and Statistical Manual of Mental Disorders, 4th ed. Washington, DC: American Psychiatric Press, 1994.
4. Frame DS Kercher EE. Acute psychosis: Functional vs. organic. Emerg Med Clin North Am 9:123, 1991.
5. Petit JR. Delusions. Handbook of Emergency Psychiatry, pp. 77–80. Philadelphia: Lippincott Williams & Wilkins, 2004.
6. Petit JR. Perceptual Disturbances. Handbook of Emergency Psychiatry, pp. 170–173. Philadelphia: Lippincott Williams & Wilkins, 2004.
7. Hockberger RS, Richards JR. Thought disorders. Rosen's Emergency Medicine, 7th ed., pp. 1430–1436. Philadelphia: Mosby, 2010.
8. Kuehl AE. Behavioral. Prehospital Systems and Medical Oversight, 3rd ed., pp. 762–773. Dubuque, IA: Kendall Hunt, 2002.

9. Battaglia J, Moss S, Rush J, et al. Haloperidol, lorazepam, or both for psychotic agitation? A multicenter, prospective, double-blind, emergency department study. Am J Emerg Med 15(4):335–340, 1997.
10. Nobay F, Simon BC, Levitt MA, Dresden GM. A prospective, double blind, randomized trial of midazolam versus haloperidol versus lorazepam in the chemical restraint of violent and severely agitated patients. Acad Emerg Med 2004; 11(7):744–749.
11. Hockberger RS, Rothstein RJ. Assessment of suicide potential by non-psychiatrists using the SAD PERSONS score. J Emerg Med; 6(2):99, 1988.
12. Callaham M. Hypoxic hazards of traditional paper bag rebreathing in hyperventilation patients. Ann Emerg Med 18(6):622–628, 1989.

Management of the Violent Patient

CHAPTER 53

James A. Temple, BA, NREMT-P, CCP

1. **What factors increase the chances of experiencing a violent patient encounter?**
   Violence can erupt almost anywhere and at any time. On occasion, there will be absolutely no warning signs and you will find yourself in the middle of an ugly situation. More likely, however, there are signs and warnings that you should notice to help take evasive action. This chapter discusses some of the factors that lead to violence.

2. **What are some common situations that can lead to violence?**
   - Patient's medical processes: diagnosed medical conditions that cause altered mental status and poor decision making may include hypoglycemia, hypoxia (which can have many causes, including our restraint method), seizures, cardiovascular accidents or head trauma, and acute psychosis.
   - Drug ingestion: cocaine, methamphetamine, alcohol, hallucinogenics, and opiates among others. The illicit drug scene is in constant flux, with new variations on old drugs, combinations of drugs, and new designer drugs. Unless you keep up with the literature and keep your ear to the streets, you may not be aware of the latest drug or drug combinations that are around. When considering chemical restraint, it is important to know what the patient has ingested in order to choose the most appropriate chemical restraint medication.
   - Personal issues: many patients who end up resorting to violence simply have lost the ability to cope, so they do what comes easiest: act out physically. Although it is easy to blame patients for their violent behavior, do not forget about your attitudes, speech, and nonverbal communication. The way you stand, hold your hands, make eye contact or not, and tone of voice just may be the last straw. If your patient picks up on these and thinks you do not really want to be there or care about their crisis, violence may be in your future. Communication is only 7% what you say; 38% is how you say it, and 55% is nonverbal. A list of some nonverbal clues can be found in Table 53.1.

TABLE 53.1: Nonverbal Communication

Nonverbal Clue	Perceived Meaning
Glancing sideways	Suspicion
Rubbing the neck	Frustration
Hands in pocket	Insecurity
Clenched fist	Defensiveness/impending aggression
Open hands	Openness
Smiling	Confidence
Upper body leaning forward	Cooperation
Stroking the chin	Evaluation
Rolling the eyes	Apathy, nonbelief

Clinical Care

3. What is the best way to approach the violent patient?

Obviously, if you know prior to patient contact that there is a scene safety issue, stay away. Allow law enforcement to secure the scene and let you know when it is safe to enter. In some systems, some personnel have dual function (police/EMS). Unless you are trained and equipped for handling scene safety issues, let the other professionals take care of it.

Once the scene is safe, approach the patient slowly and with open eyes, ears, and mind. Respect their personal space and keep about two arms-lengths away whenever possible. Speak slowly and calmly, trying not to make any sudden movements. If the patient is verbally abusive, use calm words and voice, acknowledge their concerns, answer their questions, and assure them that you are really there to help. Do not take the insults personally, although it may be difficult. If you become angry, you lose your ability to think clearly and make good decisions, which may lead to rash and inappropriate patient care.

Don't forget about the nonverbal signs you are using. Make sure you are near to and have a clear exit path. Constantly scan the scene for hazards, such as weapons or other persons coming to check out the action. A large gathering can happen quickly, so be sure to be aware of the situation as it changes.

If the situation deteriorates and you need to retreat, a code word or phrase may be used to alert all to the danger you see. One method is to call your partner by the wrong name. If you have worked together with any regularity, all should recognize what is meant and react accordingly. Another method is to ask a partner to go out and get the "green" bag, knowing full well you carry no such bag. Again, this requires communication prior to the incident but can be invaluable when faced with an erupting situation.

4. What are some signs of impending violence?

Violence can erupt at any time, so if you can predict or "sense" when it is coming your way, the healthier you will remain. You will notice that of the signs listed, more than a few can be associated with the "flight or fight" response. If you can learn to recognize the physiological indicators of impending violence, you will stay that ever-important step ahead. Signs of impending violence may include:

- Anger
- Agitation
- Chanting
- Clenched fists
- Profanity
- Flushed face
- Flared nostrils
- Darting eye movements
- Dilated pupils
- Pointing
- Pacing
- Loud outbursts

Make sure you and your crew avoid the above behaviors. These actions on your part will send the message to your patient that perhaps you are considering violence toward them and thus, they will plan a preemptive strike.

5. When should I use restraints?

Restraints should be used in situations where there is risk of injury to you, your crew, or the patient. If the patient's behavior is such that injury may occur to anyone involved, the use of restraints may be warranted. Just keep in mind local protocols regarding physical restraint. Medical control may have to be advised and actually give the order. Be familiar with your local procedure. You may wish to use restraints in any of the following situations:

- protect patients from harming themselves
- protect crew, staff, and bystanders
- allow assessment and appropriate treatment (uncooperative patients)
- protect disoriented patients from external dangers (falls, etc.)

Management of the Violent Patient

If possible, all patients who are candidates for restraint should have blood glucose and oxygen saturation checked prior to restraint.

6. What are the dangers of using restraints?
The most serious risk of restraining patients is sudden death. Research currently identifies six factors that contribute to poor outcomes from restraint:
- excited delirium
- drug overdose
- comorbid medical conditions
- recent extreme exertion
- fighting against restraints
- inappropriate restraints

7. What is excited delirium?
Excited delirium is a severe disturbance in the level of consciousness over a short period of time, manifested by mental and physiological arousal, agitation, hostility, and heightened sympathetic stimulation. It has been shown that patients who are already worked up and who now fight against restraint increase their risk for cardiac dysrhythmias, respiratory distress, and myocardial infarctions. The massive release of catecholamines over an extended period of time coupled with substance abuse and any preexisting medical conditions can lead to death while the patient is in restraint. A common presentation of excited delirium is that of a sweaty, naked person acting strangely.

8. What are inappropriate restraints?
There are many ways to effectively restrain someone; however we need do it safely. The days of sandwiching folks between long boards are over, as are the days of hog-tying people. Although effective, hog-tying or any restraint method that places people prone should never be used. Another common method is to hobble or somehow bind the feet and legs together limiting extremity movement. Again, a person who cannot get off of their abdomen may end up with respiratory compromise. Once a person is prone, respiratory effort may become impaired, especially in patients with a large pendulous abdomen. These patients are or have recently been fighting and have an increased oxygen demand; now they are in a position that can compromise their oxygen supply chain. This is called positional asphyxia and is a well-known cause of sudden death and therefore cause for legal action against emergency responders.

9. How can I use physical restraint and not endanger myself or the patient?
You can think of the restraint process in three steps: verbal, physical, and chemical. Each situation requires careful consideration as to what is the best method for the patient. The goal is to use the restraint method that is least restrictive while still allowing you to provide the care needed by the patient.

10. Starting with verbal deescalation, what does it involve?
First, speak to the patient slowly, calmly, and respectfully. Do not allow their anger, behavior, or provocations to make you angry. Tell the patient that because they are threatening responders with violence they are going to be placed in restraints. Letting them know what behaviors are not acceptable (setting limits) gives them choices and may be the key to avoiding a physical confrontation.

11. What is the next step if talking to the patient does not work?

If verbal de-escalation does not effectively control the patient, physical restraint is next. Simply put, there is strength in numbers. Use all of your available resources. Usually five persons can manage physical restraint. Although there are cases of "superhuman" strength, usually drug induced, where eight or nine persons are not enough to adequately restrain someone, these instances are rare. When faced with the need to use physical restraint, remember the following: use only the minimum amount of force necessary to control the patient.

Care should be taken when grasping clothing, given the possibility for weapons or drug paraphernalia such as needles in pockets. As always, gloves should be worn by all persons engaged in physical restraint. Direct at least one responder to control each of the four extremities and one to control the head. They should cover and control large joints. For example, holding a foot is much less effective than controlling the knee. Some patients may want to spit, so wear appropriate eye protection and maybe even a face shield. The old trick of placing an oxygen mask on the patient to prevent spitting is functional—just be sure to turn the oxygen on.

There are commercial devices available for "soft" restraint, or you can use the old standby, roller gauze, to restrain each extremity. For those who use hard restraints (handcuffs per police) or four-point leathers, always be sure to have a key available to quickly remove or adjust them should there be a sudden change in the patient's condition. Your local protocol may require the police to actually ride in the ambulance with you whenever handcuffs are used. This is especially true if patients are cuffed to the cot. Again, safety is the first priority and placing the patient prone is not an option.

12. What should I do if the patient is still out of control?

If you cannot control the patient physically, or you are concerned for their safety while they are in the physical restraint, chemical restraint is the next option. Many drugs can be used for this purpose and are commonly found in your drug box. When you proceed to chemical restraint, the risks increase as should your attention level to the patient's condition. You need to be on the lookout for possible drug interactions and not just with prescription drugs. Table 53.2 lists some common drugs used for chemical restraint. The two families of drugs most popularly used for restraint are butyrophenones (haloperidol, droperidol) and benzodiazepines (lorazepam, diazepam, and midazolam). All of these drugs can be given IV or IM,

TABLE 53.2 : Commonly Used Drugs for Chemical Restraint

Drug	Initial Dose	Onset	Peak Effect	Duration
Haldol™ (haloperidol)*	2–5 mg IM	10–30 min	30–45 min	12–38 hr
Inapsine™ (droperidol)	2.5–5 mg IV/IM	3–10 min	30 min	2–4 hr
Valium™ (diazepam)	2–5 mg IV/IM	<2 min	3–4 min	15–60 min
Ativan™ (lorazepam)*	1–3 mg IV/IM	1–5 min IV 15–30 min IM	15–20 min IV 30–60 min IM	6–24 hr
Versed™ (Midazolam)	1–3 mg IV/IM	1–5 min IV 15–20 min IM	5–30 min IV 15-30 min IM	2–6 hr

*Haldol 5 mg and Ativan 2 mg = are commonly used in combination for sedation and control.
IV = intravenously, IM = intramuscularly.

which is a definite bonus, given that the violent patient rarely will hold still long enough to allow IV access. Recently, EMS providers have started administering Midazolam, or other approved medications, via the IN or intranasal route. The medication is atomized in the nose and absorbed by the mucosa. This delivery method has been shown effective in managing violent patients, as well as decreasing risks to the provider, such as needle-sticks. Current and promising research is also looking at the efficacy of currently very expensive alternatives such as Geodon™ (ziprasidone), Risperdal™ (rispiridone), and Zyprexa™ (olanzapine) in the acute chemical restraint situation. Given the needs of EMS providers, new combinations and ideas will certainly evolve, so again, keep current on trends and literature.

13. **What are the potential dangers of chemical restraint?**
The most serious dangers of chemical restraint reside in cardiovascular and respiratory side effects. The administration of benzodiazepines may result in hypoventilation or even respiratory arrest. In addition, this class of drugs may induce moderate to severe hypotension, and paradoxically may cause agitation rather than the described sedation. Haloperidol and droperidol present special challenges in regard to side effects. Extrapyramidal symptoms may consist of dystonic reactions, motor restlessness, and Parkinsonian signs. Treatment for these symptoms is Benadryl™ (diphenhydramine) 25–50 mg IV/IM/PO (by mouth) or Cogentin™ (benztropine) 1–2 mg IM/PO. Pregnant patients should not receive Haldol™ or Inapsine™, as it has been shown to have potential detrimental effects on the fetus as it crosses the placenta. Of significant concern, however, are the cardiovascular side effects of the butyrophenones, particularly droperidol (Inapsine™). Although these dysrhythmias are rare, patients may experience premature ventricular contractions, ventricular dysrhythmias such as torsades de pointes, or bradycardia. Each patient who has been chemically restrained needs to have a cardiac monitor applied. If there is a prolongation of the Q-T interval, haloperidol and droperidol are contraindicated.

14. **How do I manage the patient who has been controlled with a taser?**
Law enforcement is continually developing new nonlethal means of controlling violent and uncooperative subjects. A taser is a gun that shoots two metal "prongs" and then delivers an electric charge intended to incapacitate the target briefly and allow control. The taser is a high-voltage low-wattage device. The voltage may be around 50,000 V; the amperage is minimal but still able to briefly incapacitate. The two prongs may penetrate up to 2 in. of material, making actual skin contact unnecessary. These prongs have fish-hook-like barbs on them, making them difficult to remove, even for responders. The best method has been to pull the skin taut around the prong and pull up to remove. This process can be somewhat painful, so beware of the potential patient reaction in the event that the prong cannot be easily removed or is in a conspicuous anatomical position, transport to an emergency department is warranted.

Although painful and effective to temporarily incapacitate, most treatable injuries from tasers involve the fall that occurs once the patient has been shocked. Remember to treat appropriately and use spinal precautions as indicated which, as a bonus, is another form of restraint.

The electric current from the taser is generally not enough to cause ventricular fibrillation. However, there have been several cases of sudden death following the use of the taser, perhaps secondary to delivery of the electric shock during the relative refractory period. During encounters with violent or potentially violent patients, it is imperative that the responder remember no two encounters will be the same. Things can change quickly and progress to violence in a heartbeat.

Clinical Care

Pearls and Pitfalls

1. Never place a restrained person in the prone position. Place them supine or in a lateral position.
2. Never leave a restrained person unattended.
3. Any patient who you would consider to be a behavioral risk should be "patted down" prior to being placed in your ambulance. The patient compartment is a difficult place to manage a patient who has a knife or other weapon.
4. Be careful when giving haloperidol or droperidol to a patient with a history of seizures or exposure to cocaine, amphetamine, or tricyclic antidepressants, as it may further lower the seizure threshold.
5. In the patient with acute cocaine ingestion who needs to be restrained, benzodiazepines are the drugs of choice.
6. Carefully watch for respiratory depression, respiratory arrest, and hypotension in any patient given a benzodiazepine for chemical restraint.

References

1. Brasic JR. *eMedicine*, Clinical safety in neurology. March 2007.
2. Wigder HN. *eMedicine*, Restraints. March 2007.
3. Stratton SJ, Rogers C, Brockett K, Gruzinski G. factors associated with sudden death of individuals requiring restraint for excited delirium. *Am J Emerg Med*, 19:187–191, 2001.
4. National Association of EMS Physicians (NAEMSP). Patient restraint for EMS systems. *Prehosp Emerg Care*; 6(3):340–345, 2002.
5. Yildiz A, Sachs GS, Turgay A. Pharmacological management of agitation in emergency settings. *Emerg Med J*; 20:339–346, 2003.
6. Whitehead S. After shock: A rational response to taser strikes. *JEMS* 30(5):56–66, 2005.
7. Savage, SS. After the zap: Taser injuries and how to treat them. *CorrectCare* summer 2005. http://www.ncchc.org/pubs/CC/tasers.html
8. Ikelheimer D. Management of the violent patient. In Emergency Medicine Secrets, 5th ed., Markovchick VJ, Pons PT, Bakes KM, eds. pp. 670–677. St. Louis: Mosby, 2011.

General Trauma Principles

Larry Mottley, MD

CHAPTER 54

1. **What is a traumatic injury?**
   Trauma may occur when an external energy source is applied to the body. The energy sources may be mechanical, thermal, or radioactive. The vast majority of traumatic injuries result from the transfer of mechanical energy. In everyday discussion, the meanings of the terms "trauma" and "mechanical injury" are identical. Thermal and radioactive injuries are discussed elsewhere.

2. **What is mechanical injury?**
   Mechanical injury, or "trauma," results when an object strikes the human body or vice versa. Energy transfer from this collision results in deformation of some or all of the body. (It may also result in deformation of the object, as in a windshield shattered by the head of an occupant.) If the energy imparted to the body is sufficient, damage to tissue will occur.

3. **What are the common types of traumatic tissue injuries?**
   Trauma to the tissue ranges from contusions (bruises), which are the result of capillary blood vessel breakage, to actual disruption of the surface and deeper layers of the soft tissue (lacerations). Skeletal tissue (bone and teeth) will fracture if sufficient force is applied. Hollow organs (e.g., gastrointestinal tract, bladder, heart) may rupture, and solid organs (e.g., liver, spleen) may fracture if sufficient force is applied to them.

4. **How is the mechanism of trauma classified?**
   Trauma is commonly divided into blunt and penetrating trauma.

5. **What is penetrating trauma?**
   Penetrating trauma is caused by external objects penetrating the exterior surface of the body and causing damage to deeper structures. In the case of bullets or other projectiles, the offending object may remain within the body. Penetrating trauma is comparatively easy to treat—you begin by finding the hole(s) and then follow the object's pathway to determine which organs may have been injured.

6. **What are the most common sites of overlooked entry wounds?**
   Both stab and gunshot wounds can be overlooked on even a moderately detailed physical exam, especially if small-caliber bullets or narrow instruments (such as an ice pick) were used. The axilla, groin, scrotum, buttocks, oropharynx, and scalp are the most common sites of missed entry wounds. There is no substitute for palpating the scalp with gloved hands to find such wounds. The back and buttocks must be examined on every patient suspected or known to have sustained a penetrating injury; the optimal time for examination of the back is when logrolling the patient onto the backboard.

7. **How can I be sure a small wound is not an entry wound?**
   You cannot always be confident that an external exam alone can identify penetrating wounds with certainty, and the patient may be unwilling to tell you or not know. One good rule is that if gun shots

Clinical Care

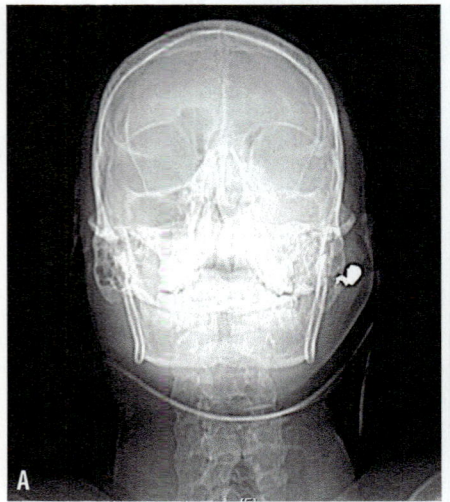 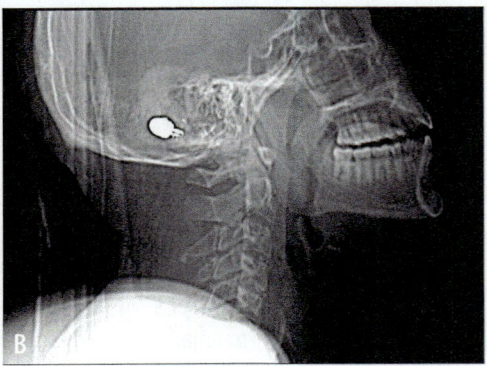

FIGURE 54.1 Front (a) and side (b) view X-rays of the skull showing a bullet. This patient walked into the emergency department with a nosebleed and a bloody ear after an altercation in which he stated he had been struck with a bat. EMS personnel reported that other victims at that same incident had been shot.

have been fired at the scene, all wounds must be X-rayed to rule out a foreign body (see Figure 54.1). Avoid making any conclusion regarding "entrance" or "exit" wounds. It is often difficult to accurately differentiate these wounds and if you label a wound you will likely find yourself called to testify about how you made that determination. It is best to just note that a wound consistent with a gunshot is present and let others determine which one was an entry wound and which one was an exit.

8. **What is blunt trauma?**
    Blunt trauma occurs when only energy is transferred to the body, and there is no penetration of the deeper tissues, although surface lacerations are not uncommon. Blunt trauma is the more challenging entity to treat: with no holes to guide you, your training, the physical exam, the mechanism of injury, your experience, and guidebooks are your guides to successful treatment.

9. **How does treatment of the trauma patient differ from that of the medical patient?**
    The trauma patient is often a patient who requires an operation to repair a life-threatening injury; therefore, a few precepts are essential. First, time is of the essence, and the time that counts is the time it takes to get to the operating room. Although it is fair to say that no one wants a surgeon, it is nevertheless true that some patients need a surgeon. For those critical patients, the role of EMS is to minimize the time spent in the field. Such patients should have a primary survey performed (correcting any abnormal findings therein), be immobilized on a long backboard, and placed into the ambulance, and be expeditiously transported to the nearest *appropriate* receiving ED. All other evaluations and treatments (if any) should take place en route.

10. **What is an appropriate ED for trauma patients?**
    There is no simple answer to this question, but there are guidelines. In a system with designated trauma centers, defined trauma patients should be brought to the nearest level 1 or level 2 trauma center, as

determined by local EMS protocols. The total prehospital time from injury to trauma center arrival should be less than 60 min and ideally, much shorter than that. In systems without designated trauma centers, the patient is generally taken to the nearest hospital. Because time to the operating room is the important measure, however, it may be appropriate for either online or offline medical control to direct such patients to specific hospitals based on operating room availability, such as a level 3 trauma hospital. Such decisions should be made based on predefined criteria.

11. **What do I do if a trauma patient demands to go to a nontrauma center?**
    This is a very difficult question and often puts the prehospital provider in a difficult situation. The following position has been taken by the New York State Department of Health:

    > As always, the Department's first concern is to ensure the best care for each patient while protecting the right of the patient to choose the provider of that care or, indeed, to choose not to accept care at all.
    > It is essential that such a decision by a patient be an informed decision. Informed consent is a guiding ethical and legal principle of medical care that the Department vigorously supports.
    >
    > It is axiomatic that a patient cannot make an informed judgment unless he or she fully understands the risks and benefits of the course of treatment suggested by the provider. In the major trauma patient, this is often not possible. Several factors interfere with the normal process of informed consent. First, the patient's injuries may result in an alteration of the patient's mental status. Such an alteration may result either directly from an injury to the head or indirectly due to injury to other areas of the body resulting, for example, in shock or extreme pain. Obviously, a patient with an altered mental status is unable to make an informed judgment, nor is the prehospital provider trained to determine the patient's capacity to do so.
    >
    > Second, the time constraints required to effectively treat trauma patients are extreme. Effective trauma care is measured in minutes. The nationally recognized principle of the "golden hour" of trauma care requires that optimum patient care can be achieved if the patient reaches definitive trauma center care as expeditiously as possible. The time required to list and to explain the risks and benefits of the various transport alternatives in a meaningful manner would prevent the patient from receiving this optimal care.
    >
    > Third, and perhaps most important, informed consent requires that the patient be informed of the suggested and alternative courses of action, and the risks and benefits of each. Yet, in the prehospital setting, the provider is a certified emergency medical technician, not a licensed physician. The scope of training of an EMT does not include knowledge of the complications, alternatives, or even the likely outcome of a particular course of action, much less the range and likelihood of reasonably known complications. Thus, because the information needed to make an informed judgment in the prehospital setting is unavailable, an informed judgment—by definition—cannot be made.
    >
    > In the absence of informed consent, the provider should follow the course of action of a reasonable and prudent EMT. Such course of action is clearly laid out in the State Emergency Medical Service Basic Life Support protocols. All EMTs are required to follow these protocols.
    >
    > Finally, it is important to remember that the decision made by the EMT is the hospital destination. Once at the appropriate hospital, the patient will be cared for by a licensed physician, who can accurately determine the capacity of the patient to make an informed judgment and provide the information necessary for that informed judgment to be made.
    >
    > For the reasons just outlined, it is the position of the Department that trauma patients, as defined in the State Emergency Medical Service Basic Life Support protocols, be transported in accordance with those protocols, even if the patient objects.

This nicely summarizes the issues faced by the EMT. Each EMS system should have a policy in place describing how this situation should be handled by the EMT.

12. **Can trauma center patients be accurately identified in the field?**
    Usually, but not always. Although EMS providers can accurately identify patients whose abnormal vital signs identify them as trauma center candidates, some trauma patients have vital signs that are initially normal. Traditionally, the mechanism of injury has been used as an indirect indicator of severe trauma. Recent data have cast doubt on at least some of these mechanism-of-injury criteria in blunt trauma.

13. **Suppose my patient's blood pressure was low the first time it was taken and is now normal?**
    There is very good evidence that even a single occurrence of hypotension in the field is associated with a quadrupling of mortality compared to patients who had never been hypotensive. Such patients should be transported to a trauma center.

14. **What other factors enter into the trauma triage equation?**
    Patients at higher risk of complications or patients who are more difficult to assess should be brought to a trauma center. Trauma recommendations now recognize that the patient's age, chronic illnesses, and EMT judgment are factors to consider in borderline cases Examples include the elderly and the very young and patients with comorbid factors such as diabetes or pregnancy.

15. **If EMT judgment is as good as any other method of identification, why do we have written trauma triage guidelines?**
    If paramedic discretion is the basis for trauma triage, every mistriage can be questioned and the individual paramedic held to account. Written trauma triage guidelines allow you to use agreed-upon criteria as a strong basis for your hospital destination decision.

16. **How long is too long to remain on the scene?**
    In a situation that does not involve entrapment or other difficult extrications, 10 min or less is the ideal time frame. We often may not know scene arrival time to the minute; however, a useful operational parameter points out that by the time you ask yourself, "How long have I been on scene?" you have been on scene too long.

17. **What interventions should be performed on scene?**
    The airway should be assessed and opened if not patent while maintaining cervical spine precautions. High-flow oxygen should be administered. An oral or nasopharyngeal airway, supraglottic airway, or endotracheal tube should be placed if the airway is unstable and there are no contraindications. Breathing should be assessed and assisted if less than 10 breaths per minute. Circulation should be assessed by palpating the pulse at the carotid and radial pulses. Cardiopulmonary resuscitation should be started if the patient is apneic and pulseless. Finally, the patient should be placed on a backboard (or other spinal immobilization device), loaded into the ambulance, and started en route to the hospital. *All* other interventions—including IV placement, cardiac monitoring, and secondary assessment—should be performed while en route to the appropriate hospital.

18. **Should I use rapid sequence intubation (RSI) if the patient will not tolerate placement of an endotracheal tube?**
    Regrettably, the published literature argues strongly that prehospital RSI is associated with significantly worse outcomes, and frequent occurrences of hypoxia, even on intubations perceived as "easy" by

the paramedics. At this time, there is ample evidence that standard basic life support/advanced life support (BLS/ALS) airway support is most appropriate for these patients.

19. **How useful is the oxygen saturation monitor in the trauma patient?**
Oxygen saturation monitors make the EMT feel better but not the patient. The sicker the trauma patient, the less useful the O_2 saturation monitor becomes. Oxygen saturation monitors are notoriously unreliable in shock states, which are marked by peripheral vasoconstriction. Bad data are worse than no data at all because they may prevent you from using alternative means of patient assessment. Remember: the treatment for hypoxia is oxygen, not (necessarily) intubation. All trauma patients should be given 100% O_2 by nonrebreather mask or via an appropriate airway device when indicated.

20. **How long should an on-scene basic life support unit wait for a responding paramedic unit?**
Generally speaking, not long at all. Given that definitive treatment is surgery, the BLS unit should not wait once the patient has been packaged for transport. In the rare patient with an unstable airway (obstruction, tension pneumothorax, or apnea), the BLS unit should wait for advanced life support (ALS) to arrive only if the ALS unit's estimated time of arrival is *clearly shorter* than the travel time to the hospital.

21. **Is fluid replacement for the hypovolemic patient still the standard of care?**
Yes, but a great deal of research has been unable to determine the effectiveness of fluid resuscitation prior to surgical control of bleeding. Further, there has been active investigation as to the best resuscitation fluid to use: larger volumes of Ringer's lactate, normal saline, or smaller volumes of 3% saline. Currently, there is no clear "best fluid," or, indeed, whether any IV fluids at all should be administered. In the absence of a clear answer, the local community standard should be followed.
In any case, there is no controversy in external bleeding. In such cases, when the bleeding site is known and controlled, aggressive IV resuscitation is clearly indicated.

Pearls and Pitfalls

1. Trauma results from the transfer of energy from an object to the victim's body.
2. Penetrating injury is often easily overlooked, particularly in areas of the body such as the scalp, axillae, groin, scrotum, buttocks, and under the breasts of women.
3. Blunt force trauma often results in internal injuries that are difficult to detect clinically and must be suspected based upon the mechanism of the injury.
4. The basic pathology of trauma is hemorrhage and while external bleeding can be controlled in the field, definitive care of internal injury can only be provided at an appropriately staffed and equipped hospital (trauma center).
5. On-scene time should be kept as short as possible with most, if not all, interventions provided en route to the hospital.

References

1. Baxt WG, Berry CC, Epperson MD, et al. The failure of prehospital trauma prediction rules to classify trauma patients accurately. Ann Emerg Med 18:1–8, 1989.

2. Bickell WH, Wall WJ, Pepe PE, et al: Immediate versus delayed fluid resuscitation for hypotensive patients with penetrating torso injuries. N Engl J Med 331:1105–1109, 1994.
3. Blackwell TH. Prehospital care. Emerg Med Clin North Am 11:1–14, 1993.
4. Rosen P: Multiple trauma. In Emergency Medicine Secrets. 5th ed., Markovchick VJ, Pons PT, Bakes KM, eds., pp. 563–567 Philadelphia:Elsevier Mosby, 2011.
5. New York State Department of Health EMS Rules & Regulations. See http://www.health.ny.gov/nysdoh/ems/publaw.htm
6. Mattox KL, Bickell W, Pepe PE, et al. Prospective MAST study in 911 patients. J Trauma 29:1104–1112, 1989.
7. Schmidt J, Moore GP. Management of multiple trauma. Emerg Med Clin North Am 11:29–52, 1993.
8. Walls RM. Airway management. Emerg Med Clin North Am 11:29–52, 1993.
9. Committee on Trauma—American College of Surgeons: Resources for Optimal Care of the Injured Patient, 2006.
10. Shapiro NI, Kocszewski C, Harrison T, et al. Isolated prehospital hypotension after traumatic injuries: A predictor of mortality? J Emerg Med 25(2):175–179, 2003.
11. Franklin GA, Boaz PW, Spain DA, et al. Prehospital hypotension as a valid indicator of trauma team activation. J Trauma 48(6):1034–1037, 2000.
12. Pinto FC, Capone-Neto A, Prist R, et al. Volume replacement with lactated Ringer's or 3% hypertonic saline solution during combined experimental hemorrhagic shock and traumatic brain injury. J 60(4):758–763, 2006.
13. Sasser SM, Hunt RC, Sullivent EE, et al. Guidelines for field triage of injured patients. Recommendations of the National Expert Panel on Field Triage. MMWR Recomm Rep 58(RR-1):1–35, 2009.

Head Trauma

Will Chapleau, EMT-P, RN, TNS

CHAPTER 55

1. **What is the single most important observation to make when evaluating a patient who has sustained head trauma?**
   The patient's level of consciousness and what it has done over time. Specifically, you want to determine what the level of consciousness was at the time of the trauma, what it was immediately after the trauma, and what has it done since. A decreasing level of consciousness is the earliest and most important sign of increasing intracranial pressure. A patient who was knocked out as a result of the head trauma and is now awake is much less worrisome than a patient who was awake initially and is now becoming unresponsive. The level of consciousness provides one of the best and earliest clues to the potential severity of the injury.

2. **The books all teach about checking the pupils. Where does that fit in?**
   Checking the pupils is an important part of the physical examination. A dilated pupil is an ominous finding suggesting increased intracranial pressure and brainstem herniation. Unfortunately, pupillary dilatation is a late sign of increased intracranial pressure. Therefore, the ideal is to recognize the subtle change in level of consciousness that indicates increasing intracranial pressure before the pupil dilates and the diagnosis becomes apparent to all. In addition, dilatation of a pupil must be evaluated within the context of the trauma sustained and the other findings of the physical examination. A dilated pupil with a normal mental status does not indicate increased intracranial pressure. The pupil can be dilated as a result of a direct blow to the globe causing traumatic mydriasis, which on close observation is seen as an irregular rather than a perfectly round pupil.

3. **What are the common causes of increased intracranial pressure after head trauma?**
   The brain is enclosed within the confines of the rigid skull. Therefore, anything that occupies space inside the skull will cause an increase in intracranial pressure. Space can be taken up by hematomas in the subdural, epidural, or intracerebral locations or by diffuse swelling of the brain tissue.

4. **You mentioned herniation of the brain as a complication of increased intracranial pressure. Can you give a little more detail?**
   As the pressure inside the cranium increases, the brain is compressed by the hematoma or swelling. Eventually, the pressure will become so great that either the intracranial pressure will exceed the ability of the vascular system to perfuse the brain or the brain will be pushed through some of the small openings in the skull. Both these complications lead to permanent neurologic damage or death.

5. **How can I tell the difference between subdural, epidural, and intracerebral hematomas clinically?**
   It is almost impossible to tell the difference between these various hematomas without performing computed tomography. There are differences, though, relative to the nature of the bleeding. Subdural

hematomas are venous bleeds and can develop slowly. Patients presenting with seizures or other level of consciousness changes should be evaluated for recent or remote history of possible head injuries. Epidural bleeds are arterial. The classic history for a patient with an epidural hematoma is that the patient loses consciousness at the time of the trauma, then wakes up and has a "lucid" period. Some time later, usually minutes to hours, the patient loses consciousness again. Intracerebral hematomas can present with loss of consciousness or neurologic abnormalities related to the area of the brain that is injured. Unfortunately, there is significant overlap in the presentation of all these entities, and clinical differentiation is virtually impossible.

6. **How can I tell the difference between a patient who has sustained a serious head injury and one whose altered mental status is from alcohol ingestion?**
   This can be extremely difficult. The intoxicated patient frequently is a victim of head trauma for a variety of reasons, including falling, driving while intoxicated and getting into a crash, or being assaulted. Unfortunately, many of these patients will present with altered mentation, which could be from the alcohol or could be from the trauma. The guiding principle should be to assume the worst possible injury consistent with the mechanism and treat the patient accordingly. This means that many patients whose only problem ultimately turns out to be alcohol intoxication will undergo cervical spine immobilization and, in some cases, endotracheal intubation in the field and computed tomography of the brain in the emergency department.

7. **How should I describe the patient who has a head injury?**
   There are many terms that are commonly used to describe the patient who has an altered level of consciousness. These terms include comatose, lethargic, stuporous, semicomatose, unresponsive, and so forth. Because these terms mean different things to different people, the best way to describe the patient is to relate how the patient responded to a stimulus. For example, "the patient followed my verbal commands correctly," or " the patient did not follow any verbal commands but pushed my hand away in response to a sternal rub," or " the patient had no response to any stimulus."

8. **What about the Glasgow Coma Scale (GCS)?**
   This is a scoring system that attempts to quantify the patient's level of consciousness in an objective fashion by assigning point scores to various observations. This has the advantage of yielding reproducible results rather than depending on a variety of terms that may mean different things to different observers. The GCS is scored as follows:

Eye opening	4—spontaneous eye opening
	3—eye opening to command
	2—eye opening to painful stimulus
	1—no eye opening
Verbal response	5—oriented and answers appropriately
	4—confused conversation
	3—inappropriate responses
	2—incomprehensible
	1—none

Motor   6—follows commands
         5—localizes pain
         4—withdrawal from pain
         3—decorticate (flexion) posturing
         2—decerebrate (extension) posturing
         1—no motor activity

For pediatric patients, the verbal score of the GCS is modified to reflect age-appropriate responses.

9. **How does the GCS relate to my patient clinically?**
   Rescoring the GCS over time and obtaining a series of results can help determine if the patient is improving or deteriorating. In addition, a severe head injury is defined as a score equal to or less than 8, a moderate head injury as a score between 9 and 12, and a minor head injury as a score greater than 12. It should be noted, however that a patient who is dead still has a score of 3.

10. **If I think someone has a serious head injury, what should the management be in the field?**
    First, assess the mechanism of injury for the potential presence of a spine injury. If there is concern about spine trauma, the spine should be immobilized. Supplemental high-flow oxygen should be provided and the patient's blood pressure maintained to assure cerebral perfusion. If the mental status is decreased or there is concern about increased intracranial pressure, airway management should be performed to protect the airway, help assure oxygen delivery, and potentially permit hyperventilation. Maintain ventilations at 10 breaths per minute, the oxygen saturation above 90%, and the systolic blood pressure (SBP) at 90 mmHg.

11. **I've heard that head-injured patients should no longer be hyperventilated. Is that true?**
    Yes, to a certain extent. Routine hyperventilation of a patient with a head injury is not recommended because it causes vasoconstriction and can actually decrease cerebral perfusion. Recent studies have shown that the optimal ventilatory rate for the adult head-injured patient is 10 breaths per minute. On the other hand, if a patient is showing signs of increased intracranial pressure and herniation, mild to moderate hyperventilation can still be used to buy some time during transport. Mild to moderate hyperventilation can be accomplished by bagging the intubated adult patient at a rate of 20 breaths per minute.

12. **Is there anything else that can be done in the field to decrease intracranial pressure?**
    When spinal immobilization does not prevent it, the head of the patient can be elevated approximately 30°, although the benefit of this to reduce intracranial pressure has recently been questioned. In addition, diuretics such as mannitol and furosemide can be administered according to local protocol to help decrease the intracranial pressure.

13. **What are some minor head injuries?**
    One of the most common injuries confronted in the prehospital setting is scalp laceration. Although not usually serious, it can be a source of major blood loss. The scalp is extremely vascular, and failure to control hemorrhage from a "simple" scalp laceration can lead to hypovolemic shock. Bleeding from the scalp can usually be controlled by digital pressure. The one problem that arises is when there is concern

about a potential skull fracture in association with the laceration. In this situation, pressure can be applied to the intact scalp and skull around the injured area and in this fashion control the hemorrhage.

14. **Is it true that IV infusion rates should be restricted in head-injured patients?**
In trauma patients in general, the rate and volume of resuscitation fluids has been reduced. In the case of traumatic brain injury, however, it is important to maintain a BP of at least 90 mmHg systolic. Thus IV fluid administration titrated to maintain a systolic BP of 90 mmHg is appropriate in the setting of traumatic brain injury.

15. **OK, why is it so important that I maintain both the oxygen saturation and BP above 90 in the traumatic brain-injured patient?**
Several studies have shown that even a single episode of hypoxia or hypotension will lead to increased morbidity and mortality. These secondary insults will further exacerbate the primary traumatic injury and are potentially correctable if they occur before the arrival of EMS and preventable with appropriate care after EMS arrival.

Pearls and Pitfalls

1. The most important observation in a patient with suspected traumatic brain injury is the patient's level of consciousness and how it has changed over time since the injury.
2. A common, and potentially fatal (for the patient), mistake is to ascribe altered mental status to concomitant alcohol use rather than a potential traumatic brain injury.
3. A "simple" scalp laceration can lead to significant blood loss; therefore, such bleeding must be controlled.
4. Even a single episode of hypoxia (SaO_2 less than 90%) or hypotension (systolic BP less than 90 mmHg) can result in increased morbidity or mortality in the patient with TBI and should be corrected immediately if found and, ideally, prevented.
5. Hyperventilation of the patient with possible traumatic brain injury is not recommended unless clinical signs (dilated pupil, abnormal posturing) of herniation are present.

References

1. Chesnut RM. The management of severe traumatic brain injury. Emerg Med Clin North Am 15:581–604, 1997.
2. Eisenberg HM. Aldrich EF, eds. Management of head injury. Neurosurg Clin North Am 2:251–501, 1991.
3. Feldman Z, Kanter MJ, Robertson CS, et al. Effect of head elevation on intracranial pressure, and cerebral blood flow in head-injured patients. J Neurosurg 76:207–211, 1992.
4. Newton E. Head trauma. In Markovchick VJ, Pons PT, Bakes KM (eds): Emergency Medicine Secrets. 5th Ed. Philadelphia, Elsevier Mosby, 2011, pp 581–586.
5. Teasdale G, Jennett B. Assessment of coma and impaired consciousness: A practical scale. Lancet 2:81–84, 1974.
6. Brain Trauma Foundation Guidelines for Prehospital Management of Traumatic Brain Injury, 2007.

Spinal Cord Injuries

Will Chapleau, EMT-P, RN, TNS

CHAPTER 56

1. **What do I need to know about immobilization?**
   How often do you actually see a patient "immobilized"? With absolutely no patient movement? In reality, you have rarely seen such a thing, yet you use that term in documentation. What is actually occurring is *spinal motion restriction (SMR)*. The patient's movement has been restricted in such a manner that the possibility of further injury is lessened. This motion restriction is accomplished by the use of various pieces of equipment, teamwork, and patient education. SMR, as always, depends on local protocol and routine.

   From an intervention standpoint, little or nothing changes. Picture yourself, however, as a defendant in a case involving a spinal cord injury. The patient involved in the litigation is the once-intoxicated noncompliant individual you really did try to help. Now visualize the attorney demonstrating how the patient was "moving" while immobilized. By use of patient and receiving-staff testimony, several eyewitnesses, an on-scene amateur video, and a simple demonstration using your equipment and a model, the plaintiff's attorney will show you in fact *lied* on your documentation. The patient was never immobilized, but rather *was* moving.

   Now imagine a completely different scenario. Your defense attorney begins the cross-examination. She points out your numerous attempts to comfort and console the patient. Your counsel directs the jury toward your efforts to educate the patient about the risk of movement. She additionally demonstrates how you *restricted the patient's motion* following local protocol and the standard of care. Although you were unable to control this violent patient completely (through no fault of your own), you clearly restricted the patient's motion in an effort to limit and/or prevent injury. The change in terminology may appear insignificant, but the adjustment might well make a substantial difference in the outcome of the lawsuit.

2. **Is this much ado about nothing?**
   SMR has been a very hot topic for some time now. There has been a great deal of discussion and some research about whether there is a need to restrict the vast numbers of patients who currently find themselves on backboards in the United States. Some protocols in select EMS systems currently allow prehospital personnel to determine whether SMR is indicated. The following is a compilation from several of the more common protocol approaches to this dilemma.

   SMR may not be indicated when **all** the following criteria are met.

   1. The patient is an adult.
   2. The patient is able to communicate in such a manner that there is no possibility of misunderstanding or misinterpretation.
   3. The patient is pain free, meaning there is no subjective complaint of neck pain and no objective finding of tenderness on palpation.

Clinical Care

4. The patient has no neurologic complaints or deficits (i.e., paresthesia or paraplegia).
5. The patient has no alteration in mental status, either from trauma or from ingestion of any substance that might interfere with his or her interpretation of pain.
6. The mechanism of injury does not suggest spinal cord injury (SCI).
7. The patient does not have any other major, distracting injury.

It is not difficult to see that using this protocol is still significantly limiting and thus results in the continued use of SMR for most patients.

3. How about the patient with penetrating neck trauma? Do I have to apply SMR devices in these cases?

As a general rule, no. With victims of shootings and stabbings, if no spinal cord injury is found initially, they are usually not going to develop one. This is because of the difference in mechanism of injury between blunt and penetrating injury and the forces and energy involved. With blunt injury, significant force and energy are applied to the vertebral column and spine, resulting in disruption of the integrity of the supporting structures of the vertebral column. Thus, even if a cord injury did not occur at the time of the trauma, the lack of structural integrity of the spinal column could permit movement of damaged vertebrae and subsequent SCI if spinal motion restriction is not used. With penetrating neck trauma, on the other hand, damage is limited to the path of the penetrating object and usually does not cause structural support disruption. Thus, subsequent neurologic injury is very rare.

4. What is the current thinking on the use of the rigid spine board?

There are studies that suggest that our current approach to SMR using the rigid spine board might actually be detrimental to a segment of our patient population. There is consensus that the long spine board is extremely uncomfortable and that there is a correlation between excessive time spent on the board and additional complications such as the development of decubitus ulcers.

Is there an alternative to the rigid spine board? At present, there are several alternatives to the board, and more are currently under development. Without doubt, the trend is to achieve SMR with the recognition that it can be accomplished with a measure of comfort and no further harm. Full-body vacuum splints are one approach that meets a direct need. Obviously, protocol adjustments will meet selected concerns, as will additional education and training for the provider. As for the majority of potentially complex extrications, the various devices available on the market today are still, for the most part, subservient to the rigid spine board for at least the initial phase of activity. With further research and development, the rigid spine board dilemma may one day give rise to discussions on the most comfortable way to achieve SMR.

5. What clinical signs and symptoms should I look for that suggest SCI?

First, evaluate the mechanism of injury to see if it has the potential to produce a spinal column or cord injury. Next, determine what complaints the patient voices. Any complaint of numbness, tingling, pins and needles, weakness, or paralysis should be presumed to be due to a spinal injury until proven otherwise. The physical examination will, of course, provide important information as well. Evaluate the patient for sensory abnormalities and motor function. As before, any abnormal findings should be presumed to be resulting from a spinal cord injury. The presence of priapism (persistent erection) is thought to be pathognomonic of SCI. Patients with very high cervical cord injuries may develop respiratory compromise.

6. I've heard about spinal shock. What should I do about it?

Spinal shock is often confused with neurogenic shock. Neurogenic shock refers to dilatation of the peripheral arteries due to disruption of the sympathetic nervous system caused by injury to the spinal cord. In these patients, blood pressure (BP) drops, whereas the pulse rate appears normal or slow. These patients often have other injuries and shock should be considered to be hemorrhagic in origin and treated as such until proven otherwise. Spinal shock refers to a temporary loss of motor and sensory function due to damage or "shock" to the spinal cord. These patients should be treated as the symptoms call for, with care given to limit movement that could make the injury worse. Generally, these patients are given a fluid challenge during their prehospital transport. If hemorrhage is ruled out and the blood pressure (BP) has not improved after 2 or 3 L of crystalloid, vasopressors may be used to support BP.

7. When there is airway compromise, what is the best method of intubation?

When confronted with an SCI patient in need of a patent airway, there is little question that time is of the essence. SCI patients with a high cervical injury or progressive secondary cord injuries are at great risk for the development of respiratory compromise. The prudent provider should always maintain a watchful eye for progressive changes in neurologic findings that may suggest pending respiratory embarrassment. Research suggests that the method of airway management most familiar to the provider will be that which is used. Further discussion points out that careful oral intubation (with appropriate personnel, in-line stabilization, and rapid-sequence medications) when necessary does not appear to create additional neurologic complications or deficits. In fact, given the experience base of today's provider, it may be the preferred method. The following is an outline of one approach that may be used to secure the airway of an SCI patient with respiratory compromise.

1. Manual stabilization and motion restriction to maintain neutral positioning (throughout procedure).
2. Preoxygenation with a bag-mask, oral airway, and cricoid pressure
3. Sedation and paralysis (as indicated by patient presentation and if permitted by local protocols).
4. Removal of the anterior portion of the cervical collar (posterior portion left in place).
5. Oral intubation with direct visual visualization of the vocal cords (cricoid pressure as needed).
6. Confirmation of tube placement.

Note that alternative methods of airway management that do not cause extension, flexion, or lateral motion are equally acceptable. Other management techniques that do not require direct visualization include blind nasotracheal intubation, digital intubation, and the lighted stylet (i.e., the TrachLight). Supraglottic airways may also be considered. In the patient in whom respiratory arrest has not occurred but a patent airway must be provided, nasotracheal intubation may be appropriate. Care must be taken to insure that patient movement and any *relative* contraindications have been taken into consideration. The key factors that are the underlying framework for successful airway management are teamwork and flexibility on the part of the providers.

8. What is a neutral position, and does it change from patient to patient?

A neutral position is when the eyes are at a 90° angle to the spine. The head is neither flexed nor extended, and the spinal column's natural "in line" position is maintained. In adult and pediatric populations, the ability to achieve a neutral position changes depending on the relationship between the occipital region of the skull and the patient's shoulders. Ask several associates to lie supine on the floor. Carefully examine the relationship between their shoulders, their occiput, and the floor. Note that some will rest their heads in a neutral position, without aid. Some, however, will need padding behind the occiput to maintain the head in the correct position (eyes at a 90° angle to the spine). The pediatric patient (depending on age and size) is most often the direct opposite of the adult. This is because infants and children have disproportionately larger heads when compared to the body. Thus, padding the pediatric patient's body under the shoulders and upper chest brings the head into a neutral position.

9. **Is there such a thing as secondary cord injury?**
   Yes. When discussing insult to the spinal cord, the conversation is often limited to the initial trauma. Recent research points to secondary cord injury resulting from ischemia and posttraumatic cell membrane changes as a significant concern. When the neutral position is achieved in any patient, there is a maximal amount of space available for the cord within the spinal canal. This space is reduced as the patient extends or flexes. If we consider normal anatomy, it is quite simple to see that any disruption or displacement could and does create a compromise in blood flow. This compromise in blood flow, in combination with edema and a failure to achieve neutral positioning, may be the cause for significant *additional* progression of the injury.

10. **Is there anything else that can be done to minimize this secondary injury?**
    Clinical experience and research indicate that spinal cord injuries benefit from appropriate oxygenation (the treatment of hypoxia), and assuring adequate perfusion by maintaining SBP above 90 mmHg

11. **Isn't the use of steroids in the field controversial?**
    Although a couple of studies have shown improved outcomes when high doses of methylprednisolone are given within 8–24 hours of injury, use of steroids in both the hospital and prehospital arena has become controversial. One position paper recommends against the use of steroids prehospital in patients with acute spinal cord injury and that the use of steroids should be up to the trauma surgeons and neurosurgeons that will be caring for the patient.

12. **Are there any additional concerns that should be addressed? What is SCIWORA?**
    Yes, age-related index of suspicion. In the pediatric population, an insult known as SCIWORA (spinal cord injury without radiologic abnormality) exists. In these cases, children present with signs of spinal cord damage, yet after arrival to the hospital, no spinal fracture can be demonstrated on radiographic study. From the perspective of care delivered in the field, these children are treated exactly the same as all others with evidence of spinal cord injury.

Pearls and Pitfalls

1. The procedure used by prehospital providers to prevent further or initial spinal cord damage is SMR, rather than spinal immobilization. It is virtually impossible to actually immobilize a patient.
2. Spinal shock and neurogenic shock are often used as interchangeable terms—they are not the same.
3. Patients with penetrating trauma in the vicinity of the spinal column generally do not need spinal motion restriction unless they present with neurologic complaints or findings.
4. Steroids for patients with SCI have become controversial. In general, starting them in the field is not recommended.

5. In order to NOT apply SMR, a patient must have a completely normal mental status, be able to communicate effectively, have no subjective neck pain or objective neck tenderness, have no neurologic complaints or findings, and have no distracting injuries. An abnormality in any one of these criteria necessitates the application of spinal motion restriction.

References

1. Anderson D, Hall E. Pathophysiology of spinal cord trauma. Ann Emerg Med 22:987–992, 1993.
2. Bracken MB, Shepard MJ, Collins WF, et al. A randomized, controlled trial of methylprednisolone or naloxone in the treatment of acute spinal-cord injury. Results of the Second National Acute Spinal Cord Injury Study. N Engl J Med 322:1405–1411, 1990.
3. Criswell J, Nolan J. Emergency airway management in patients with cervical spine injuries. Anaesthesia 49: 900–903, 1994.
4. Davis J, Phreaner D, Hoyt D, Mackersie R. The etiology of missed cervical injuries. Trauma J 34(3):342–346, 1993.
5. Diliberti T, Ronald W. Evaluation of the cervical spine in the emergency setting: Who does not need an x-ray? Orthopedics 15(2):179–183, 1992.
6. Hadley M, Zabramski J, Browner C, et al. Pediatric spinal trauma: Review of 122 cases of spinal cord and vertebral column injuries. Neurosurg J 68:18–64, 1988.
7. Spivac JM, Weiss M, Cotler J, Call M. Cervical spine injuries in patients 65 and older. Spine 19(20):2302–2306, 1994.
8. Tator H, Fehlings M. Review of the secondary injury theory of acute spinal cord trauma with emphasis on vascular mechanism. Neurosurg J 75:15–26, 1991.
9. Lemons VR, Wagner FC Jr. Respiratory complications after cervical spinal cord injury. Spine 19(20):2315–2320, 1994.
10. Bledsoe BE, Wesley AK, Salomone JP. High dose steroids for acute spinal cord injury in emergency medical services, Prehosp Emerg Care 8:313, 2004.
11. Klevens MJ, McNamara R. Cervical spine and spinal cord trauma. In Emergency Medicine Secrets, 5th ed., Markovchick VJ, Pons PT, Bakes KA, eds., pp. 574-580. St Louis: Mosby, 2011.

Neck Trauma

Nicholas C. Johnson, MD

1. **What are the major causes of anterior neck trauma?**
   Neck trauma can be divided into penetrating or blunt injuries. Penetrating injuries are more common and are associated with greater morbidity and mortality than blunt trauma. The majority of penetrating trauma is due to gunshots and stabbings, but also can be due to miscellaneous projectiles. Gunshot wounds are more likely to result in serious injury and death than stabbings. Blunt trauma overall is less common due to the protection afforded by the head, clavicles, and shoulders but when it occurs it is most commonly due to motor vehicle collisions and assaults.

2. **The neck is densely populated with important structures that can be injured in trauma. How can these structures be categorized?**
   Vascular (arterial and venous), pharyngoesophageal (upper digestive tract), and laryngotracheal (airway) are the major categories of structural elements. Of course, there are many other structures in the neck that can be injured, but these are the most important and commonly encountered injuries in prehospital management (the spinal cord is discussed separately in Chapter 56 of this book).

3. **Which structures carry the highest mortality when injured?**
   Vascular injuries have the highest rates of mortality, followed closely by injuries to the airway. Esophageal injuries are less likely to be immediately life threatening but can cause death in the subacute phase due to infection.

4. **Which structures are most commonly injured?**
   Major vessels (most commonly jugular and common carotid arteries) 23–40%, pharyngoesophageal 8–10%, laryngotracheal 8–10%, and various neurologic structures 6%.

5. **How are the areas of the neck categorized anatomically?**
   Traditionally, anatomists have divided the neck into "triangles" based on borders made up by various neck muscles. Unfortunately, these triangles are cumbersome to learn and difficult to apply clinically. From a clinical standpoint, the neck is divided into "zones," which are more helpful in predicting injury and guiding treatment. (See Figure 57.1.)

6. **Where is zone I and what does it contain?**
   Zone I extends from the sternal notch and clavicles to the cricoid cartilage and contains the vertebral and carotid arteries; subclavian, jugular, and brachiocephalic veins; lung apex; esophagus; trachea; thoracic duct (containing lymphatic fluid); and spinal cord.

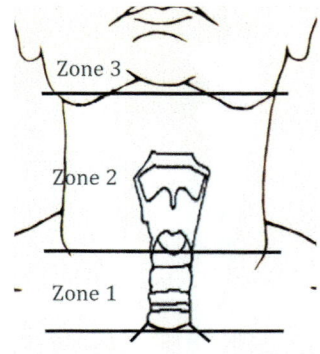

FIGURE 57.1 Zones of the neck.

7. **Where is zone II and what does it contain?**
   Zone II extends from the cricoid cartilage to the angle of the mandible and contains the vertebral and carotid arteries, jugular vein, esophagus, larynx, and spinal cord.
8. **Where is Zone III and what does it contain?**
   Zone III extends from the angle of the mandible to the base of the skull and contains the carotid and vertebral arteries, pharynx, and spinal cord.
9. **How does identifying the zone of the neck change its management?**
   In the prehospital setting, knowing the zones is important to help one predict the potential structures that could be injured to be prepared for complications en route. Hospital protocols vary, but the zone of injury may help to determine whether a patient will undergo surgical exploration or a more conservative approach with imaging and observation.
10. **What type of vascular injuries can be expected in neck trauma?**
    With penetrating neck wounds, the most common vascular injuries include laceration or transection (complete disruption) of the vessel, whereas blunt injuries will more commonly lead to aneurysm formation, dissection, or thrombosis (clot formation)
11. **What are the signs and symptoms of major vessel injury in the neck?**
    Bleeding obviously comes to mind when there is injury to any vessel. Additionally, look for signs of an expanding hematoma, which can indicate bleeding from a large vessel that is still contained in the neck or within the vessel (like an aneurysm). One can also listen over the neck for a bruit. A bruit is the sound of blood being pumped through a damaged vessel and sounds like a "whoosh" with each heartbeat. Although it would be a very late and ominous finding, one can also look for tracheal deviation, which would indicate an expanding hematoma which is displacing the trachea away from the bleeding vessel. In some cases, an injury to a blood vessel in the neck can compromise circulation to the brain with the result that the patient presents with the symptoms and signs of a stroke.
12. **When evaluating a patient with anterior neck trauma, what are the priorities in management?**
    The ABCs—airway, breathing, and circulation This should be the protocol with every patient every time but especially with neck trauma.
13. **What are the signs and symptoms of airway injury in the neck?**
    Look for signs of respiratory distress such as tachypnea, hoarseness, gurgling respirations, or coughing up blood. One may also see air bubbling from a bleeding neck wound. One may feel or hear subcutaneous emphysema, which is air that has leaked from the airway under the skin, and feels like bubblewrap popping when palpated with your fingertips (crepitus) and sounds like crackling when auscultated with a stethoscope.
14. **What is the preferred method of securing the airway in the patient with neck injury?**
    Orotracheal intubation, with or without repetitive strain injury, is usually the most effective means of securing the airway. However, beware that if the larynx or trachea has been lacerated, introducing the tube may lead to complete transection of the airway with recoil of the trachea into the chest cavity. This will make further airway management nearly impossible outside the hands of a thoracic surgeon.

In these select cases, patients can usually be ventilated via a bag-mask, even though the neck may distend with each positive pressure squeeze of the bag. An incision into the neck can be fatal if the trachea is transected and retracts into the chest.

15. **What should one expect in the airway management of a patient with neck trauma?**
    A complete disaster. Management of these airways is fraught with complication. Have backup airways ready. If there is penetration of the larynx there is most likely bleeding into the airway, which will make direct visualization of the cords very difficult. Have suction at hand. The airway may also be obscured in the event that there has been damage to a vessel in close proximity to the airway. An expanding hematoma from the injured vessel may cause external compression, distortion of the anatomy, and displacement of the airway, again making direct visualization of the cords very difficult. If you are able to effectively ventilate and oxygenate a patient, unless there is evidence the airway will become rapidly compromised, the better part of valor may be to place the patient on a nonrebreather bag reservoir mask or ventilate the patient via bag-mask and transport to an emergency department where definitive airway management can be done in a controlled environment.

16. **How do I manage bleeding from a neck wound?**
    Injury to the major vessels of the neck can lead to rapid exsanguination. Place direct pressure over the site of bleeding from the vessel; do not place a clamp blindly in the neck in an attempt to control bleeding. Sometimes a gloved finger must be placed into the wound to gain direct pressure on an artery.

17. **What are the causes of respiratory distress in a patient with anterior neck trauma?**
    In addition to the aforementioned direct laryngeal injury and compression of the airway by an expanding hematoma or edema, remember that the apex of the lung is in zone I of the neck and extends above the clavicle in some patients, particularly those with chronic obstructive pulmonary disorder, so there can be direct lung injury, simple pneumothorax, tension pneumothorax, and hemothorax as possible causes.

18. **How do I manage the cervical spine in these patients?**
    Standard cervical spine precautions should be considered the ideal for all patients with blunt neck trauma. Unfortunately, due to associated injuries, this may not always be possible. Patients with bleeding into the airway, expanding hematomas, and other neck injuries may insist on either sitting up, or being positioned in some way other than that appropriate for standard cervical spine protocols. They are usually doing this for a reason: their airway is compromised when lying flat on their back with a hard collar compressing them. Additionally, serious anterior neck injuries (i.e., expanding hematoma or bleeding vessels) may be missed or unable to be treated with a cervical collar in place. Deviation from standard cervical spine protocol may be considered on a case-by-case basis in these instances based on likelihood of cervical spine injury and based on local protocols.
    As a general rule, cervical spine precautions are not needed for patients with penetrating neck injury unless the patient has neurologic complaints or findings on exam.

19. **What are the signs and symptoms of pharyngeal/esophageal injury?**
    Generally, these injuries are silent, but can present with hematemesis (vomiting blood), dysphagia (difficulty swallowing), odynophagia (painful swallowing), or crepitus on palpation secondary to subcutaneous emphysema or cartilage fractures. Again, these injuries are usually not immediately life threatening but have a survival rate of only 64% if not treated within 24 hours.

20. **Aside from the ABCs, what head, eyes, ears, nose, and throat physical exam findings should I look for in patients with neck injury?**

    Look at the pupils. The sympathetic chain of nerves controls pupillary dilation and if severed, the pupil on the affected side will be constricted. This is important because for most of its course, this chain of nerves runs along the carotid artery, so pupillary constriction can suggest underlying carotid injury if it is not already obvious. The tongue (or one of its large feeding blood vessels) can also be lacerated in zone III injuries, causing a very enlarged or displaced tongue, which can lead to airway obstruction.

21. **What neurological findings can be found in patients with anterior neck injury?**

    Just about any of them. Patients with anterior neck injury have multiple possible mechanisms for neurologic dysfunction. Lower cranial nerve pathways can be directly disrupted by penetrating trauma. Approximately 25–30% of patients with carotid and vertebral artery injury will present with lateralizing stroke findings due to decreased cerebral perfusion from the affected artery. Spinal cord injury due to disruption, swelling, or compression of the spinal cord can occur as well.

Pearls and Pitfalls

1. Patients with penetrating injuries of the neck have a high likelihood of vascular injury and should be taken to a trauma center.
2. Hemorrhage from penetrating neck wounds should be controlled by direct finger pressure.
3. All patients with neck trauma should receive high-flow oxygen and early intubation for any signs of upper airway obstruction.
4. Hoarseness and crepitus with subcutaneous emphysema or hemoptysis are signs of laryngeal trauma.
5. Trauma to the carotid or vertebral arteries may cause a stroke.
6. Emergent transport to a trauma center is essential, as airway compromise can occur suddenly.

References

1. Murphy P, Colwell C. Prehospital management of neck trauma. Emerg Med Serv 29(5):53–60, 2000.
2. Asensio JA, Valenziano CP, Falcone RE, et al. Management of penetrating neck injuries: The controversy surrounding Zone II injuries. Surg Clin North Am 71(2):267–296, 1991.
3. Mandavia DP, Qualls S, Rokos I. Emergency airway management in penetrating neck injury. Ann Emerg Med 35(3): 221–225, 2000.
4. Barkana Y, Stein M, Scope A, et al. Prehospital stabilization of the cervical spine for penetrating injuries of the neck—Is it necessary? Injury 31(5):305–309, 2000.
5. Thompson EC, Porter J, Fernandez L. Penetrating neck trauma: an overview of management. J Oral Maxillofac Surg 60(8):918–923, 2002.

CHAPTER 58

Thoracic Trauma

Jeffrey P. Salomone, MD, and Joseph A. Salomone, MD

1. **What is meant by thoracic trauma?**
   The thorax is enclosed within the rib cage and contains many essential organs including the heart, lungs, trachea, esophagus, and great vessels. In addition, the upper abdominal organs, particularly the spleen and liver, lie in the lower thoracic cage. Any trauma to the chest has the potential of injuring any of these major organs. In addition, any injury below the nipple line anteriorly or below the inferior border of the scapula posteriorly can injure both chest and abdominal organs. With the exception of the skull and the brain, nowhere else in the body is there such a collection of organs so vital to maintaining life functions.

2. **What are the deadly dozen?**
   The deadly dozen refers to the 12 possible major injuries to the thoracic organs. The immediate threats to life are airway obstruction, open pneumothorax, tension pneumothorax, massive hemothorax, and cardiac tamponade. Potential threats to life include traumatic aortic rupture, flail chest, bronchial disruption, myocardial contusion, diaphragmatic tear, esophageal injury, and pulmonary contusion.

3. **What should I look for when I examine the chest?**
   First, it is important to get an overall impression of the patient's condition. Observe the patient for signs of respiratory distress. Then look at the chest to evaluate the rate, depth, and symmetry of chest wall expansion as well as for obvious external signs of injury. Note if there are any segments of the chest wall that have paradoxical motion, indicating a flail segment. Also look for any penetrating wounds that might represent entry or exit wounds. Next, place your hands on the patient and palpate the ribs and chest wall to check for subcutaneous emphysema and bony crepitus. Finally, if the noise level in the area permits, auscultate the chest for the presence or absence of breath sounds as well as any abnormal sounds such as stridor or wheezing. Do not forget that any chest wall findings such as penetrating wounds or possible rib fractures located below the level of the nipples anteriorly or the tip of the scapulae posteriorly should be considered to be potential abdominal wounds as well.

4. **Is monitoring the respiratory rate really all that helpful?**
   Close monitoring of the respiratory rate in a patient who has sustained thoracic trauma can be an invaluable aid in recognizing early signs of developing respiratory insufficiency, particularly in cases involving longer transport times. A gradually increasing respiratory rate is indicative of developing hypoxia and can provide a clue to deterioration in the patient's condition. Thus, it is important to carefully count (not estimate as is often done) the respiratory rate as part of the early assessment of the patient and repeat the measurement frequently, as time permits.

5. **How about when I examine the abdomen and pelvis?**
   Observe the abdomen, flank, and back for obvious penetrating wounds. Just as lower chest–penetrating wounds may also have injured upper abdominal organs, upper abdominal wounds may also traverse the

diaphragm and involve the lower chest. Then palpate the abdomen, looking for tenderness, especially over organs such as the liver and spleen. Remember that early in the course of many injuries, abdominal examination can be unremarkable in the face of significant trauma. The presence of alcohol, spinal cord injury, or other distracting painful injuries such as long bone or pelvis fractures can be misleading and mask findings of tenderness.

6. **How do I treat thoracic trauma?**
   The mainstay of prehospital treatment of thoracic trauma really revolves around the basics. A patent airway is essential. Airway obstruction should be treated as it is discovered. Active airway management may be necessary. High-flow oxygen should be administered to all trauma patients, particularly those with chest injury, via a nonrebreather bag reservoir mask. Oxygen saturation should be monitored with a pulse oximeter. The patient's circulatory status should be assessed and adequate control of obvious external hemorrhage obtained. Placement of one or more IV lines should be accomplished while en route. A brief secondary survey for other potential injuries can be performed rapidly with immobilization of fractures, if necessary. Early notification of the receiving hospital is important to allow for trauma team activation and adequate preparation to receive the patient. Prehospital management of all thoracic injuries is essentially the same regardless of the specific injury, with the exception of tension pneumothorax.

7. **How do I diagnose tension pneumothorax and treat it?**
   Tension pneumothorax is a true life-threatening emergency. It should be treated as soon as it is diagnosed. Tension pneumothorax develops when air enters the pleural space through a laceration of the lung, a bronchial tear, or a wound in the chest wall and cannot escape. As more air enters the space, pressure builds and eventually shifts the mediastinum toward the opposite side, collapsing the vena cava and decreasing blood return to the right side of the heart as well as compressing the other lung, compromising its ability to function. Diminished blood return causes a drop in cardiac output, resulting in hypotension and tachycardia. Tension pneumothorax is diagnosed by the absence of breath sounds over the involved hemithorax, hypotension, and tachycardia. Subcutaneous emphysema is often palpated and may be massive. Tracheal shift away from the affected side may or may not be apparent (it is often a late sign).

8. **How do I treat tension pneumothorax in the field?**
   Treatment is immediate decompression of the tension pneumothorax to relieve the pressure and improve venous return. Decompression is achieved using a 14-gauge 2-in Angiocath. The needle is introduced into the second intercostal space at the midclavicular line or the 4th or 5th intercostal space in the midaxillary line. Entry of the needle into the involved hemithorax will result in a sudden rush of air through the needle as the tension is decompressed. Vital signs should normalize quickly. Remain alert for recurrence of the tension and decompress again if symptoms return. Failure of the vital signs to normalize may occur with concomitant hypovolemic shock. If the patient is intubated, another sign of tension pneumothorax is greater backpressure or decreased compliance to bagging.

9. **What do I do for the other injuries?**
   Rapid transportation is the most important therapy. Administer high-flow oxygen to all patients with suspected chest or abdominal injuries. Massive hemothorax will require large-volume resuscitation, preferably with blood and blood products at the hosptial, and surgery. Cardiac contusion and tamponade may improve with administration of a relatively small fluid bolus. Flail chest and pulmonary contusions

Clinical Care

may require airway management and positive pressure ventilation in order to maintain an adequate oxygen saturation.

10. **Is giving fluid really bad?**
    Yes and no. Recent research has questioned the use of aggressive fluid resuscitation in penetrating chest trauma. The concept is that as blood pressure increases, the rate of bleeding in the noncompressible chest vessels increases or the higher pressure dislodges tenuous clots. Although this research has been questioned, the downside of "overresuscitation" is noteworthy, however, and fluid resuscitation should probably be tempered to the minimal amount necessary to maintain adequate perfusion. Fluid therapy should be titrated to maintain a blood pressure of 90 mmHg systolic. Continuous aggressive administration of crystalloid after reaching a blood pressure of 90 mmHg systolic may also be harmful to patients with large pulmonary or myocardial contusions.

11. **What are the indications for a "slash" thoracotomy?**
    There is no indication for this procedure in the field. Also known as an emergent thoracotomy, this heroic surgical procedure is rarely successful. The indications are penetrating trauma to the chest with witnessed loss of vital signs. Treatable findings are cardiac tamponade or isolated cardiac puncture wounds. Success rates are low and related to the time between loss of vital signs and thoracotomy. In the setting of blunt trauma, thoracotomies are rarely helpful and usually not indicated. A patient found in the field in traumatic arrest due to blunt trauma will stay that way. If vital signs are lost during transport, a "slash" thoracotomy on arrival to the emergency department may be indicated in cases of penetrating trauma to the chest or abdomen. Isolated head-injured patients will not benefit from thoracotomy.

12. **How does a stab wound to the left chest injure the spleen?**
    Remember that the spleen and liver lie in the lower chest. During exhalation, the diaphragm can rise as high as the nipple line. Any of these abdominal structures can be injured with a stab wound or gunshot wound to the respective lower part of the chest.

Pearls and Pitfalls

1. Trauma to the lower chest may also involve the upper abdominal organs such as the liver and spleen.
2. Penetrating trauma to the upper abdomen may also involve the lower chest.
3. Tension pneumothorax is a life-threatening emergency and requires immediate needle decompression.
4. Simple pneumothorax causes pain and shortness of breath but does not require needle decompression.
5. An increasing respiratory rate may be the earliest sign of a patient who is developing hypoxia and respiratory insufficiency after thoracic trauma.

References

1. Jackimcyzk K. Blunt chest trauma. Emerg Med Clin North Am 11:81–96, 1993.
2. Marx JA. Penetrating abdominal trauma. Emerg Med Clin North Am 11:125–135, 1993.
3. Pepe PE, Mosesso VN Jr., Falk JL. Prehospital fluid resuscitation of the patient with major trauma. Prehosp Emerg Care 2002 6(1):81–91.
4. Barton ED, Epperson M, Hoyt DB, Fortlage D, Rosen P. Prehospital needle aspiration and tube thoracostomy in trauma victims: a six-year experience with aeromedical crews. J Emerg Med 1995 13(2):155–163.

5. Boyd M, Vanek VW, Bourguet CC. Emergency room resuscitative thoracotomy: When is it indicated? J Trauma 1992 33(5):714–721.
6. Brion S, Chang JC. Chest trauma. In Emergency Medicine Secrets, 5th ed., Markovchick VJ, Pons PT, Bakes KM, eds., pp. 596–602. St. Louis: Mosby, 2011.
7. Wolf SJ. Thoracic trauma. In The Paramedic, Chapleau W, Burba A, Pons PT, Page D, eds., pp. 415–437. Boston: McGraw-Hill, 2008.

Abdominal Trauma

Kelly Bookman, MD, and Lawrence Bookman, DO, FACEP

CHAPTER 59

1. **What mechanisms are considered "high risk" for significant blunt abdominal trauma?**
   High-speed motor vehicle collisions, rollover motor vehicle incidents, falls from a height of 6 feet or higher, blast injuries (blunt trauma associated with penetrating trauma), significant damage to vehicle, prolonged extrication time at the scene, death of another occupant in the vehicle, bent steering wheel, and ejection from vehicle are all high-risk mechanisms.

2. **What mechanisms of injury occur during blunt trauma?**
   The mechanisms of organ damage during blunt trauma are deceleration, compression, and shear. Deceleration causes abdominal contents to be damaged by a sudden change in velocity. Compression causes abdominal organs to be trapped between other structures, which results in rupture or burst injuries. Shear injuries occur when part of an organ can move while another part of the same organ is fixed (i.e., ligamentum teres wounds of the liver).

3. **What mechanisms of injury are associated with penetrating trauma?**
   The mechanisms of injury during penetrating trauma result from the dissipation of energy and tissue disruption along the path of the offending projectile. Injuries result in localized tears or contusions of involved organs along the path of the penetrating object, the magnitude of which depends on the penetrating object (knife or bullet), the force of penetration, and the trajectory.

4. **What information is necessary to provide to emergency department trauma care providers upon arrival after a blunt trauma?**
   You should paint a picture of the mechanism of injury that produced the trauma. The staff in the ED (nurses, emergency physicians, and trauma surgeons) should have a clear idea of exactly what happened to the patient. In cases of assault, describe what the patient was struck with and to what part of the body. If the patient fell, document how high the patient was and what the patient landed on. If the incident involved a car crash, describe the size of the vehicle, the speed and direction of impact, the visible damage to the patient's vehicle, the use (or nonuse) of lap and shoulder restraints, air bag deployment, the condition of the steering wheel, dashboard, and windshield, and the patient's location in the vehicle and after impact (i.e., was the patient ejected?). If photographs are allowed in your system, a picture of the vehicle is worth a thousand words.

5. **What information should I provide to the ED after penetrating trauma?**
   If the patient was a victim of penetrating trauma, report on the nature of the penetrating injury – gunshot wound versus stab wound. If known, describe the caliber of gun, the type of gun (high vs. low velocity), the trajectory of the projectile and the number and location of wounds. If the weapon was a knife, describe the size of the knife if possible, blood loss at the scene, and the number and location of wounds. If the knife is available for viewing at the scene, knowing the length and depth of blood on the blade can be helpful.

6. **Which organs are most likely injured in blunt abdominal trauma?**
   Blunt trauma usually involves solid organs such as the liver, spleen, and kidney. Hollow organs such as the bladder or bowel may rupture if compressed during the traumatic event. Signs of pain, distention, guarding, rebound, and rigidity are findings consistent with massive internal bleeding. It is important to remember that in abdominal trauma these symptoms may develop later in the course and if the patient is examined shortly after the traumatic incident, these signs may be absent, even in the face of significant intra-abdominal injury.

7. **Which organs are most commonly injured in penetrating trauma?**
   Penetrating trauma often injures a hollow viscus such as the stomach or intestines. Penetrating trauma may also involve the solid organs, major vascular structures, the diaphragm, heart, lungs, or spinal cord. These injuries may be very benign looking in their external appearance but can be catastrophic to the patient if unrecognized and untreated. All penetrating trauma must be evaluated in the ED.

8. **What is the most serious result of injury to solid organs or blood vessels?**
   The most serious result of injury to the solid organs or blood vessels is uncontrolled hemorrhage and ultimately exsanguination and death. The liver and spleen are highly vascular and can bleed profusely. Intraperitoneal hemorrhage can continue unchecked as the potential capacity of the peritoneal cavity exceeds the total blood volume.

9. **What problems result from injury to the hollow organs?**
   Rupture or perforation of the hollow organs (stomach, small and large intestines, gallbladder, and urinary bladder) can result in spillage of contents into the peritoneum cavity or retroperitoneal space, ultimately leading to infection, sepsis, and death.

10. **What do I look for when I examine the abdomen in a trauma patient?**
    Expose the patient and observe for evidence of penetrating trauma, bruising, distention, and other wounds. Abrasions, contusions (i.e., seatbelt sign), lacerations, or penetrating injuries should increase the suspicion of intra-abdominal injury. Abdominal distention, the presence of bluish discoloration of the skin in the periumbilical region (Cullen's sign) or flank (Grey–Turner's sign), and patients minimizing their movement to minimize pain may all be indicators of intra-abdominal injury. Palpate for tenderness, especially in the right and left upper quadrants, suggesting liver and spleen injuries, respectively. Palpate the pelvis and gently compress the iliac crests and pubic rami to look for tenderness and instability, indicating the likelihood of a pelvic fracture. Remember to repeat the abdominal exam serially if the mechanism of injury is consistent with possible significant trauma or if vital signs deteriorate.

11. **Which patients may have an unreliable or equivocal abdominal examination?**
    Patients with altered level of consciousness from intoxication, drug effects, or head injury are more challenging to assess for abdominal trauma. Patients with spinal cord injuries may have significant intra-abdominal pathology but no pain due to the interruption of sensory fibers. The young child or elderly patient may also present with minimal findings. On the other hand, patients with lower rib fractures and pelvic fractures may have tenderness in the upper and lower abdomen, respectively, without intra-abdominal injury.

12. **Do auscultation and percussion of the abdomen contribute significantly to the prehospital evaluation of the patient with suspected abdominal trauma?**
    Auscultation for bowel sounds or abnormal vascular sounds is difficult at best with the noise typically encountered in the prehospital setting and adds little to abdominal assessment. To truly determine that

Clinical Care

the patient has diminished bowel sounds, auscultation for several minutes is necessary—time that is better spent packaging the patient and initiating transport. Percussion to elicit pain may indicate peritonitis, but absence of pain does not exclude pathology.

13. **What are peritoneal signs?**
Peritoneal signs are clinical signs of irritation of the pain sensory nerves of the peritoneum, including pain that is elicited with palpation or percussion of the abdomen or with patient movement. Rebound tenderness is elicited by gentle deep palpation and rapid withdrawal of the hand with a positive finding being increased or elicited pain upon withdrawal of the examiner's hand. Patients may also have indirect tenderness, complaining of pain in a different location when one quadrant is palpated. They may also have both voluntary and involuntary guarding, resulting from tensing up of abdominal muscles.

14. **What is referred pain?**
Referred pain is pain that a patient feels in a part of the body that is remote to the injury site. This may be noted in cases of abdominal trauma when blood from a damaged organ irritates the diaphragm above. For example, an injured spleen can manifest as pain in the left shoulder (Kerr's sign). Similarly, an injured liver may present as pain in the right shoulder. Kidney damage may present with flank or groin pain and pancreatic injury may cause midthoracic back pain. Always pay attention to the possibility of intra-abdominal injury if a patient complains of pain in these classic areas without signs of external trauma to those areas.

15. **What if my patient is pregnant?**
All pregnant women involved in trauma need ED evaluation, particularly if the fetus is viable as the patient will need fetal monitoring for contractions. Remember that the fetus' blood flow depends on maternal blood flow; therefore, always attend to the mother first as the best care for the fetus is appropriate management of the mother. Signs of shock in the pregnant female may develop late in the course secondary to the physiologic increase in maternal blood volume during pregnancy. In the third trimester, it is important to keep the mother in a modified left lateral decubitus position to remove pressure on the inferior vena cava from the gravid uterus and help facilitate venous return to the heart.

16. **What if my patient is pediatric?**
Children are more susceptible to intra-abdominal injury because of the elasticity of the child's lower rib cage and the relatively large size of the abdominal cavity. Therefore you need to have a low threshold for bringing a child in to the ED for evaluation, even if the mechanism may seem unconcerning for an adult. Remember that children look good until they look bad. You should never be falsely reassured by normal vital signs in a child.

17. **What are some specific treatment issues with penetrating trauma?**
Cover open wounds with a dry sterile dressing and apply pressure if there is significant external bleeding. If there are abdominal contents protruding from an open wound, do not replace them back into the abdomen. Instead, cover the viscera with a normal saline–soaked dressing and then cover that with a bulky dry dressing. If there is an impaled object, stabilize it with bulky dressings and leave it in place.

18. **What interventions have been shown to be the most useful for the abdominal trauma patient in the prehospital setting?**
The key factors in the survival of severely injured abdominal trauma patients are limited to rapid transport to an appropriate trauma facility and aggressive airway control. Most recent studies show that patient evacuation should not be delayed to provide prehospital advanced life support interventions.

19. How do I fluid resuscitate the abdominal trauma patient?
Recent data about the best approach to treating "the trauma patient" recommend distinguishing between the mechanism of injury (blunt, penetrating, or thermal), the anatomic site of involvement (thoracic or abdominal, extremity, head injury) and the extent of that specific process (hemodynamically stable, unstable, or moribund). Traditionally, the approach to hypotension from internal hemorrhage has been to attempt to restore normal systemic blood pressure as soon as possible, even in the prehospital setting. The combination of a pneumatic antishop garment (PASG) or medical antishock trousers (MAST) and aggressive IV fluids was the standard of care up into the 1980s. Use of the PASG diminished dramatically after one study in the late 1980s that showed that there was no patient benefit to its use and perhaps worse outcomes. Recently aggressive IV fluid resuscitation has come under question as to its benefit prior to surgical control of hemorrhage. The specific concerns raised include acceleration of ongoing hemorrhage caused by the elevated blood pressure, mechanical dislodgement of clots being formed at the injury site, and dilution of clotting factors by the large volume of IV fluid. Therefore, each EMS system must have a protocol that describes the acceptable use of crystalloid fluid resuscitation in cases of traumatic injury. Current recommendations for fluid management of the trauma patient are to try to maintain systolic blood pressure at 80–90 mmHg, unless the patient has a concomitant traumatic brain injury, in which case a systolic blood pressure of at least 90 mmHg should be maintained.

Pearls and Pitfalls

1. Trauma of the lower chest should be considered to also have caused injury to the organs of the upper abdomen until proven otherwise.
2. Clinical signs of abdominal injury may be delayed until peritoneal irritation has developed, thus misleading the unwary prehospital provider.
3. Clinical signs of abdominal injury may be blunted or absent in patients with altered levels of consciousness (for any reason) or patients with spinal cord injury.
4. Peritoneal and retroperitoneal cavities are large enough to allow a patient to exsanguinate into them.
5. Although it is true that you are dealing with two patients when caring for an injured pregnant female, the best care for the fetus is appropriate management of the mother.

References

1. Fowler R, Pepe P. Prehospital care of the patient with major trauma. Emerg Med Clin N Am 20:953–974, 2002.
2. Wohlauer MV, Moore E. Abdominal trauma. In *Emergency Medicine Secrets*, 5th ed., Markovchick VJ, Pons PT, Bakes KA, eds., pp. 602–607. St. Louis: Elsevier, 2011.
3. Franklin G, Boaz P, Spain D, et al. Prehospital hypotension as a valid indicator of trauma team activation. J Trauma 48(6):1034–1039, 2000.
4. Parks J, Elliott A, Gentilello L, Shafi S. Systemic hypotension is a late marker of shock after trauma: A validation study of Advanced Trauma Life Support principles in a large national sample. Am J Surg 192:727–731, 2006.
5. Pepe PE, Mosesso VN Jr., Falk JL. Prehospital fluid resuscitation of the patient with major trauma. Prehosp Emerg Care 6:81–91, 2002.

Pelvic Trauma

CHAPTER 60

Jeffrey P. Salomone, MD, and Matthew Bitner, MD

1. **How can pelvic fractures be identified in the prehospital setting?**
   Except in rare circumstances when a victim has an open pelvic fracture with exposed bone ends, these fractures are often difficult to diagnose in the prehospital setting. A conscious patient may complain of pelvic pain, and pelvic tenderness may be elicited on palpation. More convincing evidence of a pelvic fracture is noticeable instability of the bony structures and crepitus when the pelvis is gently compressed. If instability is noted, the exam should not be repeated, as each compression of the pelvis may result in additional internal blood loss.

2. **How are pelvic fractures classified?**
   Pelvic fractures are classified into three types: pubic rami fractures, acetabular fractures, and pelvic ring fractures. Fractures of the pubic rami represent some of the most common pelvic fractures and are rarely unstable or associated with significant internal hemorrhage. Acetabular fractures usually occur when a force is applied to the femur, driving it into the hip joint. These injuries may be associated with internal hemorrhage and may require orthopedic surgery to stabilize the hip joint and regain function. Pelvic ring fractures tend to be the most worrisome, as they can be associated with both instability of the pelvis and potentially life-threatening internal hemorrhage.

3. **What are the types of pelvic ring fractures?**
   Although it is not universally used, the most commonly used system for classifying pelvic fractures is based on the mechanism of injury (Young and Burgess classification). The three major mechanisms are lateral compression, anterior-posterior compression, and vertical shear. Lateral compression injuries are the most common injury pattern seen, accounting for the majority (60–70%) of pelvic ring fractures. Lateral compression injuries are commonly found in side-impact collisions, pedestrians struck from the side by a vehicle, or when a person falls from a significant height, landing on their side. Anterior-posterior compression injuries account for about 15–20% of pelvic fractures and are unique in that they commonly involve disruption of only ligamentous structures (and possibly a few other small fractures such as pubic rami fractures). These fractures, also known as "open-book" fractures, result from forces being applied to the anterior and posterior aspects of the pelvis, such as when a victim is trapped between a vehicle and a brick wall. Vertical shear injuries to the pelvis, accounting for only 5–15% of pelvic fractures, occur when there is an asymmetrical vertical force applied to one of the hemipelvises. This often occurs when patients fall from a significant height or are ejected from a motor vehicle or motorcycle.

4. **What is an "open-book" pelvic fracture and why is it a serious problem?**
   An open-book pelvic fracture is a term commonly used to describe an anterior-posterior compression injury. As when you open a book and the two pages widen, in an anterior-posterior compression injury there is disruption of the sacroiliac (SI joints and the pubic symphysis), which results in widening or opening of the pelvic ring. This in turn increases the potential volume of the pelvis. This is a serious problem

because there is usually significant internal hemorrhage associated with the fracture and the resultant larger volume of space permits more blood loss before sufficient pressure builds up to tamponade the bleeding vessels.

5. **What is the most life-threatening condition potentially resulting from pelvic fractures?**
The prehospital provider must always associate pelvic fractures with the potential for life-threatening hemorrhage. Not only are there several major arteries that travel over the pelvic rim as they descend into the pelvis, but there are also large veins that may also be torn with any disruption in the pelvic structure. In addition to bleeding from injury to both pelvic arteries and veins, hemorrhage may also emanate from the marrow cavity of the fractured pelvis itself. Although not all pelvic fractures will result in severe internal hemorrhage, shock does represent a major cause of morbidity and mortality in patients with pelvic fractures, especially those of the pelvic ring. However, forces required to generate pelvic fractures may also result in the potential for massive internal hemorrhage from other organs as well, including the liver, spleen, kidney, and other internal structures.

6. **What other conditions may be associated with pelvic fractures?**
With significant trauma to the pelvis, all structures that lie within the ring may be subject to damage from either the forces that produced the fracture or from displaced bone fragments. Although hemorrhage represents the greatest immediate threat to life, sharp bone ends may result in injuries to the rectum, components of the urinary system, including the bladder and urethra, and internal reproductive organs in the female, and the scrotum and penis in males. The forces that produce a pelvic fracture may produce injuries to other parts of the body, including the brain, long bones, and structures in the thorax (lungs and aorta).

7. **How can severe hemorrhage from a pelvic fracture potentially be controlled in the prehospital setting?**
The prehospital care provider who is concerned about internal hemorrhage associated with a pelvic fracture should focus first on rapid packaging of the patient and expeditious transport to the closest appropriate facility capable of caring for such an injury, typically a Level I or II trauma center. Although this action may be sufficient in an urban setting with short transport times, when faced with longer transport times, the prehospital care provider has several options that may potentially help to control internal hemorrhage. One of the best options is use of the pneumatic antishock garment (PASG), indicated if a pelvic fracture is suspected and the patient is hypotensive (systolic blood pressure less than 90 mmHg). The garment is applied and then both leg compartments and the abdominal compartment are inflated. The pressure applied by the PASG may tamponade bleeding. For interfacility transports when a fracture has already been diagnosed, a pelvic binder, described below, should be considered. Finally, if neither device is available, a bedsheet, wrapped around the pelvis centered at the level of the greater trochanters and hip joints, may help stabilize fracture fragments.

8. **What is a pelvic binder?**
A pelvic binder is a commercially manufactured device for splinting/stabilizing a pelvic fracture. At the present time, three similar products are on the market: the pelvic binder, the T-POD (trauma pelvic orthotic device), and the SAM Pelvic Sling. Each device wraps around the pelvis and can be tightened to compress and splint a pelvic fracture. Because of the circumferential compression, the volume of the pelvis may be returned to normal, thereby decreasing the potential space for blood to collect. Although each device has

been studied in the in-hospital setting, no published studies exist showing improved outcome when used in the prehospital setting. When a pelvic fracture has been documented by X-ray, a pelvic binder may be considered if the patient is hemodynamically unstable.

9. **How can EMS personnel best move a patient with an unstable pelvic fracture?**
For the patient with a pelvic fracture that has unstable fracture fragments, each movement (such as turning with even a careful log-roll maneuver) may result in additional internal hemorrhage or injury to intrapelvic structures. These patients may be best splinted with the use of a scoop stretcher. Because this device splits in half, each half may be carefully slid underneath the patient and reconnected, resulting in a minimal amount of patient movement. A recent publication by Krell et al. suggests that the scoop stretcher was also associated with less movement of the spine compared to a standard long spine board.

Pearls and Pitfalls

1. Repeated exams of an unstable, compressible pelvis may lead to increased intra-abdominal hemorrhage.
2. Major internal hemorrhage is the most life threatening complication of pelvic fracture.
3. The forces applied to a patient that caused a pelvic fracture will commonly result in other major trauma as well.
4. Shock in patients with a suspected pelvic fracture may be treated in the field with a PASG or MAST (medical antishock trousers) suit as well as a bedsheet wrapped and tied snugly around the pelvis at the level of the hips.

References

1. American College of Surgeons. Abdominal trauma. In American College of Surgeons Committee on Trauma. Advanced Trauma Life Support for Doctors Student Course Manual, 8th ed., pp. 111–126. Chicago, IL: American College of Surgeons, 2008.
2. American College of Surgeons. Musculoskeletal trauma. In American College of Surgeons Committee on Trauma. Advanced Trauma Life Support for Doctors Student Course Manual, 8th ed., pp. 187–210. Chicago, IL: American College of Surgeons, 2008.
3. National Association of Emergency Medical Technicians. Musculoskeletal trauma. In PHTLS: Prehospital Trauma Life Support. 7th ed., Salomone JP, Pons PT, McSwain NE, Jr., eds., pp. 333–353. St. Louis, MO: Elsevier, 2011.
4. Kobziff L. Traumatic pelvic fractures. Orthop Nurs 25(4):235–241, 2006.
5. Koval K, Zuckerman J. Handbook of Fractures. New York: Lippincott Williams & Wilkins, 2002.
6. Krell JM, McCoy MS, Sparto PJ, et al. Comparison of the Ferno Scoop Stretcher with the long backboard for spinal immobilization. Prehosp Emerg Care 10(1):46–51, 2006.
7. Salomone JA, Salomone JP. Abdominal trauma, blunt. I: eMedicine Specialties: Emergency Medicine. (Accessed on June 5, 2011 at http://www.emedicine.com/emerg/topic1.htm)

Interpersonal Violence

Debra Houry, MD, MPH

CHAPTER 61

1. **Child abuse, intimate partner violence, elder abuse: are these health issues?**
   Yes. For these individuals experiencing abuse, injuries and illnesses as consequences of the abuse will affect their lives more frequently than most other medical conditions. In addition, several thousand individuals will die each year as a result of injuries from abuse. Interpersonal violence has tremendous health implications and is a signficant public health issue in the United States today.

2. **How common is child abuse?**
   Almost one million cases of child maltreatment are confirmed by child protective service agencies annually. Approximately 1500 children die each year as a result of abuse and children under the age of 4 years account for more than 75% of these fatalities. Up to 10% of pediatric emergency department (ED) visits are a result of child abuse.

3. **What are the categories of child abuse?**
   Child abuse can be divided into (a) physical abuse (also known as nonaccidental trauma or NAT), (b) emotional and psychological abuse, (c) sexual abuse, and (d) neglect. Of these, neglect is the most common and accounts for over 60% of cases, although most cases of maltreatment that you will encounter in the field will involve physical or sexual abuse.

4. **Why does child abuse occur?**
   Abuse of children is thought to have a multifactorial etiology. The three major factors are "right parent, right child, right day." Parents who abuse their children were often abused themselves and are poorly equipped to deal with day-to-day stress. Isolated parents with no support systems have an increased risk of being abusers. Children who require extra attention are at increased risk for abuse: fussy infants, developmentally delayed or physically disabled children, hyperactive children, or children with chronic diseases. Other factors associated with abuse include drug or alcohol abuse in the family, socioeconomic disadvantage, and increased stress due to financial problems, unemployment, and so forth.

5. **You are called to see a 6-month-old with a probable femur fracture. What historical factors should make you suspect child abuse?**
   The key to identifying physically abused children correctly is that the history of the injury is inconsistent with your physical examination. In this case, a nonambulatory child has no plausible way of fracturing his or her femur. Knowledge of basic developmental milestones (i.e., the age at which children roll over, sit up, and walk) is useful in matching injury with history.
   Other clues to child abuse include a history of minor trauma with extensive physical injury, injuries with no explanations, a history that changes over time, and delay in seeking treatment for a significant injury.

6. **What should I look for in examining a child in whom I suspect abuse?**
   First and foremost, examine the entire child if possible. (In older children, modesty and respect for the child's privacy may prevent you from performing a complete exam.) Bruises or injuries to the back and

buttocks are commonly seen in abused infants and may be missed if a diaper is not removed and a complete exam is not performed. Look for bruises, burns, bony tenderness or deformities, and facial and mouth injuries. You may see old, healing injuries or other injuries that are not consistent with the mechanism.

7. **Children get bumps and bruises all the time. I cannot suspect child abuse in every kid I see.**
   You are right. Some bruises should raise your suspicion of child abuse, however. Patterned bruises (from a strap, a loop or cord, or a hand), linear bruises, bruises in different stages of healing, and bruises in nonambulatory infants are possible indications of abuse. In addition, bruises from physical abuse often occur in atypical places: cheeks, neck or trunk, upper legs, or genitalia. Accidental bruises usually occur over a bony prominence such as the knees, tibias, elbows, chin, or forehead.

8. **What about trauma from burns? What are the characteristics of abusive burns?**
   Burns are frequently seen in abused children. Suspicious burns are those that are symmetric (both hands or feet), have clear lines of demarcation (e.g., the leg or arm was held in hot water), or are patterned (from a cigarette, iron, stovetop burner, and so forth). Splash burns and small superficial burns from touching hot objects are less likely to be associated with abuse.

9. **What is "shaken baby syndrome"?**
   Children who are victims of shaken baby syndrome are usually younger than 2 years (most are younger than 6 months). The child is forcibly and repeatedly shaken, resulting in intracranial injuries such as hemorrhage. Over 1000 cases are reported each year and close to one-third of these cases are fatal. Often, EMS is called because of an unresponsive child or a child with seizures.

10. **When should neglect be suspected?**
    EMS providers are the only health care workers who routinely evaluate patients in their home; this gives them the opportunity to observe their patient's living conditions. Neglect should be suspected when the home is unsanitary (with garbage, animal, or human excrement present) or has sleeping and living arrangements that are cold, dirty, or inadequate. There may be evidence of poor child supervision or supervision by another child. Neglected children are frequently undernourished and dirty, demonstrate poor personal hygiene, and may be inadequately dressed for the weather.

11. **What is the appropriate management of an abused child?**
    First and foremost, attend to the child's medical needs. Police intervention may be required if the parents of a child known or suspected to be abused are refusing care or transport of their child. Carefully document the home conditions, interactions between child and parent, all injuries, and your suspicion of abuse. Communication of your concerns to the hospital staff is critical. In addition, all states require that suspected child abuse be reported to a child welfare agency or the district attorney's office immediately. Check your local protocol regarding how this report should be filed.

12. **What is the definition of intimate partner violence?**
    Intimate partner violence (IPV) occurs between two persons currently in a relationship, or who have previously been in a relationship. This is not limited to married couples but also includes dating violence and same-sex couple violence. Partner violence can include emotional, physical, or sexual violence.

13. **What are the risk factors for partner violence?**
    Partner violence occurs in all socioeconomic classes and in all races. Women who are younger than 30 years of age and single, divorced, or separated may be at increased risk. Women with depressive

symptoms, suicidal thoughts, and drug or alcohol abuse may also have an increased assoication with intimate partner violence. It is unclear, however, if some of these "risk factors" lead to partner abuse or are a result of living in an abusive situation.

14. **What about male victims?**
Men can certainly be victims of partner violence, although most studies have demonstrated higher rates of violence against females. Men who are victims of partner violence have similar risk factors as female victims including drug or alcohol abuse and mental health symptoms. One study reported that men who present to the ED with injuries inflicted by their female partners have a high rate of partner violence perpetration.

15. **I know some of the women I treat have been battered by their partners. Why won't they tell me?**
Women may not reveal the abuse for a number of reasons. They may be embarrassed and humiliated that this is happening to them. There may be cultural or religious beliefs that lead the woman to believe that this is normal or to be expected. She may be worried about involving the police or she may have had bad experiences with the legal system previously. Perhaps her abuser has threatened to harm her, her children, or other loved ones if she discloses the abuse to others, or she may believe that no one can help her. In addition, it is important to discuss this issue in private; battered women may be afraid to disclose the abuse when their abuser is present.

16. **Are there some clues to partner violence that may be present in a patient's history?**
Most important, a history that is inconsistent with the physical exam findings should raise your suspicion for IPV. Also consider partner abuse in patients with threatened miscarriages (due to abdominal trauma), suicidal ideations or attempts, patients who are depressed or who show evidence of drug and alcohol abuse, and patients with frequent calls for chronic pain complaints. Victims may also use 911 services and may present more often on the night shift, as their partners may prevent them from accessing care.

17. **Describe the physical exam clues that may be present in a victim of PV.**
Common injury patterns include injuries to the face, neck, throat, chest, breasts, abdomen, and genitals. Any injury that does not fit the history obtained is also suspicious for abuse. Other suspicious physical exam findings include evidence of sexual assault or frequent, recurrent sexually transmitted diseases.

18. **How can I increase my recognition of partner abuse?**
First, ask about partner violence. Any woman with an injury should be specifically asked who injured her. Second, raise your level of suspicion in women without injuries. Remember the clues that might be present in the history or physical exam. If you think there may be partner abuse, ask about it.

19. **Give some examples of inappropriate comments or questions to ask women regarding partner violence.**
EMS personnel should be conscious of how they inquire about partner violence. Asking questions in a judgmental, accusatory, or humiliating way only compounds a difficult situation. Many victims are embarrassed about their situation and by blaming the victim you are continuing their humiliation. Common examples of statements or questions to avoid include the following. "What did you do that made him so mad?" "Why didn't you tell anyone?" "I wouldn't let anyone do that to me." "Why don't you just leave?"

Clinical Care

20. What do I do if my patient has an injury caused by her partner?

First, treat her injuries. Second, document her history and injuries carefully. Third, communicate your findings or suspicions to the hospital staff. Many hospitals have protocols to help victims access community resources and shelters if needed. In addition, mandatory reporting of partner violence to the police is required in some states. Some EMS agencies will provide a card with an IPV assistance telephone number on it (without any other identifier) to the victim. Although some patients will not use it, others may save the card and use it in a time of crisis. This "unidentified" telephone number is also safer to give the patient in the event the abuser was to find the card.

21. Name the types of elder abuse.

Abuse of the elderly includes physical and sexual abuse, emotional abuse, neglect, and material exploitation.

22. What historical information should make you concerned about elder abuse?

Similar to child abuse, an injury in an elderly person that is inconsistent with the history given should cause concern. Abused elders often delay in seeking medical care, miss medical appointments, or appear fearful of their caregivers.

23. What are the physical indications for elder abuse?

Multiple injuries in various stages of healing, inconsistent injuries, burns or bruises that are patterned or are in unusual locations, or decubitus ulcers (from not being moved or rotated).

24. What are the signs of neglect in an elderly person?

Elderly persons who are unkempt, dirty, or unshaven; those who have soiled, torn, stained, or bloody clothing; and those with evidence of malnutrition or dehydration may be victims of neglect.

25. You are called to see a debilitated, frail woman who is bedridden and aphasic. What attitudes or actions on the part of the caregiver would make you suspicious of abuse?

Elderly victims of abuse are frequently abused by their caregiver. Abusive caregivers may have an attitude of anger or indifference toward the elder; they may seem overly concerned about the cost of the medical care; or they may try to limit the victim's interaction with medical providers.

26. What is "self-neglect"?

Self-neglect is seen in a competent individual who is capable of caring for himself or herself yet refuses to do so or in an individual who is disabled yet refuses to accept assistance in basic activities of daily living. As long as the person retains decision-making capabilities and competence, he cannot be forced to accept assistance or placement into nursing facilities.

27. Do I have any legal responsibilities when caring for an abused patient?

Although the legal response varies, every state has legislation that provides for the protection of abused patients, prosecution of the perpetrators of abuse, and legal protection for those who are mandated to report suspected abuse. In many states, suspected elder abuse must be reported to adult social services in similar fashion to cases of suspected child abuse.

Pearls and Pitfalls

1. Always consider abuse in a child or elderly person if the mechanism of injury told to you by the caregiver doesn't make sense.

2. Remember to conduct as thorough a physical examination as possible. If you do not look for patterns of injury or old injuries, you may not diagnose abuse.
3. Some victims of partner violence will not disclose abuse unless you ask.
4. Women are most commonly the victims of IPV; however, IPV directed against men is not uncommon.

References

1. Abbott J, Johnson R, Koziol-McLain J, et al. Domestic violence against women: Incidence and prevalence in an emergency department population. JAMA 273:1763–1767, 1995.
2. Chang DC, Knight V, Ziegfeld S, et al. The tip of the iceberg for child abuse: The critical roles of the pediatric trauma service and its registry. J Trauma 57:1189–1198, 2004.
3. Department of Health and Human Services (DHHS) (US), Administration on Children, Youth, and Families (ACF). Child maltreatment 2003 [online]. Washington, DC: Government Printing Office; 2005. Available from: URL: www.acf.hhs.gov/programs/cb/pubs/cm03/index.htm. Accessed June 5, 2011.
4. Houry D, Kemball R, Rhodes KV, Kaslow NJ. Intimate partner violence and mental health symptoms in African American female ED patients. Am J Emerg Med 24:444–50, 2006.
5. Jones J, Dougherty J, Schelble D, et al. Emergency department protocol for diagnosis and evaluation of geriatric abuse. Ann Emerg Med 17(10):1006–1015, 1988.
6. Markenson D, Foltin G, Tunik M, et al. Knowledge and attitude assessment and education of prehospital personnel in child abuse and neglect: Report of a National Blue Ribbon Panel. Ann Emerg Med 40:89–101, 2002.
7. Muelleman RL, Lenaghan PA, Pakieser RA. Battered women: Injury locations and types. Ann Emerg Med 28(5):486–492, 1996.
8. Muelleman RL, Burgess P. Male victims of domestic violence and their history of perpetrating violence. Acad Emerg Med 5:866–870, 1998.

Thermal Burns

CHAPTER 62

Jeffrey S. Guy, MD, MSc, MMHC

1. **How do most adults and children get burned?**
   Nearly three-fourths of all unintentional burn deaths are as a result of house fires. Of this group, children and the elderly are the most likely victims. Alcohol and drug intoxication have been reported as contributing factors in as high as 40% of all house fires. Children are often burned from playing with matches, cigarette lighters, and other ignition devices. Injuries from accidental and intentional scalding are also common forms of burns in children. Approximately 20% of burns in children are the result of intentional burning or child abuse. The majority of children that are abused by burning are between the ages of 1–3 years old. The most common form of burn child abuse is forcible immersion.

2. **How are the layers of the skin related to the depth of injury?**
   The epidermis, or outermost layer of the skin, is damaged when a minor, first-degree injury such as sunburn occurs. This injury will heal quickly due to the regeneration of epithelial cells. The dermis, or second layer of the skin, contains appendages and organs such as nerve endings, hair follicles, sebaceous glands, and sweat glands. Consequently, when damaged, as in a second-degree burn, blisters form, and the tissue is hypersensitive and very painful. If infection is prevented, second-degree wounds usually heal within 3 weeks. Full-thickness, or third-degree burns, affect the epidermis, dermis, and subcutaneous tissue. These burns are often leathery, charred, and firm. Because the epithelial, or regenerative cells, are damaged these wounds do not heal spontaneously. Regeneration from the wound border, which causes severe scarring, or skin grafting is needed.

3. **Is there such an injury as a fourth-degree burn?**
   Yes. A fourth-degree injury not only destroys the three layers of the skin but also damages the deep underlying structures such as muscle and bone (Figure 62.1). This type of deep injury usually happens as a result of electrical injury or prolonged exposure to a heat source (e.g., a lower leg pinned under the exhaust pipe of a motorcycle for an extended time). Repair of this type of injury is sometimes impossible, and amputation may be required.

4. **What is the role of applying ice for treating a thermal burn?**
   Ice should never be applied to a burn. The initial priority after moving the patient to an area of safety and establishing airway, breathing, and circulation is to stop the burning process. To stop the burning, remove all of the patient's clothing and jewelry. Clothing may continue to smolder and jewelry may maintain residual heat and continue to burn the patient. Next, stop the burning process by application of copious amounts of room-temperature water. The application of ice may actually make any thickness burn worse by making the burn larger and deeper.

5. **How does ice make the burn worse?**
   A full-thickness burn has three zones. The central portion of the burn is called the *zone of coagulation*. In the zone of coagulation the burned tissues are necrotic and not capable of repair or healing. The outermost

Thermal Burns

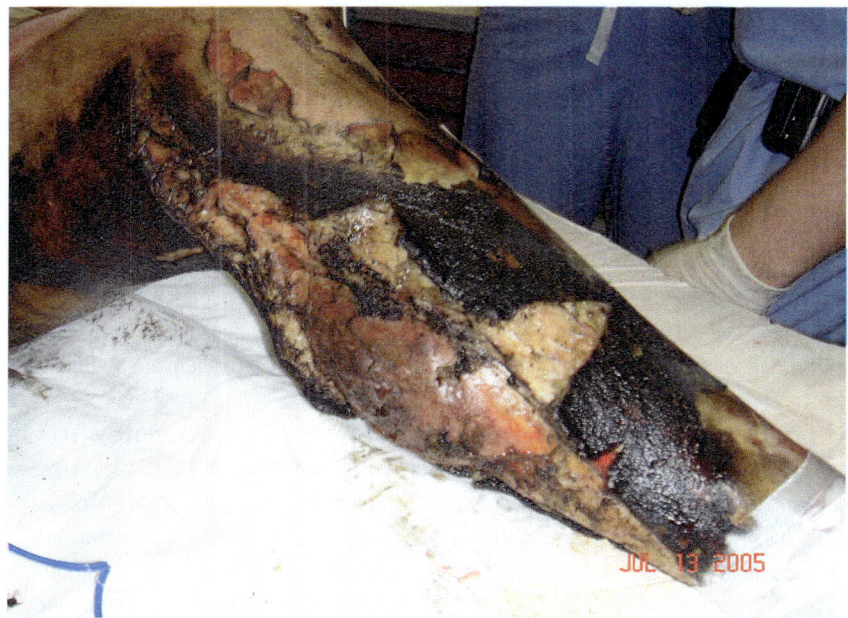

FIGURE 62.1 Fourth-degree (full-thickness) burn with extensive destruction to subcutaneous fat and muscle. (Photo courtesy of the author.)

zone is the *zone of hyperemia* and this zone has minimal cellular injury. This zone is characterized by increased blood flow from an inflammatory reaction secondary to the injury. In between these two zones is a region called the *zone of stasis*. The cells of this region are injured but are not irreversibly damaged. If they are provided with adequate blood flow and oxygen, these cells are capable of repair and healing. However, deprived of adequate blood flow and oxygen, these cells will die, and this region of tissue will die and become part of the zone of coagulation. When ice is applied to tissue, the blood vessels of that tissue will constrict, decreasing blood flow and decreasing oxygen delivery. The ice-induced vasoconstriction increases tissue damage in the vulnerable zone of stasis and thus increases the area of coagulation.

6. **Doesn't ice help provide pain relief?**
Ice does produce some relief of pain, but a more appropriate analgesic for the treatment of burn-related pain is a narcotic medication such as morphine. Preventing air from contacting the burn may also provide some relief of the patient's pain. In the case of partial-thickness burns, thousands of nerves are exposed. When air currents in the environment contact those exposed nerves the patient experiences pain. Therefore, keeping the burns covered will prevent air from contacting those nerves and hence reduce pain. Typically, the burns can be covered with a dry sterile dressing or burn sheet. Often wet dressings are placed on the burns. For certain types of chemical burns this is an appropriate method of dressing the wounds. However, wet dressings placed on a patient with large burns risks predisposing the patient to hypothermia.

Clinical Care

7. **What are some of the considerations and methods to secure an endotracheal tube in a patient who has burns to the face?**
   The most-dreaded and feared complication when caring and transporting a burn patient is the loss of the airway. Following burns to the face or inhalation of smoke, the patient's face as well as the upper airway will undergo considerable swelling and edema. A patient that can be intubated shortly after thermal injury may be difficult or impossible to intubate in a reasonably brief period of time. Therefore, the prehospital provider must take every precaution and measure to place and secure an endotracheal tube before the swelling occurs. Following a partial- or full-thickness face burn, the outer layer of the skin, the epidermis, will peel away. Therefore, any adhesive tape used to secure an endotracheal tube will also peel away and the tube will no longer be secured. Once the epidermal layer peels off, the remaining burned tissue weeps fluid that further prevents adhesives from sticking to the face. Therefore, methods to secure an endotracheal tube cannot rely on adhesive means. To secure the endotracheal tube adequately, the provider must rely on mechanical ties. Typically, one can use umbilical or cotton tape to tie an endotracheal tube in place. To provide additional security one should use two ties. One tie should circle the head above the ears, and the second tie should go around the head below the ears. In the absence of cotton ties, an adequate substitute is to use IV tubing to wrap around the head and secure the tube. Commercial devices are also available to secure endotracheal tubes that do not rely on adhesive means. Endotracheal dislodgement or accidental extubation is most likely to occur when moving or transferring the patient. Confirm correct placement of the endotracheal both before and after moving the patient into and out of an ambulance or moving from ambulance cot to hospital bed.

8. **Your unit is dispatched to an industrial setting for a patient who has chemical burns. When you arrive, the plant safety officer tells you that the patient has received a burn on the chest with sulfuric acid. What are some of the unique aspects to treatment of chemical burns?**
   The initial priority in the treatment of any emergency is scene and responder safety. This concept may almost be a cliché to some, but a cavalier attitude will result in further injury to the patient, unintentional injury to providers and bystanders, and contamination of emergency vehicles and hospital emergency departments (EDs). If required, don appropriate protective clothing and equipment. The patient's clothing is contaminated and should be handled as such. A common error is to transport the patient while he or she is still wearing the contaminated clothing or to carry the chemical laden clothes into the hospital ED, risking exposure to everyone in the receiving ED to the same chemical hazard. Make sure that the patient is as decontaminated as much as possible at the scene. Rapid decontamination is vital to reduce the magnitude of tissue destruction. If there is any particulate matter present, brush that material away. Remove any clothing, jewelry, or shoes. The best method to provide rapid decontamination is to irrigate the patient with large amounts of water. A common mistake is to stop irrigating after only a few liters of water or once the decontamination process starts to get messy. Strong acids are capable of contaminating large amounts of water. For example, 10 mL of 98% sulfuric acid will reduce the pH of 12 L of water down to 5.0. In the case of this patient, if the prehospital provider irrigates the affected area with a couple of 1-L bottles of water or saline, little has been done to decontaminate the patient, but now the area of the patient exposed to acid has actually been enlarged. Patients exposed to acid need to be irrigated with large amounts of water and care must be taken to control and drain the irrigant. If at all possible, measure the pH of the irrigation fluid flowing off the patient as an indicator of the effectiveness of the irrigation.

If the pH of the runoff fluid is 5.0 (neutral is 7.0) this would indicate that further decontamination is required. Neutralizing agents and chemicals are to be discouraged. Often, chemicals used to neutralize an acid or base generate heat during the neutralization reaction, thus adding a thermal injury to the chemical damage. Additionally, many neutralizing agents are often designed for the purpose of neutralizing equipment and machines, not personnel. Therefore, one should consult with medical control or a poison control center prior to applying a neutralizing agent.

9. **When I arrived on the scene, the plant safety officer told me to report to the cold zone. Can you tell me what that is?**

   Another element of treating victims of chemical burns or hazardous materials is to limit the spread of hazardous materials. To prevent the accidental spread of hazardous materials, the National Institute of Safety and Health (NIOSH) and the Environmental Protection Agency (EPA) have developed the use of control zones. Prehospital providers and rescue personnel should perform specified rescue or life-support activities in the specified zone. The three zones are best understood as three concentric circles, although in reality they are likely quite irregular in shape. The innermost zone is the hot zone, and the hot zone is the area immediately adjacent to the spilled chemical or hazmat incident. The objective of the rescuers in this region is to evacuate the injured patient prior to decontamination and with no patient care. The warm zone is the next region, and this is where patients should be decontaminated and a primary assessment and spine immobilization performed. Responders and providers working in both the hot and warm zones must wear personal protective equipment (PPE) appropriate for the chemical hazard. The outer zone is the cold zone, where rescue equipment and personnel are staged. In the cold zone, prehospital providers can deliver definitive care to the injured patient.

10. **Your unit is dispatched to a structure fire. You arrive and find that fire fighters have rescued a 21-year-old female from the fire. The patient is a young female who has already had her burned clothing removed. She has deep burns to the front of her chest, entire (circumferential) left arm, and entire (circumferential) left thigh. How would you quantify the magnitude or size of the burn?**

    In order to appropriately triage and fluid resuscitate a burn patient, the prehospital provider needs to estimate the extent of the patient's burns. The conventional method for reporting the size of burns is as a percentage of the patient's total body surface area. The most commonly used method of estimating burn size is the "rule of nines." This method uses the principle that for adults, major body regions are approximately 9% of the total body surface area. (Figure 62.2) Applying the rule of nines to the patient in the above scenario:

Anterior chest	=	9% total body surface area (TBSA)
Entire left arm	=	9% TBSA
Entire left thigh	=	9% TBSA
Total burn	=	27% TBSA

    The proportion of the major body regions of children is significantly different than adults. For example, infants have proportionally large heads and smaller legs. As the child grows, the legs proportionally become large and the head becomes proportionally less of the child's TBSA. Because these proportions change as the child grows, the rule of nines is not applicable to children. Other tools used to estimate

Clinical Care

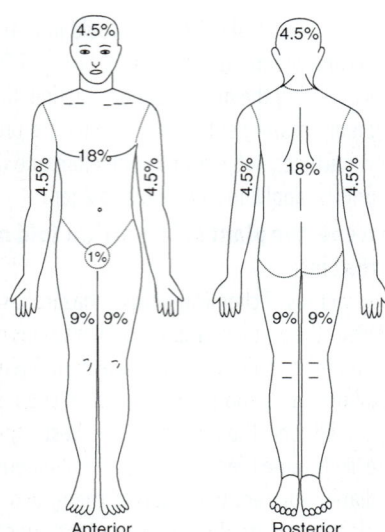

FIGURE 62.2 For purposes of estimating the extent of burns in adults, the "rule of nines" is used.

burn size in children include a Lund–Browder chart. This tool uses diagrams and reference tables to determine burn size.

Lund–Browder Chart
(relative percentage of body surface area affected by growth)

Age in Years	0	1	5	10	15	Adult
A-head (back or front)	$9^{1}/_{2}$	$8^{1}/_{2}$	$6^{1}/_{2}$	$5^{1}/_{2}$	$4^{1}/_{2}$	$3^{1}/_{2}$
B-1 thigh (back or front)	$2^{3}/_{4}$	$3^{1}/_{4}$	4	$4^{1}/_{4}$	$4^{1}/_{2}$	$4^{3}/_{4}$
C-1 leg (back or front)	$2^{1}/_{2}$	$2^{1}/_{2}$	$2^{3}/_{4}$	3	$3^{1}/_{4}$	$3^{1}/_{2}$

11. **Does it really matter if we estimate the extent of burn in the prehospital setting?**
    Yes, but not at the expense of delaying transport. Accurate estimation of TBSA burned is necessary first to determine appropriate prehospital destination and later to help guide the initial fluid resuscitation. Several simple methods can be used to determine the TBSA, most commonly the Rule of 9s already mentioned.

12. **What is the Lund–Browder Chart?**
    Probably the most accurate of the various burn charts but the hardest to use. Save this one for the ED or the intensive care unit.

13. **Besides the depth and extent of the burn, is there anything else I should be looking for when I evaluate a burn?**
    Yes, look at the shape of the burn for any recognizable patterns such as cigarette marks, clothing irons, or forced immersion. Recognizable shapes and patterns are an important clue to the possibility that the burns were not accidental but rather the result of abuse (Figure 62.3).

Thermal Burns

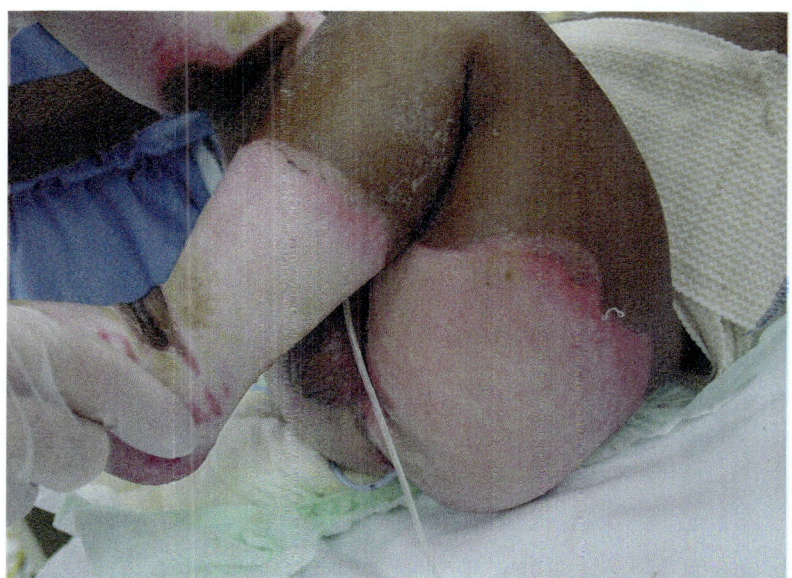

FIGURE 62.3 Third-degree burns in a child following a forcible-immersion scald burn. (Photo courtesy of the author.)

14. What is the clinical significance of a circumferential third degree burn of a limb or chest?

Circumferential third-degree burns of a limb are a surgical emergency. Following a full-thickness burn injury, the layers of the skin will become thick and nonelastic, much like leather. Additionally the burn will contract. Simultaneously, the tissue deep to the skin (fat and muscles) will start to become edematous and swell. The nonelastic nature of the burns makes no allowances for the deeper swelling and results in pressure on the arteries and veins of the extremity. The venous pressure is typically very low (e.g., 5–7 mmHg), and the veins are easily compressed and occluded. The pressure of the blood inside the arteries is much higher (e.g., mean arterial pressure of 60 mmHg); therefore, the arteries remain open pumping blood into the collapsed veins. This causes worsening of the swelling to the point where eventually the pressure increases enough that the arteries also become compressed. This creates limb ischemia. To avoid this complication, the patient requires an emergent operation called an escharotomy within a few hours following a circumferential burn of the extremity to split open the leatherlike eschar and allow for swelling (Figure 62.4).

A circumferential full thickness burn of a chest can similarly create a life-threatening respiratory condition. As the burn eschar contracts and the underlying tissue swells, the compliance of the chest wall dramatically decreases to the point where the patient will develop respiratory embarrassment. This situation is similar to having leather belts tightened around one's chest to the point where one is not capable of inhaling a breath. If the patient is being ventilated with a bag and endotracheal tube, pulmonary compliance can decrease to the point where the patient cannot be mechanically ventilated. Escharotomies made on the chest wall will allow it to expand with inspiration.

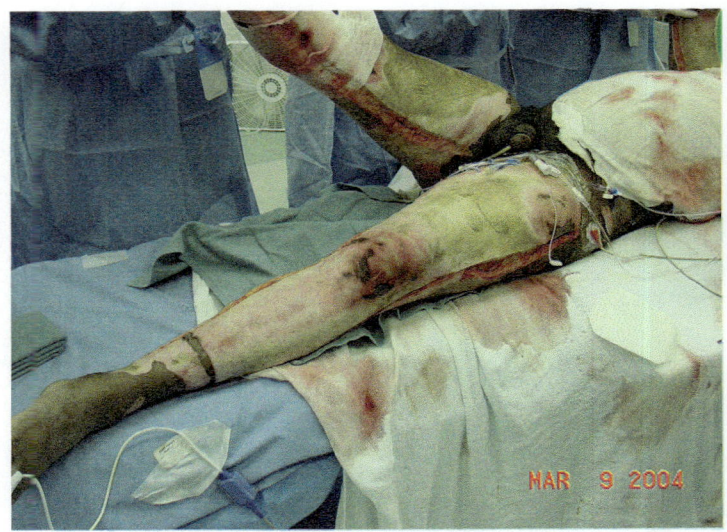

FIGURE 62.4 Circumferential third-degree burns of the legs with escharotomies. (Photo courtesy of the author.)

15. **Your unit is called to a construction site where a crane operator accidentally came into contact with some overhead high-tension wires with the boom crane. The patient is complaining of numbness in both of his hand and arms. You observe deep, full-thickness burns on both of his palms as well as the sole of his left foot. What are some of the unique considerations of treating patients with electrical burns?**

Electrical burns can be very misleading to the untrained provider. A patient may often have only small areas of visible burns to the skin and hence seem to have suffered only minor injuries (Figure 62.5). However, when one experiences an electrical injury, the current enters the body and travels through the tissues deep to the skin to another point on the body where the electrical current exits from the body. As the current passes through the body, it creates significant tissue damage. By evaluating cutaneous or skin injuries only, the provider will underestimate the magnitude of the injury.

When a patient is injured in an electrical incident, the muscles may become damaged, releasing potassium and a molecule poisonous to the kidneys, myoglobin (Figure 62.6). The release of potassium from the damaged muscle may produce a dangerous condition of elevated potassium (hyperkalemia). Hyperkalemia increases the likelihood of complications from pharmacological-assisted intubation with the depolarizing muscle relaxant, succinylcholine. To prevent a patient from going into renal failure, the patient should be vigorously fluid resuscitated.

In addition, many large muscle groups will experience sustained muscle contraction known as tetany. The magnitude of these contractions is capable of causing dislocations (most commonly of the shoulders), fractures of long bones as well as bones of the spine. For these reasons, patients who have suffered an electrical injury should undergo full spine immobilization. Other acute complications from electrical injuries include: cardiac dysrhythmias or conduction abnormalities, intracranial hemorrhage, and spinal cord injuries.

Thermal Burns

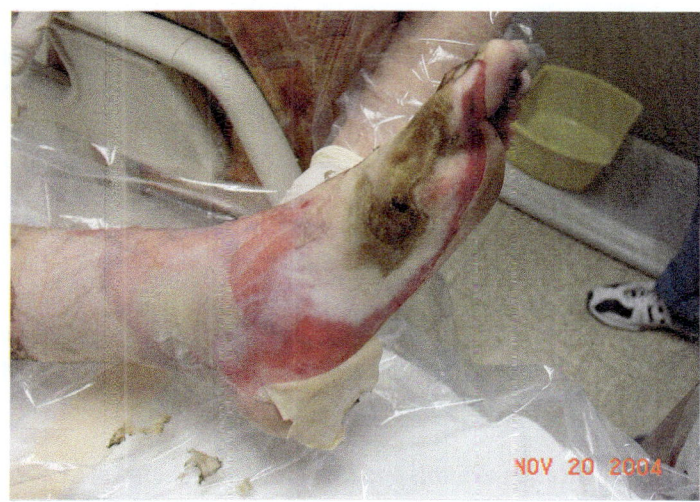

FIGURE 62.5 Full-thickness electrical contact burn of the foot. (Photo courtesy of the author.)

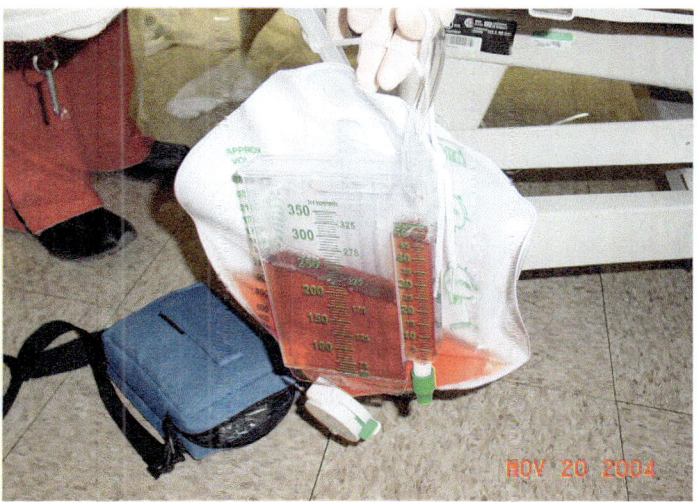

FIGURE 62.6 Red-coloration from myoglobin in the urine in a patient following electrical injury. (Photo courtesy of the author.)

Patients who have electrical injuries may also sustain large areas of cutaneous burns without having conducted electrical current through the body. These types of injuries are commonly the result of electrical arc flash injuries. Electrical arc flash injuries occur when an electrical flash, similar to a bolt of lightning, superheats the air around the patient as much as several thousand degrees. This can cause extensive burns to the patient and even ignite or melt the victim's clothes.

Clinical Care

16. Do patients commonly get burns of the respiratory tract?

No. The respiratory tract is very efficient at cooling down (or warming up) the air we breathe. Consequently, the trachea, bronchi, and alveolar sacs are quite well protected from heated air. Superheated air saturated with water—steam—is a whole different situation. Because the water can carry as much as 200 times more heat than air, steam can cause significant damage to air passageways and lung parenchyma. The respiratory complications of burns generally result from inhaling the toxic products of combustion, resulting in pneumonia or pulmonary edema. Respiratory complications are the major cause of death in thermal injuries. Half of the patients will be dead at the scene.

17. How do you manage inhalation injuries in the field?

All patients with burns should receive high-flow oxygen (preferably humidified) via nonrebreather by reservoir mask or endotracheal tube. Patients with the signs and symptoms of inhalation injury and upper airway obstruction such as stridor should be intubated before edema in the upper airway causes total obstruction.

18. Describe the classification of burns and its impact on prehospital care.

The classification of burns may seem purely academic, but it is not. These classifications can help the prehospital provider and the receiving ED with appropriate triage and destination decisions. According to the American Burn Association (ABA), major burns should be treated at a burn center; moderate burns can be adequately managed in a general hospital; and minor burns are treated on an outpatient basis.

Classification of Burns

Minor Burn Injuries	Moderate Uncomplicated Burn Injuries	Major Burn Injuries
Partial-thickness burns over < 10% adult total body surface area (TBSA) or < 5% TBSA in patients <10 or >50 years of age.	Partial-thickness burns over 10–20% adult TBSA or 5–10% TBSA in patients <10 or >50 years of age.	Partial-thickness burns over >20% adult TBSA or >10% TBSA in patients <10 or >50 years of age.
Full-thickness burns of ≤ 2%	Full-thickness burns of <2–5% TBSA	Full-thickness burns involving ≥5% TBSA
No functional or cosmetic risk to areas of specialized function, such as the eyes, ears, face, hands, feet, or perineum	No functional or cosmetic risk to areas of specialized function, such as the eyes, ears, face, hands, feet, or perineum	All burns involving eyes, ears, face, hands, feet, or perineum that may result in functional or cosmetic impairment
	All burns in immunocompromised or debilitated individuals	All inhalation injuries
	Suspected inhalation injury	High-voltage electrical burns
		All burns complicated by fractures or other trauma

19. What are some of the home remedies used on burns? Are they acceptable?

Many bad and some good home remedies are used on burns. Anything from butter to toothpaste or lard to bacon fat has been put on burns. Regretfully, these home remedies usually just contaminate the wound and make it impossible to assess the depth of injury. Petroleum jelly, burn cream, and antibiotic ointments are also used and, although contamination is not as bad, visual assessment remains difficult and in most cases these remedies will be removed immediately upon arrival to the hospital at a cost of increased discomfort for the patient. Clean water is still the best home and prehospital treatment.

20. Describe priorities in the care of a minor burn.

(a) Be sure the mechanism of injury correlates with the visible injury. Don't overlook the potential for something more serious, such as child abuse.
(b) Stop the burning process, or immerse the burned area in cool clean water.
(c) Do not apply any ointments or home remedies.
(d) Leave blisters intact.

21. How much fluid is needed to begin resuscitation of the burn-injured patient?

Large, even massive, amounts of intravenous fluids are needed to resuscitate the severely burned patient. The Parkland formula is the most universally accepted formula used to initially guide fluid resuscitation:

4 mL Ringer's lactate/kg body weight/% TBSA burned in the first 24 hours
$1/2$ administered in the first 8 hours
$1/2$ administered in the next 16 hours

The foregoing amount calculated is for use over 24 hours; thus, massive volume infusion in the prehospital setting is almost never needed.
A simpler formula is recommended by the ABA for prehospital use:

Over 15 years of age: 500 mL per hour
5–15 years of age: 250 mL per hour
Under 5 years of age: no IV

22. I have heard something called the "Rule of 10s" for fluid administration. What is that all about?

The Rule of 10s was developed by the military. The hourly requirement for fluid replacement in a burn patient can be approximated by multiplying the %TBSA burned by 10 mL. This formula works well for patients who weigh between 40 and 80 kg. For every 10 kg of body weight over 80 kg, add 100 mL to the calculated hourly volume.

23. How should pain be addressed?

The pain associated with burns can be excruciating. Covering the wound and elevating the extremities will begin to help. However, appropriate amounts of narcotics such as morphine are typically needed to manage the pain. To provide an appropriate amount of analgesia will often require large doses of narcotics that may exceed standard protocols. Be sure to monitor the blood pressure and respiratory status.

Clinical Care

24. Is hyperbaric oxygen useful in burns?

The use of hyperbaric oxygen (HBO) therapy in the management of the burn victim is controversial. Carbon monoxide (CO) toxicity with associated burn injury is different from an isolated CO inhalation. Treatment of carbon monoxide toxicity is removal from the source and administration of oxygen. When breathing room air (i.e., 21% oxygen), the body will eliminate half of the CO in 250 minutes. When the patient is placed on 100% oxygen, the half-life of the carbon monoxide–hemoglobin complex is reduced to 40–60 minutes and it is further reduced to approximately 20 minutes in a hyperbaric chamber. However, it is often hazardous to place patients with a large burn into an HBO chamber, as any complications are difficult, if not impossible, to manage inside a chamber. Also with the large amount of mucus plugging in a patient with severe smoke inhalation, the lungs can be damaged when returning back to normal pressures.

25. What is the difference between a surgical intensive care unit and a burn ICU? Does it matter where the patient is admitted?

Both surgical ICUs and burn ICUs are staffed by highly qualified specialists. Burn patients are very labor intensive and require specialized nursing and therapy that are not available in nonburn centers. The objectives in the treatment of the burned patient is not only to save life and limb but to return the patient back to a functional status. Without the specialized nurses and therapists, patients may survive but will not be able to resume a normal life style.

Injuries Requiring a Referral to a Specialized Burn Facility after Initial Assessment and Treatment at an ED

Partial thickness burns >10% TBSA

Burns that involve the face, hands, feet, genitalia, perineum, and major joints

Full-thickness burns

Electrical burns, including lightning injury

Chemical burns

Inhalation injury

Circumferential burns of the extremity and chest

Burn injury in patients with preexisting medical disorders that could complicate management, prolong recovery, or affect mortality

Hospitals without qualified personnel or equipment for the care of children should transfer burned children to a burn center with these capabilities

Any burn patient with concomitant trauma (e.g., fractures) in which the burn injury poses the greatest risk of morbidity or mortality. However, if the trauma poses the greater immediate risk, the patient may be treated in a trauma center initially until stable before being transferred to a burn center. Physician judgment will be necessary in such situations and should be in concert with the regional medical control plan and triage protocols.

Adapted from American Burn Association. Criteria for Burn Center Referral. www.ameriburn.org. Accessed November 11, 2011.

Pearls and Pitfalls

1. Early intubation is crucial to avoiding airway compromise from edema after burn injury to the face, neck and airway.
2. Large-volume fluid resuscitation is generally not needed in the prehospital setting except in cases of delayed or prolonged transport.
3. Use of cool or cold water to stop continued burning or to provide comfort can lead to hypothermia.
4. Narcotic analgesics will be necessary to relieve pain in burn patients.
5. Burns in recognizable shapes and patterns suggest abuse and intentional injury.
6. Looking only at the obvious wounds from an electrocution injury may lead to underestimating the severity of the injury.

References

1. Bromberg BF, Song IC, Walden RH. Hydrotherapy of chemical burns. Plast Reconstr Surg 35:85–95, 1965.
2. Chadwick DL. The diagnosis of inflicted injury in infants and young children. Pediatr Ann 21:477–483, 1992.
3. Hight DW, Bakalar HR, Lloyd JR. Inflicted burns in children: Recognition and treatment. JAMA 242:517–520, 1979.
4. Leonard LG, Scheulen JJ, Munster AM. Chemical burns: Effect of prompt first aid. J Trauma 22:420–423, 1982.
5. Mozingo DW, Smith AD, McManus WF, et al. Chemical burns. J Trauma 28:642–647, 1998.
6. Olshaker JS, Tek D. Environmental emergencies. Emerg Med Clin North Am 10:211–475, 1992.
7. Robinson MC, Del Becarro EJ. Increasing dermal perfusion after burning by decreasing thromboxane production. J Trauma 20:722–725, 1980.
8. Rosen CL, Adler JN, Rabban JT, et al. Early predictors of myoglobinuria and acute renal failure following electrical injury. J Emerg Med 17:783–789, 1999.

Pediatrics

SECTION VI

Chapter 63
Assessment of the Pediatric Patient — 417
Katie M. Bakes, MD

Chapter 64
Field Approach to Infants and Children — 422
Julie Scadden, NREMT-P, PS

Chapter 65
Seizures in Children — 429
Jeffrey J. Messerole, PS

Chapter 66
Respiratory Distress in Infants and Children — 439
James A. Temple, BA, NREMT-P, CCP

Chapter 67
Pediatric Trauma — 450
Robert W. Schafermayer, MD, FACEP, FIFEM, FAAP

Chapter 68
Child Abuse and Nonaccidental Trauma — 456
Nicholas C. Johnson, MD

Assessment of the Pediatric Patient

Katie M. Bakes, MD

CHAPTER 63

1. **What is the best way to begin the assessment of the pediatric patient in the field?**
   The pediatric assessment triangle (PAT) emphasizes the three important elements in field assessment of the pediatric patient: appearance, work of breathing, and circulation to the skin (see Figure 66.1, page 440). A child's anxiety and fear of strangers makes their evaluation difficult under the best of circumstances. This fear is only heightened by illness or injury. Unless there is a clear life-threatening situation present, taking time to assess a child from a distance of a few feet can minimize the child's fear and make subsequent evaluation less frightening. Try to put yourself at or below the eye level of the child. A great deal of information can be gathered by simply assessing a child's behavior and appearance before touching him or her. Whenever feasible, a child should not be separated from his parents or other familiar adults. It is always a good idea to examine children in a "toes-to-head" format rather than the traditional "head-to-toes" approach, as this is less threatening to the child, and whenever possible, examine the area of concern last, after you have established trust.

2. **How are vital signs different in children?**
   Vital signs are of paramount importance in children just as in adults. However, the normal ranges for children vary by age. In general, as the child grows, the heart rate and respiratory rate decrease and blood pressure increases, approaching normal adult ranges around the age of 12. For example, a pulse of 150 beats/min, respirations of 45 breaths/min and a blood pressure (BP) of 73/45 mmHg would be perfectly normal in a 2-month-old infant but constitute profound shock in a 10-year-old child. A general rule of thumb is that the average systolic BP for children ages 1–10 years is $90 + (2 \times age)$ and the lower 5th percentile is $70 + (2 \times age)$. A systolic BP less than 60 is abnormal for an infant. Normal pulse oximetry and temperature ranges are the same as for adults.

3. **What are some unique features of the pediatric airway?**
   Compared to the adult airway, the pediatric airway is more anterior and cephalad, more flexible, and narrower. The pediatric airway is also more funnel-shaped with the criccid being the narrowest part and providing a natural seal, which obviates the need for a cuffed tube for children under the age of 8 years. The epiglottis is large and omega-shaped, necessitating the use of a straight blade during intubation to lift it up to visualize the vocal cord. The tongue and adenoid tissues are also more prominent in children.

4. **What is the priority in managing the pediatric airway?**
   If the child is maintaining his or her airway despite the presence of audible stridor, leave them in a position of comfort and do not instrument or agitate them. Trying to forcefully alter the position of a child with an impending upper airway obstruction could lead to rapid deterioration and the need for an emergent surgical airway. Any maneuvers or inspection should be done in a controlled hospital setting.
   In the pediatric population, being proficient at bagging is more important than knowing how to intubate. Good bagging necessitates using the "EC" technique: E with the middle, ring, and pinky fingers placed

along the jaw line and the thumb and index finger forming a C around the mask. Furthermore, bringing the face up to the mask instead of pushing the mask down toward the face will prevent one from easily compressing or kinking the child's upper airway. Say "squeeze, release, release" to yourself as you bag to time the ventilation rate appropriately, as overbagging is a common cause of barotrauma in the pediatric population.

5. **What is unique about the head of infants and young children that impacts their care when they are critically ill or injured?**
Children younger than 3 years old have a relatively large occiput compared to older children and adults. This difference causes flexion of the neck and subsequent airway obstruction when the child is lying on a flat surface. Hence, gentle extension of the neck using a head–tilt–chin lift maneuver opens the airway. Infants may require that a towel be placed under their shoulders for proper airway axes alignment. If cervical spine trauma is suspected, a jaw thrust replaces the head tilt so that spinal precautions are maintained. Children with respiratory distress or who require bag–mask ventilation will breathe more effectively with these maneuvers.

6. **What are the most common dysrhythmias seen in children?**
Dysrhythmias are generally uncommon in children. Supraventricular tachycardia (SVT) is the most common pediatric dysrhythmia, with heart rates in infants greater than 220 beats/min. Older children and adolescents in SVT will generally have a heart rate over 180 beats/min. Because of their ability to tolerate tachycardia well, children in SVT are usually stable initially and can remain so for the duration of hospital transport in the urban or suburban setting.
The most common *immediately life-threatening* dysrhythmia is sinus bradycardia and is usually the result of hypoxia. Any child demonstrating sinus bradycardia and signs of shock requires aggressive attention to oxygenation with high-flow oxygen and bag–mask ventilation if needed. Bradycardia that does not respond to increased oxygen delivery mandates epinephrine therapy.

7. **How should I interpret tachycardia in the pediatric patient?**
Tachycardia is a frequent finding in children. Pain, fever, anxiety, and fear often lead to substantial increases in heart rate. However, tachycardia is often the first sign of serious illness such as sepsis, severe dehydration, or hemorrhage. Any elevation of heart rate, especially in the absence of confounding factors such as those above, should alert the EMS provider to the presence of a potentially serious illness or injury. Hypotension is a very late and ominous finding in shock in children. As children exhaust their considerable ability to increase cardiac output by increasing heart rate, they are very close to cardiovascular collapse as their ability to increase cardiac contractility is quite limited.

8. **Where are the best places to feel for pulses?**
Infants' pulses are best felt in the brachial or femoral artery areas, whereas children's pulses are more readily palpated in the carotid and femoral artery areas. When a neonate is in shock, pulses should be palpated in all four extremities, as this may provide a clue to an underlying cardiac defect such as a coarctation of the aorta in which lower extremity pulses are often weaker.

9. **How should I assess circulation in the pediatric patient?**
Capillary refill (CR) time is assessed by pressing a thumb to the bottom of the foot, kneecap, or forearm for 3 seconds and then releasing. A normal CR time is less than 3 seconds and anything over this may indicate a state of shock. Diminished urine output, tachypnea, and altered mental status are signs of compromised end-organ perfusion.

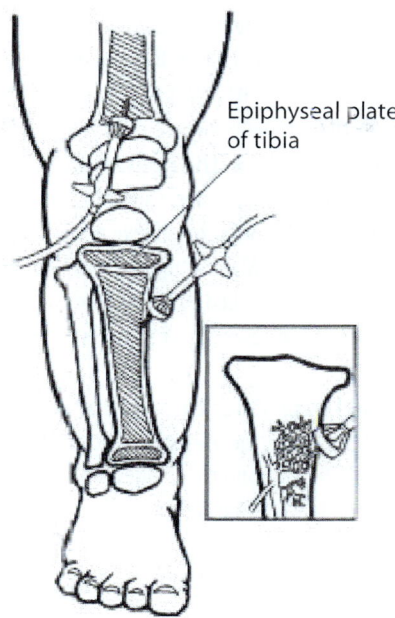

FIGURE 63.1   Intraosseous infusion into the tibia or femur.

10. **How should I approach circulation support in the field?**
    Intravenous access is often difficult to obtain in children. Scoop and go with critical pediatric patients and try IV access en route, but do not wait for an IV to transport. Consider intraosseous access in critical patients. The upper part of the tibia is the preferred site. (Figure 63.1) For the tibia, the needle is directed toward the foot to avoid the growth plate at the knee.

11. **What are signs of respiratory distress in children?**
    Nasal flaring and mild retractions (usually supraclavicular) may be subtle in children and should be carefully assessed from a distance. As distress heightens, grunting and substernal or intercostal retractions develop, with or without abdominal breathing. Finally, central or perioral cyanosis and altered mental status herald an impending respiratory arrest.

12. **Is the examination of the abdomen different in children?**
    No. However, remember that the abdominal musculature in children is thinner, thus the organs are less protected. Furthermore, with the shorter bony thorax, the liver and spleen are not completely covered by the ribs. Use gentle pressure to examine the abdomen and palpate the liver and spleen. Deep palpation is rarely necessary and will often give misinformation, as the normal child will resist these efforts. Try distraction techniques, leaving the child on the parent's lap or in their arms. If intense stranger anxiety exists, consider having the parent palpate the abdomen while you observe.

13. **How is assessment different in the pediatric trauma victim?**
    The child's body is like a dart, with any impact likely resulting in head injury. For example, Waddell's triad occurs when a child is struck by a motor vehicle, usually first on the lower extremity, sustaining a

femur fracture, then abdominal or chest trauma and finally concomitant head injury. Also, because the bony structures of children are more pliable than those of an adult, intrathoracic or intra-abdominal injury may be less apparent externally. The EMS provider should always be suspicious of significant injury in the setting of a high-risk mechanism.

14. **How do I protect the cervical spine in the injured child?**
Because of the anatomic differences of a young child's head and neck, some variation is required to protect the child's cervical spine. In order to achieve a neutral position, place one or two folded blankets under the back and shoulders. Many ambulances are not equipped with appropriately sized cervical collars for children. Two tightly rolled towels placed on either side of child's head with tape securing the forehead and chin and towels to a spine board provides improvised spinal motion restriction.

15. **What information should I note about the scene of any pediatric patient?**
In a home, note the state of the home, the presence of other children, and the degree of safety and supervision of those children. If there is concern for ingestion, get information about what medications and household chemicals are in reach of the child, including over-the-counter medications, vitamins, and herbal remedies. At any scene of injury, and if the patient's condition allows, attempt to visually reenact the events of the injury.

16. **How do I assess pain in children?**
Because young children have limited or no vocabulary, and they may become unwilling to respond to strangers when injured or ill, other clues to pain become important. Tachycardia is common, as are changes in facial expression. Guarding of an injured or painful body part may go unnoticed if you are not looking for them. Children tend to be able to understand much more than they can express verbally. For younger children, scales using pictures of painful expressions can help children indicate the severity of their pain (see Figure 63.2).

17. **What do I do if a parent refuses the transport of an ill or injured child?**
Parents have the right to refuse medical care, even lifesaving care for their child. However, there are legal limits on this right. If the child appears critically ill or injured, your duty is to get the child to appropriate medical care. The medical director or medical control for your EMS system has the responsibility to aid in deciding which patients need transport for emergency care. If the parents physically attempt to prevent you from treating the child, enlist the help of law enforcement to create a safe environment in which to work so that you can focus on the care of the child. Consider that a parent

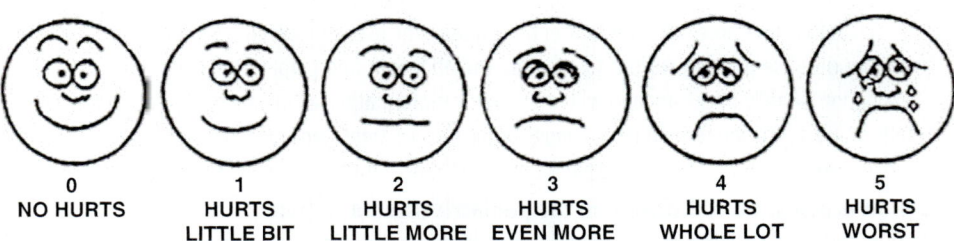

FIGURE 63.2   Pediatric pain rating scale. (Wong-Baker FACES Scale)

may be refusing care because the child is the victim of abuse. All medical personnel are mandated by law to report their suspicions of child abuse to the authorities.

Pearls and Pitfalls

1. The key to assessing a child is using the PAT, which evaluates three elements: the overall appearance of the child, the work of breathing, and the child's circulation.
2. When examining a child, use a "toes-to-head" approach rather than the traditional "head-to-toes" format and evaluate the area of concern last.
3. Be familiar with the differences in normal vital signs based on the patient's age.
4. If a child is maintaining their airway, regardless of the presence of abnormal sounds such as stridor, resist the urge to manage the airway with intubation.
5. The most common life-threatening cardiac dysrhythmia is sinus bradycardia and is usually the result of hypoxia.

References

1. American College of Pediatrics; American College of Emergency Physicians. Patient- and family-centered care and the role of the emergency physician providing care to a child in the emergency department. *Ann Emerg Med* 48(5): 643–645, 2006.
2. Fuchs S, Gausche-Hill M, Yamamoto L, eds. APLS: The Pediatric Emergency Medicine Resource, 4th ed. Sudbury MA: Jones and Bartlett, 2004.
3. Erickson TB, Thompson TM, Lu JJ. The approach to the patient with an unknown overdose. *Emerg Med Clin North Am* 25:249–281, 2007.
4. Gausche M. Effect of out-of-hospital pediatric endotracheal intubation on survival and neurological outcome: a controlled clinical trial. *JAMA* 283(6): 783–790, 2000.
5. Orenstein JB. Prehospital airway management. *Clin Pediatr Emerg Med* 7(1):31–37, 2006.
6. Barkin R, ed. Pediatric Emergency Medicine: Concepts and Clinical Practice, 2nd ed. St. Louis: Mosby, 1997.
7. Fleisher GR, Ludwig S, eds. Textbook of Pediatric Emergency Medicine, 6th ed. Philadelphia: Lippincott Williams & Wilkins, 2010.

Field Approach to Infants and Children

Julie Scadden, NREMT-P, PS

CHAPTER 64

1. **Why should children not be assessed and treated as if they were small adults?**
   Children have many unique features in anatomy, physiology, and psychosocial development that can affect assessment and treatment of each age group.

2. **Why are pediatric EMS calls more stressful than adult calls?**
   Only about 14% of 911 calls are for pediatric patients. Historically, there has been little pediatric-specific education provided on a regular basis and tensions can be high simply because the patient is a child. The tendency for prehospital providers to identify with the patient (e.g., thinking that he or she looks like one's own child or neighbor), may further increase the provider's anxiety.
   Depending on the age and development of the child, they can be frightened, anxious, and unable to communicate to you what the problem is. The child's developmental level, previous experience with the health care system, culture, and nature of the emergency are just a few of the factors that will determine the patient's and family's response.

3. **What in pediatric anatomy and function can create challenges for prehospital professionals?**
   Although children and adults have body systems that perform the same functions, there are growth differences in those body systems that create challenges in children not seen in adults. For example, a child's airway is smaller, with a relatively larger tongue than an adult's. Secretions or swelling from illness or trauma can more easily block a child's airway. Due to the flexibility of a child's upper airway anatomy, hyperextending the neck of an infant or child can cause airway occlusion.

4. **What is the Pediatric Assessment Triangle?**
   The Pediatric Assessment Triangle (PAT) is a tool for the rapid, initial assessment of any child, whether the child has an injury or an illness (See Figure 66.1, page 440). The three components of the PAT all reflect the child's overall physiologic status:
   - Appearance—reflects the adequacy of ventilation, oxygenation, brain perfusion, body homeostasis and central nervous system (CNS) function.
   - Work of breathing—reflects the child's attempt to compensate for abnormalities in oxygenation and ventilation and is an indicator for the effectiveness of gas exchange.
   - Circulation to skin—determines the adequacy of cardiac output and core perfusion or perfusion of vital organs. An important sign of core perfusion is circulation to skin.

5. **What does the TICLS mnemonic stand for?**
   TICLS is a method for pediatric assessment. The most important characteristics of appearance can be summarized in the "tickles" (TICLS) mnemonic:
   T—tone
   I—interactiveness

C—consolability
L—look/gaze
S—speech/crying

6. What are the "sniffing position" and "tripoding"? How do they help breathing?

The sniffing position and tripoding are both body positions assumed by patients in respiratory distress, usually visualized as you enter the scene. A child in the sniffing position will appear to be pushing their nose toward the ceiling and is trying to align the axes of the airways to improve patency and increase airflow. Children with severe upper airway obstruction are most often seen in this position. Tripoding is seen in the child who refuses to lie down and sits leaning forward with outstretched arms on their knees or another surface, attempting to stretch the torso and create the optimal use of accessory muscles of respiration.

7. How is circulation assessed?

Although the PAT provides important visual clues pertaining to the circulation to the skin, further hands-on evaluation of heart rate, pulse quality, skin temperature, capillary refill time, and BP will provide additional information in evaluating the adequacy of perfusion.

1. *Heart rate* can vary depending on the age of the child. Although tachycardia can be a sign of hypoxia or poor perfusion, it can also be caused by other conditions such as fever, anxiety, pain, and excitement. Interpretation of heart rate should be done within the context of the overall history, PAT, and initial assessment.

2. *Pulse quality* should be assessed by palpating the brachial pulse, located medial to the biceps in the antecubital fossa. If peripheral pulses cannot be felt, central pulses, such as the femoral pulse in infants and young children or the carotid pulse in an older child or adolescent, should be assessed.

3. *Skin temperature and capillary fill time (CFT) may illuminate circulatory issues not obvious in other ways.* Children with normal circulation may have cool hands and feet; however, the skin should be warm above the wrists and ankles. Normal CFT is less than 2–3 seconds and should be checked in a fingertip, toe, heel, or on the pads of the fingertips. Keep in mind that peripheral perfusion may vary in some children, and environmental factors (such as a cold room) may make it difficult for an accurate CFT assessment. CFT must be evaluated as part of an overall assessment that includes the PAT, heart rate, pulse quality, and blood pressure (BP).

4. *BP* may be difficult to determine in children for a number of reasons, including lack of patient cooperation, inappropriate cuff size, and problems remembering age-appropriate normal values.

8. How helpful is BP in determining shock in a child?

A fall in BP is a *late* finding in children due to their great ability to increase their systemic vascular resistance, which shunts blood to central circulation. BP can be maintained until as much as 50% of intravascular volume is lost. During the period when tissue perfusion is poor but *before* the BP has fallen below normal for age (compensated shock), vital organs such as the heart, kidneys, liver, and brain are suffering insults; thus, the BP is often not useful or illuminating.

9. How can pain be accurately assessed in pediatric patients?

Assessing pain has come to be considered to be a vital sign in all age groups, including children. Assessment for, and treatment of, pain in the prehospital setting helps to relieve distress of both the child and family. It can also facilitate communication, physical assessment, and transport.

The ability to recognize pain improves with the age of child; therefore, age must be taken into consideration when assessing for pain. Crying and agitiation in an infant who will not be consoled when held by the caregiver may be due to hunger, hypoxia, or pain; therefore, it is necessary perform further assessments and identify the source of the pain prior to administering analgesia.

Visual analogue scores are helpful in assessing the need for pharmacologic relief of pain in older children. The Wong–Baker FACES scale is an example. See Figure 63.2, page 420.)

10. How should pain be managed in the pediatric patients?

Managing pain in the pediatric patient must include methods that will relieve anxiety and reduce the perception of pain. It is imperative for the prehospital provider to remain calm and provide quiet reassurance to both parent and child. Distraction with toys and games, keeping the caregiver with or holding the child, and music are all techniques that can help lessen the perception of pain. A 12% to 25% sucrose solution before a painful procedure as well as sucrose pacifiers for neonates are known to reduce pain perception. Pharmacological methods include the use of opiates, benzodiazepines and nitrous oxide. Preferred routes of administration for analgesic and anxiolytic drugs are through inhalation and transmucosal (e.g., sublingual, rectal) routes. The fastest drug administration route is intravenous, which also provides the most effective and controllable method.

11. What are the best sites for IV access in pediatric patients? When should IO access be used?

The best I.V. sites in infants and neonates are the scalp, hands, antecubital fossa, and saphenous vein at the ankle or feet. The hands, antecubital areas, and external jugular veins are the best sites in toddlers and older children.

Intraosseous (IO) needles provide rapid and effective entry into the venous circulation and should be used in any critically ill child requiring immediate drugs or fluid and when peripheral IV access cannot be rapidly obtained. The availability of a secure IV line or an obvious extremity deformity in the same bone as the planned insertion site should contraindicate the use of IO. In addition, insertion of an I.O. line is extremely painful and is ideally only performed in patients with altered mentation.

12. What types of intravenous fluids are best for pediatric patients?

Crystalloid fluids (almost always 0.9% Sodium Chloride) administered in a 20 mL/kg bolus (up to 60 mL/kg) are normally recommended to improve perfusion, and should be based upon continuing assessment and vital signs.

13. How is a neurologic assessment carried out in a pre-verbal or non-verbal child?

Various pediatric equivalents of the Glasgow Coma Scale exist for the pediatric age group. The best way to assess mental status in infants and toddlers is to evaluate their general level of consciousness: Is the child alert, responsive, and aware of surroundings? Does the child recognize his or her parents? Is the child appropriately afraid of emergency medical services (EMS) personnel for age group?

14. What is "AVPU" and how is it used?

AVPU is loosely based on the Glasgow Coma Scale (GCS) and assessed during the hands-on ABCDE (airway, breathing, circulation, disability, exposure) evaluation. The AVPU system can be used to quickly determine level of consciousness and to assess for major changes in level of consciousness throughout transport. Each letter is a measure of the level of consciousness: A—alert, V—responsive to verbal stimuli, P—responsive to painful stimuli, U —unresponsive.

The PAT and AVPU should be used in concert to evaluate both cortical and brainstem functions.

Field Approach to Infants and Children

15. **Describe the approach to a critically ill or injured child in the field.**
    - Stay calm. If you manage the ABCs well (airway, breathing, circulation), nothing will be overlooked and all vital functions of the child will be evaluated and maintained.
    - Managing the airway effectively is paramount. Use noninvasive means first (head positioning, chin lift/jaw thrust, suctioning, an oral airway if unconscious, bag–mask ventilation), followed by oral intubation (if child is <12 years old), or rarely, needle cricothyrotomy. Use cervical spine precautions when indicated.
    - Ensure adequate oxygenation and ventilation.
    - Check peripheral perfusion. If abnormal, obtain vascular access and begin a 20-mL/kg normal saline bolus.
    - Note the child's mental status and pupillary size and reactivity.
    - Keep the patient warm: use blankets, overhead lights, and turn the heat up in the ambulance. Undress only what is necessary to examine the patient.
    - Transport the patient to the most appropriate facility with pediatric expertise.

16. **List the steps for managing a pediatric patient with altered level of consciousness (ALOC).**
    Assertive management is paramount in treating pediatric patients with altered mentation as follows:
    1. Open the airway, using appropriate spinal stabilization if head or neck injury is suspected. Suction as needed to relieve potiential obstruction from vomitus or secretions. If no gag reflex is present, insert an oropharyngeal or nasopharyngeal airway.
    2. Ensure adequate breathing, administer 100% oxygen (O_2) using a nonrebreathing mask. Assist or provide ventilation using 100% oxygen via an appropriately sized bag–mask device if patient:
       (a) is cyanotic,
       (b) has an oxygen saturation of less than 90% on 100% O_2 using a nonrebreather mask,
       (c) is breathing at a rate too slow for age or if respiratory effort is shallow or irregular. Airway management should be considered in any child with inadequate breathing to protect the airway and avoid aspiration. Place the patient on an electrocardiogram monitor and pulse oximeter via local protocol.
    3. Safeguard circulation by establishing an IV and obtain a blood sample to measure glucose. Use isotonic fluid at a keep-vein-open rate unless the child is showing signs of shock.
    4. Perform a bedside blood glucose test. Glucose should only be administered to children with documented hypoglycemia.
       Administer IV glucose or IM (intramuscular) glucagon if the bedside glucose test shows hypoglycemia as follows:
       - <40 mg% in a newborn—give D10W, 2 mL/kg IV or IO (intraosseus)
       - <40 mg% in infant—give D10W, 5 mL/kg IV or IO bolus (one part D50W, four parts sterile water or normal saline)
       - <60 mg% child <2 years old: Give D25W, 2 mL/kg IV or IO bolus (one part D50W, one part sterile water or normal saline)
       - <60 mg% child >2 years old: Give D50W, 1 mL/kg IV or IO bolus

Any child with known diabetes and hypoglycemia who is conscious with a gag reflex can be given oral glucose.

5. Narcotic overdose is an unlikely cause of ALOC in children but is an important consideration in teenagers. Naloxone (Narcan), 0.1 mg/kg, repeat as necessary, to a maximum dose of 2 mg, should be considered in any child with an altered level of consciousness and depressed respirations.
   - Caution should be used when giving naloxone to a depressed newly born child of a narcotic-addicted mother. Aggressive administration may induce acute withdrawal symptoms and seizures.

17. **What special modifications for prehospital assessments may be needed for children with special health care needs?**

    EMS response for children with special health care needs (CSHCN) is generally initiated in a time of crisis when the caregiver has exhausted all their options and the child has not responded. Other situations may include equipment failure, an exhausted or panicked caregiver, or caregivers new to caring for the child.

    The following special modifications should be implemented when assessing the CSHCN:
    - Determine the child's baseline status by asking their caregiver what is "normal" for that child.
    - Ask the caregiver's opinion on what might be wrong or how the child is "acting differently."
    - Ask what approaches work best for interaction with the child.
    - When the child is physiologically stable, complete the focused history.
    - Be patient with the patient and caregiver. Children may be slow to answer questions or unable to talk. Always talk directly to the child when possible, not the caregiver, when asking questions. Unless absolutely necessary, do not allow the caregiver to answer for the child.
    - Remember that illnesses normally considered mild can be life threatening in some children with special health care needs.
    - Check for medical alert tags, forms, or cards with information about the child's medical problems when a caregiver is not present.
    - Listen to the caregiver's concerns and take them seriously; they know what is "normal" for the child and what is not.
    - Determine from the caregiver what therapies or interventions they have already attempted in response to the child's emergency.
    - Try to transport the child to the medical facility that is familiar with their ongoing medical care, keeping in mind local EMS protocols on treatment and transport decisions. If there is a question, consult medical direction on-line.

18. **What are "acyanotic defects" and how are they treated in the prehospital setting?**

    Acyanotic defects affect cardiac function and are normally congenital in nature. Abnormalities such as ventricular septal defects and artial septal defects are associated with left-to-right shunts and obstruction to ventricular outflow, thus causing oxygenated blood from the left side of the heart to mix with deoxygenated blood from the right side of the heart. Children with these issues can develop congestive heart failure quickly and may need to be treated with medications until surgery can be performed to correct the underlying problem.

Field Approach to Infants and Children

Treatment for acyanotic defects in the prehospital setting includes assessment and management of ABC. Treatment involves placing the patient in their position of comfort, oxygen therapy, cardiac monitoring, appropriate airway interventions, and IV access with fluid resuscitation as directed by local protocol or on-line medical control. Transport should be to the facility most familiar with the child's medical history and long-term treatment plan, if possible.

19. How can I become more familiar with the care of critically ill children?
- Request clinical rotations in a pediatric emergency department, visit a pediatric intensive care unit, or ride as an observer with a pediatric specialty transport service whenever possible.
- Attend courses targeting pediatric education such as PALS (Pediatric Advanced Life Support), APLS (Advanced Pediatric Life Support), PEPP (Pediatric Education for Prehospital Providers), or EPC (Emergency Pediatric Care).
- Attend targeted Emergency Medical Services for Children (EMS-C) prehospital care courses; contact your state's EMS division for availability.
- Use self-paced instructional programs, such as video workbooks or interactive videodisk technology, to reinforce other training and experience. Contact your state's EMS division or the National EMS-C Resource Center for information.

20. What aids are available to help in the field care of children?
- Use of a preprinted sheet with drug doses, equipment sizes, and vital signs based on age or weight has been shown to improve speed and accuracy.
- A length-based emergency tape (i.e., Broselow tape), which provides accurate and rapid dose determination, as well as equipment sizes based on the child's length.
- Personal digital assistants with programs that provide algorithms, drug and IV fluid calculators, and metric conversion programs have become popular.

21. What are some general tips?
- Assess the scene for hints of abuse, neglect, or ingestions.
- Weight estimate in kg = $2 \times$ (age in years $+ 4$).
- Minimum systolic BP = $70 + (2 \times$ age in years). Do not delay treatment or transport to obtain BP.
- Limit your examination to the essentials, using a toe-to-head approach to increase compliance.
- Airway stabilization coupled with initial efforts at optimizing ventilation and oxygenation should be initiated prior to loading the child for transport; all else may be done in the ambulance.

Pearls and Pitfalls

1. Infants ages 0–6 months are obligate nose breathers; therefore, it is vital to clear secretions from the nose of an infant 6 months of age and under.
2. The general appearance of a child is the most important clue when assessing severity of illness or injury and the need for treatment and response to therapy.
3. Assume that the infant or child who is quiet and pale but making eye contact is not very sick.
4. A "normal" BP frequently exists in compensated shock in children until the bottom drops out of the BP.

5. Remaining on scene to start an IV or obtain a thorough history in a critically ill infant or child is a common pitfall. Getting the critical child to definitive care is of paramount importance.
6. Do not assume that the child with a physical disability is also cognitively impaired.

References

1. American Academy of Pediatrics: Pediatric Education for Prehospital Professionals Provider Manual, 2nd ed. Sudbury, MA Jones and Bartlett, 2006.
2. American Heart Association. American Heart Association guidelines for cardiopulmonary resuscitation and emergency cardiovascular care. Part 13: Pediatric basic life support. Circulation 122;S862–S875, 2010. Part 14: Pediatric advanced life support. Circulation 122;S876-S908, 2010.
3. Argall JA, Wright N, Mackway-Jones K, Jackson R. A comparison of two commonly used methods of weight estimation. Arch Dis Child. Sep;88(9):789–790, 2003.
4. Adirim TA, Smith E. SCOPE—Special Children's Outreach and Prehospital Education. Sudbury, MA: Jones and Bartlett, 2006.

Seizures in Children

Jeffrey J. Messerole, PS

CHAPTER 65

This chapter is dedicated to the author's son, Jordan. His seizures helped me better understand an affliction as old as medicine itself, and yet still in about 7 out of 10 seizures the cause is unknown. Having responded to my own home for a 911 call for a child having a seizure, I can tell you there is nothing more frightening than finding your child unresponsive, convulsing, and not knowing why it is occurring, or what exactly should be done to resolve it.

1. **What is the cause of a seizure?**
   The brain contains billions of nerve cells (neurons). They communicate with each other through electrical charges that fire on and off in an organized fashion. When some of these neurons begin to abnormally fire together, a wave of electrical energy travels through the brain. This massive uncontrolled discharge (MUD) of neurons causes the seizure. Several factors determine the type and seriousness of the seizure and include whether the discharge is limited to a small portion of the brain, or both hemispheres, as well as the length and frequency of the MUD. Fortunately most seizures are short lived and are often over by the time the EMS provider arrives. Most simple one-time seizures do not require medical intervention, but repeated seizures without cessation, known as status epilepticus, are a true life-and-death emergency. Seizures can be a sign of something very serious. Further assessment after the seizure is required to find a correctable cause. Whatever the underlying cause, the treatment for the more serious types of seizures is similar. During this MUD of neurons it should be noted that the brain's use of both oxygen and sugar increases and can lead to hypoxia and hypoglycemia.
   Seizures can occur any time the brain is injured, irritated, or deprived of nutrients. The causes can be divided up into those that occur in the head, those that occur outside the head, and those with no known cause (idiopathic). See Table 65.1 for common causes of seizures.

2. **What is epilepsy?**
   Having a single seizure does not mean that a child has epilepsy. Epilepsy is the name for seizures that happen more than once without a known treatable cause. Epilepsy includes a family of different syndromes. Recurring seizures of the same type, with diagnostic electroencephalogram findings, defines the epilepsy syndrome. Because it is difficult to diagnose the specific type of epilepsy, many children go undiagnosed or are told they have a seizure disorder. Epilepsy is said to account for about 25% of the seizures for all ages. Epilepsy affects the very young and the very old. Epilepsy can occur at any age, but it is estimated that it affects more than 360,000 children under the age of 15, and more than 90,000 have severe seizures as the result of their epilepsy that cannot be adequately controlled.

3. **How prevalent are seizures in children?**
   Seizures are a common childhood neurological disorder. Approximately 4–10% of children have a seizure for no known reason and without recurrence. Each year, about 150,000 children and adolescents have

TABLE 65.1 Common Causes of Seizures

Causes	Examples
Intrinsic central nervous system disorders	Brain tumors, lesions, cysts, cardiovascular accidents, head injuries
Infections/Infectious Diseases	Meningitis, encephalitis, otitis media
Extrinsic metabolic disorder	Hypoxia, hypercapnea, hypoglycemia, hyperglycemia, liver or renal failure, electrolyte imbalances, failure to take seizure medication, fever
Unknown	Idiopathic epilepsy

their first seizure and 25% of them are found to have epilepsy, 25% are found to have a treatable cause, and 50% remain unknown or idiopathic.

4. Are there different types of seizures?

A seizure occurring for the first time is a sign of something potentially more serious. In 1981 and 1989 the International League against Epilepsy developed a classification system for seizure disorders (Table 65.2). This description allows EMS providers to classify the type of seizure activity either described to them or that they have had the opportunity to witness. A description of the type of seizure activity assists the physician in determining the need for diagnostics such as lab studies, lumbar punctures, computed tomography, or magnetic resonance imaging and which type of antiseizure medication may be appropriate.

Seizures can be classified into two types: partial or generalized. (See Table 65.2.) Partial seizures begin with a focal onset, meaning that those neurons discharging are limited to only one part of the brain. Partial seizures can further be divided into simple and complex.

Seizures can also be generalized, meaning that all the neurons of both hemispheres of the brain are involved. This type of seizure can further be divided into categories describing the clinical appearance of the seizure. Those categories include absence, tonic/clonic, atonic, or myoclonic.

5. What are the signs and symptoms of a seizure?

Diagnosing a particular type of seizure is difficult and requires close observation and a description of the muscle activity that occurred at the onset of and during the seizure. If the seizure activity has ceased before your arrival, the signs and symptoms may be subtle and include things such as incontinence of urine or feces, tongue biting, or a postictal state of consciousness where the child may be confused or would rather rest or sleep than stay awake to answer questions. If you do witness the seizure, the signs and symptoms you observe will assist in identifying the type of seizure.

6. What do the various types of seizures look like?

Partial seizures may cause periods of automatic, repetitive behavior and altered consciousness. The behaviors may be activities such as buttoning and unbuttoning a shirt multiple times and are often not remembered by the patient.

Simple partial seizures begin in one part of one hemisphere and *do not* affect the level of consciousness. The simple partial seizure may consist of any task the brain is capable of doing, such as the jerking or

TABLE 65.2: Classification of Seizures According to Type

1. Partial (Focal, Local) Seizures

Simple partial seizures (consciousness not impaired)

    With motor signs

    With somatosensory or special sensory symptoms (simple hallucinations such as tingling, light flashes, buzzing)

    With autonomic symptoms or signs (e.g., epigastric sensation, pallor, sweating, flushing, piloerection, and pupillary dilatation)

    With psychic symptoms (disturbance of higher cerebral function) (e.g., déjà vu, distortion of time sense, fear). Note: these rarely occur without impairment of consciousness.

Complex partial seizures (with impairment of consciousness)

    With simple partial onset followed by impairment of consciousness

    With impairment of consciousness at onset

Partial seizures evolving to secondarily generalized seizures (may be tonic/clonic, tonic, or clonic)

    Simple partial seizures evolving to generalized seizures

    Complex partial seizures evolving to generalized seizures

    Simple partial seizures evolving to complex partial seizures and then evolving to generalized seizures

2. Generalized Seizures (Convulsive or Nonconvulsive)

    Absence seizures (impairment of consciousness alone or with mild clonic, atonic or tonic components, automatisms, and/or autonomic symptoms or signs)

    Atypical absence

    Myoclonic seizures

    Clonic seizures

    Tonic/clonic seizures

    Atonic seizures

3. Unclassified Seizures

twitching of just one extremity, or hand, or finger, abnormal sensation of one part of the body, flushing of the skin, nausea, an intense fear, hallucinations, or a feeling of déjà vu.

Complex partial seizures begin in one part of one hemisphere and do affect the level of consciousness. There usually is an aura, which is the feeling or sense that a seizure is about to occur, followed by confusion, an intense fear, laughter, hallucinations, or a feeling of déjà vu, which is accompanied by lip smacking, fumbling, wringing of the hands or fluttering of the eyes, or unconsciously walking or running. The aura preceding a seizure is thought to represent an initial symptom produced by the onset of the seizure activity and is often described as a foul odor or taste. Complex partial seizures last several minutes and are accompanied by a postictal state; the child appears awake during the seizure. Seizures are often mistaken for a psychotic event because of the bizarre behavior exhibited during the seizure.

Both simple and complex partial seizures may spread and involve both hemispheres resulting in a generalized tonic/clonic seizure.

Generalized seizures involve both hemispheres of the brain, and generally cause a loss of consciousness. They are categorized by the type of muscle movements involved and include absence, tonic, tonic/clonic, myoclonic, and atonic.

Classic absence seizures are commonly referred to as petit mal seizures. An absence seizure is typically seen in children and, like all generalized seizures, there is no aura. Absence seizures present as a brief staring spell lasting 3–30 seconds. The child will stop whatever activity they are doing, and there may be some eye fluttering, mild lip movements, or twitches. The child is unresponsive to even strong stimuli. The child normally does not fall to the ground, recovery is quick, and there is no postictal period following the absence seizure. The child has no remembrance of the seizure and is often embarrassed.

With **tonic seizures** the child just stiffens up, both arms are raised over their head, and the legs become stiff. Facial muscles tighten into a grimace, as if someone is pulling on the cheeks. If the child is standing, he or she may lose balance and fall. These seizures typically do not have a postictal state, but if several are close together the child may complain of being tired. Tonic seizures usually last less than 20 seconds, and the child remains conscious during the stiffening of the muscles.

A **generalized tonic/clonic or grand mal seizure** describes the type of muscle activity seen with this type of seizure. Tonic refers to continuous stiffening of the extremities and clonic refers to the rhythmic jerking of the muscles. Tonic/clonic seizures are among some of the most frightening and dramatic seizures to witness. The child has an immediate loss of consciousness, may produce a loud cry, fall to the ground, and begin this initial stiffening of the muscles followed by the violent rhythmic jerking of the muscles. Tongue biting is common during this phase of the seizure, and blood may be seen coming from the mouth. Facial muscles are drawn and fixed to one side, secretions cannot be swallowed, and drooling may be excessive. Tonic/clonic seizures affect all muscles including those of respiration. During the stiffening and violent rhythmic jerking of muscles, the child will not be breathing adequately and depending on the length of the seizure may become severely hypoxic, hypercapneic, and hypoglycemic in addition to a host of other metabolic problems associated with the violent excessive muscle activity. The muscle contractions may be so violent that the child fractures a long bone or dislocates a shoulder. The child may also become incontinent of urine and feces. These seizures usually last from 1–3 minutes but can last as long as 30 minutes. There is a postictal state following the seizure activity where the child will want to sleep and is difficult to keep awake. During this phase the child must rest and replenish the stores of energy consumed by the seizure. There is usually no memory of the seizure.

Myoclonic seizures typically occur in the morning shortly after awakening and often involve the arms and shoulders and present as quick startlelike jerks. If the myoclonic jerk is violent enough, the child may drop things or fall to the floor. There is no loss of consciousness during these seizures. Often, the child has become accustomed to the myoclonic jerks and never mentions them to their parent. The age of onset for juvenile myoclonic epilepsy is as young as 6 years, although most seizures begin between the ages of 12 and 18 years of age. There are some forms of myoclonic seizures that can begin in infants as young as 3–6 months of age. Some triggers of myoclonic seizures include sleep deprivation, psychological stress, alcohol use, or photic stimulation while staring into a strobe light, watching TV, or playing a video game. It is a lifelong syndrome that can usually be well controlled.

Atonic seizure, as the name implies, means lacking muscle tone. The eyelids may droop, the head may nod, and the child may drop what he or she is holding and suddenly fall to the ground, often landing headfirst. These seizures have also been called "drop attacks." There usually is no loss of consciousness as they only last about 15 seconds. Because of the potential for serious head injury these children are often seen wearing a helmet. They begin early in childhood and may last well into adulthood.

7. **What is status epilepticus?**

    Several definitions of status epilepticus exist. A seizure lasting more than 30 minutes or two or more seizures without regaining consciousness between the seizures are considered status epilepticus. Some experts would advocate shorter time frames. Status epilepticus carries a 30% mortality rate and the longer the seizure activity persists, the more likely the development of serious life threats such as hypoxia and hypoglycemia plus a host of other metabolic problems associated with the violent excessive muscle activity. Aspiration, bodily injury, or cardiac arrest can also occur with status epilepticus, making it a true life-or-death emergency. Status epilepticus requires aggressive airway management and the administration of antiseizure medications, sometimes at higher-than-normal doses, to stop the seizure activity.

8. **What role does a fever play in seizures?**

    Seizures caused by fever are termed febrile, from the Latin word *febris*, which means fever. Febrile seizures are very common, and occur in 3–5% of all children. One in 25 children will have a febrile seizure before age 6, and more than one-third of these children will have additional febrile seizures before they outgrow them. Febrile seizures are rare in children less than 6 months old and usually are not seen in children older than 6 years of age. They usually occur within 24 hours of the onset of fever. It is not certain whether it is how fast the temperature rises or how high the temperature must get before a child has a febrile seizure. Typical febrile seizures cause tonic/clonic motor activity lasting 1 or 2 minutes with rapid return of consciousness.

    Febrile seizures usually occur only once during any given illness. Repeated febrile seizures during the course of an illness point to a more serious problem such as encephalitis, an abscess, or meningitis; signs for those illnesses should be sought.

    Children with febrile seizures have only a 0.9% chance of developing epilepsy. Febrile seizures can be classified as simple, complex, and atypical and are caused by an infection in children who are otherwise neurologically normal. Febrile seizures are commonly associated with viral infections and vary in length and presentation. Table 65.3 lists the classification of febrile seizures. Although they can be frightening to parents, the majority of febrile seizures are harmless. During a febrile seizure, there is a small chance

TABLE 65.3:   Classification of Febrile Seizures

Type	Onset
Simple	Last less than 15 minutes and do not recur within 24 hours
Complex	Last less than 15 minutes; recurs more than once in 24 hours, seizures in which only one side of the body is affected
Atypical	Prolonged seizure activity exceeding 15 minutes, multiple seizures during the same febrile illness

TABLE 65.4: Risk factors for developing febrile seizures

Family history of febrile seizures

High temperature

Parental report of developmental delay

Neonatal discharge at an age greater than 28 days (suggesting perinatal illness requiring hospitalization)

Daycare attendance

Presence of 2 of these risk factors increases the probability of a first febrile seizure to about 30%.

Maternal alcohol intake and smoking during pregnancy has a 2-fold increased risk.

---

that the child may be injured by falling or may choke from food or saliva in the mouth, but generally these seizures are not life threatening.

There is no evidence that febrile seizures cause brain damage. Large studies have found that children with febrile seizures perform as well on intellectual tests as do their siblings who do not have seizures. Most children recover completely from even prolonged febrile seizures. Febrile seizures tend to run in families. In a child with a febrile seizure, the risk of febrile seizure is 10% for the siblings and almost 50% for the siblings if a parent had febrile seizures as well. Although clear evidence exists for a genetic basis of febrile seizures, it remains unclear as to how it is passed on genetically. Table 65.4 lists the risk factors for developing febrile seizures.

9. What does the assessment for a seizure include?

The assessment begins with a SAMPLE history, a thorough description of how the seizure started, what the seizure activity looked like, and how long it lasted in order to help determine the type of seizure.

S—Signs and symptoms include looking for the evidence of actual seizure activity if the episode has stopped prior to your arrival. Is there evidence of tongue biting? Is the child incontinent of urine or feces? Is the child in a postictal state or is there some other etiology for their unresponsiveness? Head and spine injury may be present if the child fell and manual c-spine immobilization should be performed.

A—Is the patient allergic to any medications, foods, animals, or plants? An allergic reaction may be the cause of the apparent seizure and as a paramedic you may give appropriate medications should the seizure reoccur.

M—Does the child take medications for seizures and have they been taken? A common cause for a seizure is noncompliance with medications. Taking the medications often makes them feel no better and sometimes makes patients feel worse. Forgetting to take them or a rapid withdrawal will lead to seizures. Common antiseizure medications are listed in Table 65.5. Is the patient taking any drugs such as cocaine or amphetamines that may cause seizure activity?

P—Pertinent past medical history to include a history of seizures, epilepsy, febrile seizures, diabetes, recent head injury are important to note and will assist in establishing a history of seizures or a condition likely to cause a seizure.

L—Last oral intake may suggest the likelihood of a full stomach and the potential for vomiting and aspiration. It may also indicate the need to check a blood sugar in the patient with diabetes.

E—Determining what events lead up to the seizure activity are important. Did the child complain of an aura? Younger children may not be able to communicate the presence of an aura and may just suddenly run up to the parent or caretaker prior to the onset of seizure activity. Did the seizure start or affect one part of the body more than the others? The establishment of an aura and the seizure affecting only one part of the body defines a seizure with a focal onset, as seen with complex partial seizures. A generalized seizure affects the entire brain at its onset and usually is not associated with an aura. Did the child experience a recent head injury? Is the child diabetic and has he or she taken insulin but not eaten or been more active than normal? Has the child been exposed to a toxic substance, and is the scene safe? Often the child is confused or does not remember the seizure, so family member, or bystanders may need to be asked these important questions.

TABLE 65.5: Common Antiseizure Medications

Phenytoin (Dilantin)
Phenobarbital
Ethosuximide (Zarontin)
Carbamazepine (Tegretol)
Valproic acid (Depakote or Depekene)
Clonazepam (Klonopin)
Clorazepate (Tranxene)
Felbamate (Felbatol)
Fosphenytoin (Cerebryx)
Gabapentin (Neurontin)

A rapid head-to-toe examination looking for injuries that may have occurred if the patient fell to the ground, experienced violent muscle jerking, or tongue biting is essential following the termination of the seizure activity.

Pulse oximetry should be measured to determine the presence of hypoxia. Patients with generalized tonic/clonic seizures do not breathe normally during their seizures and depending on how long the seizures last, they may become hypoxic and hypercapneic. Pulse oximetry is of little value and highly inaccurate if obtainable at all during an actual seizure. Pulse oximetry should be initiated after the seizure activity has stopped.

A blood sugar should be obtained in all patients with an altered mental state. Assuming that the confusion is a postictal state may lead to the hypoglycemia going undiagnosed and untreated, which can result in permanent brain injury.

10. **What is the treatment for a seizure?**
Although most seizures require no special treatment other than close observation, seizures that alter the level of consciousness or cause severe muscle jerking may need advance level care. The goal of seizure treatment is to stop any active seizure activity, support the ABCs, determine a possible treatable cause, lower the body temperature if it is elevated, and ensure that hypoglycemia does not exist. Treatment for seizures should begin, like the treatment of all patients, with the ABCs

A—Secretions are often heavy and swallowing may not occur during a tonic–clonic seizure, putting the child at risk for choking and aspiration. Vomiting may also occur if the child has a full stomach. EMS providers need to place the patient on their side to assist in drainage of secretions and remain alert for the need to suction. Children in a postictal state may have trouble maintaining their airways. Items should not be placed in the mouth to prevent tongue biting, as they may cause teeth to be broken off or cause an airway obstruction. A nasopharyngeal airway is most appropriate to assist keeping the airway open.

B—Breathing is inadequate for the duration of a tonic/clonic seizure and administering supplemental oxygen at 15 L/min via a nonrebreather mask is appropriate. After the seizure stops, assess the rate of breathing, as the child's respirations may be shallow during the postictal state and positive pressure ventilation may be required initially until the postictal state resolves. The need to intubate the child is rare and is usually based on respiratory depression from multiple doses of antiseizure medications or status epilepticus.

C—Check the child's pulse, as seizurelike activity may occur from cardiac arrest resulting from hypoxia or hypovolemia. IV access may be difficult during the tonic/clonic phase of the seizure but should be attempted once the activity stops. Arms should not be held down during the seizure as fractures may occur from the violent muscle jerking.

Blood sugar should be checked following cessation of seizure activity. Hypoglycemia may be the cause of the seizure. Excessive muscle and brain activity during a tonic/clonic seizure can utilize a tremendous amount of sugar, making the child hypoglycemic. If hypoglycemia is found, administer D25 appropriately based on the child's weight. D25 is prepared by mixing D50 1:1 with sterile water, which can be given at a dose of 0.5–1 g/kg IV/IO.

If the child has a fever, rectal administration of acetaminophen suppository, if available and allowed per protocol, will help to reduce the fever. Reducing the fever raises the seizure threshold in children with epilepsy and should be a priority.

If the child seizes in your presence or continues to seize, antiseizure medication administration is appropriate. Benzodiazepines are the first line drugs of choice, should be administered IV, and include diazepam (Valium), lorazepam (Ativan), or midazolam (Versed). Table 65.6 outlines the particular properties of each medication. If IV access is unobtainable, diazepam may be given rectally by inserting the barrel of the syringe into the rectum about 3 cm and instilling the medication. Remove the syringe and hold the cheeks together allowing the diazepam to be absorbed. Rectal diazepam may take longer to reach a therapeutic level but will last longer because of continued absorption. Keep in mind that the use of benzodiazepines may cause hypotension and respiratory depression. Respiratory arrest has been reported with multiple doses of benzodiazepines.

If the child develops respiratory arrest, aggressive airway management is required to prevent cardiopulmonary arrest. The need to intubate children is a highly debated topic in medical circles. Intubation is appropriate in the following situations:

- Respiratory arrest after administering anticonvulsants in a child who did not respond to several minutes of bag–mask ventilation
- A concern for increased intracranial pressure after the seizure activity has stopped as demonstrated by posturing, dilated pupil, or abnormal breathing pattern

TABLE 65.6: Benzodiazepines Used to Treat Seizures

Drug	Advantages	Disadvantages	Dose
Diazepam (Valium)	■ Rapid IV onset ■ May be given rectally ■ Widely available ■ Inexpensive	■ Short duration of about 20 minutes ■ Apnea common when given IV ■ Irritating to veins	■ 0.1–0.3 mg/kg IV/IO ■ 0.2–0.6 mg/kg rectally
Lorazepam (Ativan)	■ Rapid IV onset ■ Duration of 4–6 hours	■ Requires refrigeration	■ 0.1 mg/kg IV/IO (not to exceed a single 4-mg dose)
Midazolam (Versed)	■ May be given IV, IM, intranasal ■ Rapid onset of action	■ Short duration of about one hour	■ 0.1 mg/kg IV/IO ■ 0.2 mg/kg IM ■ 0.2–0.3 mg/kg intranasal (maximum single dose of 4 mg any route)

■ Status epilepticus not terminated by benzodiazepines
■ Hemodynamic compromise

Successful treatment of seizures is based on recognizing that a seizure has occurred, looking for a treatable cause, and initiating general treatment for all seizures to include protection of the patient, supporting their ABCs, ensuring adequate oxygenation and supplying oxygen when indicated, determining the presence of hypoglycemia and administering dextrose to correct it, determining the presence of a fever and controlling body temperature, and, if necessary, administering anticonvulsant medications.

Pearls and Pitfalls

1. Blood glucose should always be checked in children who have had a seizure, as hypoglycemia may be the cause of or result from seizure activity. Assuming that confusion after a seizure is a postictal state may lead to hypoglycemia going unrecognized.
2. If a seizure occurs in your presence, closely observe and document the onset and progression, as this will assist in identifying the type of seizure.
3. Complex partial seizures often involve bizarre behavior that may be mistaken for a psychiatric abnormality.
4. Febrile seizures do not result in any demonstrable brain injury.
5. Cervical spine restrictions should be considered for any child who fell as a result of a seizure.
6. A common cause for seizures is noncompliance with antiseizure medications.
7. Benzodiazepines used to stop a seizure may cause respiratory depression and hypotension.

Pediatrics

References

1. Reiser RC. Seizures, In Aghababian R, ed. Essentials of Emergency Medicine, pp. 97–116. Sudbury, MA: Jones and Bartlett, 2006.
2. Bledsoe B, Porter R, Cherry R. Cardiology. In Essentials of Paramedic Care, 2nd ed., pp. 1211–1224, Upper Saddle River, NJ: Pearson Prentice Hall, 2007.
3. Dalton TM, Limmer D, Mistovich J, Werman H. Seizures and seizure disorders. In Advanced Medical Life Support, 3rd ed., pp. 355–375, 20Upper Saddle River, NJ: Pearson Prentice Hall, 2007.
4. Dieckmann R. Medical emergencies. In Prehospital Education for Prehospital Professionals, 2nd ed., pp. 100–106. Sudbury, MA: Jones and Bartlett, 2000.
5. Ralston M, Hazinski M. Pediatric Advanced Life Support Provider Manual. Dallas, TX: American Heart Association, 2006.
6. Stone KP. Pediatrics. In Nancy Caroline's Emergency Care in the Streets, 6th ed., Pollak A. (ed) pp. 41–42. 44. Sudbury, MA: Jones and Bartlett, 2008.

Websites visited May 2011:
www.webmd.com/epilepsy/epilepsy-in-children
www.aafp.org/afp/20000901/1109.html
www.emedicinehealth.com/seizures_in_children/article_em.htm
www.meddean.luc.edu/lumen/MedED/pedneuro/epilepsy.htm
www.nlm.nih.gov/medlineplus/seizures.html
www.epilepsyfoundation.org/
http://www.ninds.nih.gov/disorders/febrile_seizures/detail_febrile_seizures.htm
http://www.emedicine.com/EMERG/topic376.htm

Respiratory Distress in Infants and Children

CHAPTER 66

James A. Temple, BA, NREMT-P, CCP

1. **What are some of the anatomical differences between the adult and pediatric respiratory systems, and how do they affect my assessment and treatment of the pediatric patient?**
   Let us begin with the most obvious difference, the relatively large tongue. The tongue dominates the oropharynx of infants and children. The most common cause of airway obstruction is the tongue, and this is especially true in the pediatric population. Any condition that produces an altered mental status may place the pediatric patient at risk for obstruction. Pay close attention to airway positioning. In the supine patient, maintain the "sniffing" position. This can be done by using the head-tilt chin lift, taking care not to hyperextend the neck, as the cartilaginous rings of the trachea are not completely formed, and may collapse under hyperextension. One way to maintain proper airway position for an unconscious child is to place a towel under the shoulders aligning the airway axes.

2. **Are there any physiologic differences between the adult and pediatric respiratory systems?**
   Young children, especially infants, are obligate nose breathers. Any secretions or congestion in the nasopharynx may cause respiratory distress and should be carefully suctioned using a bulb syringe. Special care should be exercised when suctioning pediatric patients to avoid inducing bradycardia.
   The diaphragm in young children is comprised of muscle fibers that are more prone to fatigue than the diaphragm of adults. Pediatric patients have tremendous compensatory capabilities, but due to immature musculature, they can tire quickly and crash rapidly. The diaphragm is the primary muscle of respiration and in very young patients there are only minor contributions by the accessory muscles of respiration. Another consideration is the fact that any abdominal distention will impair diaphragmatic excursion and interfere with the efficiency of respiratory effort. This is important to remember in trauma assessment and especially when assisting ventilations without a definitive airway.

3. **How can I quickly and accurately assess a pediatric patient with respiratory distress?**
   The ability to gather pertinent information quickly without having to use any of your monitoring equipment is an invaluable skill. This "across-the-room assessment" is best accomplished by using the Pediatric Assessment Triangle or PAT (Figure 66.1). This rapid observational assessment takes no longer than 30 seconds and gives you the "down and dirty" information you need to make sound clinical decisions.

4. **What should I be looking for in the "appearance" part of the PAT?**
   The most important observation you will make is the general appearance of the child. Remember, if a child appears ill, chances are they are in need of timely medical care. By observing the general appearance, you can determine the severity of the illness, what therapy is appropriate, and if that therapy is effective. The EMS has traditionally used mnemonics to help with memory. We are going to add another one to your arsenal. When assessing the child's appearance, consider using the TICLS mnemonic.

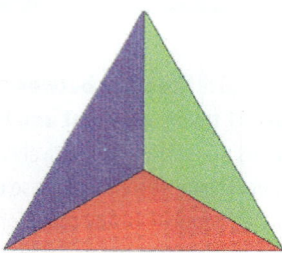

FIGURE 66.1   Pediatric Assessment Triangle (PAT).

T: Tone
I: Interactiveness
C: Consolability
L: Look/gaze
S: Speech/cry

Pay special attention to how the child interacts with the environment around them. Do they react appropriately to light? Do they smile or brighten to a familiar object or relative? Do they make eye contact with you? This is an important finding, as the child with a blank, vacant stare likely has serious physiological problems that require rapid intervention.

5. **What is meant by "work of breathing" in PAT?**
When assessing the work of breathing (WOB) side of the triangle, again, initially, you do not need any equipment. WOB is a more accurate way to assess oxygenation and ventilation than respiratory rate, pulse oximetry, and auscultation of lung sounds. You will be observing for signs of increased work of breathing, which may include:
   (a) Positioning
      (i) Sniffing: an attempt by the child to align the axes of the airways, thus improving air flow. This position is usually the result of upper airway obstruction.
      (ii) Tripod: a child who presents leaning forward on his or her extended arms is trying to maximize accessory muscle use in an attempt to increase tidal volumes.
   (b) Accessory muscle use.

(c) Retractions: these children are trying to recruit all the power in their small muscles to pull air into their lungs. You may see inward incursion of the skin and soft tissues in the supraclavicular, intercostal, and substernal areas, and even see muscles in the neck heaving to move air. An ominous form of retractions seen in infants is "head-bobbing." As infants inhale, they extend their necks and upon exhalation, the head falls forward. As you may expect, this is a sign of severe hypoxia requiring rapid intervention.
(d) Nasal flaring: during moderate and severe hypoxia, children may flare and open their nostrils in order to make them larger during labored inspiration. This occurs reflexively and can be easily noted if you are looking for it.

6. **How about the circulation part of PAT?**
The third piece of the PAT is circulation to skin. This evaluates cardiac output and perfusion, of which oxygenation and ventilation play vital roles. The child who is adequately oxygenating and perfusing should not show any signs of pallor, mottling, or cyanosis. Remember the body's response to shock is shunting, and by directing blood away from the periphery, the skin may become pale or mottled and cool to the touch. Cyanosis is an easily recognized sign of compromise, but you need to take into account the time and severity of the condition it took to produce the cyanosis.

7. **When do I use my stethoscope and other respiratory assessment equipment?**
Once you have formed an initial impression using the PAT, you will need to use the more traditional methods of respiratory assessment. Listen to both lungs with your stethoscope. Get a good history from a caregiver or someone who is somewhat familiar with the child. Take a complete set of baseline vitals, including pulse oximetry. Remember that cold extremities from environmental exposure or shunted circulation may give falsely low oxygen saturation readings, and do not forget that carbon monoxide will give false high pulse oxygen readings. If all of your assessment findings point to respiratory distress and you have that "gut" feeling that something bad is going on, do not let the pulse oximetry reading change your mind. As always, treat the patient, not the machine.
More recently, technology has given us prehospital waveform capnography. If you are able to measure the exhaled CO_2 of the nonintubated patient, you are way ahead of the curve. It is extremely helpful to know if your patient is retaining CO_2. Do you have to increase the rate of ventilations or decrease the tidal volume? This tool allows the prehospital provider to be more confident in dealing with pediatric respiratory distress and can give information on when to manage the airway and ventilation.
Your assessment skills, observational abilities, and use of the PAT will usually give you the information to determine whether the child is "sick or not sick," and just how quickly you need to intervene.

8. **What are the "big-time" signs of respiratory distress found in children and infants?**
As mentioned in the foregoing discussion of the PAT, a lethargic infant who does not make eye contact and presents with a pale color should propel you to the hospital. Conversely, the child who is interactive, carries on a conversation, and smiles at you means much less anxiety for the provider.
Tachypnea is the most common sign of respiratory distress in children. Tachypnea can have many causes. If the cause is hypoxia or hypercapnea, intervention is required. If the cause is fear, anxiety, or pain, you must be able to rule out hypoxia and hypercapnea. Remember that the respiratory rate is only part of the assessment picture.
Are there noisy respirations? Does the child present with stridor, a high-pitched sound heard upon inhalation from an airway obstruction? Does the child exhibit grunting at the end of the expiratory phase? This is indicative of a reflexive attempt to increase "auto-peep" and keep the alveoli

open for the next inhaled breath. When fluid is present in the lower airways, the child will exhale against a partially closed glottis in an effort to keep the alveoli from collapsing. This is a worrisome finding requiring further investigation and intervention. Does the child present with a prolonged expiratory phase? This is usually accompanied by wheezing. Think about what wheezing is telling you. Wheezing means air is going in and coming out. Wheezing is manageable most of the time. We need to be concerned when the wheezing goes away without any therapy from us, and the patient deteriorates. This is known as a "silent chest" and indicates no air movement. This is a dire emergency requiring airway management and pharmacologic intervention, such as in-line beta-agonist nebulizer therapy. This in-line nebulizer is attached between the bag–mask device and the ETT tube, and with each assisted ventilation, you deliver the medication directly into the lungs. This can truly be a lifesaving intervention. You must be able to differentiate between stridor and wheezing, as the patient with croup does not usually receive beta-agonist therapy.

9. **What are the signs of impending respiratory failure?**
Be alert for mental status changes, as they may appear early. Note how the child reacts to the environment during your PAT evaluation. This parameter should be continuously monitored, as changes may be subtle. A listless, noninteractive child is in critical condition. Evaluate the WOB. Do you see marked retractions, head bobbing, decreased lung sounds, or a decrease in respiratory effort? Do you notice "seesaw" breathing? This is characterized by alternating chest and abdominal excursion. The chest moves inward, and the belly moves out and vice versa. This is an easily identified and significant finding of significant distress. Is there pallor, mottling, or cyanosis present? Finally, bradycardia is a most ominous finding in the pediatric patient indicating impending arrest. These are all serious findings, with cyanosis being an extremely late sign, indicating failing compensatory mechanisms.

10. **What are the general management principles for children with respiratory distress?**
    - Any child who is short of breath should receive supplemental oxygen, whether it is via blow-by, cannula, or face mask, regardless of the pulse-oximetry value.
    - Prepare for assisted ventilation and airway management. Many providers have specialized pediatric equipment bags that includes a pediatric resuscitation tape (Broselow tape). This eases the calculation of medical dosing and endotracheal tube (ETT) size based on the length of the child (Figure 66.2).
    - Whenever you are going to control an airway, it is imperative that you prepare a back-up plan and alternative devices prior to initiating the procedure. This saves valuable time in the event the procedure was not successful. Alternatives to ETT include bag mask ventilation, or in the case of the apneic and unresponsive child the appropriately sized supraglottic airways, such as the King LT airway device, Air Q, the Combitube blind airway device, or even nasal/oral pharyngeal adjuncts with bag–mask ventilations, which have been shown to work very well in children.
    - Allow the child to assume the position of comfort. Pay special attention to the sniffing position when positioning lethargic or unresponsive infants. Do not attempt to lay children with fever, drooling, and cough supine, as they will adamantly resist lying flat and will become more hypoxic.
    - Do all you can to reduce anxiety and avoid agitation of the child. This may include holding off on starting an IV if it is not absolutely necessary. This may also be accomplished by keeping someone or something familiar close to the child.

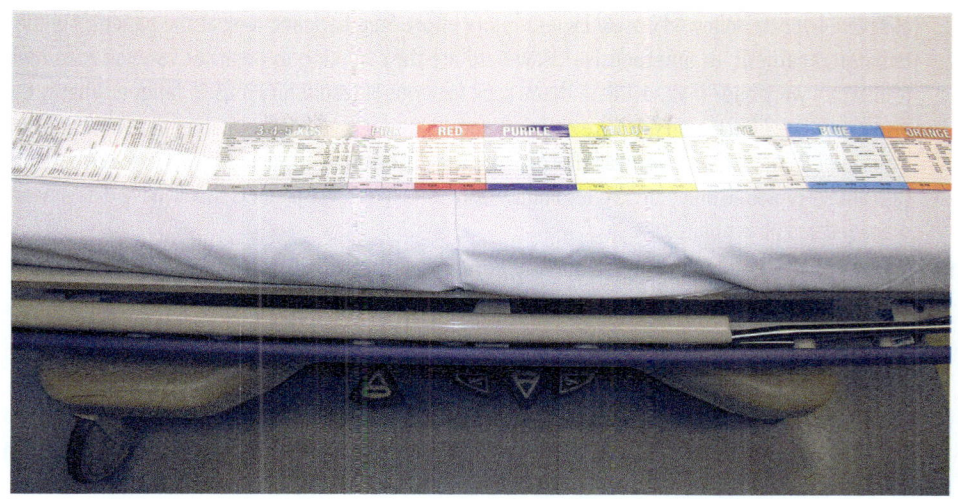

FIGURE 66.2 Broselow tape.

- Attempt the simple airway and ventilatory management techniques first. Most pediatric patients can be managed by adequate bag–mask and facemask ventilation. If you can achieve good chest rise and fall, acceptable capnography, and pulse oximetry, advanced airway management may not be warranted or even advised.
- Children compensate very well but not for very long. Once they have used their small but mighty reserve tanks, they crash rapidly. With this in mind, be aware of transport times and any special considerations such as "is there a facility with a pediatric emergency room or one capable of providing appropriate pediatric care in your system?"

11. **When does a child with respiratory distress require definitive airway management and ventilation?**
   There is no black-and-white answer. What worked on the last call may not work on the next one. It all comes back to your assessment skills and your use of the PAT. Mental status is usually the first indicator

of severe hypoxia, followed closely by respiratory effort. Step back and look at the patient. Are they lethargic, apathetic, or unresponsive? How hard are they working to breathe? Can you ease their respiratory workload? If so, ventilate them. Look for signs of respiratory muscle fatigue. What is the respiratory rate? Decreased rates are ominous and suggest impending respiratory arrest. What is the heart rate? Remember, bradycardia is the pediatric response to system failure. In most pediatric patients, the cause of profound bradycardia is respiratory distress/failure. These patients should have their airways managed and be ventilated.

12. **What are the keys to effective airway management in children?**
    - Success begins with proper positioning. If necessary, place a towel under the shoulders of younger children to align the axes of the airway, being wary of hyperextension. If the child is sitting up, be sure to check the airway for obstruction from hyperflexion.
    - When ventilating without a definitive airway in place, remember to use the Sellick maneuver (cricoid pressure) to decrease the amount of air entering the esophagus, which will eventually result in gastric distension, vomiting, and the potential for obstruction or aspiration. This maneuver may also help facilitate ET intubation. Take into consideration the immaturity of the pediatric airway, and be careful of how much pressure you use with this procedure. It is all too easy to compress the immature cartilage of the pediatric airway and actually obstruct the trachea.
    - If adequate chest excursion and oxygenation can be maintained with simple bag-mask ventilation, don't be hasty with intubation. ETT placement has inherent risks, most notably bradycardia in pediatric patients. In addition, the fact that most prehospital providers do not intubate enough pediatric patients to feel comfortable can add up to unexpected delays and complications. In a recent study of pediatric airway management, it was shown that ET intubation may actually be detrimental to some of our patients. Research is ongoing as to the effectiveness of pediatric prehospital intubation.
    - Recently, a new class of emergency airways has been developed, the supra-laryngeal or supraglottic airway. These include the laryngeal mask airway and the King LT, both of which are blindly inserted and reside in the supralaryngeal space. They are reliable and easily placed by the trained provider. Be sure to use the appropriately sized airway adjunct. Again, if a pediatric patient can be adequately ventilated using these devices, intubation may not be needed or recommended.
    - When intubation is deemed the appropriate course of treatment, most placements will be orotracheal. Nasotracheal is possible but is made extremely difficult by the high and anterior position of the vocal cords and the abrupt and acute angle (almost 90 degrees) at the nasohypopharyngeal junction. Remember the following points regarding pediatric intubation:
        - Position the child appropriately, aligning the airway axes.
        - Have a back-up plan and necessary equipment out and ready.
        - Tube size can be estimated by the size of the patient's little finger, calculated by the following formula: 4+ (age in years/4), or use the length-based pediatric resuscitation tape. The use of a cuffed ET tube may be beneficial to reduce the chance of a glottic air leak. Any air that gets out around the tube will decrease tidal volumes and not be available for gas exchange.

Respiratory Distress in Infants and Children

- Ventilation should be performed with an appropriate size bag-mask device. Tidal volumes are usually 10–15 mL/kg. Consult local protocols for ventilation rates, as most evidence currently points to lower ventilation rates, paying close attention to waveform capnography data.
- Straight blades (Miller) are preferred due to the child's small oral space and the blade's ability to directly lift up the large floppy epiglottis.
- Due to the airway anatomy it may not be easy to visualize the tube passing through the cords, the cardinal sign of successful intubation. That being said, it is imperative you use secondary means of confirmation. Which should include at least 2 of the following:
- Auscultation of the chest and epigastrium
- Equal chest expansion
- Adequate heart rate
- Waveform end-tidal CO_2 within acceptable parameters
- Pulse oximetry
- After confirmation of successful placement, if your patient becomes difficult to ventilate (poor compliance) or bradycardia develops, use the following mnemonic to quickly diagnose and correct the situation:
    - D: Displacement—has the tube moved up / down?
    - O: Obstruction—mucus, foreign body plugging the tube
    - P: Pneumothorax
    - E: Equipment failure—air leak, tube too small

13. **What are the signs and symptoms of croup and what is the best management strategy?**
Croup is the most common cause of upper-airway infection seen in children. Croup is a viral infection usually found in patients ranging from 6 months to 4 years of age and occurs most commonly in the late fall and early winter. Croup produces subglottic edema near the cricoid cartilage, the narrowest portion of the pediatric airway. The typical croup presentation is a small child with a recent history of an upper respiratory infection (URI) and cold symptoms. They usually exhibit worsening distress, accompanied by a "barky" hoarse cough, fever, and stridor. The good news is that very few of these patients will require prehospital intubation. Remember, stridor is indicative of some degree of upper respiratory obstruction. The onset of croup is slower than that of epiglottitis. (Table 66.1)

TABLE 66.1: Comparison of Croup versus Epiglottitis

Croup	Epiglottitis
Age 6 months–4 years	Age 3–7 years
Slow onset	Rapid onset
Patient may lie or sit upright	Patient prefers to sit upright
Barking cough	No barking cough, possible inspiratory stridor
Lack of drooling	Drooling, pain during swallowing
Low-grade fever	High fever

Management of the child with croup includes allowing the child to assume a position of most comfort, oxygen administration (humidified if possible), and transport with minimal agitation, as that may exacerbate the obstruction. Given the season in which croup is found, the time the patient spends in the cool damp air on the way to the ambulance is actually quite therapeutic. Pharmacological intervention is aimed at decreasing airway edema. This can be accomplished with nebulized racemic epinephrine. It constricts precapillary arterioles, thereby decreasing airway edema; as always, be aware that along with the benefits, racemic epinephrine also can cause tachycardia and hypertension. Generally, racemic epinephrine administration is reserved for those with moderate to severe respiratory distress. (Table 66.2)

TABLE 66.2: Description of the Severity of Symptoms in Croup

Mild	Moderate	Severe
Occasional barking cough	Frequent cough	Frequent bark cough
No stridor at rest (SAR)	Audible SAR	Inspiratory/expiratory SAR
Mild/no retractions	Visible retractions	Obvious retractions
No agitation	Little agitation	Severe agitation

14. **What are the signs and symptoms of epiglottitis and what is the best management?**

Epiglottitis can be a dire emergency, requiring rapid identification and intervention. In comparison to croup, epiglottitis is usually a bacterial infection producing significant supraglottic edema. The danger here is that the edema occurs above the laryngeal opening, making visualization and placement of advanced airway adjuncts difficult if not impossible in field settings. Historically, most epiglottitis was caused by *Hemophilus influenza* (H.flu), however, the H.flu vaccine has significantly decreased the number of annual cases of epiglottitis. Other bacteria can also cause this condition but are not usually as severe or rapidly progressing. Most children with epiglottitis are 3–7 years old who present with no warning symptoms. The classic presentation is that of a young child who wakes in the middle of the night with a high fever and drooling due to the painful process of trying to swallow secretions through the edema. These children will present sitting upright, maybe even leaning forward (tripod) in an attempt to pull in more air. Placing this patient supine has been associated with immediate respiratory arrest. Young children can progress from mild supraglottic edema to complete obstruction very quickly. Keeping this in mind, management is aimed at minimizing agitation, providing oxygen, and managing the airway only if the patient becomes unresponsive and cannot be adequately ventilated with a bag–mask device. Transport should be initiated quickly but so as to not further agitate the patient. By introducing a laryngoscope blade or anything else into the supraglottic region, you run the risk of increasing the edema, and causing complete airway obstruction.

15. **What is RSV?**

Respiratory syncytial virus (RSV) has been shown to be the leading cause of lower respiratory infections (LRI) in the pediatric population. Most children will develop bronchiolitis or pneumonia with an RSV infection. Children between 2–8 months of age are at greatest risk for contracting RSV. A common progression of RSV begins with a 1–2 day history of URI symptoms, followed by cough, wheezing, rales, and a low-grade fever. In the prehospital setting, these children are commonly seen with vague symptoms per the caregivers. It is important to note the hydration status of these patients, as poor oral intake may lead to dehydration. Prehospital management of the RSV patient is mainly supportive with administration of oxygen. As you may find wheezing and rales, refer to local protocols regarding β-2 agonist administration.

16. **Isn't asthma in children a relatively mild disease?**
    Absolutely not. Asthma is a disease of small airway inflammation. This inflammatory process also leads to mucosal edema, copious secretions, and bronchoconstriction. Almost 5 million children suffer from asthma, and the mortality rate is rising. Half of pediatric asthma deaths occur outside of the hospital. The length of the asthma attack in over half of the patients who die is 2 hours, with some being less than 1 hour. We, as prehospital providers, are going to see these children, and we need to be ready. An asthma attack can have many causes, or triggers. Some of the more common triggers are URIs, exercise, emotional stress, exposure to cold air, and even passive exposure to smoke. This is by no means a comprehensive list but a listing of the more common causes. Although it is very important to get a good history from someone at the scene, remember, the last thing you want your dyspneic patient to do is to expend energy and interrupt respiratory effort to give you a long medical history. Use closed-end questions with a nod or shake of the head for answers. A pen and paper also works well. Along with the usual EMS history questions, try to ask the following questions of the patient or their family which may help identify a severe attack:

    (a) Have you previously been intubated?
    (b) Have you been admitted to the intensive care unit (ICU)?
    (c) Have you been to the emergency department more than three times in a year?
    (d) Have you used more than one metered dose inhaler canister within the last month?
    (e) Have you used your bronchodilators more frequently than every 4 hours?
    (f) Are you getting worse despite aggressive home therapy?
    (g) Does this attack feel like the one that caused you to be intubated or admitted to the ICU?

    "Yes" answers to the above questions coupled with your assessment findings of distress should be cause for concern and aggressive intervention.

17. **How can I recognize asthma?**
    Common signs and symptoms of an asthma attack include tachypnea, tachycardia, increased WOB, and expiratory wheezing. The really difficult work for the asthmatic is to expel air from the bronchioles. The bronchospasm, mucus, and secretions promote air trapping, leaving carbon dioxide in the alveoli and making less oxygen available for diffusion. As previously mentioned, wheezing means air is moving in and out of the lungs. If wheezing is present on both inspiration and exhalation, the attack is progressing and requires aggressive intervention. If the patient's mental status decreases, they appear extremely fatigued or the wheezing dissipates, it is suggestive of impending respiratory failure.

18. **What should I do to treat the patient with an acute asthma attack?**
    Management of the asthmatic patient should be directed towards reversing the bronchospasm, drying up the secretions, and improving oxygenation. Releasing the bronchospasm may be accomplished by the use of a β-agonist, such as albuterol. In children with severe episodes, consider continuous nebulized albuterol therapy, if recommended per local protocol. More recently, prehospital management of an acute asthma attack includes the use of DuoNeb (ipratropium and albuterol). The added benefit to using

DuoNeb is you get the bronchodilation of the albuterol plus the anticholinergic benefit of drying the secretions. You may have DuoNeb premixed or simply combine albuterol and ipratropium. Ipratropium should not be administered to children under 5 years old or anyone with glaucoma. If no relief is realized with these inhaled medications, you may consider subcutaneous or intramuscular (IM) injection of epinephrine if protocols allow. ET intubation and assisted ventilation are indicated for the patient in impending or actual respiratory failure.

19. Are foreign bodies a problem in children?
Foreign body aspiration should be suspected in children and infants who develop sudden onset of respiratory distress associated with gagging, coughing, stridor, or wheezing. Coins, marbles, balloons, hot dogs, hard candies, raisins, nuts, and grapes are frequently aspirated. The symptoms often reflect the location of the lodged object. Drooling and gagging will be present with an esophageal obstruction. A foreign body in the trachea may cause complete or partial obstruction. Complete obstruction will be manifest by no air movement or lung sounds. Patients with an incomplete obstruction will often present with coughing, crying, or stridor while still being able to speak. The presentation is very important when deciding whether or not to intervene. If the obstruction is incomplete, management includes oxygen administration, allowing the position of comfort, minimizing agitation, and rapid transport. Relief of an airway obstruction should be attempted only if signs of complete obstruction are present, including ineffective cough (loss of sound), increasing dyspnea with stridor, cyanosis, or decreased mental status including up to and including unresponsiveness. In children less than 1 year of age, five back blows with the head dependent are followed by five chest thrusts. In children older than 1, abdominal thrusts are indicated. If the infant or child becomes unresponsive, and the obstruction still exists, attempt bag–mask ventilation. If this is unsuccessful, attempt to visualize the foreign body with direct laryngoscopy and to remove it with Magill forceps. If you are still unsuccessful, attempt bag–mask ventilations and intubation. Intubation may actually facilitate movement of the object down into a bronchus, which is not ideal, but the airway is now open and the patient can be oxygenated and ventilated using the other lung. In extreme cases, you may need to perform a needle cricothyroidostomy, or another type of surgical airway procedure, if the foreign body is above the planned surgical opening.

Pearls and Pitfalls

1. Normal appearance and increased WOB = respiratory distress. Abnormal appearance and increased or decreased WOB = respiratory failure.
2. Seriously ill children will benefit most from rapid transport to an appropriate receiving facility.
3. Do NOT wait until you find cyanosis to begin supplemental oxygen and other therapy. If you do find cyanosis, it should always be taken seriously and attacked with ventilatory support.
4. A prolonged inspiratory phase is associated with upper-airway obstruction, such as croup or a foreign body obstruction, whereas prolonged expiratory times are indicative of lower-airway disease, such as asthma and bronchiolitis.
5. Intubation should not be done electively in the field for a child who can be ventilated adequately with a bag mask.
6. All that wheezes is not asthma.

References

1. Brownstein D, Fuchs S, Diekmann RA, eds. Pediatric Education for Prehospital Professionals, 2nd ed. American Academy of Pediatrics, Sudbury, MA: Jones and Bartlett, 2006.
2. Blumen IJ, ed. APLS: The Pediatric Emergency Medicine Course, 2nd ed. Elk Grove Village, IL: American Academy of Pediatrics/American College of Emergency Physicians, 1993.
3. Associates in Emergency Medical Education. PALS Provider Manual. Lutz, FL: 2005.
4. Eckstein M. Out-of-hospital pediatric airway management. Ann Emerg Med 44(2):181–182, 2003.
5. Gausche M, Lewis RJ, Stratton SJ, et al. Effect of out-of-hospital pediatric endotracheal intubation on survival and neurological outcome: A controlled clinical trial. JAMA 283(6):783–790, 2000.
6. Gompf SG. Epiglottitis. eMedicine, Accessed November 11, 2011
7. Sharma G. Asthma. eMedicine, Accessed November 11, 2011
8. Defendi GL. Croup. eMedicine, Accessed November 11, 2011
9. Leader S, Kohlhase K. Recent trends in severe respiratory syncytial virus (FSV) among US infants, 1997 to 2000. *J Pediatr.* Nov 2003;143(5 Suppl):S127–32
10. Priestly MA. Pediatric respiratory failure. eMedicine, Accessed November 11, 2011
11. American Heart Association. 2010 Guidelines for Cardiopulmonary Resuscitation and Emergency Cardiovascular Care.
12. Rachelefsky G. Inhaled corticosteroids and asthma control in children: assessing impairment and risk. Pediatrics. Jan 2009;123(1):353–66.

Pediatric Trauma

Robert W. Schafermayer, MD, FACEP, FIFEM, FAAP

CHAPTER 67

1. **What is the most common cause of death in children?**
   Trauma is the most common cause of death in children between the ages of 1 and 14 years. Beyond infancy, motor vehicle crashes—as an occupant, cyclist, or pedestrian—are the most common cause of death, followed closely by penetrating injuries (primarily gunshot wounds). Traumatic injury is more common in summer and occurs more frequently to boys than to girls. Children from low socioeconomic settings also appear to be at higher risk. Falls, burns, and drowning occur more frequently in children than in adults.

2. **What is the Pediatric Assessment Triangle and how does it help me evaluate children?**
   The Pediatric Assessment Triangle is a concept where the health care provider assesses the appearance of the child, the breathing, and the circulation. (See Figure 66.1, page 440.) In assessing appearance, one is looking for mental status, muscle tone, and body position as well as interactiveness, consolability, gaze, and speech or cry. In assessing breathing, one is checking the respiratory rate, visible movement of the chest/abdomen, and effort, as well as abnormal airway sounds, abnormal positioning, retractions, or nasal flaring. In assessing circulation, one is checking the child's color for the presence of pallor, mottling, or cyanosis as well as pulse rate, its quality, capillary refill, and blood pressure. Based on the results of the assessment, the health care provider has a better sense of whether the child is normal, sick, or has signs of respiratory distress/failure or shock and can plan their interventions.

3. **Aren't cervical spine injuries uncommon in children?**
   Actually, they are more common than you might think. Studies have demonstrated that children account for 1–10% of all cervical spine injuries. Therefore, any child with a history of significant trauma should be immobilized in the field prior to transport simultaneously with resuscitative efforts. The injury could be a fractured vertebra or it could be spinal cord injury without radiographic abnormality (SCIWORA). Although this cannot be diagnosed in the field, it is a reminder that one must not only consider pain, bony tenderness, and muscle spasm but also neurologic function. Ask the child to hold the arms up off the ground or stretcher for a count of 5 and do the same for the legs. If there is any weakness or other signs of spinal cord injury, place the child in spinal protocol.

4. **What are the common causes of cervical spine injury in children?**
   Spine injury may result from moderate to major motor vehicle collisions, from falls greater than 8–10 feet, trauma above the clavicles, trauma associated with neurologic findings including loss of consciousness and altered mental status, diving injuries, and multisystem trauma. In addition, any child who complains of neck pain in association with minor trauma should be immobilized.

5. **How do I immobilize a child?**
   In larger children, immobilization can be achieved using pediatric-sized rigid cervical collars such as the stiff-neck or Philadelphia collar. Smaller children should be immobilized with a Kendrick extrication

device-type board if available. Blanket rolls are also an option. Because of a proportionally larger occiput, small children are difficult to immobilize in an anatomically correct position. Therefore, efforts should be made to align the external auditory meatus of the ear with the anterior line of the shoulders using padding placed under the back and shoulders. Infants can also be successfully immobilized in a pediatric car seat if available.

6. **What are the signs of airway obstruction in children?**
Airway obstruction is usually manifest by hoarseness, stridor, high-pitched voice, chest and abdominal retractions, grunting, nasal flaring, and drooling. Children who are speaking normally or crying vigorously are unlikely to have an obstructed airway. Cyanosis may be seen if the obstruction causes hypoxia.

7. **When should I insert an airway in a child?**
Airways should be used only in comatose or semicomatose children or in children requiring bag–mask ventilation, as the risk of vomiting and aspiration is somewhat higher in children. Nasal airways are better tolerated in the patient with an intact gag reflex. Appropriate airway size can be estimated by measuring the airway against the side of the child's face. An oral airway should extend from the corner of the mouth to the angle of the jaw. A nasal airway should extend from the corner of the mouth to the tragus of the ear. One can also use one of the length-based equipment sizing tapes, such as the Broselow tape. In children, oral airways should not be inserted backward and rotated as in the adult due to the risk of trauma to the teeth and mouth. Instead, the tongue should be pulled forward and the airway inserted in the physiologic position.

8. **How does intubation differ in children of different ages?**
Field intubation of children has a lower success rate when compared to adults. Nasotracheal intubation is very difficult in children because of the acute angle of the nasopharynx and the anterior and superior position of the larynx, and it should probably not be attempted. Oral intubation is the procedure of choice for comatose children in whom bag–mask ventilation has failed or who are at substantial risk for aspiration. Laryngoscope blade size can be estimated based on the child's age:

- Newborn–18 months, #1 blade
- 18 months to 10–12 years, #2 blade
- 12 years and up, #3 blade

A straight blade is generally recommended for children younger than 2–3 years old because their larynx is typically anterior and high.

Endotracheal (ET) tube size can be estimated by using a tube the size of the child's little finger or by the equation: $(age/4) + 4$ or by using a length-based equipment tape. Children younger than 8 years old should be intubated only with uncuffed tubes due to the normal physiologic narrowing at the cricoid cartilage, which should adequately prevent aspiration. Children who are 8 years and older require a cuffed tube. As a final note, confirmation of tube placement using multiple methods is required and always includes auscultation over the stomach in addition to both axillae, as esophageal intubation can mimic tracheal intubation by transmitting false breath sounds to the lungs. If available, end-tidal CO_2 detectors or monitors should be used to confirm proper tube placement.

9. **What if intubation is unsuccessful?**
If bag–mask ventilation and endotracheal intubation are unsuccessful, needle cricothyroidostomy can be performed with the approval of medical control. The space between the cricoid cartilage (Adam's

apple) and thyroid cartilage is palpated. This is the cricothyroid membrane. A 12- or 14-gauge IV catheter can be inserted through this space by entering the skin and angling the needle 45° downward toward the lungs. The needle should be aspirated continuously until air is returned. An adapter from a #3 or #3.5 ET tube can be attached to the end of the catheter, and the child may be bagged through this. Alternatively, if pressurized oxygen is available (25–50 psi), a Y connector can be attached to the catheter and oxygen line. The third unused port is then occluded for 2 seconds to permit inflation of the lungs and released for 4–5 seconds to allow for exhalation. This type of ventilation can be used only for 30 to 40 minutes before the buildup of carbon dioxide becomes toxic. Unless absolutely necessary, this procedure should not be attempted in children with significant neck trauma because the procedure becomes exponentially more difficult with any distortion of the anatomy.

10. **I hear wheezing so it must be asthma, right?**
Although it is likely that the patient has asthma, not every wheezing patient has asthma. It is essential to remember that aspiration of a foreign body, as well as infections and cardiac causes, can result in wheezing. Unfortunately, not all children will have a witnessed or obvious history of choking or swallowing an object or bite of food, thus making the diagnosis often difficult. A foreign body must always be suspected whenever an otherwise well infant or child presents with sudden onset of shortness of breath and unilateral wheezing on auscultation.

11. **What are the injuries associated with severe chest trauma? What signs should alert you to them?**
As in adults, chest trauma in children can produce tension pneumothorax, open pneumothorax, and, less commonly, flail chest, in addition to a number of other complications that cannot be diagnosed or treated in the prehospital setting, such as pulmonary contusion. General signs of critical chest injury include asymmetry of chest wall movement, retractions, nasal flaring, grunting, asymmetry of breath sounds, crepitance, rib deformity, and chest wall abrasions. All patients with significant chest or head trauma should receive high-flow oxygen by mask.
It is important to remember that external evidence of chest injuries is often lacking in children owing to the compliance of their chest wall. Ribs in children tend to bend rather than break. Thus, internal injury such as pulmonary contusion is a more common injury than rib fractures or flail chest.

12. **What is the most important finding that will help me recognize significant pulmonary injury?**
An important clue in the detection of respiratory compromise is an increasing respiratory rate. Careful initial and repeated determination of the patient's respiratory rate can help provide early recognition that the patient's respiratory status is compromised or deteriorating.

13. **Does shock manifest itself differently in children compared with adults?**
Unlike adults, in whom blood pressure can be used as a reliable measure of shock, children frequently will not demonstrate hypotension until they have lost 40% of their blood volume. Tachypnea can be an early sign of shock. Tachycardia is a much more sensitive indicator of shock in children, although confounding factors such as fear, pain, fever, and hypoxia can also produce a rapid heart rate. Circulating volume can be quickly assessed by checking capillary refill. The nail bed or thenar eminence (at the base of the thumb) can be compressed for 5 seconds and then released. With adequate circulating blood volume, color should return within 2 seconds. A table of age-based pediatric vital signs can also be very

helpful (Table 67.1). Roughly, the upper limit of normal for pediatric heart rates is 180 beats/min for neonates, 150 beats/min for infants 1 year old; 150 beats/min from 1 to 3 years old; 125 beats/min from 3 to 7 years old; and 110 beats/min from 7 to 14 years old. Heart rates that exceed these maximums should be considered signs of significant hypovolemic shock. A quick estimation of minimum normal blood pressure in children can be made with this equation: $(2 \times \text{age}) + 80$.

TABLE 67.1: Pediatric Vital Signs (range of normal)

	Heart Rate		Respiratory Rate		Systolic Blood Pressure (mmHg)
	Low	High	Low	High	
Newborn infant	120	180	30	60	>60
Infant 1–12 months	100	150	24	60	>70
Toddler (1–3 years)	90	150	22	40	>80
Preschooler (3–5 years)	80	125	22	30	>80
School age (6–12 years)	70	110	16	30	>80
Adolescent (13 years and over)	60	100	12	20	>90

14. **What if an IV line is difficult to place?**
Placing an IV line can be particularly difficult in children. The easiest sites for placing a percutaneous IV line are the antecubital fossa, the interdigital vein of the dorsum of the hand between the fourth and fifth digits, and the greater saphenous vein at the ankle. Access should be attempted on scene only if transport time is greater than 15 minutes. An unstable child is probably better served by rapid transport with IV access attempts made en route only. If no venous access is possible and the child is in desperate need of fluids, an intraosseous line may be placed, whether by standing order or on the order of medical control. These lines are easier to insert in children younger than 6 years of age and are extremely painful. Thus, it is generally reserved for the child who clearly needs fluid emergently and has an altered mental status. An intraosseous needle or 16- or 18-gauge ½-inch bone marrow needle should be used. The puncture is made one finger width distal to the tibial tuberosity (the insertion of the patellar tendon) on the anterior aspect of the tibia. The leg is placed in a 30° flexed position, and the needle is introduced with the bevel up. The needle should be directed toward the foot at a 45–60° angle to the surface of the tibia. Placement should be confirmed by aspiration of bone marrow. When flushed, the line should flow easily without swelling around the site. If the line appears to be in good position, fluid and medications can be infused through it effectively. The line must be discontinued when adequate venous access has been established.

15. **How do I give IV fluids to a child?**
Any child with evidence of shock should receive prompt fluid resuscitation. The initial recommendation is to administer a bolus 20 mL/kg of isotonic fluid, either lactated Ringer's or normal saline. The appropriate volume of fluid should be run wide open or bolused using a 50-mL or 60-mL syringe. If the child's clinical picture or vital signs fail to respond to this initial bolus, a second and third bolus, also at

20 mL/kg, can be given. It should be noted that the total blood volume for a child is 80 mL/kg. Therefore, any child who fails to respond to three fluid boluses should be assumed to be in severe hypovolemic shock and will likely require red blood cell transfusions and immediate surgical intervention. Heart rate, respiratory rate, blood pressure, and mental status should be followed closely during transport. If the child's weight is not available from individuals on the scene, a Broselow tape may be used to estimate the child's weight using the child's height (length) (See Figure 66.2, page 443.) For children one year of age or older, you can roughly estimate weight with the following formula:

$$\text{wt in kg} = (\text{age} \times 2) + 8.$$

16. How is the Glasgow Coma Scale (GCS) modified for children?

In addition to observing pupillary response and movement of extremities, you should perform a brief mental status examination for all pediatric trauma patients. This may be as simple as asking the child his name. An adequate response to questioning is sufficient to establish appropriate mentation. This process is more difficult in the nonverbal or preverbal child. The AVPU mnemonic (**A**lert, responds to **V**ocal stimuli, responds only to **P**ainful stimuli, **U**nresponsive) can, in the primary survey, be used without alteration; however, the verbal and motor portions of the GCS require modification for these patients. (The eye-opening response is unchanged.) The motor response is only slightly modified: A score of 6 is associated with *spontaneous intentional movement*, and a score of 5 is *localized withdrawal to pain*. The entire verbal-response scale is modified as follows:

Appropriate words or social smile, normal gaze (i.e., looks at an object and follows it when moved)	5
Cries but consolable	4
Persistently irritable or inconsolable	3
Restless, agitated	2
None	1

17. How does the small size of children affect outcome after a traumatic event?

Physiologically, children have less subcutaneous tissue and relatively thin skin when compared with adults. In addition, small body size increases the ratio of surface area to body mass. Because of these differences, children are much more prone to hypothermia than their adult counterparts. Great care should be taken in the field to avoid hypothermia by using ambulance heaters, blankets, and warmed intravenous fluids. Exposure should be minimized, as hypothermia and shivering greatly increases oxygen consumption. With falling body temperature, body tissues become refractory to treatment, the central nervous system becomes depressed, and coagulation becomes impaired. Children who present with extreme hypothermia to the point of coagulopathy have only a 50% survival rate.

18. What concerns should I have in a child with a seatbelt sign?

A true seatbelt sign is bruising or ecchymosis along the mid to lower abdomen, depending on how and where the seatbelt was applied and whether the child slid down during impact. The associated injuries include not only the usual intra-abdominal solid organ injuries but also possible bowel-wall perforation and lumbar spine flexion fracture. The child should be properly immobilized, transported to an appropriate hospital, and watched for any early signs of shock.

Pearls and Pitfalls

1. Practice and use your assessment skills. They are important to your decision making in the care of the child and, by recognizing early signs of compromise, may prevent a respiratory or cardiac arrest.
2. Assess the work of breathing by looking for retractions; nasal flaring, head bobbing, grunting, or lethargy and grunting respirations are ominous.
3. Do not wait for cyanosis; assess respiratory effort, get the patient on oxygen and check pulse oximetry.
4. Recognize shock in its early stages; look for tachypnea and tachycardia; as shock progresses you will note delayed capillary refill and altered mental status.
5. If the child is hypotensive, administer oxygen, transport rapidly, start your vascular access enroute and give fluid as a bolus.

References

1. Wesson DE, ed. Pediatric Trauma: Pathophysiology, Diagnosis, and Treatment. New York: Taylor and Francis Group, 2006.
2. Waltzman ML, Mooney DP. Major trauma. In Textbook of Pediatric Emergency Medicine, 5th ed., Fleisher GR, Ludwig S, Henretig FM, eds., pp. 1349–1360. Philadelphia: Lippincott Williams & Wilkins, 2006.
3. Dieckmann RA, Schafermeyer RW. Emergency medical services. In Pediatric Emergency Medicine: A Comprehensive Study Guide, 2nd ed., Strange GR, Ahrens WR, Lelyveld S, Schafermeyer RW, eds., pp. 773–787. New York: McGraw-Hill Companies Inc., 2002.
4. Tepas JJ, Fallat ME, Moriarty TM. Trauma. In APLS: The Pediatric Emergency Medicine Resource, 4th ed., Gausche-Hill M, Fuchs S, Yamamoto L, eds., pp. 268–323. Sudbury, MA: Jones and Bartlett, 2004.
5. Burg J, Fleisher GR. Prehospital care of the injured child. In Pediatric Trauma: Prevention, Acute Care, Rehabilitation, Eichelberger M. ed., pp. 99–112. St. Louis: Mosby Yearbook, 1993.
6. Graneto JW, Solgin DF. Transport and stabilization of the pediatric trauma patient. Pediatr Clin North Am 40:365–380, 1993.
7. Meyer P, Carli P. Transport of the severely injured child. Int Anesthesiol Clin 32:149–170, 1994.
8. Polhgeers A, Ruddy R. An update on pediatric trauma. Emerg Med Clin North Am 8:267–290, 1995.

Child Abuse and Nonaccidental Trauma

Nicholas C. Johnson, MD

CHAPTER 68

1. **What are the four categories of child abuse?**
   Physical abuse, sexual abuse, psychological abuse, and neglect
2. **How many children are the victims of abuse each year?**
   There were approximately 700,00–900,000 cases of abuse confirmed by Child Protective Services (CPS) in 2009, although this number is thought to be a gross underrepresentation of the incidence of true abuse in the United States due to lack of reporting and inability to confirm some cases. CPS investigated approximately 3.6 million suspected cases of abuse and almost 1700 children died from documented child abuse in 2009.
3. **What is the prehospital role in child abuse?**
   In nearly all states, prehospital personnel are mandated reporters of child abuse; that is, they are legally obligated to report suspected child abuse. EMS providers have a very unique and important role in prevention and treatment of child abuse, as they are often the only medical providers given access to a home. The home environment can provide significant insight into a child's social and family situation and raise suspicion of abuse when it might not otherwise be suspected.
4. **What if I report suspected child abuse, and I am wrong?**
   In nearly all states, those who report child abuse in good faith are immune from prosecution in criminal and civil trials. Alternately, in nearly all states, those mandatory reporters who "knew" or "should have known" abuse was occurring and did not report it, can be penalized by loss of license, fine, or criminal prosecution.
5. **What historical clues might raise suspicion for abuse?**
   - Injury with inconsistent or suspicious history (i.e., inability to explain injury, inconsistent story, injury blamed on third party)
   - Delay in seeking care
   - Injury inconsistent with developmental milestones (i.e., a two-month-old cannot roll over, a 10-month-old cannot climb stairs)
   - Lack of parental concern about injuries, or overconcern about trivial injuries
   - Lack of parental concern about a child in pain
   - Lack of parental trust of health care providers
6. **How does one recognize that abuse is or may be occurring?**
   In the absence of obvious objective evidence or reports of abuse, presentations may be subtle and require knowledge of developmental milestones (i.e., Can a two-month-old roll off a changing table? What is the appropriate weight for a 4-year-old?), a baseline suspicion during any pediatric call, and keen observation.

Child Abuse and Nonaccidental Trauma

Recent studies involving prehospital personnel show that most do not feel adequately trained and prepared to recognize and report suspected child abuse. Another study showed that in confirmed cases of child abuse by medical examiner, only 25% were suspected by EMS providers at the scene.

7. **What physical signs might one see that should raise the suspicion of child physical abuse?**
   Signs of child abuse can vary widely and are often quite nonspecific. They need to be taken in context with the explained mechanism for injury, the social situation, and other available information. Injuries unusual in accidental trauma which may be apparent to prehospital personnel include:
   - Bruising on the ears, cheeks, neck, buttock, thighs, torso, and genitals, or bruising in any child who is not "upright" and therefore cannot fall
   - Any patterned bruising (i.e., in the shape of an object, fingers, belt, rope, etc.)
   - Burns from cigarettes, ropes, or immersion (i.e., immersed in hot water)
   - Bites
   - Multiple sites of injury

8. **What are signs of neglect?**
   Signs of neglect noted by prehospital providers may include inappropriate hygiene or dress, severe diaper rash, failure to thrive (i.e., noticeably undersized or underweight, abnormal behavior, delayed development), lack of supervision, or abandonment.

9. **A recent panel of experts in EMS and CPS (Child Protective Services) convened to define the responsibilities of prehospital personnel in cases of suspected abuse and neglect. What are these responsibilities?**
   Gather information (scene survey, observe patient/family interaction, assessment of mechanism of injury), provide appropriate medical care, recognize suspected child abuse and neglect (obtain education, be open to possibility of abuse), provide interventions, document and report (preserve evidence, learn what and how to report), integrate with CPS, and engage in prevention activities.

10. **What are the consequences of child abuse?**
    Other than the obvious risk of death and physical and emotional pain of the child, children who are victims of abuse are more likely to develop behaviors that put their health at risk; these include smoking, alcoholism, drug abuse, eating disorders, severe obesity, depression, suicide, sexual promiscuity, and certain chronic diseases. Abuse in early childhood can cause the brain to form improperly and lead to physical, mental, and emotional problems including attention deficit hyperactivity disorder, sleep disturbances, and panic disorder. While 25% of cases of shaken baby syndrome result in death, nonfatal consequences include blindness, cerebral palsy, and cognitive deficits. Children who are abused are twice as likely to be physically abused as adults.

Pearls and Pitfalls

1. Prehospital personnel are legally obligated to report suspected child abuse.
2. A mechanism of injury not compatible with the child's age and development milestones is suspicious for child abuse.
3. Lack of appropriate parental concern is suspicious for abuse.
4. When in doubt report the suspicion so that an appropriate investigation can be done.

References

1. Markenson D, Foltin G, Tunik M, et al. Knowledge and attitude assessment and education of prehospital personnel in child abuse and neglect: Report of a national blue ribbon panel. Ann Emerg Med 40:89–101, 2002.
2. Lonergan, GJ. Uniformed Services University of the Health Sciences, Child abuse referral and education (CARE) network [online]. 2007 Feb 17. [Cited 2007 Feb 17.] Available from http://rad.usuhs.mil/rad/home/peds/abuse.html
3. Markenson D, Tunik M, Cooper A, et al. A national assessment of knowledge, attitudes, and confidence of prehospital providers in the assessment and management of child maltreatment. Pediatrics 119(1):103–108, 2007.
4. King BR, Baker MD, Ludwig S: Reporting of child abuse by prehospital personnel. Prehosp Disaster Med 8(1):67–68, 1993.
5. Graham SD, Olson LM, Sapien RE, et al. Adequacy of EMS data collection during pediatric cardiac arrest: Are EMTs getting the whole story? Prehosp Emerg Care 1(1):28–31, 1997.
6. Markenson D, Foltin G, Tunik M, et al. Knowledge and attitude assessment and education of prehospital personnel in child abuse and neglect: Report of a national blue ribbon panel. Ann Emerg Med 40:89–101, 2002.
7. Centers for Disease Control and Prevention. National Center for Injury Prevention and Control. Child maltreatment: fact sheet [online]. Atlanta, GA. 2006 Sep 7. [Cited 2007 Feb 16]. Available from http://www.cdc.gov/ncipc/factsheets/cmfacts.htm

Special Situations

SECTION VII

Chapter 69
Water Emergencies 461
Lee W. Shockley, MD, MBA

Chapter 70
Decompression Illnesses 465
Jeffrey J. Messerole, PS

Chapter 71
Wilderness Emergency Medical Services 473
Paul S. Auerbach, MD, MS, FACEP, FAWM, and Laura W. Kates, MD

Chapter 72
Lightning 479
Lee W. Shockley, MD, MBA

Chapter 73
Bites, Stings, and Envenomations 484
Richard C. Dart, MD, PhD

Chapter 74
Tactical Emergency Medicine 488
David Q. McArdle, MD, and Tamra D. Glore, RN, BSN, CPHM

Chapter 75
Hazardous Materials 503
Michael G. Stanley, M.Ed, EMT-P

Chapter 76
Technical Rescues 508
Michael G. Stanley, M.Ed, EMT-P

Water Emergencies

Lee W. Shockley, MD, MBA

CHAPTER 69

1. **What is drowning? Near-drowning? Submersion incident?**
   "Drowning" is defined as death by suffocation after submersion. The term "near-drowning" is open to misinterpretation and is not preferred. The terminology recommended by the American Heart Association and the European Resuscitation Council is "submersion incident." A person who suffers adverse affects from being submersed in water has experienced a submersion incident; this may or may not result in a fatal outcome.

2. **How common are submersion incidents?**
   There were 3443 unintentional drownings (deaths) in the United States in 2007, not including drownings in boating-related incidents. Worldwide, there may be as many as 500,000 deaths from drowning. There is a bimodal age distribution in submersion deaths: children younger than 4 years old are the victims in nearly half (highest rate in children 1 to 2 years old) and young adults, age 15 to 25 (related to risk-taking behavior and alcohol use).
   There are some identified risk factors for submersion incidents:
   - Male gender: 80% of drownings in the United States are males.
   - Children: the second leading cause of injury-related death for children is from 1 to 14 years.
   - Race: the overall age-adjusted drowning rate for African Americans is 1.4 times higher than for whites; this is most likely due to primarily socioeconomic factors.
   - Alcohol: 25–50% of adolescent and adult deaths associated with water recreation also involve alcohol use.
   - Boating: 70% of boating fatalities are caused by drowning.

3. **What is the sequence of events in a submersion incident?**
   Mammals must breathe to survive. Through force of will, we can hold our breath for a period of time. The duration of breath holding is quite variable among individuals and circumstances. Eventually, however, a "breakpoint" is reached at which a powerful involuntary drive forces inhalation. If this gasp occurs underwater, the result is aspiration. Water enters the lungs and "washes out" surfactant, resulting in alveolar collapse, atelectasis, intrapulmonary shunting, ventilation–perfusion mismatch, pulmonary edema, hypoxia, and the acute respiratory distress syndrome. Hypoxemia, in turn, produces effects in all of the tissues throughout the body.

4. **What is "dry drowning"?**
   Ten to twenty percent of drowning victims do not have evidence of a significant volume of aspirated water in their lungs at autopsy. These have been called "dry drownings." The phenomenon has been attributed to severe laryngospasm. Recently, however, this notion has been questioned. Dry drownings more likely represent death by sudden cardiac standstill (as associated with patients with long-QT syndrome). The percentage of drowned victims with otherwise normal heart and lungs who do not have

penetration of liquid into their airways is less than 2%. Whether fluid is aspirated into the lungs or not would seem to be an important determinant of survival. "Wet" versus "dry" drowning probably does not matter. First, it is nearly impossible in the prehospital environment to establish whether aspiration has taken place or not. Second, the success of the resuscitation is much more dependent upon the rapid reversal of hypoxia rather than whether the drowning was "wet" or "dry."

5. **Does it make a difference whether the person was submersed in fresh water or salt water?**
In theory, aspiration of hypertonic fluids (saltwater) can lead to massive pulmonary edema and hypertonic serum; hypotonic fluids (freshwater) can lead to intravascular volume overload, dilution of serum electrolytes, and hemolysis. However, aspiration of more than 11 mL/kg is necessary before blood volume changes occur; aspiration of more than 22 mL/kg is necessary before electrolyte changes occur. Most drowned victims aspirate less than 4 mL/kg. Aspiration of as little as 1–3 mL/kg of either freshwater or saltwater can lead to significant impairment of gas exchange in the lungs. Therefore, the distinction between freshwater and saltwater drowning is not significant. It is the amount of water aspirated, not the tonicity, which most greatly determines the effects on the lungs.

6. **What are some of the comon signs and symptoms of submersion incidents?**

Common Symptoms and Signs of Submersion Incidents by Organ Systems

Pulmonary		Gastrointestinal	
Symptoms	**Signs**	**Symptoms**	**Signs**
■ Coughing	■ Apnea	■ Nausea	■ Gastric distention
■ Choking	■ Hypoxia	■ Vomiting	■ Aspiration
■ Dyspnea	■ Cyanosis		
	■ Tachypnea		
	■ Rhonchi		
	■ Rales		
	■ Wheezing		
	■ Pulmonary edema		
	■ Aspiration pneumonia		

Central Nervous System		Cardiac	
Symptoms	**Signs**	**Symptoms**	**Signs**
■ Lethargy	■ Altered mental status edema	■ Palpitations	■ Dysrhythmias
■ Coma	■ Increased ICP[a]	■ Chest pain	■ Cardiac arrest
	■ Decreased Glasgow coma scale score		■ Hypotension
			■ Cardiac ischemia
			■ Immersion syndrome

Renal	Hematologic
Signs	**Signs**
■ Acute renal failure[b]	■ Acidosis (lactate)
	■ Coagulopathy
	■ DIC[c]

[a]ICP: intracranial pressure.
[b]As a result from hypoxia, acidosis, or rhabdomyolysis.
[c]DIC: disseminated intravascular coagulation.

7. What is "immersion syndrome"?

Immersion syndrome is sudden cardiac death on submersion in very cold water (at least 5°C less than body temperature). It is likely a result of vagal stimulation and subsequent cardiac arrest. It may be related to the mammalian dive reflex. There is great individual variability in the strength of this reflex in human beings, and it is probably strongest in small children.

8. Speaking of cold water, is hypothermia an issue in submersion incidents?

Yes. Water has 25 times the ability to conduct heat, as does air. Heat can be lost quickly through the skin, and cold water that is swallowed or aspirated can lead to very rapid core cooling. Significant cerebral cooling is likely in these patients, even before circulatory collapse. This may have a protective effect through decreasing the oxygen demands of the brain and probably accounts for the rare cases of recovery in victims submerged under very cold water for 30 minutes or more.

Patients who are profoundly hypothermic may appear to be dead. Therefore, it is generally considered prudent to continue resuscitation efforts until the victim has been warmed to a core temperature of at least 33–35°C (91.4°F–95 °F).

9. What is "postimmersion syndrome"?

Postimmersion syndrome has also been called "secondary drowning." It is a respiratory distress syndrome that develops hours or days after the initial resuscitation. It may occur in up to 5% of submersion patients. The etiology is likely multifactorial, including hypoxia, loss of surfactant, transalveolar fluid shifts, and aspiration of contaminants. Therefore, everyone who has been a victim of a submersion incident should be transported to the hospital for evaluation and observation, regardless of how good they may initially or currently look.

10. How should I attempt to rescue a drowning person?

If the victim is awake, flotation devices, a pole, or ropes may be extended. Boat rescue is another option. It is frequently best, however, to use the boat to support the victim in the water rather than risk capsizing by pulling the victim in. Swimming rescue is the most dangerous of all to the rescuer. It should only be attempted by rescuers who are trained in water rescue.

Prompt rescue breathing is the most important treatment for submersion victims. If it can be safely accomplished while the patient is being extricated from the water, it should be. There is no need to clear the patient's airway of aspirated water. The Heimlich maneuver may be used only if it is suspected that solid foreign matter is obstructing the airway. Routine immobilization of the cervical spine is probably not necessary unless there is a history of diving, use of a water slide, signs of trauma, or signs of alcohol intoxication. If any of those conditions are present, however, the patient should be suspected of having suffered occult trauma and should be treated accordingly.

Due to buoyancy, in-water chest compressions are ineffective. However, they may be provided once the patient has been extricated, if necessary. Early intubation and the usual advanced cardiac life support (ACLS) guidelines are recommended. Patients should have their wet clothing removed and wrapped in blankets to prevent further hypothermia. All submersion victims, regardless of how minimal their resuscitation, require monitoring and transportation to a medical facility.

Pearls and Pitfalls

1. Protect the spine if there is a history of diving or trauma.
2. All submersion victims should be transported to an ED for evaluation.
3. Hypothermia is commonly associated with submersion incidents.
4. Up to 50% of submersion incidents occur in young males and involve alcohol.
5. Prompt rescue breathing is the most important treatment for submersion victims.

References

1. American Heart Association. 2010 American Heart Association Guidelines for Cardiopulmonary Resuscitation and Emergency Cardiovascular Care. 122(Suppl. Pt. 12.11). S847–S848, 2010.
2. Bierens JJ, Knape JT, Gelissen HP. Drowning. Curr Opin Crit Care 8(6):578–586, 2002.
3. Brenner RA, Trumble AC, Smith GS, et al. Where children drown, United States, 1995. Pediatrics 108(1):85–89, 2001.
4. Centers for Disease Control and Prevention. Water injuries fact sheet. http://www.cdc.gov/HomeandRecreational Safety/Water-Safety/waterinjuries-factsheet.html. Accessed June 5, 2011.
5. Lunetta P, Modell JH, Sajantila A. What is the incidence and significance of "dry-lungs" in bodies found in water? Am J Forensic Med Pathol 25(4):291–301, 2004.
6. Modell JH, Bellefleur M, Davis JH. Drowning without aspiration: Is this an appropriate diagnosis? J Forensic Sci 44(6):1119–1123, 1999.
7. Newman AB. Submersion incidents. In Wilderness Medicine, 4th ed., Auerbach PS, ed., pp. 1340–1365. St. Louis: Mosby; 2001.
8. Orlowski JP, Szpilman D. Drowning. Rescue, resuscitation, and reanimation. Pediatr Clin North Am 48(3):627–646, 2001.
9. Parkes MJ. Breath-holding and its breakpoint. Exp Physiol 91(1):1–15, 2006.
10. Smith DJ. Diagnosis and management of diving accidents. Med Sci Sports Exerc 28:587, 1996.
11. Weinstein MD, Krieger BP. Near-drowning: Epidemiology, pathophysiology, and initial treatment. J Emerg Med 14:461, 1996.

Decompression Illnesses

Jeffrey J. Messerole, PS

CHAPTER 70

1. **What are dysbarisms? Is that the same as decompression illness (DCI)?**
   Dysbarisms are medical conditions that result from exposure to increased ambient pressure through volume-pressure changes within the air-filled cavities in the body and from increased dissolution of gases, particularly nitrogen, in body tissues. Decompression illness (DCI) is one form of dysbarism. DCI results from the formation of small bubbles of nitrogen gas in the blood and tissues.

2. **So it's all physics, right?**
   Well, certainly an understanding of physical laws is important in appreciating the mechanisms of dysbarism. Some of the laws of physics that are important include:
   Pascal's law: a pressure applied to any part of a liquid is transmitted equally throughout.
   Boyle's law: at a constant temperature, the absolute pressure and the volume of gas are inversely proportional. As pressure increases the gas is compressed and the volume is reduced; as the pressure is reduced the gas volume increases (see Figure 70.1).
   Charles' law: at a constant pressure, the volume of a gas is directly proportional to the change in the absolute temperature.
   Dalton's law: the total pressure exerted by a mixture of gases is equal to the sum of the pressures (partial pressures) of each of the different gases making up the mixture, with each gas acting as if it alone was present and occupied the total volume.
   Henry's law: the amount of a gas that will dissolve in a liquid at a given temperature is directly proportional to the partial pressure of that gas.
   The *general gas law* combines these concepts to predict the behavior of a gas when the factors change. The formula for expressing the general gas law is:

   $$P_1 * V_1/T_1 = P_2 * V_2/T_2$$

   where

   P_1 = initial pressure (absolute)
   V_1 = initial volume
   T_1 = initial temperature (absolute)
   P_2 = final pressure (absolute)
   V_2 = final volume
   T_2 = final temperature (absolute)

3. **What else do I need to know about the physics?**
   Seawater is obviously denser than air (nearly 800 times more dense). On the surface, we experience one atmosphere (atm) of pressure (760 mm Hg at "standard conditions": temperature = 68°F (20°C), air density = 0.075 lb/ft³ (1.29 kg/m³), and relative humidity = 0%). To lower the atmospheric pressure to $1/2$ atm, one

Special Situations

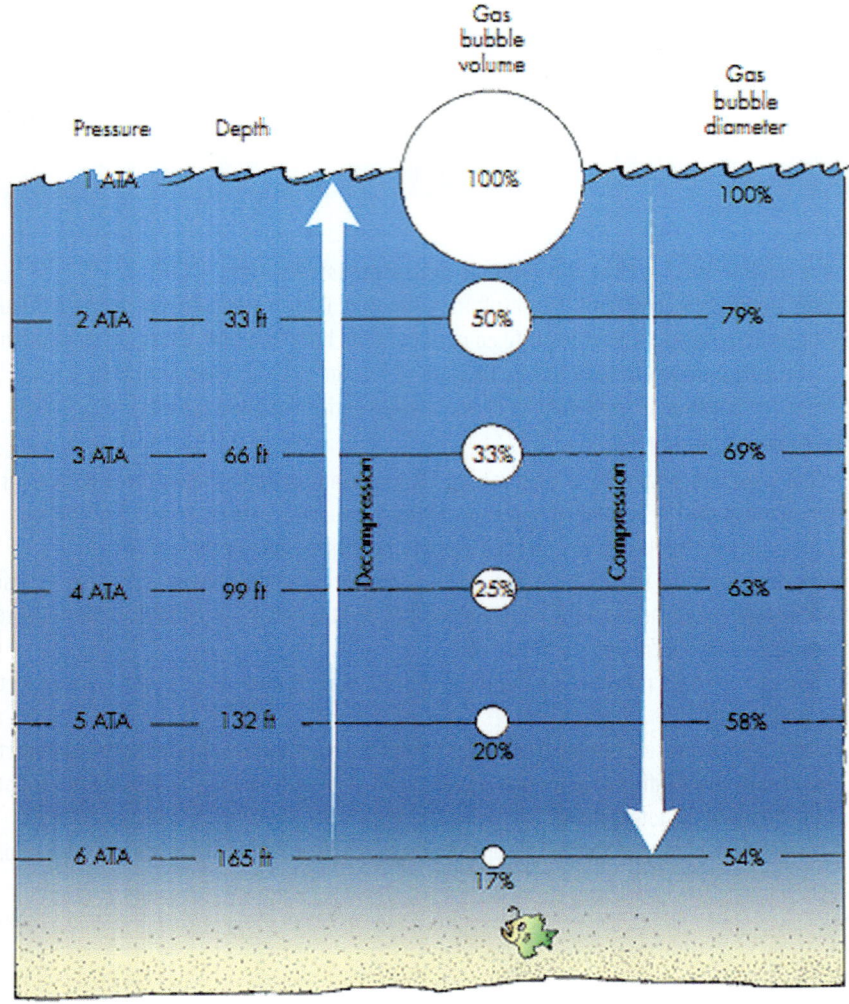

FIGURE 70.1 Boyle's law. From Kizer KW, Diving medicine, in Wilderness Medicine, 5th ed., Auerbach PS, ed. St. Louis: Mosby, 2007. Used with permission.

would have to ascend to 18,000 feet. However, to double the pressure (2 atm), one needs to only descend 33 feet in seawater (fsw). Each additional 33 feet of depth adds another atmosphere of pressure.

4. **So dysbarism is a scuba-diving problem, right? I don't dive and I live in a state that doesn't border an ocean.**
Not exactly true, and not so fast. It is true that free divers (breath-holding divers), are not at risk for DCI because they are not absorbing increased levels of nitrogen. However, they can suffer from other dysbarisms, such as mask squeeze, sinus squeeze, and pulmonary barotrauma. Free diving occurs in every state in the union and dysbarisms have been known to happen even in shallow diving in swimming

pools. Furthermore, the popularity of diving is growing and your patients may return from a diving vacation with serious dysbaric illnesses that need your attention.

5. **How do I make sense of all of the various dysbarisms?**
   It helps to classify dysbarisms in terms of when they occur during the dive. There are disorders of descent (increasing pressure), disorders of depth, and disorders of ascent (decreasing pressure).

Disorders of Descent	Disorders of Depth	Disorders of Ascent
Middle ear barotrauma	Nitrogen narcosis	**EXCEED NO DECOMPRESSION LIMIT**
	Oxygen toxicity	Decompression illness (DCI Types I and II)
External ear barotrauma		**RAPID ASCENT**
Inner ear barotrauma		Arterial gas embolism (AGE)
Barosinusitis		Pneumothorax
("sinus squeeze")		Pneumomediastinum
Facial barotrauma		Subcutaneous emphysema
("mask squeeze")		Alveolar hemorrhage
		Alternobaric vertigo
		Barodentalgia
		Gastrointestinal barotrauma
		Pulmonary edema

6. **Is it just a matter of when the symptoms begin?**
   Although that is an important thing to note, there is more to the history. The onset of symptoms may be somewhat variable. For example, arterial gas embolism (AGE) typically manifests itself immediately upon surfacing; however, the symptoms of decompression illness (DCI) may begin upon surfacing or may be delayed several hours.
   This is a suggestion for a focused dive history which will help you make your way through the differential diagnoses:

Focused Dive History

- When was the first onset of symptoms?
- What type of equipment was used? Compressed air, mixed gas, enriched air, rebreather? What was the source of the gas?
- Did the dive approach or exceed decompression limits? Was a dive computer used?
- What were the number, depth, bottom time, total time, and surface intervals for all dives in the 72 hours preceding symptoms (the dive "profiles")?
- Were decompression stops used? Was in-water decompression attempted?
- What was the time delay from the last dive to air travel?
- Did the diver experience difficulty with ear or sinus equilibration? Did the pain occur on descent or ascent?

Special Situations

- Was the diver intoxicated? Dehydrated? Working strenuously?
- How long after the dive did symptoms present? Were they present at surfacing? Delayed? Progressive?
- Is a medical history of ear or sinus infections or abnormalities present? Emphysema or asthma? Coronary artery disease? Patent foramen ovale? Neurologic illness?

7. **Tell me about the disorders of descent.**
   They are caused by the increasing pressure of water against air-filled structures of the body during descent. The most common is middle ear barotrauma (MEBT), also known as barotitis or "ear squeeze." It is experienced by 30% of novice scuba divers and 10% of experienced divers. If the diver does not increase the pressure behind the tympanic membrane (by "equilibrating" through forcing air through the eustachian tube), the tympanic membrane becomes bowed inward and painfully stretched (see Figure 70.2). If that situation is allowed to continue, the result is typically tympanic membrane rupture. The ruptured tympanic

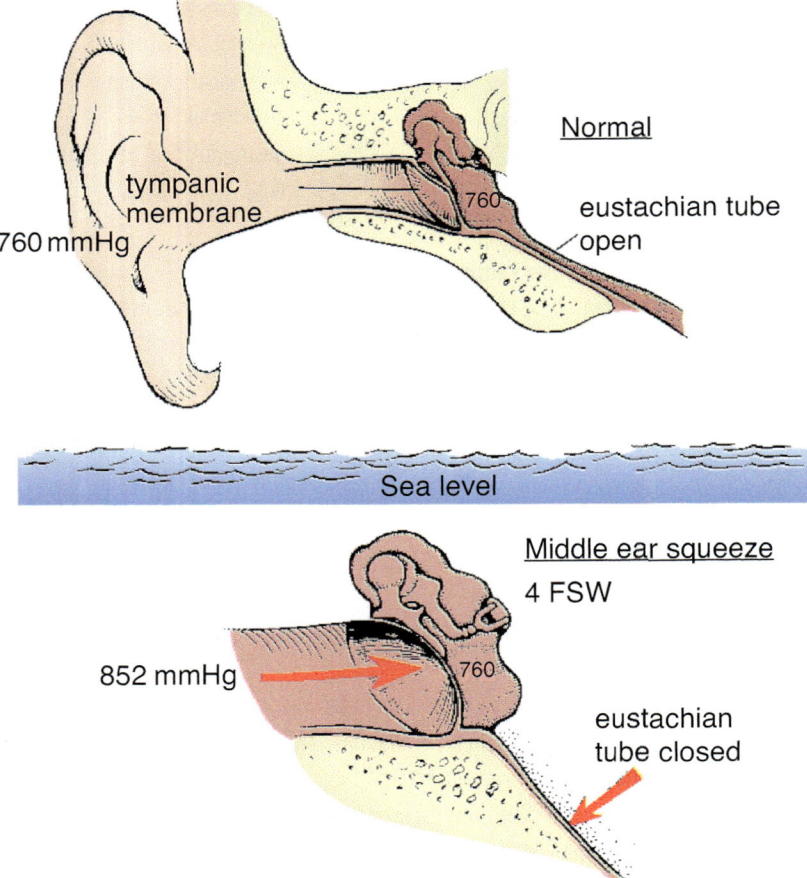

FIGURE 70.2 Anatomy of the ear and middle ear trauma. From Kizer KW, Diving medicine, in Wilderness Medicine, 5th ed., Auerbach PS, ed. St. Louis: Mosby, 2007. Used with permission.

membrane may expose the middle ear to cold water, causing caloric-induced nystagmus, vertigo, nausea, and vomiting.

External ear barotrauma (EEBT) is less common than MEBT. It comes about when there is some obstruction to the external ear canal (cerumen or foreign bodies). This is why divers should not use ear plugs.

Inner ear barotrauma (IEBT) is also much less common than MEBT. Initially, the mechanism is similar to MEBT. However, sudden equilibration of pressure in the middle ear or a vigorous Valsalva maneuver may rupture the round window and may cause hemorrhage into the inner ear or tearing of the labyrinthine (Reissner's) membrane. The symptoms and symptoms of IEBT include hearing loss, severe vertigo, nausea, tinnitus, and fullness in the affected ear. severe nystagmus, positional vertigo, ataxia, and vomiting.

Sinus squeeze acts in a similar fashion. The pain of maxillary barosinusitis may be felt primarily in the upper teeth.

Mask squeeze is due to a failure of the diver to equilibrate the pressure within their mask upon descent. It can cause very impressive facial edema and bruising as well as subconjunctival hemorrhages.

8. **How about the disorders of depth?**

The most common is nitrogen narcosis, also called the "rapture of the deep." An interesting property of nitrogen is that it has general anesthetic effects at increased pressures. The symptoms include euphoria, a false feeling of well-being, confusion, loss of judgment or skill, disorientation, inappropriate laughter, diminished motor control, and tingling and vague numbness of the lips, gums, and legs. The initial symptoms mimic mild intoxication; as it progresses, however, judgment and coordination are impaired. Finally, loss of consciousness may result.

Nitrogen narcosis is depth dependent. Some divers speak of "Martini's law" as a rule of thumb: for every additional atmosphere of pressure (33 fsw), the physiological effect of nitrogen is roughly equivalent to drinking one alcoholic beverage (hence the "Martini" part). Therefore, a dive to 99 fsw or more may have a significant intoxicating result.

At partial pressures exceeding 1.6 atm absolute for extended periods of time, oxygen can be toxic to the central nervous system (CNS) or lungs. Symptoms of CNS oxygen toxicity may be remembered by the mnemonic VENTIDC:

V: Visual symptoms (tunnel vision or blurred vision)
E: Ear symptoms (tinnitus)
N: Nausea or spasmodic vomiting
T: Twitching and tingling symptoms (small facial muscles, lips, or muscles of the extremities)
I: Irritability, confusion, agitation, and anxiety
D: Dizziness, clumsiness, incoordination, and unusual fatigue
C: Convulsions

It is unlikely, however, that sport divers will have the duration of exposure that will make this a significant problem.

9. **What are the disorders of ascent?**

As the diver ascends the surrounding pressure from water decreases. This can cause two problems: gases trapped within an enclosed space expand (Boyle's law) and gases in solution may come out of solution and form bubbles (Henry's law).

The first mechanism can cause barodentalgia (toothache from an abscess or newly placed filling), gastrointestinal barotrauma (gastric or intestinal distention), or alternobaric vertigo (the result of an inability to equalize pressure within the middle ear during ascent; the patient experiences a profound but transient sense of vertigo that may be associated with nausea and vomiting).

Air trapped within the lungs during ascent (often the case in a panicked diver who makes a rapid, uncontrolled ascent) can cause pulmonary barotrauma. This may result in any combination of five conditions: arterial gas embolism (AGE), AGE, pneumothorax, pneumomediastinum, subcutaneous emphysema, and alveolar hemorrhage. The most severe of these is AGE. AGE is the second leading cause of mortality of sport divers after drowning, accounting for approximately 30% of diving-related deaths. Coronary and cerebral artery air emboli are associated with the most serious consequences. Alteration of consciousness is common in AGE. Therefore, a scuba diver who surfaces unconscious or who loses consciousness within 10 minutes of reaching the surface should be assumed to be suffering from AGE. The other mechanism of ascent dysbarism involves the formation of nitrogen bubbles and is the cause of DCI. The microbubbles can cause mechanical obstruction, ischemia, and tissue hypoxia as well as inflammation, platelet aggregation, and thrombosis. A patent foramen ovale may be a risk factor for increased susceptibility to DCI because bubbles in the venous circulation may not be prevented from entering the arterial circulation by the vasculature of the lungs. The clinical manifestations of DCI have been divided into two categories, Type I and Type II. Type I DCI affects the musculoskeletal system, skin, and lymphatic vessels (so-called "pain-only" DCI). Type I DCI is also called "the bends." It is manifest most commonly as joint pain, especially the elbow and shoulder. Type II DCI involves any other organ system (such as the CNS, the inner ear, and the lungs).

10. To make this simple, I'll just send every dive injury to a hyperbaric chamber for recompression therapy, right?

Hold on there. Not every dysbarism requires the resources of and treatment in a hyperbaric chamber. By sending everybody, you may be using resources unnecessarily (not to mention exposing the patient to the potential expense, risk, and discomfort of a transfer that could be substantial).

Diving disorders that do or that do not require recompression therapy are divided as follows:

Diving Disorders that Require Recompression Therapy	Diving Disorders that Do Not Require Recompression Therapy
DCI Type 1	Middle ear barotrauma
DCI Type 2	External ear barotrauma
AGE	Inner ear barotrauma
Possibly contaminated air (carbon monoxide poisoning)	Barosinusitis
	Facial barotrauma
	Nitrogen narcosis
	Oxygen toxicity
	Pneumothorax
	Pneumomediastinum
	Subcutaneous emphysema

Alveolar hemorrhage
Alternobaric vertigo
Barodentalgia
Gastrointestinal barotrauma
Avascular osteonecrosis

Fortunately, help is just a phone call away. Duke University maintains a 24-hour hotline (the Diver Alert Network or DAN) at +1-919-684-8111 or +1-919-684-4DAN (collect). The calls are answered at the switchboard of Duke University Medical Center. Tell the operator you have a diving emergency. The operator will either connect you directly with DAN or have someone call you back at the earliest possible moment. The DAN Web site is http://www.diversalertnetwork.org/

11. **Okay, give me a case to try.**
Sure. A twenty-year-old woman making her first open water scuba dive (compressed air) descends to 60 fsw and spends 20 minutes on the bottom. She makes a rapid, uncontrolled ascent to the surface after an unfortunate encounter with a barracuda. At the surface, she is unconscious and breathing rapidly; she is tachycardic and hypotensive.

12. **What's your differential diagnosis?**
First, it appears to be a disorder of ascent. It could be barotrauma or DCI. DCI is less likely because she did not exceed the no-decompression limits for her dive (at 60 feet, this limit is 60 minutes). The immediate onset also goes against DCI. Immediate unconsciousness upon surfacing in a panicked manner is characteristic for AGE.

13. **What are your initial resuscitation measures?**
Of course, it all starts with airway, breathing, and circulation. High-flow oxygen is particularly important. Intubate the patient if you can and establish intravenous access. If there is evidence for tension pneumothorax, the patient may require needle decompression. Depending upon her cardiovascular status, she may need volume resuscitation, vasopressor support, or cardiopulmonary resuscitation.
Transportation decisions will depend upon the facilities available. In-water recompression is dangerous and should not be attempted in an unconscious diver. Time is of the essence: patients with AGE who are recompressed within 5 minutes of surfacing face a mortality rate of 5%, with an extremely low risk of morbidity among the survivors. However, if recompression is delayed by 5 hours or more, the mortality rate climbs to 10% with 50% of the survivors suffering morbidity. Therefore, if there is a medical facility that has a hyperbaric chamber and can offer recompression therapy nearby, that would be optimal. Otherwise, she should be transported to a facility where she can be stabilized prior to transfer to a recompression chamber. Rapid ground transportation is best but if air transportation is necessary, the flight crew should try to limit their altitude and be aware that her condition may deteriorate even further during the flight.

Pearls and Pitfalls

1. With rapid air travel, DCI can be seen at locations quite distant from the ocean.
2. A good history will differentiate between disorders of descent, depth, and ascent.
3. Be aware of the indications for emergent recompression in a hyperbaric chamber.

Special Situations

4. Use the 24/7 Diver Alert Network (DAN) for questions and advice.
5. A diver who surfaces unconscious or becomes unconscious within 10 minutes of surfacing should be assumed to have AGE until proven otherwise.

References

1. Brylske A. A brief history of diving: Evolution of the self-contained diver (part 2). Dive Training 4:20–26, 1994.
2. Butler BD, Hills BA. The lung as a filter for microbubbles. J Appl Physiol 47(3):537–543, 1979.
3. Bynny RL, Shockley LW. SCUBA diving and dysbarisms. In Rosen's Emergency Medicine: Concepts and Clinical Practice, 7th ed., Marx JA, et al., eds., pp. 1903–1916. Philadelphia: Mosby Year Book, 2009.
4. Cales RH, Humphreys N, Pilmanis AA, Heilig RW. Cardiac arrest from gas embolism in scuba diving. Ann Emerg Med 10(11):589–592, 1981.
5. Francis TJR, Gorman DF. The pathogenesis of the decompression disorders. In The Physiology and Medicine of Diving, 4th ed., Bennett PB, Elliott, eds. Philadelphia: WB Saunders, 1993.
6. Green SM., Rothrock SG, Green EA. Tympanometric evaluation of middle ear barotrauma during recreational scuba diving. Int J Sports Med 14(7):411–415, 1993.
7. Strauss MB, Borer RC Jr. Diving medicine: contemporary topics and their controversies. Am J Emerg Med 19(3):232–238, 2001.
8. Tomassoni AJ. Cardiac problems associated with dysbarism. Cardiol Clin 13(2):266–271, 1995.
9. U.S. Navy. U.S. Navy Diving Manual, Revision 4, Naval Sea Systems Command, United States Navy, 1999. (The manual may be downloaded from the Internet at http://www.vnh.org Accessed November 11, 2011

CHAPTER 71

Wilderness Emergency Medical Services

Paul S. Auerbach, MD, MS, FACEP, FAWM, and Laura W. Kates, MD

1. **What is wilderness medicine?**
   According to the Wilderness Medical Society (WMS), "Wilderness medicine focuses on medical problems and treatment in remote areas. It includes aspects of physiology, clinical medicine, preventive medicine, and public health." For the purpose of emergency medical services (EMS) personnel, there are four qualities that define wilderness medicine:
   - An austere environment
   - Prolonged time to definitive care requiring modifications to traditional prehospital protocols
   - Integration of rescue and medical skills
   - Environmental threats

2. **What is the difference between wilderness EMS and urban EMS?**
   Rapid response, stabilization, and transfer to an advanced care facility comprise the focus of traditional urban EMS training systems. The physical remoteness, environmental exposure, challenging geography, and often extended periods of time needed for rescue and stabilization require special training and define wilderness EMS. Traditionally, urban EMS is reactive and protocol driven, whereas wilderness EMS requires improvisation, innovation, and extended protocols. In urban EMS, patient extrication is typically the responsibility of fire department personnel, who typically hand off patients to the EMS providers who begin providing medical care. In wilderness EMS, patient extrication is often technically difficult and time intensive, requiring simultaneous administration of medical care by providers skilled in both medical and rescue skills.

3. **How are wilderness emergency medical technicians (WEMTs) different from regular EMTs?**
   The US Department of Transportation (DOT) is responsible for creating EMT curricula. The National Registry of Emergency Medical Technicians was inaugurated in 1970 to serve as a national certifying body for EMTs. Standardized tests are used to certify and recertify EMTs at the state level or into the National Registry.
   There is no national standard or formal certification exam for WEMT designation. The WEMT curriculum is based on the DOT EMT curriculum and establishes an approach to emergency care in wilderness settings that is based on recommendations from the Wilderness Medical Society, Wilderness EMS Institute (WEMSI), National Association of Search and Rescue (NASAR), National Ski Patrol, National Outdoor Leadership School (NOLS), and other groups. Typically, a WEMT course includes 45–100 hours of classroom didactic time, 10 hours of emergency department time, and an additional 48–80 hours of clinical training, as opposed to nonwilderness EMT courses that require approximately 120 hours of classroom and ambulance ride-along time. WEMT courses include a minimum of 22 hours of training on medical conditions related to the environment. In contrast, a typical EMT course includes only 3–10 hours

addressing environmental emergencies. Other unique aspects of the WEMT curriculum include added training on extended patient care, rescue techniques, special equipment, and providing care for injuries unique to remote outdoor situations.

4. What procedures can be performed by WEMTs?

The procedures performed by a WEMT are determined by both the state protocols under which a WEMT practices, as well as his or her level of training. Because there is no national standard for WEMT training, different states and health care systems have a variety of policies regarding what actions health care providers may and may not take given their levels of training. It is the responsibility of all health care providers to know the standard of care for their level of training, what procedures may be performed, and the protocols and policies of their system.

Key elements in WEMT training include technical skills and authority to perform the following:

- Airway management, including endotracheal intubation
- Needle thoracostomy for tension pneumothorax
- Shock management, including intravenous fluid therapy
- Use of military antishock trousers, although this is experiencing decreased use except for pelvic fracture stabilization
- Oxygen administration
- Medication administration, including epinephrine for allergic reactions; antibiotics for certain circumstances; acetazolamide, nifedipine, and furosemide for altitude sickness; and pain medications for injuries
- Field rewarming techniques
- Field reduction and splinting of fractures and dislocations

5. What employment opportunities and experiences are available for WEMTs?

Wilderness EMT skills are useful for anyone who spends a substantial amount of time in wilderness areas, but can also open new opportunities for employment. Some possibilities include:

- National and state park ranger, such as the ParkMedic program in Yosemite National Park
- Adventure travel
- Search and rescue
- Forest service worker
- Disaster medicine/relief work
- Work in rural/wilderness areas
- Military

6. Are standards for wilderness (e.g., mountain, water) rescue teams different around the world?

Wilderness rescue teams vary tremendously around the world. In the United States, most teams are composed of volunteers, with a wide range of qualifications and skills from first aid to paramedic, and are under the jurisdiction of national parks, state parks, or county sheriffs. In Canada, mountain rescue teams are coordinated by the military. In Europe, most teams are staffed with full-time physicians and paramedics. In many of the most remote areas of the world, there is no organized system of wilderness emergency care, so travelers and expeditions are required to be self-sufficient.

7. **What questions must be answered when assembling a team for a rescue?**
Wilderness rescue requires coordinated and thorough preparation with consideration of the following:
Environment/Geography
    - What time of day is it and will it be? (Are you prepared for a night rescue?)
    - What are the anticipated weather (environmental) conditions, and are you prepared for them?
    - Is a helicopter, boat, or other specialized rescue vehicle(s) needed or available?
    - Is the weather acceptable for air rescue?

Victims
    - How long ago did the accident occur?
    - What is the number of victims?
    - What are their injuries?
    - How many people are in the victim's party?
    - How well prepared are they?
    - Does anyone in the party have medical experience or training?

Rescue Personnel
    - Do you have a location, or is this a search and rescue?
    - Is a "hasty" team (a smaller, less equipped team sent ahead to provide initial care or to search and rescue while the main team prepares and follows) needed? If so, has it been deployed yet?
    - Are all team members prepared?

Are the Rescuers at Significant Risk?
    - Are all team members trained for this type of rescue?
    - Who is on the medical team?
    - Who is on the evacuation team? Is the number of team members adequate? (For instance, 16–20 litter carriers are typically necessary for a ground evacuation of 1–3 miles over level terrain).
    - Is the team equipment organized and divided up adequately?
    - How urgent is the situation?
    - Will multiple agencies be involved?
    - Are communications coordinated between the different agencies?

8. **Who is responsible for search and rescue?**
Search and rescue (SAR) are the responsibilities of national and state parks, sheriffs, state conservation offices, or other government agencies, depending on the location and jurisdiction. National and state parks do not have a "duty to rescue." In addition, there is sometimes significant controversy about when rescue missions should be attempted and who should pay for them. The prevailing opinion is that a call for help cannot ethically be dismissed.
    - As mentioned in question 4, most rescues are done by volunteer groups.
    - 90% of mountain rescues are done on foot.
    - 95% of rescues are performed without physicians present.
    - Only Yosemite and Grand Teton National Parks use helicopters extensively.

Special Situations

- Only Denali National Park uses fixed-wing aircraft extensively and helicopters occasionally.
- Only Yosemite, Grand Teton, and Mount Rainier National Parks have rangers specifically trained in technical rescues, advanced medical care, and helicopter operations.
- Many backcountry and climbing areas are outside parks. Rescues in these areas are by local fire and rescue departments, with or without the benefit of special training or technical skills.

9. **What special knowledge is needed for searches and rescues (e.g., mountain, high angle, cave, ocean)?**
   - Understanding equipment (ropes, slings, carabiners, harnesses, helmets, litters, litter harnesses, haul systems, personal flotation devices, throw rings and bags, and litter patient packaging equipment) used in SAR operations, including their maintenance and care
   - Basic radio communication and signaling
   - Basic helicopter and fixed-wing operation and procedures
   - Understanding search-and-rescue procedures
   - Knowledge of the Incident Command System and its use in SAR
   - Basic rope handling and knot-tying skills
   - Advanced skills as needed for specific circumstances, including water SAR, white-water rescue, avalanche SAR, technical or vertical (rock) techniques, or cave training
   - Interpersonal skills and the ability to deal with field death and inform family and friends of a death.

10. **What are some examples of scenarios likely to require "extended" rescue and emergency care?**
    Mountain, wilderness, rural, white-water, air–sea, cave, and avalanche rescue, as well as expedition and disaster medicine and most search and rescue missions. The terms "extended rescue" and "extended emergency care" refer to medical care and rescue efforts beyond the first, or "golden," hour.

11. **What government agencies are responsible for search and rescue?**
    Federal SAR activities are either under the supervision of the US Air Force (for inland regions), the Aerospace Rescue and Recovery Service (responsible for federal aircraft incidents,) or the US Coast Guard (supervises coastal regions and all maritime and ocean searches). At the state level, there is significant variety in SAR supervision, because it is often under the jurisdiction of law enforcement agencies. All states have legislation that provides support to local governments during emergencies. During a nationally declared disaster, the Federal Emergency Management Agency (FEMA) assumes responsibility for SAR activities. The Department of Health and Human Services runs the National Disaster Management System (NDMS), which develops and dispatches Disaster Medical Assistance Teams (DMAT) that can be rapidly deployed to nationally declared disaster areas.

12. **What are the four phases of SAR?**
    - Locate
    - Access
    - Stabilize
    - Transport

13. **How many SAR missions occur each year in the United States?**
    Specific numbers are not reported. It is estimated that more than 100,000 SAR missions occur annually.

Wilderness Emergency Medical Services

14. **What are factors that may cause someone to need to be rescued (and, therefore, to require the services of a WEMT)?**
    Any one, or a combination, of the following may produce a situation that results in the need to be rescued, stabilized, and treated.
    - Improper clothing or footgear
    - Fatigue
    - Dehydration
    - Hypo- or hyperthermia
    - Overextension of abilities
    - Lack of physical conditioning
    - Inadequate food
    - Inadequate planning
    - Inadequate leadership
    - Itinerary confusion
    - Inadequate recognition of environmental, physical, or mental factors
    - Inadequate preparation for weather conditions
    - Lack of navigational proficiency (getting lost)
    - "Invincible" mind-set
    - Injury, illness, or exposure to an adverse environmental condition or event

15. **Is an EMS provider on a trip liable for care rendered during that trip?**
    The question is, "Is the provider acting as a designated health care provider, or is the provider merely a person on the trip who happens to be an EMS provider?" If the provider is the latter, then he or she is not duty bound to assist others in need. If he chooses to help, he is not invariably protected from liability by a Good Samaritan law. Although a Good Samaritan law provides protection for medical personnel voluntarily assisting within the scope of their skills at an emergency scene, it is important to note that the provider is held to the full capabilities commensurate with his or her training. If an EMS provider is acting as the trip medical support, then he or she is liable to provide care at the accepted standard of care. In addition, because EMTs and almost all EMS providers act under a physician's supervision, the doctor under whom the EMT is working may also be liable for his or her actions.

16. **What are some unique ethical dilemmas associated with wilderness EMS?**
    - How much risk will you accept for yourself and your team when planning a SAR (e.g., going out in a snowstorm looking for a child) and treating victims in the wilderness?
    - If a rescuer becomes injured, who will you treat first? The original victim or the rescuer?
    - If a limited amount of supplies is available, who gets treated?
    - How will the care affect others in the group (e.g., leaving scuba divers in the water in order to deliver a diver with decompression sickness to a hyperbaric chamber)?
    - In a remote and prolonged care situation, how do the relationships of people in the group affect their choices for care and decisions regarding the group?

    More so than in urban situations, a serious emergency in a wilderness area stresses many unique aspects of relationships and decision-making capabilities. From a survivalist point of view, it is necessary to take care of rescuers and teammates before caring for victims. Many potential circumstances can influence this decision. Therefore, one must think about potential circumstances in advance and plan appropriate ways to incorporate a productive reaction to ensure the survival and optimal outcome for rescuers, the team, and patients.

17. **Where can I get more information about wilderness medicine and wilderness EMS?**
    Wilderness Medicine Organizations
    - The Wilderness Medical Society, 2150 S 1300 E, Suite 500, Salt Lake City, UT; 84106; (801) 990-2988
    - The International Society of Mountain Medicine
    - The International Society of Travel Medicine
    - The Divers Alert Network

    Search and Rescue Organizations
    - The Mountain Rescue Association
    - The National Association for Search and Rescue
    - The National Ski Patrol

    Wilderness EMT Training Programs
    - The Wilderness Emergency Medical Services Institute
    - The National Outdoor Leadership School, Wilderness Medicine Institute

    There are many companies and colleges that offer WEMT courses. Check in your region for programs near you.

Pearls and Pitfalls

1. WEMT designation requires specialized training in rescue techniques, use of special equipment, and extended patient care in remote areas.
2. WEMTs must work very closely with all SAR personnel to ensure the safety of the patient and all team members.
3. The four phases of SAR are locate, access, stabilize, and transport.
4. A unique ethical dilemma for the WEMT is how much personal risk is acceptable to accomplish the rescue.

References

1. Auerbach PS, ed. Wilderness Medicine, 6th ed. Philadelphia: Mosby Elsevier, 2012.
2. Cooper DC, LaValla PH, Stoffel RC. Search and rescue. In Auerbach PS, ed., Wilderness Medicine, 6th ed. Philadelphia, Mosby Elsevier 2012, p. 687.
3. Langer CS, Baine JG. Medical liability and wilderness emergencies. In Auerbach PS ed., Wilderness Medicine, 6th ed. Philadelphia, Mosby Elsevier 2012, p. 2105.
4. Hubbell FR. Wilderness emergency medical and response systems. In Auerbach PS ed., Wilderness Medicine 6th ed. Philadelphia, Mosby Elsevier 2012, p. 674.
5. Iserson KV, Heine CE. The ethics of wilderness medicine. In Auerbach PS, ed. Wilderness Medicine, 6th ed., p. 2170, Auerbach PS, ed. Philadelphia, Mosby Elsevier 2012, p. 2113.
6. Johnson L. An introduction to mountain search and rescue. Emerg Med Clin N Am 22:511, 2004.
7. Russell MF. Wilderness emergency medical services systems. Emerg Med Clin N Am 22:561, 2004.
8. Sholl JM, Cursio EP. An introduction to wilderness medicine. Emerg Med Clin N Am 22:265, 2004.

Lightning

Lee W. Shockley, MD, MBA

CHAPTER 72

1. **How big of a problem is lightning?**
   Well, as you are reading this there are 2000 active thunderstorms worldwide right now. Each day there are up to 8 million lightning flashes in the earth's atmosphere; there are as many as 100 cloud-to-ground strikes per second. There are between 50 and 300 deaths in the United States annually from lightning strikes; four to five times that number of victims sustain nonlethal injuries. Lightning is the second most common storm killer in the United States (behind flash floods). Overall, the odds of becoming a lightning victim are about 1 in 240,000. However, if you are one of them, it is a big problem.

2. **Are there any particular risk factors for lightning strike victims?**
   Yes; they are:
   - Exposure to thunderstorm conditions
   - Either being the tallest object in near vicinity or being in contact with the tallest object
   - Being outdoors:
     - In open fields
     - Under trees
     - Around or on water
     - Operating tractors or road equipment
     - On golf courses
   - Summer (approximately two-thirds of the lightning flashes in the United States happen in June, July, or August)
   - Afternoons (approximately two-thirds of the lightning flashes in the United States happen from noon to 6:00 p.m. local time).

3. **What is lightning and how does it develop?**
   Lightning is a very high voltage unidirectional current impulse (technically, not really direct current or alternating current). The amount of energy released may be up to 2 billion volts and 300,000 peak amps (there is more electrical energy in a single lightning bolt than is produced by all of the electrical generators in the United States at that instant). However, because the duration of the strike is so short (0.1–1 millisecond), there is only enough total electrical energy to light a single light bulb for about a month, if it could be harnessed. This energy is dissipated as light, heat, sound, and radio waves.
   For lightning to develop, there must be a charge separation. This typically begins with hailstones and raindrops settling with various rates within a convectively active cloud. Charged particles become stripped off and the cloud becomes a dipole (negatively charged base and a positively charged cloud top). A tripole

phenomenon is also possible with a negatively charged base and roof and a positively charged center. In either case, the cloud acts like a large battery or capacitor.

The lightning strike begins with a "stepped leader," an ionized plasma channel that extends downward in a series of zigzag, short, stepped branches. Simultaneously, there is a rising, positively charged "pilot stroke" coming up from the ground. The pilot stroke and the stepped leader meet at 50–100 meters above the ground, creating a connection that initiates the "return stroke." The return stroke is the high-voltage, high-current, high-velocity rising discharge that we think of as the lightning bolt. Before the plasma channel dissipates, there is an average of four to five return strokes through it. The plasma channel is also extremely hot—up to 8000–50,000°C (by comparison, the surface of the sun is about 6000°C).

4. What are mechanisms of injury from lightning strikes?
- *Direct strike.* In this case, the electricity is conducted directly through the victim. It carries the highest rates of death and injury.
- *Contact.* The victim is touching an object that gets struck (e.g., touching a fence that is struck at some distant point).
- *Side flash or "splash."* A portion of the lightning bolt energy "jumps" from an object and catches the victim in its circuit (e.g., a tree is struck; most of the energy is conducted to the ground through the trunk, but a side flash strikes a person standing close by).
- *Step voltage.* The lightning strikes the ground and spreads underground until it is dissipated. If a victim is standing with one foot closer to the impact point than the other, the charge underground can create an induced current that travels up one leg and down another. This mechanism probably accounts most often for multiple victims from a single strike.
- *Blunt, or direct, trauma.* The victim is thrown by the strike. Injuries result from implosion/explosion forces along the lightning pathway or from debris or muscle contractions. Burns from clothing or jewelry also occur.

5. What is the "flashover phenomenon"?
Given the short duration of a lightning bolt, current is often conducted over the skin without penetration. When this happens, it significantly lowers the mortality of a direct strike victim from 85% with signs of penetration to 40% without.

6. Why is lightning different from other high-voltage injuries?
The average lightning strike has 10–20 million volts, and the figure may be as high as 2 billion volts. The duration of the shock is very brief, however, only 1/10,000th–1/1,000th of a second, so much less energy is delivered. Lightning is direct current (DC) as opposed to alternating current (AC). The path of lightning tends to stay along the outside of the victim, vaporizing sweat and moisture, causing the classic "feather burns" (See Figure 72.1) and blowing off clothes. A small amount of energy may "leak" internally and cause cardiac arrest, seizure, muscular contractions, or neurologic dysfunction, but it does not cause the extensive tissue destruction seen with AC electrical injuries.

7. What is keraunoparalysis (Charcot's paralysis)?
This "lightning paraplegia" is characterized by the inability of the victim to move his or her extremities. It is accompanied by cool, pale skin, and diminished peripheral pulses. The pathophysiology likely stems from severe vasoconstriction from the hyperadrenergic state and often resolves.

Lightning

8. Is it safer to be in a car during a thunderstorm? It's the rubber tires that insulate the car, right?

It is safer to be inside a car. However, it has nothing to do with the tires. Think about it. The lightning bolt just struck through thousands of feet of air. Six inches of rubber would not be adequate insulation. The car is safer not because of the tires but because of the metal body. In effect, the car's metal shell acts as a Faraday cage; it appears that the lightning energy travels around the outside of the vehicle before striking the ground.

9. Am I safe inside a building during a storm?

Actually, not 100%. Although being inside a building does reduce your risk compared to being outside, there are numerous cases of lightning injuries occurring indoors, usually this happens when the house or phone line is struck (particularly if the person is on the phone at the time and there is a faulty ground).

10. What is the immediate life-threatening consequence of being struck by lightning?

Although there are numerous injuries associated with lightning strike, the most immediate is cardiac arrest. The victim is exposed to an instantaneous, massive electrical discharge, typically causing asystole.

11. What sort of long-term damage can lightning victims experience?

Eye disorders, including cataracts; hearing problems, as half the victims have their eardrums ruptured; psychiatric disorders, such as anxiety, depression, posttraumatic stress disorder, and the imagined ability to predict lightning strikes or other delusions; and neurologic deficits, such as balance problems, memory difficulties, or impairment of other functions. Seventy to 75% of victims have some medical sequelae.

12. If a victim is not killed and has no external signs of trauma, do they still need follow-up and medical evaluation?

Absolutely. The sequelae above are not limited to those who suffer cardiac arrest or have external signs of trauma. All persons unfortunate enough to have been struck by lightning should have a thorough medical evaluation and follow-up.

13. I have been taught that at multiple casualty incidents (MCI), I should allocate resources to victims who are not breathing and not moving *only after* I have taken care of those with signs of life. Is that rule applicable in a lightning strike MCI?

No. Lightning strike is the one exception to the usual MCI triage rule. In most non-lightning-related incidents involving multiple casualties, victims who appear dead are deemed low priority, and care is preferentially directed at the living. In contrast, when dealing with multiple casualties from a lightning strike, the first priority should go to those who are not breathing and not moving. The reason is that only those individuals who present in cardiac arrest are at high risk of dying. Those who have not already arrested have little chance of dying and will likely recover; therefore, in this case the first priority goes to "the dead." Bystander cardiopulmonary resuscitation (CPR) doubles survivability from about 24% without CPR to 50% with CPR. Thus, initial care is directed at resuscitating the dead, in reverse of the standard practice with MCI.

14. I'm treating a farmer who was found unconscious in his field after a thunderstorm. He has no recollection of what happened. How can I tell if he was struck by lightning?

Quick, put down this book and go look at his skin and look in his ears. His memory of the events won't help; in fact, it is said that 100% of direct strike victims have amnesia. However, arborescent superficial erythema

Special Situations

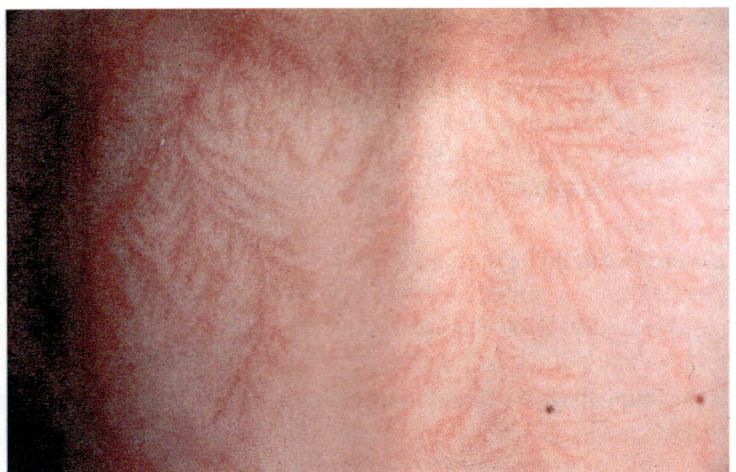

FIGURE 72.1 Arborescent superficial erythema on the back of a lightning strike patient. From Price TG, Cooper MA: Electrical and Lightning Injuries. In, Marx, JA, et al (eds.). Rosen's emergency medicine: concepts and clinical practice. Volume 2, 7th ed. Philadelphia: Mosby/Elsevier, 2010, p. 1898. Copyright Mosby/Elsevier. Used with permission.

(known as Lichtenberg's flowers, ferning, arboration, or fractals) is pathognomonic for lightning (Figure 72.1). Unfortunately, it is seen in only seen in 20% of confirmed cases and it fades away over hours. It is not a true burn but the effect of a strong electromagnetic field on wet skin. In addition, there may be partial thickness linear or punctate burns in moist areas. The ears? Tympanic membrane rupture occurs in 50% of victims. Tinnitus is also common and usually resolves in hours to days. Seven to 12% of victims experience temporary hearing loss and a few have permanent hearing loss.

Pearls and Pitfalls

1. Rescuers should not become victims. (Lightning does strike twice in the same place; move the resuscitation to a place of safety if necessary.)
2. Start with the ABCs (actually CABs); Bystander CPR
3. Assume the presence of spinal injury and search for occult trauma.
4. Lightning MCI priority goes to the "dead."
5. Reduce lightning risk by:
    (a) Avoiding: thunderstorms, being the tallest "target," holding a "lightning rod," touching conductors
    (b) Seeking shelter indoors or in a car
    (c) Staying away from groups (especially people who know CPR—they are your potential rescuers)
    (d) Keeping your feet together and crouching down to reduce your strike potential.

References

1. Brigham PA. Lightning injuries revisited. Ann Emerg Med 26(4):528–529, 1995.
2. Cherington M, Mathys K. Deaths and injuries as a result of lightning strikes to aircraft. Aviat Space Environ Med 66(7):687–689, 1995.
3. Cherington M. Lightning injuries. Ann Emerg Med Apr 25(4):517–519, 1995.
4. Cooper MA, Andrews CJ, Holle RL. Lightning injuries. In Wilderness Medicine, 5th ed., Auerbach PS, ed., pp. 67–108. St. Louis: Mosby-Year Book, 2007.
5. Fontanarosa PB. Electrical shock and lightning strike. Ann Emerg Med Feb 1993; 22(2 Pt 2):378–387.
6. Lightning-associated deaths—United States, 1980–1995. MMWR Morb Mortal Wkly Rep 47(19):391–394, 1998.
7. O'Keefe Gatewood M, Zane RD. Lightning injuries. Emerg Med Clin North Am 22(2):369–403, 2004.
8. Price TG, Cooper MA: Electrical and Lightning injuries. In Rosen's Emergency Medicine: Concepts and Clinical Practice, 7th ed., Marx JA, Hockberger RS, Walls RM, eds., pp. 1893–1902. Philadelphia: Mosby/Elsevier, 2009.
9. Zimmermann C, Cooper MA, Holle RL. Lightning safety guidelines. Ann Emerg Med 39(6):660–664, 2002.

Bites, Stings, and Envenomations

Richard C. Dart, MD, PhD

CHAPTER 73

1. **You are with a group hiking in the mountains when one member is bitten by a snake. What do you do?**
   Keep calm. Leave the snake alone. Examine the bite site. Nearly all venomous snake bites in the United States involve one or two puncture wounds.

2. **How can you tell if a snake is poisonous?**
   There are two types of venomous snakes in the United States: pit vipers and coral snakes. Pit vipers include rattlesnakes, copperheads, and cottonmouths. They are marked by triangular heads and a "pit" on their head looking like an extra nostril. The rattlesnake has rattles on the tail.
   The coral snake is a brightly colored red-, black-, and yellow-ringed snake. The color combination is similar to that of the harmless king snake, which mimics its dangerous cousin as a defense mechanism. The coral snake is red, yellow, and black, as in the saying, "Red on yellow, Kill a fellow. Red on black, venom lack." (This applies in the United States only.)

3. **What are the signs of pit viper envenomation?**
   Pit viper bites can develop three types of effects: local, coagulation, and systemic. Local effects include puncture marks and swelling at the bite site. Coagulation effects (platelets, prothrombin time) usually develop after an hour or so and are discovered when blood tests are performed. Systemic effects indicate a severe bite and include weakness, lightheadedness, nausea, diarrhea, decreased blood pressure, and shock.

4. **What can we do before reaching the hospital?**
   There are no proven first aid measures. Do NOT incise, suck, or otherwise treat the bite! These measures can worsen the injury and cause infection. Tourniquets should not be used. Splint the affected extremity, place the limb below heart level, remove any rings or other constrictive devices, keep the patient calm, and evacuate as rapidly as possible to a medical facility. Mark the extent of swelling with a pen directly on the limb for later reference.

5. **How do I determine if it is a dry bite?**
   About 25% of pit viper bites are "dry," meaning that no venom was injected. A dry bite is determined only by observing the patient for several hours. If no effects develop, then it was a dry bite. A dry bite cannot be determined in the prehospital arena.

6. **What if a rattlesnake-bite patient has systemic signs such as hypotension?**
   Hypotension is likely caused by loss of fluid into swollen areas and is initially treated in the same manner as hypovolemic shock. A large-bore IV should be started in the unbitten extremity and 0.9% normal saline, 20 mL/kg, infused rapidly. Definitive treatment is provided by antivenom, which is administered only in the ED.

7. **What if the snake was small or a baby rattler?**
   Small rattlesnakes are capable of envenomating. The crucial issue is whether there are visible bite marks. If so, then the patient should be managed as any pit viper bite.

8. **What is significant about Gila monster bites?**
   There are two venomous lizards in the world: the Gila monster and the Mexican beaded lizard. Both reside in the southwestern United States. They deliver venom by chewing and holding on to the victim. It is often difficult to get them to release the bitten hand. Place the lizard on the ground and it may release voluntarily. Fire is not recommended. Injuries usually are related to the trauma of the bite, although systemic effects similar to those of mild Crotalidae bites have been described. Treatment is supportive.

9. **How dangerous is a scorpion sting?**
   Most scorpions found within the United States are not dangerous. The exception is the *Centruroides* scorpion found in Arizona, New Mexico, southeastern California, and southern Nevada. Also known as the bark scorpion, *Centruroides* scorpions are small and yellow-brown. In adults, the main effect of their venom is local pain with minimal swelling. In children, the venom can produce systemic effects of hyperexcitability, increased salivation, tachypnea, muscle twitching, myoclonic jerks, and ultimately respiratory failure. Care is supportive with close attention to the airway and transport to a medical facility.

10. **A surfer accidentally steps on a stingray and is stung. What is the treatment?**
    Stingray, scorpion fish, stonefish, catfish, oldwife fish, lionfish, rabbitfish, ratfish, stargazer fish, surgeonfish, toadfish, and the weeverfish are all venomous fish. Symptoms include severe pain at the sting site; pain radiating up the limb; numbness at the puncture site; systemic intoxication with paralysis and problems with vision, speech, and gait; malaise; nausea; and vomiting. Shock and respiratory depression occur very rarely. Many of these fish poisons are unstable in heat and become nontoxic when exposed to increased temperatures. Treatment is to first to address the airway, breathing, and circulation, then place the affected extremity in water heated to 42°C (or as hot as can be tolerated without scalding) for 30–90 minutes. Stonefish antivenom is available in the United States through Sea World in San Diego, California, and Cleveland, Ohio.

11. **A child comes running down the beach toward you, screaming that a shell bit her. She appears agitated and ill and seems to be deteriorating in front of you. What stung her? What is the treatment?**
    The cone shell is an attractive, colorful mollusk found in Hawaii and throughout Indo-Pacific waters. It is a highly venomous creature with a paralytic poison similar to tetrodotoxin or curare. Symptoms start with burning pain at the site of injection, followed by numbness around the site, which may spread. Double vision, difficulty speaking, blurry vision, itching, nausea, vomiting, and muscle weakness may follow. The paralysis may be incomplete, with only muscle weakness, or may be complete. Symptoms may resolve or rapidly worsen. No specific treatment is available.

12. **What is the treatment for jellyfish stings?**
    The true "jellyfish" is only one of three classes of coelenterates, but their stings are all treated the same, as are the stings of the sea anemone and the fire coral. For patients in severe pain or exhibiting signs of cardiovascular collapse, the primary goal is EMS activation and provision of advanced cardiac life

support. Vinegar (acetic acid) may be poured over the site for at least 30 minutes to reduce further discharge of the stingers. The tentacles should not be handled because of the risk of EMS personnel being stung as well. There is antivenom available for the box jellyfish, found in Australia.

13. **What happens with Hymenoptera (bees, wasps, hornets, and ants) stings?**
    The honeybee kills more people (50–100 people per year) in the United States than any other animal. Two types of reactions occur. Anaphylaxis is the most common cause of death and is addressed elsewhere in this book. The second is a toxic reaction from the venom itself. Depending on the number of stings (over 500 stings is considered serious), symptoms can include pain and swelling at the site, nausea, vomiting, diarrhea, lightheadedness, headache, fever, malaise, muscle spasms, swelling elsewhere on the body, syncope, or seizures.

14. **How should a bee's stinger be removed?**
    Care should be taken to not squeeze the stinger, because the venom sac is still attached and this maneuver may inject more venom. Instead, it should be scraped off the victim with a scalpel blade of similar device as soon as possible to minimize the amount of venom injected.

15. **Are tick bites significant?**
    Yes. Ticks are associated with many diseases, such as tick paralysis, Lyme disease, Rocky Mountain spotted fever, tularemia, Colorado tick fever, and Q fever. The diagnosis is often missed because the tick may be attached in the scalp or other hairy areas. The most important thing is to remove the tick completely, making sure that the head and mouth parts are disengaged from the skin. This can be done in a number of ways. Grasping the tick close to the skin and pulling with a slow, even pressure is probably the easiest method. Care should be taken not to jerk or twist the tick, which causes the mouth parts to break off.

16. **What are the signs of a black widow spider bite?**
    Systemic effects may begin 10–60 minutes after the bite. The main symptom is muscle pain that begins in the bitten extremity and then migrates centripetally. For example, leg pain may move to the buttocks and then become an abdominal muscle spasm that may mimic an acute surgical emergency. Upper-extremity bites may mimic myocardial infarction. Other effects include fever, nausea, headache, lightheadedness, diaphoresis, and difficulty swallowing. Initial treatment involves titrated doses of a benzodiazepine and opioid such as lorazepam and fentanyl. An effective antivenom is available.

17. **What is the most common spider bite in the United States?**
    The jumping, or *Phidippus*, spider. Fortunately, although it is rather aggressive, it is not significantly venomous. Simply washing the bite site is sufficient.

18. **Are tarantulas dangerous?**
    With the exception of some of the South American and Australian species, mygalomorphs are not particularly dangerous. The main concern is urticating hairs that detach easily and may get in the eye, causing conjunctivitis.

19. **Is there anything else I should know?**
    Consider calling your state poison center for information: 1-800-222-1222.

Pearls and Pitfalls

1. Do not attempt to suck the venom out of a snake bite.
2. Topical administration of acetic acid (vinegar) should be used for jellyfish stings.

3. Stingray stings should be treated by 30 minutes of immersion in hot water.
4. Call your regional poison center with any questions regarding bites and stings.

References

1. Boyer LV, Binford GJ, McNally JT. Spider bites. In Wilderness Medicine: Management of Wilderness and Environmental Emergencies, 5th ed., Auerbach PS, ed., pp. 1008–1010. St. Louis: Mosby, 2007.
2. Schneir AG, Clark RF. Bites and stings. In Emergency Medicine: A Comprehensive Study Guide, 7th ed. Tintinalli JE, ed. pp. 1344–1354. New York, McGraw-Hill, 2011.
3. Dart RC, Gold BS. Crotaline Snakebite. In Dart RC, ed. Medical Toxicology, 3rd ed., pp. 1559–1565. Philadelphia: Lippincott Williams & Wilkins, 2003.
4. Traub SJ, Cummins GA. Tick-Borne Diseases. In Wilderness Medicine: Management of Wilderness and Environmental Emergencies, 5th ed., Auerbach PS, ed., pp. 982–1008. St. Louis, Mosby, 2007.
5. Isbister GK. Trauma and envenomations from marine fauna. In Emergency Medicine: A Comprehensive Study Guide, 7th ed., Tintinalli JE, ed., pp. 1358–1366 New York: McGraw-Hill, 2011.

Tactical Emergency Medicine

CHAPTER 74

David Q. McArdle, MD, and Tamra D. Glore, RN, BSN, CPHM

1. **What is tactical emergency medical support?**
   Tactical emergency medical support (TEMS) is much more than Emergency Medical Services (EMS) in black or camouflage uniforms. It is a unique evolving specialty that makes occupational medicine and emergency care available to law enforcement and military special operations units. All rescue operations carry inherent risks in prehospital care such as fire, electrocution, drowning, and falls. In the tactical environment there is the added element that the caregivers may be attacked by opposing forces on the battlefield or the tactical incident. Because of this underlying threat of intentional violence directed toward rescuers, significant modifications from routine prehospital medical care have evolved. There is always a constant interplay between tactics and medicine in the tactical environment.

2. **Historically, what are the roots of TEMS?**
   Many of the major contributions to medicine ironically have resulted from war:
   - During the Napoleonic wars, Baron Dominique-Jean Larrey created the Ambulance Volante, a system that involved sending trained medical personnel into the field to provide medical care for the injured soldiers, both friend and foe alike on the battlefield.
   - Florence Nightingale is the first named camp follower acknowledged to bring nursing care to the wounded in the Crimean War.
   - Walter Reed at the end of the Spanish-American war identified mosquitoes as the vector for yellow fever. Techniques to eradicate the mosquitoes helped support the mission of building the Panama Canal.
   - Penicillin and sulfa drugs and the use of blood banking were all largely developed to support the medical needs of World War II.
   - Vietnam saw the expanded use of helicopter transport and far-forward trauma surgical care that had its roots in the Korean War and previous conflicts. Prior to the Department of Transportation in the 1960s mandating training for responders and equipment for ambulances in the United States, many injured patients were transported to the hospitals in hearses or police paddy wagons.

   The more recent history of TEMS starts with a few agencies independently integrating emergency medical service into SWAT (Special Weapons and Tactics) teams in the late 1970s and early 1980s. John Kolman, the first director of the National Tactical Officers Association, hosted the first national meeting to bring these providers together in Los Angeles in 1989. The following year, Dr. Richard Carmona, team physician for the Pima County Sheriff's office and later Surgeon General of the United States, hosted the next meeting in Tucson. At that meeting, staff from the Casualty Care Research Center at Bethesda Naval Hospital came to outline a class that they had developed. What was then known as Buddy Care for the Military was modified for law enforcement. As the major source of funding at the time was Drug

Enforcement Agency (DEA) seizure money, the program and participating teams had to use the training for drug interdiction. This program was known as Counter Narcotics Tactical Operations Medical Support (CONTOMS). It took lessons learned from previous wars for not only treating wounds but also emphasizing mission planning to prevent injuries. In its heyday, CONTOMS was operating a class a month at Bethesda Naval Hospital with the field training day conducted at Quantico, Virginia. Several classes were done regionally as well. Budget cuts just prior to September 11, 2001 would have ended the program; however, it has continued on a smaller scale as the recent war on terrorism renewed awareness of the need for this specialized branch of emergency medical care.

3. **What is a medical threat assessment?**
A medical threat assessment (MTA) is prepared by the tactical medical support group to assist a SWAT team in considering all of the possible threats that may be encountered by the team on any given mission. The most obvious question of "Where do we go if someone gets shot?" only scratches the surface.

- Regional resources need to be identified for both major and minor problems. If one of the participants requires treatment for a minor injury that cannot be easily fixed on scene, where can they be taken so that they can be quickly treated and returned to the operation?
- In the event of multiple casualties, it is usually not prudent to have the family of the victim who was shot in the same waiting room as the family of the suspect who is now requiring medical care.
- Identification of burn units, pediatric specialty care needs, and the like should be accomplished in advance. Contact numbers for each of those referral sites needs to be immediately available so that prompt notification can take place.
- Routes or even modes of transport may need to vary because of weather, construction, traffic, or even the constraints of the tactical situation itself. The closest route may come under hostile fire.

Suspects, victims, or innocent bystanders may have significant underlying pathologies that need to be addressed. Advice on deployment of equipment to mitigate environmental hazards and prevent injuries or illness may be required. Although many teams may use the same template for missions, it is important to consider that all information ages with time (time is the fourth dimension of the tactical environment). Periodic reviews are needed to ensure that contact numbers have not changed. Divert status of one of your regional resource hospitals may require a change in the game plan. Nothing should come as a surprise during a time of crisis. Highlights of an up-to-date MTA need to be included in any premission briefing.

4. **What is a tactical medic and where do they fit in the chain of survival?**
The military concept of having medical practitioners integrated into each front line unit has been slow to carry over into law enforcement. In contemporary American law enforcement, if a team has tactical medics, they are usually EMTs or paramedics borrowed from the local ambulance providers or fire department. These individuals are then provided some tactical training and are called to duty with their respective police agencies when the need arises. Recently the DEA has been successful in taking full-time SWAT officers and adding a tactical emergency medical block to the basic EMT training for agents that are being deployed abroad to high risk areas such as Afghanistan. In most police agencies, the patrol officers are still the weakest link in the chain of survival for providing emergency medical care. This has become evident in the response to homicides in progress (e.g., school shootings and workplace violence

Special Situations

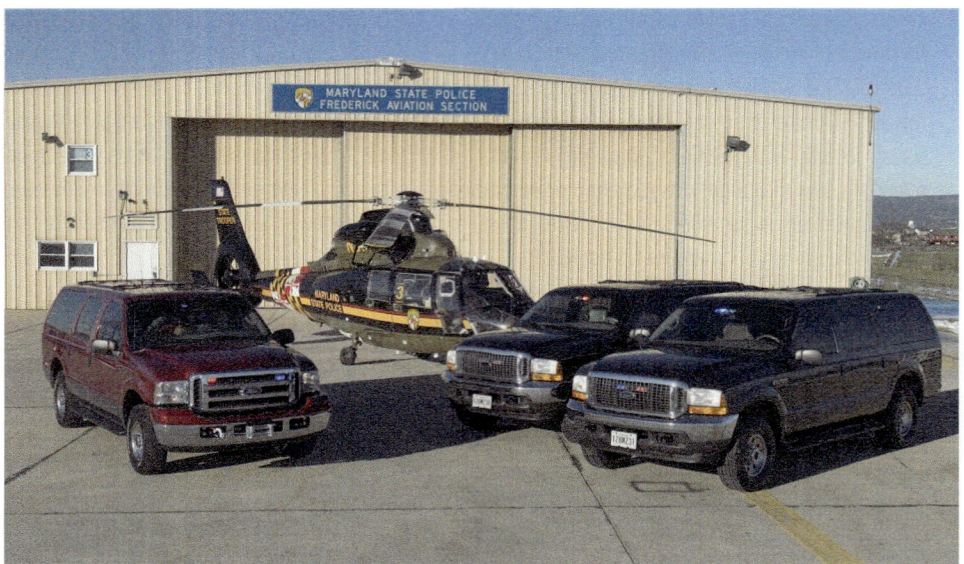

FIGURE 74.1 The Maryland State Police have a fleet of "undercover ambulances" that provide a patient transport work space similar to the access that medic troopers have in their helicopters. These unmarked vehicles help maintain operational security when the SWAT team is about to conduct a raid.

where the suspects do not wish to negotiate and are intent on killing). In these crises, the patrol officers will often lead the tactical response before the arrival of SWAT with their part-time tactical medics. Notable exceptions are the NYPD Emergency Service Unit, the Maryland State Police Medevac program (Figure 74.1), and the Los Angeles Sheriff's Emergency Service Detail, who have full-time police officers working as paramedics in the tactical realm. Vancouver, Washington police and Oklahoma City police have EMTs embedded into some of the front-line first-response units. Not only does having embedded patrol medics reduce their response time dramatically, but this capability also has a very positive impact on community policing. It helps reduce the stigma of "use of force" issues when prompt care can be rendered once the fight is over.

Only about half of the officers killed in the line of duty die from hostile action. The other half die primarily in motor vehicle accidents – many while they are roadside during traffic stops. Environmental emergencies such as being struck by lightning, carbon monoxide exposure and drowning are some of the unique hazards that may claim the life of a police officer.

Fellow officers are often the only personnel available to care for them prior to the arrival of civilian medical personnel. As many as 70% of officers have been in this position, and they often lack proper training and equipment to render care in this setting.

5. Do physicians have a role in tactical EMS?

Yes. Physicians have a role that extends well beyond just supervising training for the paramedics. Specially trained physicians can provide consultative and on-scene occupational medicine. Other midlevel providers can handle sick call issues.

6. **Who are the patients in the tactical environment?**
   In the broadest sense, we deal with the good guys, the bad guys, and the people we just are not sure about. Someone who is a "friend down" should not be a threat to us when we approach and treat them. Because we do not want the opposing forces to get access to the weapons, the radio, or the victim, we are aggressive about recovering them from this contested area and conserving unit integrity. Care must still be exercised on approach because the friend in shock may not recognize that we are friendly forces there to assist them. Someone who is a "foe down" may not want to be rescued (i.e., captured) by us, so they may resist and even attempt to kill the potential rescuer. The "everyone else" is by far the largest and most complex patient population we may have to deal with. Their actions may not be overtly aggressive or criminal, but even hostages may be sympathetic friends or associates of those who have taken them hostage. Hostage takers or criminals may attempt to hide amongst those that they previously victimized. Bystanders may have routine medical problems such as diabetic emergencies, heart attacks, or imminent child birth in an area that is controlled by a barricaded gunman. An important caveat is that just because someone wears the same uniform that we do, it does not necessarily guarantee that they are friendly forces. In numerous recent terrorist incidents, the bad guys often arrived dressed as police, soldiers, or ambulance attendants in vehicles that were used to carry large secondary explosive devices or wearing explosive vests. This is why ambulances and responding personnel may be stopped at the outer perimeter of a law enforcement emergency so that photo identification and vehicle inspection can be carried out.

7. **What are the types of missions that might be done and how does the medical plan reflect the mission needs?**
   Patrol services handle the vast majority of police work. They are the first responders to all calls for service from the community. They initiate contact with people thought to be engaged in suspicious activity or overt crimes with the bulk of these crimes comprised of traffic violations. It is imperative to remember that there is no such thing as a "routine call" in police work. The person being contacted for speeding or an illegal lane change may well be a homicide suspect with a body in the trunk. It is not paranoia to understand that a life-and-death struggle may be only around the corner for a police officer. Most calls for service are handled by a lone patrol officer or possibly with two or three backup officers if there is a perceived higher potential for violence.
   More complex missions that may require larger numbers of officers or more specialized training and equipment are handled by relatively small highly trained SWAT units. These missions may include protecting dignitaries, serving high-risk warrants, responding to barricaded suspects, and responding to hostage situations. The medical plan must reflect the underlying mission objectives.
   Dignitary protection is pretty straight forward. The main objective is to protect the principal individual. If there is an attack on the principal, the main effort will be to treat them appropriately. If the President is visiting town, the Secret Service will have a liaison agent in the designated receiving hospital and the blood bank will have the appropriate blood type available during the stay. Some high-profile criminals also need a protective detail when they are moved. However, there may also be casualties to the protective detail, supporting local law enforcement or other citizen participating in the event. Plans have to be in place to address major and minor problems that may arise during the event.
   High-risk warrants are often served by SWAT teams because the suspects may be known to have a violent history, weapons caches, or large quantities of drugs or other sensitive evidence that may be destroyed.

Special Situations

Many of the chemicals in drug labs are highly toxic, and thus a suspect and their children may need to be decontaminated prior to their removal from the scene.

A suspect is considered to be a *barricaded gunman* when he is armed, placed in a fortified position and refusing to come out in response to a lawful request. Although the suspect may pose a threat to innocent parties in a large area that he can control with his field of fire, he does not have someone with him that he is threatening. Typically, the first arriving patrol officers establish a perimeter so that the suspect cannot escape. Innocent bystanders are protected in place or evacuated. Negotiators attempt to talk the suspect out and if necessary chemical agents are used to flush the suspect from his position of advantage and the suspects are then taken into custody. If casualties occur, they are often most safely removed immediately in an armored vehicle as the most obvious avenues of approach may not be safe for responding unarmored vehicles.

Hostage situations occur when a suspect has direct control of one or more people and the hostage taker is using them as "bargaining chips" with the negotiators. Hostages may be random victims or family members of the hostage taker. The overall goal of a successful mission is to have the hostage(s) released or rescued safely from the hostage taker. Commonly negotiations will resolve a hostage situation. In the event that the commander does not feel that negotiations will be successful in saving the hostages, then a hostage rescue mission must be carried out. In a hostage rescue, even if officers are injured, the assault will press on until the hostage taker is separated from the hostages and the threat to them is over. The casualties will be picked up and dealt with subsequently. Classic hostage negotiation doctrine suggested negotiations should continue indefinitely because, prior to 9/11, persons who were crusading for a cause were thought to be amenable to a negotiated resolution. A disturbing recent trend is that hostage takers may do very irrational actions if they are given more than about 3 hours to ponder their circumstances. They have been known to blow up the buildings they are in and execute even their own children.

Another disturbing trend is the *homicide in progress*. These are typically disturbed individuals who go on a killing spree in their workplace or attack a soft target such as a school. They do not want to negotiate. They just want to kill people and possibly commit "suicide by cop." These events evolve so quickly that often the calls are handled by patrol officers before a full SWAT response can occur.

8. **What are the main differences between conventional emergency prehospital care and TEMS?**

The three most common causes of preventable death on the battlefield that need to be addressed immediately are bleeding, airway obstruction, and tension pneumothorax.

In the tactical environment the liberal use of tourniquets is appropriate to control *bleeding* (Figure 74.2). Victims often have multiple wounds. Most police officers and military personnel will have vests to protect the trunk from penetration by handgun rounds and possibly some fragments projected a distance from an explosive device. Ballistic protective head gear is seldom utilized in contemporary law enforcement. The nearly universal use of protective head gear in the military has significantly reduced head injuries. The brief application of a tourniquet to stem the bleeding of extremity wounds is considered routine. The advantage in gaining proximal bleeding control until more traditional care can be rendered is clearly better than the alternative of exposing the victim and rescuers to additional threats. Operative reconstructive surgical procedures demonstrate that tourniquets may be safely applied for duration of 2 hours without incurring irreversible damage to the extremity. Indeed, many of the limbs that require initial tourniquet application can not be salvaged. In the Vietnam War, over 2000 troops died of isolated

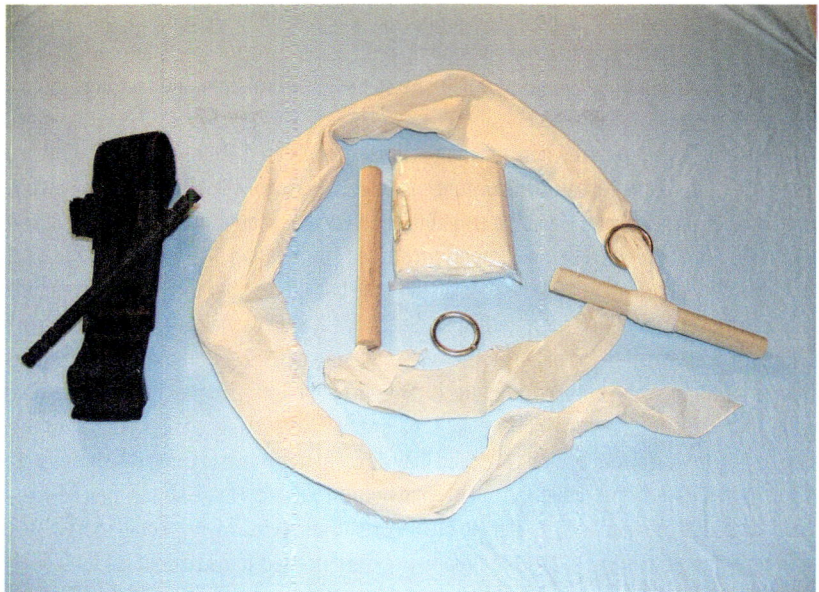

FIGURE 74.2 A very inexpensive tourniquet can be made using a small wood dowel, a metal ring, and a triangular bandage. Commercially available tourniquets should be easily applied by the officer one handed if he or she needs to preform self-rescue. These can be discreetly carried in the "sap" pocket of police uniform pants.

extremity trauma in an era when tourniquet use was not in vogue. Clearly, the benefit of briefly applying a tourniquet to prevent exsanguination far outweighs the concomitant risks.

Because of the ever present danger of an endotracheal tube being dislodged during moving, the casualty off the battlefield, *airway* management in the tactical environment relies on simple positioning, use of a nasopharyngeal airway, or cricothyroidotomy.

The most rapidly fatal yet treatable complication of penetrating chest trauma is the development of a *tension pneumothorax*. Classic training suggests there may be deviation of the trachea, distended jugular veins, and decreased breath sounds as diagnostic indicators of this dreaded complication. However, current Navy SEAL doctrine simplifies the treatment protocol by stating that "if you have a hole in your chest and are in significant respiratory distress, you deserve a well controlled hole (to treat or prevent a tension pneumothorax) in your chest." Therefore, there is a liberal use of needle decompression of all penetrating chest wounds. Because the battlefield may be a noisy, chaotic place, any physical assessments must be streamlined and performed under noise and light discipline, preferably behind good cover, so as not to give away your position and make you an easy target.

9. **What are the phases of care in the tactical environment?**
There are three phases of care in the tactical environment: care under fire, tactical field care, and casualty evacuation care. These terms are often erroneously described as hot zone, warm zone, and cold zone—a carryover from hazardous material incidents. First, zones imply geography and phases more appropriately

Special Situations

imply time lines. Second, there are no concentric circles of safety at a tactical situation. Although police will eventually establish an inner and outer perimeter, relative zones of safety are pockets behind cover. Around these islands of relative safety, rescue personnel may come under direct fire by the opposing forces.

"*Care under fire*" is the phase when a casualty is first encountered. There is a strong likelihood of the rescuer also becoming a casualty. The distance to adequate cover will determine what, if any, limited medical maneuvers are done. Cover is a structure or object that should stop the rounds that are fired at you by the opposing forces. The most important strategy for treating a victim is to get behind cover as soon as possible. Eliminating the threat or keeping the bad guys under their cover via suppressive fire may be the most prudent first short-term objective. A full 10% of battle casualties that occurred during the Vietnam war occurred to soldiers who were rendering first aid to their downed buddies. To help minimize that threat, one unique technique is the concept of *remote patient assessment*. If the victim is yelling for help, we know that his airway is patent and he has adequate perfusion to the brain to realize he is in trouble. From behind cover, you may direct him to move to cover if he is not already there and provide self-care. If he is down and not moving from an obviously fatal wound then he does not need to be recovered immediately. If you elect to break cover to aid a victim, you should coordinate that with your friendly forces so they can provide suppressive fire if needed. If the patient is a long distance from cover, the only medical maneuvers to even consider would be application of a tourniquet to stem extremity bleeding or use of a nasopharyngeal airway to increase his chance of survival while you drag him back to cover. An important note on suppressive fire: in law enforcement every round must be legally defensible. There is no "spray and pray" in law enforcement.

"*Tactical field care*" is care rendered once the victim and rescuer are behind cover or no longer under effective hostile fire. This phase is merely preparation to move off the battlefield. The duration of this phase will depend on the seriousness of the wounds and the intensity of the fight. Bleeding is controlled once again with the use of tourniquets or direct-pressure bandages. Consider establishing intravenous access with a Buff cap but fluids are *not* routinely given unless there is significant mental status deterioration that is the result of blood loss, rather than a head wound. Splinting of major fractures may be considered at this point. Advanced airway maneuvers consist of the use of a nasopharyngeal airway or cricothyroidotomy. Direct endotracheal intubation is discouraged in this phase for two reasons:

- The tube may become easily dislodged during subsequent movement and occlude the airway.
- In darkness, the use of a light may give away your position and make you a target for opposing forces.

Consideration of decompressing the chest for tension pneumothorax is balanced against the risk of opening or removing the ballistic vest that the victim may be wearing. The victim may need to be ultimately carried off the battlefield or picked up by an armored vehicle, which can provide mobile cover.

"*Casualty evacuation care*" *(Casevac)* is the phase when care begins to resemble traditional civilian ambulance care. This may be done in an armored vehicle in transit to rendezvous with a conventional ambulance, in a boat or in an off road vehicle traversing difficult terrain (Figure 74.3). Use of oxygen, cardiac monitor, and blood pressure cuff is usually started in this phase.

From a strictly medical point of view, all of these phases should be as short as possible so that the casualty can get to definitive surgical/medical care as soon as possible. From a tactical perspective this may unduly place rescuers at significant risk and must be balanced with medical care needs.

Tactical Emergency Medicine

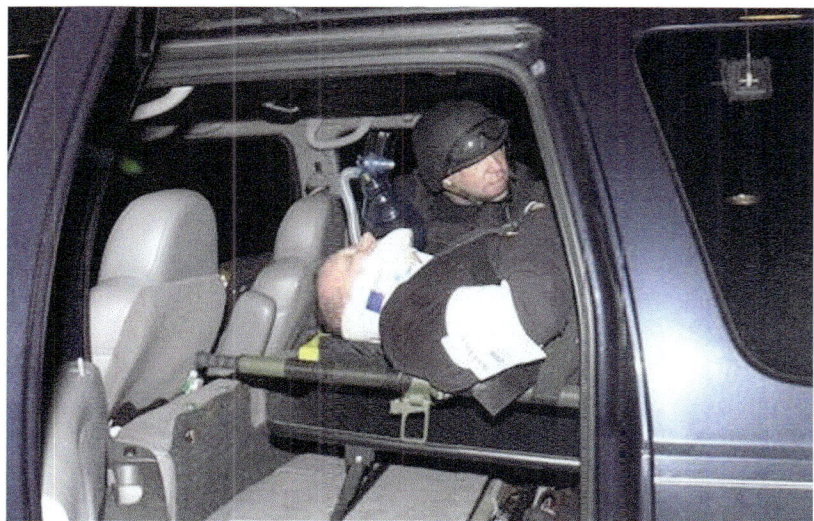

FIGURE 74.3 Maryland State Police trooper medic has access to a patient in an unmarked medical support vehicle just as he would in their helicopter.

10. **What types of medical equipment packs are used?**

   The personal equipment needed varies with the rescuer's role in the mission. Every police officer should be able to provide self-care and immediate buddy care. A tourniquet can be discretely carried in a standard uniform "sap" pocket. Some gauze roles or triangular bandages can be carried behind the breast insert on most ballistic gear. SWAT teams or other special units that use battle dress uniforms can designate which cargo pocket the individual officer will carry the equipment that should be used on him- or herself. This should include:

   - Equipment to stop bleeding. This may include a tourniquet, a roll of gauze (that may also be impregnated with a hemostatic agent) to insert into extremity wounds that are too proximal to allow the use of a tourniquet. A battle dressing that has the sterile dressing and securing bandage attached, such as the Israeli or Oakes dressings. (Figure 74.4).
   - Airway equipment would include a nasopharyngeal tube that would fit.
   - Equipment to manage a chest wound. Some occlusive dressings are designed with a one-way valve to release overpressure. A long over-the-needle catheter to decompress a tension pneumothorax is also carried by many personnel.

   Patrol officers can also carry the foregoing in something as discrete as a nylon shaving kit with a length of parachute cord to serve as a carry strap. This can be kept in the front seat office of the patrol car so that their emergency medical equipment is always immediately at hand. Personal protective equipment (Figure 74.5). should be included to protect the officer from exposure to transmissible diseases and consist of a pocket mask, gloves, and eye protection.

   Polycarbonate eyewear that is at least 2 mm thick will also afford some protection from secondary missiles created by an explosive devices or concrete debris from a near-miss gun shot.

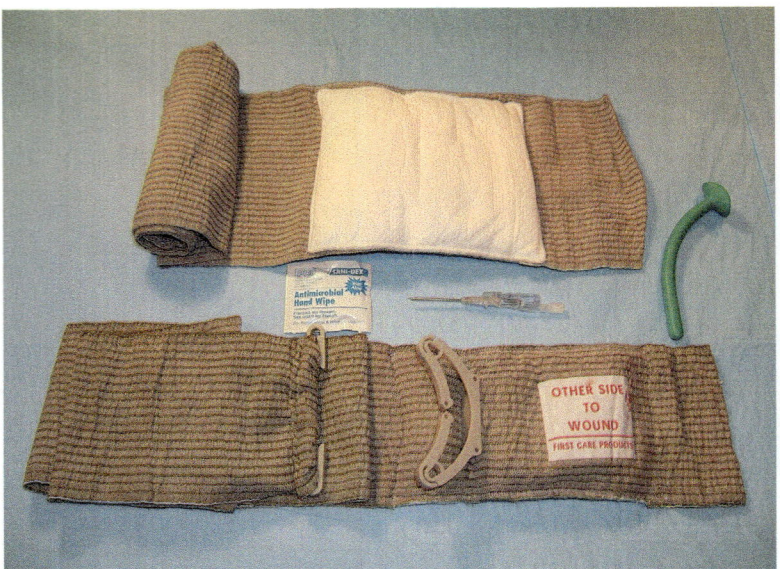

FIGURE 74.4 Front and rear view of an Israeli battle dressing. Sterile dressing is attached to one end of a bandage that can be quickly locked in place on the victim. Nasopharyngeal airway and catheter over needle for chest decompression should be available on each SWAT member for their care in the event they are injured during the mission.

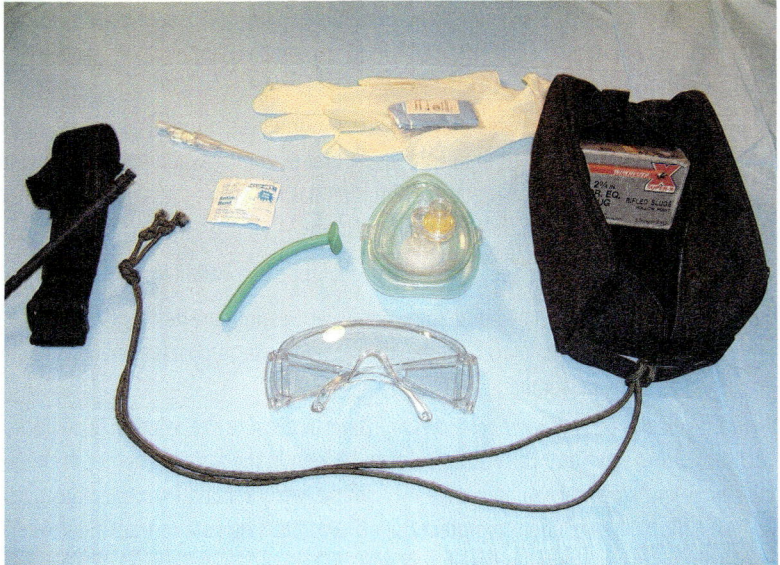

FIGURE 74.5 A shaving kit with personnel protective equipment and additional medical supplies can be carried in the front seat of a patrol car so that it is immediately available for rapid deployment.

Tactical Emergency Medicine

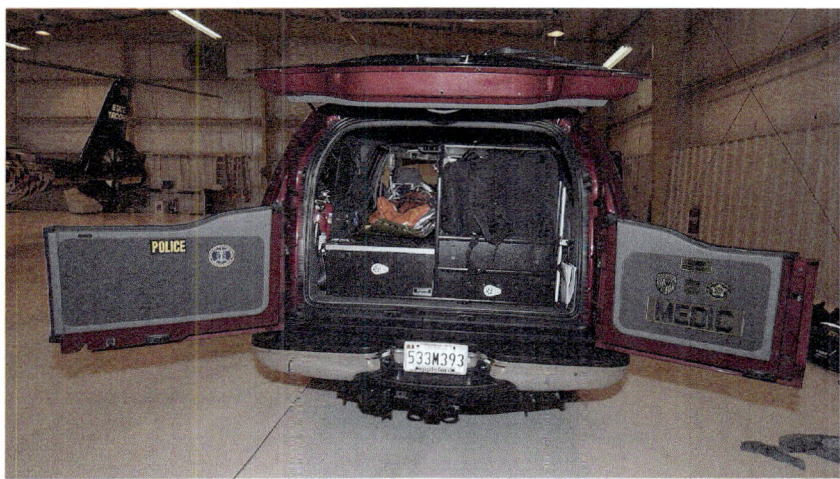

FIGURE 74.6 Large medic bags available on passenger side of vehicle for rapid deployment. Sick-call items, equipment for radiologic monitoring, air sampling, hasty decontamination, and additional advanced life support and rescue equipment available in cabinet storage.

The embedded medic should have a larger pack to carry additional supplies and more advanced equipment consistent with his or her training (Figure 74.6). In addition to laying out their equipment as do their civilian counterparts for airways and intravenous fluid loads, many tactical medics also load individual patient care packs identical to those carried for self-rescue by their SWAT team members in large plastic bags. These packets can then be tossed to officers caring for the injured behind cover positions in the event of multiple casualties. If the tactical situation is resolved, the individual officers' self-care equipment can then be used in a mass casualty situation.

Another type of kit is a "sick call bag," which is used to treat minor problems for the team members. This can include Band-Aids, antibiotic ointment, sunscreen, insect repellent, over-the-counter medications, and special items such as inhalers to meet the specific medical needs of the team members during extended operations.

11. **What important forensic topics should the tactical medic master?**

    Medical care rendered at a crime scene must not only be appropriate medically but also must be done in such a way that important forensic evidence is not destroyed or contaminated. Everyone entering a crime scene needs to be "logged in" and then submit a written statement of all observations and actions performed on the scene. Blood and other body fluids on scene may be biohazards, but they are not cleaned up until after the investigators are done processing the crime scene. A person who was struggling for life may have hair, tissue, DNA evidence, or gunpowder residue on their hands or under the fingernails. Consider placing a paper bag individually over each hand of the victim and taping that in place above the wrist as soon as practical. When you are exposing the victim, take care not to cut directly through knife or bullet holes in the garments. Any evidence you collect should be placed individually in a paper bag and subsequently identified and logged. This would include the gauze you use to wipe over a wound to inspect it.

Special Situations

12. Is it important to document entry and exit wounds?

In one classic study, physicians had a 50% chance of accurately determining whether a gunshot wound was an entrance or exit wound. For tactical medicine purposes, just document where the injuries are and what you did to treat them. If you are in life-saving mode you do not need to or have the time to make sufficiently detailed analysis of the wound to declare this is an entrance or an exit. When a victim is struck with a bullet, there will *always* be an *abrasion ring* at the *entrance* as the skin is pushed out of the way during penetration by the bullet. This is independent of the distance from the firearm. Soot is the smoke from the firearm that may be deposited on the clothing or skin if a weapon is discharged at close range. It may wipe away on gauze swabbed over the wound. Stippling is the unburned powder and debris that is imbedded in the skin and the bruising of the skin from this debris as it strikes the target from close range. These observations need to be documented in your treatment note and the gauze you used to wipe each individual wound should be separately saved for evidence.

13. What are less lethal weapons?

These are devices that fire a projectile with the intention of delivering an impact similar to a baton strike, an electrical device, or chemical agent used to temporarily incapacitate a suspect who is actively resisting detention. Any use of force must be objectively reasonable in stopping bad behavior. These weapons have been designed to fill the gap in response from close contact "hands on" restraint to the use of deadly force by instead temporarily disabling the suspect. These weapons are most typically used on suicidal parties or very agitated suspects who are felt to be too dangerous to approach. Target areas for impact weapons are generally the extremities. These may result in significant soft-tissue injuries and even fractures of the bones under the impact area. There is a greater possibility of permanently disabling and even fatal outcomes if sensitive areas such as the head are hit.

Electrical devices that deliver high-voltage/low-amperage shocks can also be incapacitating. The most commonly used chemical agents in law enforcement are cayenne-based powder (active ingredient in chili peppers), agents that create a burning sensation, and lacrimation. It is thought that the Soviets used a fentanyl-like aerosol in a hostage rescue mission in Moscow. The use of these less lethal tools has decreased the use of deadly force in many incidents, but there is always the possibility of serious injury and even death when these technologies are used. It is important that prompt medical care is available to deal with these contingencies.

14. What is sudden death in custody?

Specific technologies or techniques have been associated with the unfortunate deaths of some suspects who expire shortly after being taken into custody. These deaths are likely multifactorial in nature; however, caution must be exercised in the use of these techniques. The first modern reported cases attributed death to positional asphyxia when suspects were hog-tied in a prone position, having their legs attached to their handcuffs. One of the follow-up reports that challenged this precept showed that young healthy police recruits experienced no significant change in pulmonary function when restrained in a similar manner. Underlying medical conditions certainly play a role in some cases. Many suspects that die are chronic cocaine or methamphetamine users who get their high from catchecolamine release. After a brief fight or flight response, many of these suspects die a sudden asystolic death. Rhabdomyolysis and hyperthermia have also been implicated in some deaths. Even veterinary literature describes capture myopathy and death of animals shortly after capture. Electrical stun devices typically use amperages that are minute fractions of the energy delivery of cardiac defibrillators. Ultrasound evaluation of human subjects who consented to being energized with a electrical conductive device have failed to demonstrate any significant adverse effect on cardiac function. It is necessary to recognize that these technologies can have potential complications. It is important to have personnel trained to recognize and treat these individuals immediately.

15. **How does decision making occur in a tactical situation?**

Given the high stress environment of tactical situations, it is important to understand how decision-making occurs in these settings. Air Force Captain John Boyd was the first to describe the observe, orient, decide, and act (OODA) loop in air combat over Korea. First you must *observe* a threat. Darkness, bad weather, and distance are a few of the most common factors that limit our ability to observe. Your training and experience will then *orient* the information into a most likely scenario. An officer that sees a suspect in a high-crime area reach into his pants behind his belt when challenged will orient to the suspect going for a gun. The officer then has to *decide* from many options what to do. Do I move right for cover? Is my best cover to the left? Should I draw my weapon? Do I duck or freeze? You will then start to *act* on one of those options or some combination of actions. You then start the cycle over again as you observe what effect your actions are having on your opponent. In combat, the cycles are fast, but in more strategic planning, the same processes cycle more slowly. When you have the initiative, you have the liberty to think slightly longer without as much pressure as your opponent. You have to set realistic priorities and timelines in longer operations.

In medicine, information and action is processed in a similar manner to running a code. Who will start the IV? Who will intubate? When do we see the rhythm and what is the rhythm? By having previously agreed upon plans (SOP: standard operating procedures), arriving resources can see what actions are being done and what needs to be done. The team leader can then orchestrate the resuscitation so that most appropriate tasks are addressed first. A commander has a finite span of control in any operation. It is easy to become overwhelmed by events if the individual is attempting to address too many conflicting tasks in a rapidly evolving operation.

In the public safety sector the fire service first developed the concept of incident command to provide greater accountability of responding resources. Their response to an alarm is more predictable with operators arriving in groups on engines or trucks from established stations. These groups routinely work in small units. In the past, some groups were lost on the fire ground during building collapses and not recognized as being missing. To maximize accountability the fire service has evolved a top-down management scheme where "freelancing" is discouraged. The incident commander tightly controls who will do what, and when that will happen. This is the type of management scheme used by the former Soviet military. Information has to pass through multiple command layers, each operating in their own OODA loops, leading to slower and less flexible responses.

Police officers typically handle most of their calls alone. In a major incident, they arrive in an unpredictable time frame depending on their patrol location when the incident was broadcast. SWAT officers spend more time working as a team using small-unit tactics. In the early moments of a dynamic police emergency, such as a homicide in progress, most likely a few tactical officers will try to orchestrate the movement of the patrol officers they have with them at the time. This more closely resembles the U.S. military style where noncommissioned officers in charge of small units are expected to find and exploit the enemies' weaknesses acting under the overall commander's stated mission intent. The command structure is designed to support the exploits of those able to seize the initiative. Windows of opportunity may close if there is a delay in getting approval for numerous tasks through multiple levels of command staff. Facilitating rapid information flow and remotely controlling activities through cyberspace is the fifth dimension of the modern battle space.

16. **What type of training should the tactical medic have?**

    If you start with a medical professional (EMT, paramedic, registered nurse, nurse practitioner, independent medic or physician), they need to be selected much as any other operator on SWAT. They must be physically fit, team players with a good work record, and demonstrated ability to stay calm and think in chaotic situations. They need to be schooled in basic law with an emphasis on search and seizure and maintaining a chain of custody for evidence collected. They need to be able to write coherently because the documentation of the cases they deal with will be closely scrutinized by the legal system. If you think hospital peer review can be tough, consider that any action a police officer takes may well be the basis for an ultimate Supreme Court ruling, and that your actions as a TEMS provider will also be held to those standards. Arrest control techniques and fundamentals of hand to hand combat should be taught and practiced often. There should be an ongoing exposure to seeing detainees so that subtle body language clues that a fight is about to begin do not go unnoticed. The skills to formulate an MTA and basic mission planning with an emphasis on preventative medicine for threats in the tactical environment are essential. Team members should also be good instructors. It is important that they assist in training team and patrol members in addressing the most immediate life threats that need to be handled because the medics may become casualties or not be able to get to victims in a timely manner on the battlefield. The medics should know how to render safe any weapons they may need to handle. If they are to function as armed officers, there is a huge commitment to basic and advanced firearms training. Use of force training needs to include simulated *shoot/don't shoot* decision making on an ongoing basis. Every round fired by a police officer has to be legally, morally, and procedurally justified.

17. **What is the future of TEMS?**

    It is impossible to predict exactly how TEMS will be practiced in the future. There are numerous key points to consider in the continuing evolution of the specialty, but the need for such service remains. Most police agencies have not adequately provided combat life savers to the communities they serve. Just as bilingual officers give an added capability to resolve emergencies, so too can the law enforcement corpsmen add to the life saving combat missions that have fortunately been rare in the United States. Selected full-time peace officers, especially those with previous medical training, should be recruited for additional specialized medical training to work in this unique environment. The current Navy SEAL doctrine has been included in the recent Prehospital Trauma Life Support (PHTLS) book as a specific chapter. Officers with this very narrow focus of medical care would be a valuable first link in the chain of survival on the battlefield. All of these embedded law enforcement corpsmen equivalents also need to be capable of doing hasty decontamination. They will also need to be familiar with the management of blast injuries. Natural disasters have historically demonstrated the need for rapid regional responses to emergencies. In law enforcement there is a current shift toward regionalization of SWAT teams. This shift has been due in part to the multifactorial rise in violent criminal behavior throughout the world over the past decades, the impact of which has been blunted by increasing capability to care for severe multisystem trauma. There are radical groups that have vowed to end Western Civilization as we know it. All of these groups have access to conventional weapons and explosives; and some have, or soon will have, access to weapons of mass destruction. The events of 911 underscore the fact that terrorists are at war with us. Even without the prospect of man-made disasters, the increasing operational tempo and complexity of modern law enforcement operations clearly calls for a greater capability to provide specialized medical care in the austere environment of the battlefield. TEMS will play an integral role in community policing, disaster management and public safety.

Pearls and Pitfalls

1. Before you start an operation, develop a plan and then be prepared to modify your plans to best fulfill the mission objectives and time lines.
2. Stopping the bleeding takes precedence over starting IV fluids. Using a tourniquet may be life saving for the victim and the rescuer.
3. The "one-plus rule" applies to bleeding sites as well as to suspects. Always assume there is one more than you saw. The one you do not see will kill your patient or you. Be vigilant and recheck often.
4. Solving the tactical problem takes precedence over addressing the medical problem. You cannot be an effective life saver if you are seriously injured or dead. Consider remotely assessing the patient and coaching them in self-care.
5. "Communication problem" does not mean there are not enough radios. Often people can not exchange information effectively face to face. Say what you mean and mean what you say. Build personal relationships with key personnel before the incident.
6. "Call A CAB and go!" **C**all for backup, **A**bolish the threats (suspects, blood borne pathogens, weapons, uncapped needles) **C**ompress bleeding sites with compressive battle dressings or tourniquets, simple **A**irway maneuvers, assist **B**reathing and consider needle decompression of possible tension pneumothorax. **G**o to the nearest appropriate facility immediately. The "golden period" is the time from injury to surgical stabilization.
7. Tension pneumothorax is rapidly fatal, difficult to diagnosis, and easy to treat. Consider needle decompression if the signs and symptoms of tension pneumothorax are present.

References

1. Butler FK. Tactical medicine training for SEAL mission commanders. Mil Med 166:625–631, July 2001. This article is also available on line at www.specialoperations.com/Specialties/Medicie/Military.html
2. Rinnert KJ, Hall WL. Tactical emergency medical support. Emerg Med Clin N Am 20:929–952, 2002.
3. Heiskell LE, Carmona RH. Tactical emergency medical support: An emerging subspecialty of emergency medicine. Ann Emerg Med 23(4):778–785, April 1994.
4. Bozeman WP, Eastman ER. Tactical EMS: An emerging opportunity in graduate medical education. Prehosp Emerg Care 6(3):322–324, Jul-Sept. 2002.
5. Chan TC, Vilke GM, Neuman T, et al. Restraint position and positional asphyxia. Ann Emerg Med, 30:5, p. 578-586, Nov. 1997.
6. Ruttenber, AJ, McAnally H, Wetli CV, et al. Cocaine-associated rhabdomyolysis and excited delirium: different stages of the same disease. Am J Forensic Med Pathol 20(2):120–127, 1999.
7. Heal CS. Sound Doctrine: A Tactical Primer. New York: Lantern Books, 2000.

Special Situations

8. Heal CS. 21st century tactics: Fighting in the 5th dimension. Tactical Edge Winter:21–25, 2003.
9. Counter Narcotics Tactical Operations Medical Support (CONTOMS) Millennium Edition CD ROM and Special Extrication and Rescue Tactics (SERT) CD ROM, available at the Casualty Care Research Center of the Uniformed Services University of the Health Sciences, Bethesda, MD.
10. Sharma, N, Vancouver police deploy SWAT-tactical EMS. Tactical Edge Spring:35–38, 2000.
11. Greenburg MJ, Wipfler EJ. Medical ballistics. Tactical Edge Fall:68–78, 2006.
12. Yanor R. High Risk Life Saver Course, Tactical Response 4:11, p. 112-117, Sept-Oct. 2006.
13. Ciccione TJ, Anderson PD, Gann CA, et al. Successful development and implementation of a tactical emergency medical technician program for United States federal agents. Prehosp Disaster Med 20:1:36–39, Jan-Feb, 2005.
14. Merrick C, ed. Military medicine, Chapter 16. PHTLS: Basic and Advanced Trauma Life Support. 5th ed. St. Louis: Mosby, 2003.
15. National Association of EMTs. Prehospital Trauma Life Support, Military Edition, 7th Edition. Butler FK, Giebner SD, Salomone JP, Pons PT (eds). Mosby JEMS/ Elsevier, St. Louis, MO, 2011.
16. Officer Down Memorial Page. www.odmp.org. Accessed November 14, 2011.
17. Sztajnkrycer MD, Callaway DW, Baez AA. Police Officer Response to the Injured Officer: A Survey-Based Analysis of Medical Care Decisions. In Pre-Hospital & Disaster Medicine, Vol 22, No 4, July-Aug 2007, p. 335–341.
18. Ho J, Reardon RF, Dawes D, et al. Ultrasound Measurement of Cardiac Activity During Conducted Electrical Weapon Application in Exercising Adults, in Annals of Emergency Medicine, Vol 50, No 3, Sept 2007, p. s108.
19. Pasquier M, Pierre-Nicolas C, Vallotton M, Yersian B. Electronic Control Device Exposure: A Review of Morbidity & Mortality, in Annals of Emergency Medicine, Vol 58, No 2, August 2011, p.178–188.

Hazardous Materials

Michael G. Stanley, M.Ed, EMT-P

1. **What is a hazardous material?**
   An excellent, yet simple definition of a hazardous material is provided by hazardous material specialist, Ludwig Benner. Benner says it best when he defines a hazardous material as, "Any substance that jumps out of its container at you when something goes wrong and hurts and harms the things it touches."

2. **What kind of harm can they cause?**
   Hazardous substances can cause harm not only to people but also to wildlife and the environment. This can occur because of the substances themselves, their flammability, their reactivity, and their toxic health effects. This could affect the patient through burns, poisoning, corrosion, and asphyxiation.

3. **Will EMS providers encounter hazardous materials?**
   With industrial chemicals being produced at a rate greater than 50 billion tons each and every year, the chance that EMS providers will encounter these substances is very high. It is likely that the rescuer will respond to hazardous materials incidents in both fixed facilities such as warehouses as well as in transportation accidents or as a result of intentional release such as acts of terrorism.

4. **What are the most common types of hazardous substances encountered at an incident scene?**
   The substances that are most often present at emergency scenes are gasoline, natural gas, chlorine, and ammonia. All are very prevalent in today's society. Each also poses its own unique risk and must be approached and handled with great caution.

5. **If it is believed that hazardous materials are involved in the incident, how should the rescuers approach the scene?**
   The most important consideration should be to approach the scene cautiously and with the most information possible. If there is any indication of toxic materials relayed in the initial dispatch report, caution should immediately be exercised. It is important that the approach to the scene be made from uphill. This will prevent liquid materials from running downhill and contaminating the rescuers and response vehicles. Wind speed and direction should also be obtained from the dispatch center. By approaching from upwind, rescuers and vehicles will not encounter vapor clouds.
   The rescuer should also note that there has been a tremendous increase in clandestine drug labs. This further complicates response, as not only are there toxic substances present, other hazards such as violent individuals, boobytraps, or improvised explosive devices may be present.

Special Situations

6. What should the EMS provider do if they are first on scene of a hazmat incident?

According the National Incident Management System, the first arriving unit on scene should take command of the incident. The rescuer may make the first incident decisions that will help protect on-scene personnel and those that are still responding. Additionally, these decisions should also protect the patients and the bystanders. The first action should be to call for additional resources such as law enforcement, fire departments, additional ambulances, and hazardous-material response teams. Secondly, it is crucial that an incident perimeter be established to begin developing hot, warm, and cold zones.

7. What are hot, warm, and cold zones?

The "hot zone" is the actual contaminated area, and entry into this area is limited to team members in proper protective clothing who need to enter the area for reconnaissance, victim rescue, and mitigation of the situation. The size of the hot zone is based on the chemical involved and its particular properties and hazards. Access to the hot zone must be controlled and should be via only one entry/exit point. The "warm zone" is the area where team support services are located. Patients will be brought out of the hot zone and enter the warm zone where the decontamination area will be located. Responders working in the warm zone also need to wear appropriate personal protective equipment. Once the patients have been decontaminated, the patient will be brought to the cold zone where the EMS responder can perform an evaluation, treatment can be initiated, and transport decisions made.

8. What resources are available to help identify the problem?

A variety of resources should be available to responding prehospital providers that will assist them in their decision making. For example:

The North American Emergency Response Guidebook. This resource is required to be on every emergency response vehicle. It provides the responder with vital information for using placards to identify the chemical, what hazards are associated with it, initial patient treatment recommendations, and evacuation distances.

Binoculars. Binoculars can aid in identifying shapes of vessels and containers from a safe distance. (Remember, this should be done from uphill and upwind.) They can also be used to read product or company names and to visualize placards on shipping containers and vessels. Finally, it may be possible to estimate the number of patients and their conditions based on what can be seen through the binoculars.

Shipping papers. Shipping papers should be present whenever sufficient quantities of hazardous substances are being transported by ground, rail, air, or sea. Many times, they will have product information that can help rescuers identify the substance and provide recommendations for decontamination and treatment.

Material safety data sheets (MSDS). MSDS are required to be in fixed facilities. This enables the employee to know what chemicals they could come in contact with while at the workplace. These are invaluable resources to the rescuer and provide a wealth of information including suggestions for courses of treatment.

Regional and national databases. There are numerous resources such as Poison Control Centers, Chemtrec, and Chemtel that can be accessed by telephone in order to provide the most current and useful information available to the rescuer. In addition, a number of databases such as PoisIndex© and smartphone applications such as WISER can be accessed to provide information.

Hazardous Materials

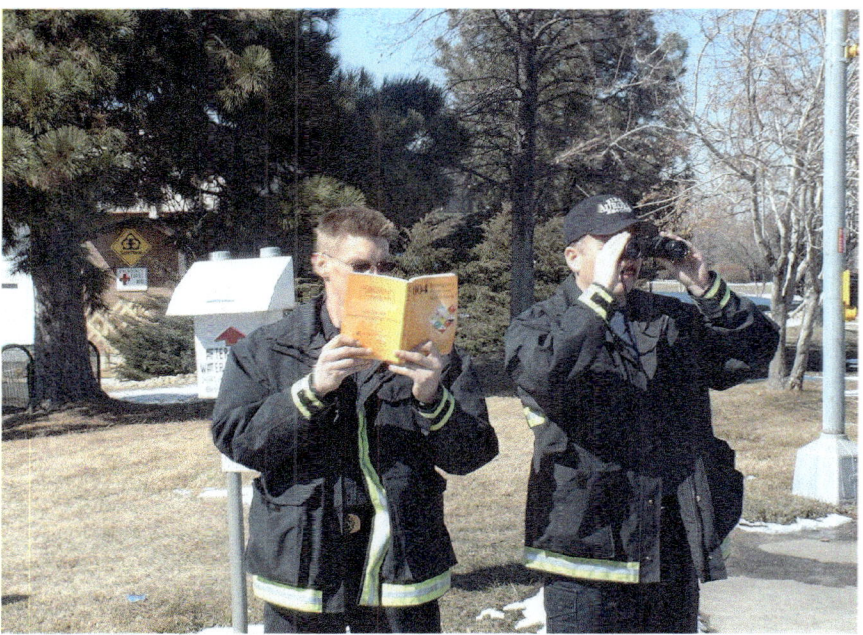

FIGURE 75.1 EMS providers should assess the incident through binoculars and use reference material whenever possible.

9. What will the role of the EMS provider be in an incident?

Unless the rescuer has received additional training, most EMS providers should operate at the awareness level. This means that the rescuer should only take part in defensive operations such as establishing perimeters and helping to identify the product.

The majority of the duties of the EMS provider at the emergency incident will revolve around patient care. The provider may be directly involved in treating the patient or may perform support functions. The prehospital provider should be prepared to take a role in the incident command structure. For example, the provider could be assigned to the position of triage officer, medical branch director, or the transport officer.

It may also be necessary for the rescuer to assist the members of the hazmat team. Prior to donning protective suits and entering the danger area, team members must have their vital signs assessed and receive a medical prescreening. After exiting the hazard zone, and removing their equipment, monitoring of the vitals should be performed. The members assigned to the team will be responsible for making the decision if rehabilitation is necessary; the team members can again take part in the incident or if further treatment and transport is necessary.

10. What type of personal protective equipment will the EMS provider need?

There should be no reason for any additional protective equipment beyond that required by the Occupational Safety and Health Administration. Prior to coming into contact with health care providers,

505

Special Situations

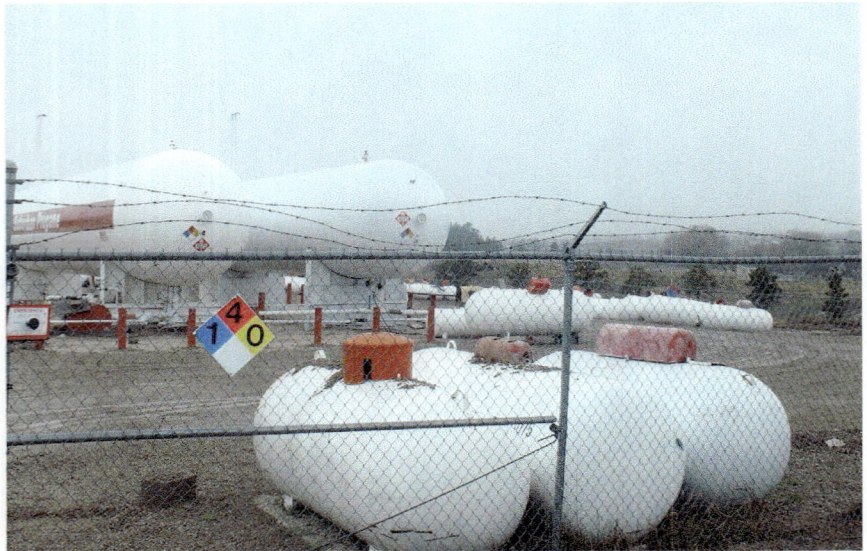

FIGURE 75.2   EMS providers should become familiar with the hazards that may be present in their response areas.

victims should at least be decontaminated with water after removing their clothes. This can remove upward of 90% of the contaminants. By using normal body substance isolation procedures, more than adequate protection should be available to the medical responder.

11. **Are there any specific medications and treatments that can be given to the exposed patient?**
    Depending on the amount, type, and concentration of the chemical that the patient is exposed to, there are several antidotes available. Unfortunately, there are several limiting factors that make this difficult — the first being that some of these antidotes are not widely available to prehospital providers. Most commonly, they are carried by hazmat units or are located at local or regional hospitals. Second, the protocols for their usage vary greatly from one locality to the next. The local policies and protocols should be consulted in this situation. Examples of specific antidotes include hydroxocobalamin for cyanide poisoning, atropine and pralidoxime (2-PAM) for nerve agent or organophosphate exposure, and high-flow oxygen for carbon monoxide toxicity.

Pearls and Pitfalls

1. Remember, slow down and take your time: the safety of the rescuer is paramount. Be part of the solution, not the problem.
2. The priorities for a hazmat incident are the same as for any other type of emergency incident:
   - Life safety
   - Incident stabilization
   - Property conservation

3. Eighty-eight percent of hazmat incidents are caused by human error resulting in a high probability of one or more patients.
4. Do not forget to suspect trauma in the patient from a hazardous material incident. Remember to notify the local hospitals as soon as possible so that they can prepare to treat victims of chemical exposure.
5. Not approaching from uphill and upwind and coming into contact with the product will result in your being contaminated.
6. Not establishing or operating within an organized command structure during the incident will complicate the response.
7. Operating in a capacity that you are not trained or equipped for may cause you to become part of the problem.
8. Not requesting additional and appropriate resources early in the incident will delay the overall management of the incident.
9. Transporting patients who have not been decontaminated will contaminate you, your vehicle, and the receiving hospital.

References

1. Benner L. Recognizing and identifying hazardous materials. National Fire Academy, Emmitsburg, MD, pp. 1–2, 1985.
2. Bledsoe B, Porter RS, Cherry RA. Paramedic Care: Principles and Practice, 2nd ed. Vol. 5, pp. 427–437. Upper Saddle River, NJ: Brady Publishing, 2006.
3. Borak J, Callan M, Abbott W. Hazardous Materials Exposure: Emergency Response and Patient Care. Upper Saddle River, NJ: Brady Publishing, 1991.
4. Christen H, Maniscalco P. Mass Casualty and High-Impact Incidents: An Operations Guide, pp. 91–100. Upper Saddle River, NJ: Brady Publishing, 1991.
5. Lesak DM. Hazardous Materials: Strategies and Tactics. Upper Saddle River, NJ: Brady Publishing, 1999.
6. Meryl-Levy J. The First Responder's Pocket Guide to Hazardous Materials Emergency Response, 2nd ed. Campbell, CA: Firebelle Productions, 2000.
7. Department of Homeland Security. National Incident Management System. Washington, DC: U.S. Government Printing Office, 2004.
8. U.S. Department of Transportation. North American Emergency Response Guidebook. Washington DC: U.S. Government Printing Office, 2008.
9. http://wiser.nlm.nih.gov/ Accessed November 12, 2011.

Technical Rescues

Michael G. Stanley, M.Ed, EMT-P

CHAPTER 76

1. **What is a technical rescue?**
   A technical rescue is one that requires specially trained personnel and special equipment and resources to complete the rescue. This could include rescues from high angles, trenches, confined spaces, building collapses, and bodies of water (Figure 76.1).

2. **What should be the most important concern when operating at an incident?**
   At any emergency incident, the first and foremost concern is the safety of the rescuers. This is even more important during technical rescue operations. Clearly, there are risks inherent to the situation at hand. If it were not for these dangerous factors, the rescue would most likely be unnecessary. Far too many rescuers who did not have either the proper equipment or the proper training have been injured or killed trying to perform a rescue they were not qualified to attempt. The key point to remember is, *do not attempt a rescue until qualified and equipped personnel arrive on scene* (Figure 76.2).

3. **Will I encounter technical rescues as an EMS provider?**
   Although these types of emergencies do not occur routinely, the potential for them to occur does exist. When they do, they typically become very resource- and equipment-intensive. Prehospital providers should take the time to contemplate what hazards are present in their jurisdictions. For example, lakes, rivers, wilderness areas, and construction sites all could potentially necessitate technical rescues. Forethought into what types of emergencies may occur can enable a smoother emergency scene.

4. **What is a risk–benefit analysis?**
   A risk–benefit analysis is a decision-making process that should be used by emergency services persons to help mitigate the incident. After assessing the scene and the hazards, the risk to the rescuer is determined. This is weighed against the benefits that would result in effecting a rescue. If the risk outweighs the benefit, rescue should not be attempted. Remember, "Risk a lot to save a lot, risk a little to save a little, and risk nothing to save nothing."

5. **What should the EMS provider do if they are first on scene of a technical rescue incident?**
   After conducting an assessment of the scene and performing a risk–benefit analysis, there are several other critical tasks that must occur. According the National Incident Management System, the first arriving unit on scene should take command of the incident. Next, a hazard zone should be established. It is imperative to keep bystanders safe and away from the incident. Historically, many incidents have been further complicated by well-meaning bystanders who themselves become victims. Once this is completed, try to identify the number of patients that may be present. It is very possible that the incident would have multiple or mass casualties, particularly in the case of building collapses. Finally, if it is safe to do so, contact should be made with the patient. Because of the hazards that are present, this may be accomplished by using loudspeakers, megaphones, or simply by yelling. Psychological first aid should be provided by comforting the patient or patient(s) and assuring them that trained help is on its way.

Technical Rescues

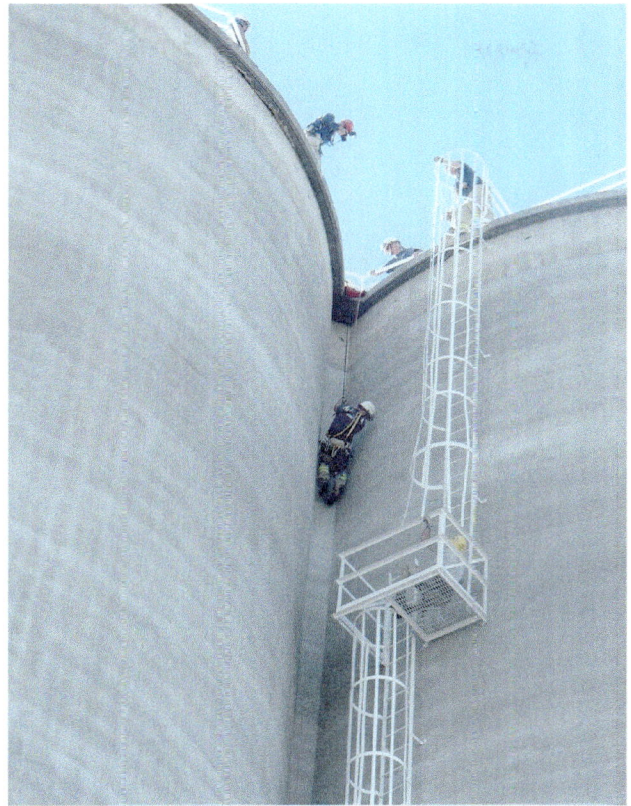

FIGURE 76.1 EMS providers should not attempt to make a rescue unless they are properly trained and equipped.

6. What resources are available to assist in the rescue?
The most likely resources to be used are local, regional, or federal technical rescue teams. Prehospital providers should educate themselves as to what is available in their community and the capabilities and resources of the responding teams. Another source of assistance may come from technical specialists at industrial sites or from construction companies that may supply heavy equipment and operators. Finally, the use of a physician on scene may be beneficial. This will become particularly relevant if the need for a field amputation is being considered.

7. What will the role of the EMS provider be in the incident?
The majority of the duties of the EMS provider at the emergency incident will revolve around patient care. The provider may be directly involved in treating the patient or may perform support functions. The prehospital provider should be prepared to take a role in the incident command structure. For example, they could be assigned to the position of triage officer, medical branch director, or transport officer.

It may also be necessary for the rescuer to assist the members of the technical rescue team. Many of these types of operations will be very time- and labor-intensive. Also, environmental conditions may also

Special Situations

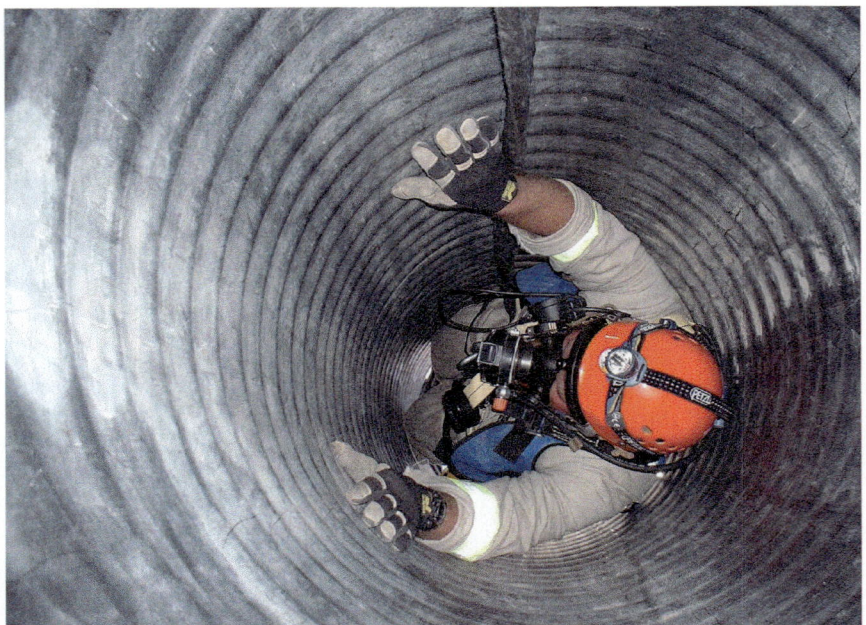

FIGURE 76.2 EMS providers should become familiar with the hazards that may be present in their response areas.

affect the rescuer. Therefore, rescuers will need to be consistently monitored for signs of fatigue. The EMS members assigned to the team will be responsible for making the decision if rehabilitation is necessary, the team members can again take part in the incident, or if further treatment and transport is necessary.

8. **What type of personal protective equipment will the EMS provider need?**
Typically, there should be no reason for any additional protective equipment beyond that required by the Occupational Safety and Health Administration. By using normal body substance isolation procedures, more than adequate protection should be available to the rescuer. On rare occasions, additional equipment such as leather work gloves, hearing protection, and hard hats may be necessary, especially when working around heavy equipment and machinery.

9. **What kind of medical care usually takes place during a technical rescue?**
As in any medical emergency, care varies widely based on the patient's injuries. Mechanism of injury, weather, life hazards, access, and extrication circumstances all enter into how a patient can be managed most effectively. Technical rescue involves everything from rescuing stranded victims with no injuries to fall victims with multisystem trauma. Just as the entrapped victim of a motor vehicle accident will receive care based on access, length of extrication, severity of injuries, and other factors, the same considerations come into play when planning for the care of the technical rescue victim. For instance, certain decisions are required when considering the care of a person who has fallen from the roof of a two-story building

and has received multiple fractures, a possible head injury, and internal injuries and requires transport to a trauma center 12 minutes away. However, when the victim is half a mile up a rocky trail at the bottom of a steep 200-foot slope, just gaining access to the patient is a challenge and planning for efficient care presents an entirely different set of problems.

10. What type of medical equipment is used in technical rescues?

In many technical rescue situations, the amount of equipment that can be carried will be limited. It is often impractical and unsafe to carry a complete advanced life support (ALS) medical kit, personal safety equipment, and the rescue equipment required to perform a technical rescue. Therefore, the paramedic on a rescue team, in conjunction with a physician advisor, must determine what types of problems are likely to be encountered and plan and equip accordingly. In general, a kit should include splints and bandages, angiocatheters, fluids and drip sets for intravenous therapy, blood pressure cuff, a stethoscope, warm and cold packs, a pocket mask, and limited medications. Saline or heparin locks can help to avoid having an IV bag and tubing hanging from the litter during extrication through brush and trees.

11. Why is no advanced airway or other ALS resuscitation equipment part of the equipment list?

As in any EMS situation, safety of the rescuers is top priority. Most technical rescues preclude the use of bag–mask devices or doing chest compressions due to the location of the rescue. A victim who might survive injuries that were sustained in close proximity to a trauma center may not survive the same injuries if they were received in a setting that requires a technical rescue.

12. Are there any specific medications and treatments that should be considered for the patients?

The overall premise of the rescue operation should be that the removal of the victim from the hazard zone should not complicate the injuries of the patient. In regards to specific medications, the need for oxygen should be prioritized. Many of these rescues could occur in low-oxygen environments or result in injuries that cause hypoxia. By administering supplemental oxygen, the hypoxic condition may be alleviated. Additional medications may be necessary to alleviate the symptoms from crush injuries or harness suspension injuries. Local protocol should always be consulted and followed. The rescuer should also monitor the electrocardiograph while treating the patient. Again, do not overlook heat- and cold-related injuries secondary to prolonged exposure.

13. Are there any technical rescues that EMS responders might be tempted to attempt that they should instead wait until trained personnel arrive?

Perhaps the two most deceiving situations are trench and water rescues. The appearance of the scene may suggest that the EMS responder can attempt to rescue the victim without apparent risk; however, this is usually not the case. If a victim has become entrapped or buried in a trench, the situation has already declared itself as one involving an unstable structure that will require appropriate shoring up. An untrained rescuer in these cases may well add to the victim count if further collapse of the trench occurs while the responder is attempting to access the patient.

Similarly, water rescues also can be extremely difficult as the risk of moving water and becoming entrapped is often not visually obvious. Currents and swirling eddies can easily sweep rescuers off of their feet and carry them along or trap them underwater near drains and culverts. A water rescue should only be attempted by trained individuals with appropriate safety equipment.

Special Situations

Pearls and Pitfalls

1. Remember, slow down and take your time. The safety of the rescuer is paramount. Be part of the solution, not the problem.
2. The priorities for a technical rescue incident are the same as for any other type of emergency incident: life safety, incident stabilization, and property conservation.
3. Do not get tunnel vision. Many other hazards such as hazardous materials or electricity may be present in combination with the other factors surrounding the technical rescue.
4. Do not forget to suspect hypothermia in the patient. There are many scenarios that could involve hypothermia secondary to prolonged exposures.
5. Allowing bystanders to attempt rescues will often serve only to increase the number of casualties.
6. Operating in a capacity that you are not trained or equipped for is an invitation for injury or worse.
7. Failing to identify the need for a body recovery versus an actual rescue can needlessly use resources and place rescuers at risk.

References

1. Browne GJ, Crist GS. Confined Space Rescue. Albany, NY: Delmar Publishing, 1999.
2. Department of Homeland Security. National Incident Management System. Washington DC: U.S. Government Printing Office, 2004.
3. Gargan JB. First Due: Trench Rescue. St. Louis: Mosby Lifeline, 1996.
4. Martinette Jr., CV. Trench Rescue: Awareness, Operations, Technician. Sudbury, MA: Jones and Bartlett Learning, 2002. www.trenchrescuebooks.com
5. National Fire Codes® Online. NFPA 1670: Standard on Operations and Training for Technical Rescue Incidents, National Fire Protection Association, 2009.
6. Roop M, Vines T, Wright R. Confined Space and Structural Rope Rescue. St Louis: Mosby, 1998.
7. Vines T, Hudson S. High Angle Rescue Techniques, 3rd ed. St. Louis: Elsevier-Mosby, 2004.

SECTION VIII

Aeromedical Transport

Chapter 77
Air Medical System Design and Configuration   515
Michael W. Brunko, MD, FACEP

Chapter 78
Aeromedical Transportation: Physiology of Altitude   526
Lee W. Shockley, MD, MBA

Air Medical System Design and Configuration

Michael W. Brunko, MD, FACEP

CHAPTER 77

1. **Historically, where did modern air medical transport (AMT) get its start?**
   Airplanes were used for mass evacuations during World Wars I and II. Helicopters were used initially in Burma in 1944 and then on a larger scale during the Korean War with Sikorsky S-51 and Bell Model 47 helicopters that were equipped with outboard stretchers, not allowing care in flight. The larger, more powerful UH-1H ("HUEY") was used during the Vietnam War, allowing casualties to receive medical attention during transport. Almost 1 million wounded soldiers were transported during Operation Dustoff in Vietnam. The advances in AMT in wartime likely contributed to improved mortality statistics: per 100 casualties, there were 4.5 deaths during World War II, 2.5 deaths during the Korean War, and less than 1 death during the Vietnam War.

2. **How did the military experience transition to the civilian application as we know it today?**
   Because of the helicopter's success in Vietnam, it gained attention after the war as a means of transport of civilians, especially for rural victims of trauma. (In the mid 1970s, 70% of trauma fatalities in the United States occurred in rural areas.) The military began to provide AMT to victims of rural traffic accidents through the Military Assistance to Safety and Traffic program, which gave rise to public programs such as the Maryland State Police (the first civilian agency to transport a critically injured trauma patient by helicopter) and the Los Angeles County Fire Department programs operating today. In 1972, the current-most representative model of rotor AMT began—the "hospital-based" helicopter. The initial program started at St. Anthony Hospital in Denver, Colorado, and primarily transported victims of trauma from the scene to the hospital. In 1980, there were 32 helicopter emergency medical services (HEMS) programs with 39 helicopters, the majority of which were developed as components of hospital trauma programs and were owned and operated by these early trauma centers. In 1990, the number of HEMS programs steadily increased to over 230 helicopter services with over 400 aircraft. By 2006, there were 270 services operating 792 rotor-wing (helicopter) and 150 dedicated fixed-wing aircraft.

3. **What systems operate AMT today?**
   Whereas most of the systems were hospital-based, not for profit, with combined rotor-/fixed-wing AMT service in 1990, there has been a shift from this traditional hospital-based model to community-based programs (not for profit and for profit) with ~60% of the current programs fitting this model. These so-called nontraditional models are operated by independent organizations who locate an aircraft and a transport team at airports, clinics, fire stations, or hospitals. The majority of these operations employ the transport teams, communication specialists, and the aviation personnel. An extension of the nontraditional model is the "hybrid" model, which has become more popular in AMT today. In the hybrid model, the AMT program is owned and operated by the air medical provider but the affiliated hospital uses and maintains control of the clinical personnel and medical director and maintains their identity on the

aircraft. All other aspects of the program's management are controlled by the air medical provider. A minority of programs are private or public service programs, such as those operated by the Maryland State Police and the Los Angeles Fire Department.

4. **What are the advantages of these new "nontraditional" and "hybrid" models?**
   With the nontraditional model, the primary advantage is that the management team is involved with all aspects of the control and direction of the transport program. Sharing of services, such as billing, communications center, and backup for aviation personnel and aircraft are another advantage. With the hybrid model, the hospital maintains control of the clinical team and also identity on the aircraft for marketing purposes. The hospitals also may find an advantage to being relieved of the majority of the financial responsibilities of the program regarding cost of aircraft, fuel, liability, and management.

5. **What are the disadvantages of these new "nontraditional" and "hybrid' models?**
   With the nontraditional model, if the air medical program does not maintain profitability, the chances are greater that the program will relocate or shut down more rapidly than a hospital-based/sponsored program, leaving the community without such service. Philanthropic support may also be limited if the service is for-profit. The hybrid model, so far, seems to be a "win-win" situation for the operator and the hospital. It is possible that an operator may also provide aviation services to a potential hospital competitor with an AMT program creating a perceived conflict, but by keeping control of the clinical staff and medical direction, the majority of these programs have been able to function without concern for competition.

6. **How do you design an AMT program?**
   First, a mission statement should be developed that encompasses the goals of the program. This usually involves assessing and evaluating the needs of a particular community for extending medical resources to that geographic area. Will the program extend to accident scenes (urban or rural), be restricted to interhospital transports, or accommodate both? Should you pursue adult, pediatric, and/or perinatal patients? You will need to evaluate how you can collaborate and interact with the current emergency medical services (EMS) systems without duplicating existing services. Of prime importance is evaluating how the program can attain maximal safety for the goals of the program, establishing experience and training requirements for both the clinical and aviation personnel. Economics of developing the program also need to be studied, with scrutiny of potential base locations, nearby competitive programs, type of aircraft used, establishment of customer relationships, opportunities for growth, and what the potential payor reimbursement will be.

7. **What types of aircraft can be used for AMT?**
   Rotor-wing (helicopters) and fixed-wing aircraft are currently used for AMT.

8. **How do you select the best rotor-wing or fixed-wing aircraft?**
   The first decision is whether the program will purchase the aircraft or lease it from a vendor/operator who has experience in AMT. This decision is quite dependent on how the program is structured, as mentioned before. The procurement of an aircraft must be carefully researched and outside expertise obtained, if necessary, to ensure that the aircraft fulfills the specific objectives of the organization's strategic business plan. When choosing the ideal aircraft, you should consider altitude/pressurization limits, range, air speed and performance (especially at higher altitudes), space and configuration of the patient care area, loading door size and location, useful load capabilities, landing zone/runway needs, and capability for instrument flight rules (IFR) in addition to visual flight rules (VFR) flight. The ideal rotorcraft for AMT is

Air Medical System Design and Configuration

economical, fast, agile, has twin engines and IFR capabilities, and is dual pilot capable; however, the actual usefulness of IFR helicopter flight depends on flying between instrument-approach-capable airports and being able to avoid icing, wind, and potential stormy weather conditions.

Helicopters are powered by single or twin engines. Twin engines generally are preferred because they provide more power and aid in the ability to transport a greater load. They also provide an additional safety measure in case one engine fails. However, twin-engine helicopters have a longer warm-up time—and thus a delayed ability to lift off promptly—and are more costly to operate than single-engine helicopters.

Fixed-wing aircraft used in AMT are generally turbine-powered, pressurized twin-engine aircraft. Jet aircraft are preferable for flights greater than 500 miles. Most fixed-wing aircraft used in AMT have IFR capability, cruise at 200–500 miles per hour, and have ranges of 1000–2500 miles.

9. **What are the advantages of rotor-wing aircraft?**
Helicopters can be based at a hospital or another location near your service area. Helicopters do not require a runway for takeoff and landing, are capable of landing in relatively small and secluded areas, and can usually be ready for takeoff in a matter of minutes. Because they can travel in a straight-line unimpeded by road characteristics or geography, they can often deliver a patient to definitive care in a shorter period of time.

10. **What are the advantages of fixed-wing aircraft?**
They have a much greater range than rotor-wing aircraft. Rotor-wing aircraft generally have a maximum range of about 350 miles, but fixed-wing aircraft can fly thousands of miles. Fixed-wing aircraft usually are able to transport a heavier load and are faster and more economical for most flight distances. Fixed-wing aircraft, which are pressurized, are preferable for the transport of patients in whom altitude changes could potentially worsen certain conditions. They also can operate with instrument flight in more weather conditions than can helicopter services without added risk. Their primary application is to move patients over great distances quickly and provide emergent transfers from frontier/rural areas to tertiary care centers.

11. **What are the disadvantages of rotor-wing aircraft?**
The use of helicopters is quite dependent on the weather, which prevents operation in many adverse conditions. The safety record of AMT helicopters has been criticized in recent years because of the higher crash rate compared to non-AMT helicopter operations.

12. **What are the disadvantages of fixed-wing aircraft?**
Fixed-wing travel is limited to travel between airports and is dependent on locations of airports in close proximity to the origination and destination of the patient. They must rely on intermediary ground ambulances or helicopters to shuttle patients from a scene or hospital to the aircraft and from the destination airport to the receiving facility.

13. **What type of medical equipment should be carried on AMT aircraft?**
    - Oxygen supplies
    - Endotracheal and rescue airway equipment
    - Cardiac monitors with defibrillator and external pacing capabilities
    - Pacemaker generators

- Mechanical ventilators
- Infusion pumps
- Immobilization equipment
- Medications that would be available in the emergency department and intensive care unit
- Manual, Doppler, and automatic blood pressure-monitoring capabilities
- Pulse oximetry and capnography- monitoring capabilities

A program that does specialty transport needs equipment that is specific to the specialty, such as an incubator and neonatal ventilator for neonatal care or transportable intra-aortic balloon pumps for cardiac care. All equipment should be lightweight, durable, compact, have extended battery capability, be easily secured, not interfere with aircraft avionics, and be able to withstand altitude, temperature, and gravitational changes without affecting performance. Equipment that relies on auscultation may be of limited use because of noise and vibrations that are common in most aircraft.

14. What types of crew configurations are used on AMT?
Most AMT programs use two medical crew members. Certain flight conditions (heat, humidity, altitude, multipatient transport) may necessitate flying with one crew member, as weight limitations are a larger factor in these circumstances.

In order of decreasing prevalence, AMT crews consist of nurse/paramedic, two nurses, nurse/physician, two paramedics, nurse/other (e.g., respiratory therapist), and one nurse only.

15. Is there an ideal crew configuration?
There is no proof that any one particular flight crew configuration is ideal. Logically, the ideal crew is adequately trained; if their experiences and backgrounds are different, they complement each other in working well as a team. The mission statement and the types of transports the program provides may dictate the crew configuration.

16. What kind of training should the flight crew have?
The flight crew's training should be optimal for the majority of transports the program provides. In general, the training and experience required of the flight crew is similar to physician-level skills and should surpass what is available from local ground emergency medical services. Because most AMT programs transport critically ill or injured adults and children from health care facilities and accident scenes, the ideally trained individual should have experience in critical care medicine, pediatrics, and emergency medical services. Special training that is common to AMT but different from other patient care areas is knowledge of flight physiology, safety, communications, survival in case of a downed aircraft, and the uniqueness of delivering patient care in limited confines. The flight crew should have training in basic life support, prehospital trauma/basic trauma life support, pediatric life support, advanced cardiac life support, trauma, and neonatal resuscitation. The crew should be competent to perform all types of intubations, rescue airway use, cricothyroidotomy, thoracostomy, peripheral and central venous line placement, pericardiocentesis, umbilical artery/vein catheterization, intraosseous insertion, ventilator, and pacemaker management, and emergency vaginal deliveries.

17. Is it possible to train a flight crew to have expertise in all potential types of AMT?
Probably not. Most AMT services realize this and train their crews to be able to adequately care for and transport most patients. Many AMT services use on-call, possibly off-site specialty crews that can be

available in a reasonably short time for flights requiring specialty services, such as neonatal services, high-risk obstetrics, and patients requiring intraaortic balloon pump devices.

18. **How do you select a service for AMT of a patient from one facility to another?**
    First and foremost, you must not decrease the level of care that the patient has already received. You must be aware of the types of AMT programs that are available and select the one that is most appropriate for the patient's injury or illness. Ideally, you should have a relationship with one AMT communication center and they should try to match you with the closest, most appropriate aircraft and medical crew that is available in your area. If the patient requires specialty services such as tertiary pediatric, invasive respiratory, or cardiovascular care, it would be helpful to select a program that is experienced with these types of problems.

    If a helicopter service turns down a request for transport because of local or intermediate weather conditions or other safety reasons, do not "helicopter shop" for another service to do the transport unless the second service has communicated with the declining service why and under what circumstances the transport was declined. There may be circumstances in which the second program can safely manage the flight, but it must be notified at the time of the request that another program has already declined it and why it was declined.

19. **When should an AMT be used instead of ground transport?**
    The choice should be based on a variety of factors. In general, the *rule of Ts* should be considered.
    - *Time* of transport is always a consideration, especially when considering the time it may take to transport a patient to a *trauma* or *tertiary* care center by air versus the time it would take to transport the same patient by ground to the local hospital. Time is especially crucial in the transport of a trauma patient in whom decreasing the time between the onset of injury and the receipt of definitive care is essential to increase the chances of survival.
    - *Time-critical* interventional care for patient conditions such as acute myocardial infarction, cardiovascular accidents (CVAs), and vascular emergencies.
    - The geographic *terrain* is a consideration. The patient may be located in an isolated area that ground transport may not be able to reach.
    - *Traffic* may dictate the use of AMT instead of ground transport.
    - AMT may be useful when advanced life support (ALS) ground units are unavailable because they are assisting other patients. Also, AMT may be required in circumstances where ALS or critical care interventions are not available from the ground providers. Guidelines based on injuries or illnesses are available to aid in the decision to use an AMT.

    The National Association of EMS Physicians has established the following "Questions That Can Assist in Determining Appropriate Transport Mode":
    - Does the patient's clinical condition require minimization of time spent out of the hospital environment during the transport?
    - Does the patient require specific or time-sensitive evaluation or treatment that is not available at the referring facility?
    - Is the patient located in an area that is inaccessible to ground transport?
    - What are the current and predicted weather situations along the transport route?

- Is the weight of the patient (plus the weight of required equipment and transport personnel) within allowable ranges for air transport?
- Is there a helipad and/or airport near the referring hospital for interhospital transports?
- Does the patient require critical care life support (e.g., monitoring personnel, specific medications, and/or equipment) during transport, which is not available with ground transport options?
- Would use of local ground transport leave the local area without adequate emergency medical services coverage?
- If local ground transport is not an option, can the needs of the patient (and the system) be met by an available regional ground critical care transport service (i.e., specialized surface transport systems operated by hospitals and/or airmedical programs)?

20. Are there any types of patients who should not be transported by AMT?

In general, only patients who require a higher level of care should be transported by an AMT service. AMT should not be used for the patient with a stable injury or illness who is not felt to be at high risk for life-threatening complications that may occur during the transport. Ground transport offers a more cost-effective means of transfer and also preserves limited AMT resources for those patients that may benefit from it. Patients who are pre-arrest or are in cardiac arrest should not be transported by AMT. Similarly, patients with serious medical conditions who have preexisting "Do Not Resuscitate" orders should probably not be transported by AMT. The combative patient who places the safety of the air medical crew at risk should not be transported. Such patients include violent prisoners, suicidal or homicidal patients, or intoxicated or head-injured patients who cannot safely be restrained. A woman who is in active labor or whose cervix is dilated 4 cm or more should not be transported by AMT unless the program has the capabilities, personnel, and equipment to not only manage an emergent delivery but also to resuscitate and care for a potential unstable neonate.

21. How should AMT be integrated with ground EMS?

All AMT should maintain relationships with the EMS agencies within their geographic service area. The AMT program should take the initiative to educate the ground medics in the following areas:

- Appropriate triage criteria for requesting AMT.
- If "autolaunch" or aerial standby is offered by the AMT, the ground EMS and fire and law enforcement providers must establish criteria in conjunction with the AMT to determine when autolaunch should be initiated by the dispatching centers.
- Locating, marking, and securing a safe landing zone for the aircraft that is used.
- Preparation of the patient for AMT.
- Safely approaching the aircraft to prevent injury.
- "Hot-load" training and criteria.
- Training and implementing plans for multicasualty incidents, disasters, and Homeland Security responses.

EMS systems should strive to assure that every patient having an emergent condition that can be addressed by a nationally recognized time-critical treatment has access to quality AMT to benefit from that treatment if logistics of distance and availability of ground transport would prevent access to such a treatment.

22. What does it cost to start up and operate a rotor-wing AMT program?
This really depends on the size of the program and specifically if you decide to operate independently or partner with an AMT provider. The average annual budget for a rotor AMT program is $2.5 million to $4 million, with approximately half of that amount dedicated to aviation costs. This amount considers the use and leasing of one or two aircraft. If the program were to purchase and operate its own helicopter, the initial cost could range from $2 million to $8 million per aircraft. The balance of the costs would be dedicated to personnel expenses and equipment and the amounts would depend on the types of staffing and equipment the program requires.

23. Who pays for the high cost of AMT?
Unlike a decade ago when AMT programs were subsidized by sponsoring hospitals, now many AMT programs have been forced to decrease their costs, which they primarily have done by merging programs into consortiums, sharing services within geographic areas, or merging into nontraditional or "hybrid programs" where many of the costs and liabilities are controlled by the AMT provider. AMT depends on a combination of revenue sources including patient billing, commercial insurance including automobile insurance, Medicare, private and publicly traded corporate financing, and philanthropy. Some programs have developed "subscription services" in which a subscriber pays an annual membership to use the AMT service at a discount or for free, but this is dependent on state laws that may limit this type of insurance. Many air medical programs are able to continue operation despite the inability to recoup the cost of operation because they receive strong local charitable donations and philanthropic contributions. A few AMT programs are subsidized by small fees that are included in a state's motor vehicle taxes.

24. How has managed care affected AMT?
It has forced the AMT industry to become more cost effective and efficient in all aspects of its operation. Ongoing use management, including educating the users of AMT, has become very important in AMT administration. Many AMT programs are contracting with managed care insurers to transport the covered patients at set rates—using a multidimensional transport team of AMT, critical care ground transport, or ALS ground transport to match the most cost-effective means of transport with the patient's medical requirements. Compared to 10 years ago, physicians and managed care plans have become more comfortable using critical care transport to transfer or "repatriate" critical patients to participating subscriber centers where costs can be saved by the insurance provider.

25. Is there any proof that AMT is cost effective?
This is a difficult question to answer. When compared to ground transport, air transport is much more expensive, but if you were to supply a comparably staffed and equipped ground ambulance over the long distances that air transport generally cover, ground transport may be less cost-effective than air medical transport. Air ambulances provide an opportunity for the rapid transport of patients with emergent conditions requiring time-dependent specialized or definitive care, especially in regard to traumatic injury, cardiac and cerebrovascular emergencies, decreasing morbidity, and mortality. Measuring the cost effectiveness, especially in regard to risk–benefit analysis, is difficult because of the broad differences in patient presentations, injuries and illnesses, and the types of transports involved. There have been some cost-effectiveness studies that show that air transport is more economical when the cost per year life saved is compared to other expensive treatment modalities that are used in medicine today.

26. Is there any proof that patient outcomes are improved when air medical transport is used?

Again, this is another difficult question to answer. There are numerous studies that show improvement in multiple trauma mortality and survival when air transport is compared to ground transport. It has been shown that there is improvement in adjusted mortality and outcomes in moderate to severe head-injury patients when air medical transport is used instead of ground transport. It is thought that a major factor in this may be related to early successful out-of-hospital intubation of these patients by the air medical personnel, although the benefits of endotracheal intubation in the prehospital setting have come into question. However, it also has been shown that there is no advantage in outcomes to using AMT in urban areas where ground transport times are relatively short. All of these studies have been criticized by both proponents and opponents of air medical transport because of the variability of injury severity, the skills of the transport personnel, and the speed of transport and capabilities of the trauma center destination. There are ongoing efforts being made to collect and analyze multicenter collaborative studies where these variables can be controlled.

As mentioned earlier, time-sensitive treatments such as acute ST segment elevation myocardial infarction (STEMI) and CVA emergent revascularization offered by specialized centers have shown improvement in cardiac, central nervous system function, and decreased mortality. Air medical transport should be a consideration where there is a need for rapid transport of a critically ill patient who may benefit from these interventions when ground services, because of geographic distance or capabilities, would be unable to accomplish the transport in a timely manner. The costs and benefits of providing air medical transport to these "time sensitive" emergencies need further analysis and many studies are currently underway to look at this.

27. How safe is AMT?

In the infancy of AMT, HEMS accidents occurred two to three times more frequently than non-HEMS accidents. These accidents were found to be three and one half times more likely to be fatal than non-HEMS accidents. Since the late 1980s, safety has taken a priority with all AMT programs in an effort to decrease these disturbing statistics. Safety committees have been developed involving all members of the air medical crews. Access to the most up-to-date weather information and outfitting the aircraft with the best safety and survival gear have become standard. As a result, in 1987–1993 EMS rotor-wing aircraft crashed less often than other turbine helicopters. The fatal accident rate was three times less than in 1980–1986. Unfortunately, the number of accidents nearly doubled between the mid-1990s and 2005. This correlates well with the HEMS industry's rapid growth rate from 2000 to 2006. The main causes of crashes were controlled flight into terrain, inadvertent operation into instrument meteorological conditions, and pilot spatial disorientation/lack of situational awareness in night operations. Because of this, the Federal Aviation Administration has established a task force for review and to guide government and industry efforts to reduce HEMS accidents. Some of the recommendations include having the larger HEMS operators focus on surveillance and certification requirements of their programs, minimal guidelines for Air Medical Resource Management to work with the National Center for Atmospheric Research to develop and implement a graphical flight-planning tool for ceiling and visibility assessment in areas where there is limited available surface observation capability, implement certification and training for the use of night vision goggles and evaluate their potential advantages, support use of flight data recorders in HEMS operations, and support voluntary implementation of the use of terrain awareness warning systems.

Air medical programs should never accept a transport based on fear of losing that transport to a competing program or because they feel pressured by the referral hospital or agency. Crew safety should always be the top priority when considering transport of a patient.

28. **Are guidelines available that ensure that certain standards for safety and care are met?**

    The primary organization responsible for the accreditation and maintenance of standards for AMT programs is the Commission on Accreditation of Medical Transport Systems (CAMTS). An AMT program can request, on a voluntary basis, that CAMTS review the program to meet the accreditation standards if the program has been in operation for at least one year. After the initial accreditation, the AMT program must undergo a reaccreditation process every three years in order to maintain CAMTS accreditation. The CAMTS accreditation standards are updated every two to three years under an ongoing consensus process with input from multiple member organizations and disciplines with expertise in critical care transport medicine and aviation. CAMTS-accredited programs have been recognized by insurance companies as conducting safer operations. Numerous managed care organizations specify that CAMTS accreditation be a prerequisite in order to contract with them. The federal government has made CAMTS accreditation a requirement for transportation contracts. Also, a number of state governments (Utah, Washington, New Mexico, Colorado, Michigan, New Hampshire, Rhode Island, and Maryland and counties in California and Nevada) require CAMTS accreditation as a condition for licensure for performing patient transport into and out of their jurisdictions. The Association of Air Medical Services, which comprises almost 90% of the AMT providers in the United States, adopted a position statement in 2005 recommending that all AMT organizations use the CAMTS standard in developing their internal operating standards regardless of their decision to pursue voluntary accreditation.

29. **Do medical directors of AMT programs have different qualifications than other EMS medical directors?**

    Yes, in some respects. The experience of most AMT medical directors originated from ground EMS medical direction. AMT medical directors must have knowledge in altitude physiology and aviation safety, the appropriate use of the AMT service, be active in educating the referral agencies in regard to the appropriate use of the service, and be actively involved in retrospective analysis of use of that service. The Air Medical Physician Association has developed a three-part dynamic core curriculum that addresses the unique requirements including clinical, aviation, safety, and administrative education for current and potential AMT medical directors. One particular difference between ground EMS and AMT medical directors is that the AMT medical director must be actively involved in patient follow-up with referring agencies and physicians because the referring parties geographically may be far away, making follow-up legally and logistically difficult.

30. **What is the medical director's primary function?**

    The medical director is primarily responsible for ensuring the quality of care of the AMT program. Other responsibilities include:
    - The authorization, review, and updating of standing orders and protocols
    - Medical training of the flight personnel, including the nurses and paramedics

- Active involvement in quality improvement and in maintaining an open line of communication to referral physicians and agencies in regard to follow-up

Depending on the geographic location of the program, the medical director may be actively involved in outreach education to rural EMS agencies and hospitals that may need the services of the AMT program.

31. **Are there any differences between the United States AMT design and the international AMT designs?**

    The primary difference is that the European systems extensively use physicians as flight crew members. Most of the programs in Australia and Europe use a physician in all transports, in particular for the resuscitation and stabilization of the patient, either at the scene or referring institution prior to transport. Depending on the location, other members of the crew may have expertise in rescue and extrication. Other differences in transport relate to the repatriation of patients from Third World countries; a patient may require a higher level of care than what is available in his or her country or may need to be returned to his or her own country. These programs must deal not only with the lack of medical care available but also with governmental and bureaucratic rules that may be involved in crossing international borders. Where most U.S. programs are single pilot, use VFR, and use single engine aircraft, many European countries and the Canadian government require dual engine, dual pilot, and IFR. Of note, Canadian HEMS have never experienced a crash.

32. **What is the future of AMT?**

    AMT programs have the capability of bringing a physician level of care to scenes or to hospitals where a lower level of care is only available and maintaining a higher level of care during transport with delivery of the patient to a tertiary facility. As mentioned earlier, there has been a significant increase in the number of programs that are not based at trauma centers or tertiary hospitals but are based at rural satellite bases such as airports, fire stations, and community hospitals. By locating AMT program bases in rural areas, the amount of time it takes to get to the patient when AMT is needed is decreased compared to AMT program aircraft that are located in metropolitan locations. A concern and challenge for AMT programs that are non-hospital based will be how to find and train clinical crew members and maintain and ensure the quality of knowledge and skills required by them in order to work in these nonurban areas. The use of AMT in these situations may occur without weighing the risk and costs of the AMT against the needs of the patient for a higher level of care and what the benefit may be for the patient.

    AMT programs' use, quality assurance/improvement, medical control, dispatch, coordination with local EMS system personnel, and destination decisions will likely need to be integrated into state EMS systems in order to improve, control, and standardize AMT availability, use, and safety.

Pearls and Pitfalls

1. AMT is a valuable and scarce resource and should be used only when necessary.
2. A "hybrid" model is the most cost-effective way to operate an AMT.
3. There is a paucity of high-quality outcome studies proving the efficacy of AMT versus ground transport.
4. AMT is the most expensive form of medical transport.

Air Medical System Design and Configuration

5. If one AMT system declines to fly because of weather, an alternative AMT system must be so informed.
6. AMT programs should be integrated into local and state EMS systems.
7. Medical directors, nurses, and EMTs in AMT programs need specialized training and expertise.

References

1. Davidoff J. History of air medical transport. In Principles and Direction of Air Medical Transport, 4th ed., Blumen I, ed., pp. 3–6. Salt Lake City, UT: Air Medical Physician Association, 2006.
2. Collier J. Air medical business models. In Principles and Direction of Air Medical Transport, 4th ed., Blumen I, ed., pp. 277–289. Salt Lake City, UT: Air Medical Physician Association, 2006.
3. Stiles T, Kinkade S, Maitlen G. Aircraft capabilities for medical transport. In Principles and Direction of Air Medical Transport, 4th ed., Blumen I, ed., pp. 572–578. Salt Lake City, UT: Air Medical Physician Association, 2006.
4. Eljaiek L, Davidoff J, Stubba W. Biomedical equipment and technology in critical care transport. In Principles and Direction of Air Medical Transport, 4th ed., Blumen I, ed., pp. 449–460. Salt Lake City, UT: Air Medical Physician Association, 2006.
5. Stocking J. Crew configuration. In Principles and Direction of Air Medical Transport, 4th ed., Blumen I, ed., pp. 36–42. Salt Lake City, UT: Air Medical Physician Association, 2006.
6. Werman H, Falcone R. Indications for air medical transport: Practical applications. In Principles and Direction of Air Medical Transport, 4th ed., Blumen I, ed., pp. 12–23. Salt Lake City, UT: Air Medical Physician Association, 2006.
7. Hankins D, Thomson D, Fullagar C. Basics of EMS Systems and Air Medical Integration. In Principles and Direction of Air Medical Transport, 4th ed., Blumen I, ed., pp. 7–11. Salt Lake City, UT: Air Medical Physician Association, 2006.
8. Yale C. Financial Concepts for the EMS Administrator. In Principles and Direction of Air Medical Transport, 4th ed., Blumen I, ed., pp. 257–269. Salt Lake City, UT: Air Medical Physician Association, 2006.
9. Gearhart PA, Wuerz RW, Lacalio AR. Cost-effectiveness analysis of helicopter EMS for trauma patients. Ann Emerg Med 30, 1997, pp. 500–506.
10. Blumen I. UCAN Safety Committee. A Safety Review and Risk Assessment in Air Medical Transport. Supplement to the Air Medical Physicians' Handbook, 3rd ed. Salt Lake City, UT: Air Medical Physician Association, 2002.
11. CAMTS. 2010 Accreditation Standards, 8th ed. Sandy Springs, SC: Commission on Accreditation Standards of Medical Transport Systems, September 2010.
12. Carrubba, C. Role of the medical director in air medical transport. In Principles and Direction of Air Medical Transport, 4th ed., Blumen I, ed., pp. 113–119. Salt Lake City, UT: Air Medical Physician Association, 2006.
13. Thomas, S. Helicopter EMS, Outcomes Research, Cost-Effectiveness and Triage. University of Oklahoma Emergency Medicine, Tulsa, OK. 2010

Aeromedical Transportation: Physiology of Altitude

CHAPTER 78

Lee W. Shockley, MD, MBA

1. **What happens to a person's physiology with ascent to altitude?**
   Atmospheric pressure is a function of altitude; as one ascends, atmospheric pressure decreases. For example, the atmospheric pressure on a standard day at sea level is 760 mmHg; the pressure is roughly half of that at 18,000 feet and only a third of that at 28,000 feet. The effects of the decreasing atmospheric pressure with altitude are manifest in volume (Boyle's law), partial pressures of gases (Dalton's law), the solubility of gases (Henry's law), and temperature (Charles' law) (see Table 78.1).

TABLE 78.1: Effects of Decreasing Atmospheric Pressure

Name	Equation	Effect of Altitude
Boyle's law	$P * V = k$ or $P_1 * V_1 = P_2 * V_2$	Gases expand in volume as pressure decreases.
Dalton's law	$P_{total} = p_1 + p_2 + \ldots p_n$	The partial pressure of a gas decreases with altitude.
Henry's law	$P = k * C$ or $e^p = e^{kC}$	The amount of a gas that can be dissolved in solution decreases with altitude.
Charles' law	$V/T = k$	Temperature lapse rate of 2°C (3.5°F) per 1000 feet

P = pressure, V = volume, T = temperature, k = constant, C = concentration, e = exponent.

What these laws and formulas really say is that with increasing altitude: (1) gas-filled structures expand, (2) the partial pressure of gases (e.g., oxygen) drops, (3) dissolved gases (e.g., nitrogen) come out of solution, and (4) ambient temperature drops.

2. **Why is it important to understand the physiologic changes that occur with altitude?**
   A patient who is transported by air may be subjected to an environment with lower atmospheric pressure than he or she would be exposed to during ground transport. Practically speaking, this means that:
   (a) Trapped gases will expand in the relatively hypobaric atmosphere. A pneumothorax that is unvented (no needle decompression, no chest tube, or a chest tube that is blocked) can increase in size or become a tension pneumothorax. Air splints can get too tight and impair circulation. The patient with an ileus or intestinal obstruction can experience worsening symptoms (aerogastralgia) or even hollow viscus rupture as gas trapped in the bowel expands. Air in endotracheal tube cuffs and intravenous tubing will expand. Gases in obstructed sinuses, ears, or abscesses will expand and can cause pain.
   (b) If the patient has a serious alveolar/arterial gradient problem (e.g., chronic obstructive pulmonary disease or pulmonary embolism) or an altered hemoglobin dissociation curve (e.g., carbon monoxide

poisoning), it may be very difficult to adequately oxygenate him or her. Anemia (less than 7.0 g hemoglobin/100 ml) may also lead to tissue hypoxia at altitude. Consider supplemental oxygen, pulse-oximetry monitoring, early intubation, or positive end expiratory pressure to maintain sufficient oxygenation. High-altitude diseases (high-altitude pulmonary edema, high-altitude cerebral edema, or acute mountain sickness) may be exacerbated by the transport at even higher altitudes.

(c) Decompression sickness can worsen at altitude because more of the dissolved nitrogen comes out of solution as microbubbles. If these patients must be transported by air (such as to a hyperbaric facility), they should be given 100% oxygen and transported at as low an altitude as possible. It may be advisable to transport the patient in a pressurized fixed-wing aircraft.

(d) The lower ambient temperature at altitude may worsen the condition of a hypothermic patient. Passive or active rewarming techniques may be necessary in-flight.

3. **If the aircraft is pressurized, will ascent to altitude still affect patients?**
It can. Although an aircraft is pressurized, it does not mean that the cabin altitude is sea level. Commercial pressurized aircraft (such as the Boeing 737 and the McDonnell-Douglas DC-9) maintain cabin altitudes of up to 8450 feet during cruise flight. Pressurization is a relative thing. The pilot can tell you at what altitude the cabin is being maintained.

4. **What should I do besides giving every patient supplemental oxygen?**
Preflight chest tubes and nasogastric tubes should be considered in patients at risk. Make certain that tubes do not become blocked or kinked. In flight, pay attention to expanding trapped gases in the medical equipment. This means continuous, careful monitoring and evaluation of patients and preparing to decompress the spaces in which trapped gas has expanded. Specifically, needle or chest-tube thoracostomy for pneumothorax or nasogastric tube insertion for abdominal distention should be available during transport and performed by appropriately trained personnel in the event that the patient's condition deteriorates. In addition, endotracheal tube cuff pressures may increase by as much as 23 cm H_2O from ground level to 8000 feet. This is well above the critical perfusion pressure of the tracheal mucosa and, if left uncorrected, can lead to necrosis of the mucosa.

5. **Are there other physiologic risks of aeromedical transportation?**
Several. There has been a case report of a patient with photosensitive seizures caused by sunlight shining through spinning helicopter rotor blades. Patients who have been recently operated on may have air trapped in the closed abdomen (laparotomy or laparoscopy) or skull (craniotomy or ventriculostomy). Expansion of that gas at altitude can cause wound separation or an increase in intracranial pressure. Helicopters tend to be noisy environments. This makes communication difficult at times without a headset and intercom. Veteran pilots may have a 10- to 20-dB loss of hearing acuity in the higher frequencies. Finally, although not specifically a physiologic stress, temperature variations within an EMS helicopter can predispose stored medications to deterioration.

Pearls and Pitfalls

1. No pneumothorax is too small to receive a chest tube prior to aeromedical transport.
2. Monitor pulse oximetry closely during the flight.
3. Watch the pressure in the endotracheal tube cuffs.

4. Open nasogastric tubes to vent if they are not already on suction.
5. Give serious consideration to other modes of transportation for patients with decompression illnesses, recent abdominal surgery, or recent cranial surgery.

References

1. Andersson N, Grip H, Lindvall P, et al. Air transport of patients with intracranial air: Computer model of pressure effects. Aviat Space Environ Med 74(2):138–144, 2003.
2. Benson NH, Low RB, Chisholm CD, et al. Air medical transport: An annotated bibliography of the recent literature. Am J Emerg Med 9:510–519, 1991.
3. Burney RE, Fischer RP. Ground versus air transport of trauma victims: Medical and logistical considerations. Ann Emerg Med 15:1491–1495, 1986.
4. Cottrell JJ. Altitude exposures during aircraft flight. Flying higher. Chest 93(1):81–84, 1988.
5. Cushman JT, Floccare DJ. Flicker illness: An underrecognized but preventable complication of helicopter transport. Prehosp Emerg Care 11(1):85–88, 2007.
6. Hansen PJ. Safe practice for our aeromedical evacuation patients. Mil Med 152:281–283, 1987.
7. Henning J, Sharley P, Young R. Pressures within air-filled tracheal cuffs at altitude—An in vivo study. Anaesthesia 59(9):919–920, 2004.
8. Madden JF, O'Connor RE, Evans J. The range of medication storage temperatures in aeromedical emergency medical services. Prehosp Emerg Care 3(1):27–30, 1999.
9. Parsons CJ, Bobechko WP. Aeromedical transport: Its hidden problems. Can Med Assoc J 126(3):237–243, 1982.
10. Thomas SH, Cheema F, Cumming M, Wedel SK, Thomson D. Nontrauma helicopter emergency medical services transport: Annotated review of selected outcomes-related literature. Prehosp Emerg Care 6(2):242–255, 2002.
11. Thomas SH, Cheema F, Wedel SK, Thomson D. Trauma helicopter emergency medical services transport: annotated review of selected outcomes-related literature. Prehosp Emerg Care 6(3):359–371, 2002.

Prehospital Skills and Interventions

SECTION IX

Chapter 79
Prehospital Interventions: What Really Works   531
Herbert G. Garrison, MD, MPH

Chapter 80
Intravenous Access   535
John Riccio, MD, and Anne Clouatre, MHS, EMT-P

Chapter 81
Prehospital Airway Management   542
Arthur Hsieh, MA, NREMT-P, and Gregory J. Chapman, BS, RRT, REMT-P

Chapter 82
Pharmacologic Agents in Airway Management   550
Jedd Roe, MD, MBA, FACEP

Chapter 83
PASG   555
Robert Suter, DO, and Jeffrey Metzger, MD

Chapter 84
Needle Decompression   560
John Riccio, MD, and Anne Clouatre, MHS, EMT-P

Chapter 85
Immobilization and Splinting   565
Will Chapleau, EMT-P, RN, TNS

Chapter 86
Prehospital Pain Management   569
Timothy Howey, BA, NREMT-P

Chapter 87
Ultrasound in the Field   574
John Kendall, MD, FACEP

Prehospital Interventions: What Really Works

CHAPTER 79

Herbert G. Garrison, MD, MPH

1. **As an emergency medical technician (EMT) or a paramedic, I am well trained and qualified to use the medications and procedures that all EMS professionals at my level of certification use. Why do I need to read this chapter?**
   Although you are obliged to follow and adhere to system protocols and medical direction, as an emergency medical services (EMS) professional you should understand the science (and the profound need for more research) for what you do for your patients in the field. Part of that understanding is knowing that many of the medications and procedures in the prehospital armamentarium are unproven in terms of their efficacy or effectiveness.

2. **What do you mean by efficacy and effectiveness?**
   The research term "efficacy" refers to the effect of an intervention or treatment on patient outcome when used in a controlled environment. The best example of an efficacy study is a randomized clinical trial in which the investigators are aware of and may control the circumstances and events that affect the study's outcome. An intervention found to be effective in a clinical trial is said to be efficacious. Interventions that are efficacious in controlled circumstances may not be effective in typical everyday situations. In contrast to efficacy, "effectiveness" describes the effect of an intervention or treatment in the uncontrolled "real" world. An effective intervention improves patient outcome when it is applied in usual and customary settings outside of a laboratory or research setting (i.e., outside the hospital when used by real paramedics and EMTs).

3. **Aren't the prehospital interventions used by EMTs and paramedics effective or at least efficacious?**
   The entire EMS system has been created and implemented with little analysis of the overall effectiveness of the tools used to manage the many conditions for which treatment is offered in the prehospital setting. This is not surprising, since one of the original constructs for prehospital EMS was moving the hospital emergency department (ED) and its treatments to the street. (A construct is a complex model, idea, or theory.) We now know that not everything that is efficacious or effective in the hospital ED translates necessarily as an effective or prudent prehospital treatment. An example is prehospital endotracheal intubation of children. Establishing an airway via endotracheal intubation in an unresponsive child is a standard treatment in the hospital. However, Dr. Marianne Gausche-Hill and her colleagues found in a controlled clinical trial of the EMS system in her community that prehospital endotracheal intubation of children is no more effective than bag-mask ventilation.

4. **Are there any prehospital interventions that do work?**
   As noted by Dr. Dan Spaite: "Despite a plethora of EMS research, only two specific interventions have been proven to impact outcome in any prehospital patient population—early CPR and early defibrillation in the setting of out of hospital, non-traumatic cardiac arrest." Since that was written, the Ontario

Prehospital Advanced Life Support (OPALS) group has demonstrated in a controlled clinical trial that paramedic-level care improves survival in prehospital patients with shortness of breath. Others argue that the EMS component of trauma care systems improves survival for the patient who has sustained severe injuries.

5. **If we don't really know for sure that many of the treatments we use routinely really work, how do medical directors for EMS systems determine what to use?**
Most medical directors rely on the recommendations of consensus guidelines produced by national groups and associations of experts, such as the American College of Emergency Physicians, the National Association of EMS Physicians, and the American Heart Association. In North Carolina, for example, medical directors can choose from a long list of optional skills and medications but usually only allow the use of procedures and medications that are recommended by published guidelines.

6. **What are the gaps in EMS knowledge?**
The gaps in EMS knowledge were made clear by a recent systematic review of the medical literature. Smith and colleagues identified 400 prehospital trials of interventions; two-thirds (67%) of the 400 trial reports concerned resuscitation and cardiac care. While resuscitation research has improved outcomes from cardiac arrest, similar progress is lacking on other prehospital conditions. As the authors point out, "The principal finding of this study is the contrast between the wide scope of the out-of-hospital field (resuscitation, airway diseases, injury, out-of-hospital medical treatments, etc.) and the lack of high-quality evidence on which to guide practice. Although taking nothing away from the quality of research in this area, cardiac arrest and acute resuscitative attempts account for only 2% of all ambulance responses.... Therefore, the majority of interventions used in the out-of-hospital environment are not based on strong evidence...."

7. **What EMS interventions require study?**
The authors of the National EMS Research Strategic Plan have compiled and prioritized an exhaustive list of core topics for which there is need for investigation. There are too many to list here and the reader is encouraged to review the entire Strategic Plan. Examples of questions in need of research answers include: What are the most effective and safe EMS airway management strategies? Which EMS treatments, including destination decisions, are effective for acute cardiac ischemia? Does out of hospital therapeutic hypothermia mitigate brain injury? How can EMS professionals best recognize and manage pain? Which patients, if any, require spinal immobilization? Which patients with injuries should be routed directly to a trauma center? What are the best strategies for reducing errors and improving patient safety? What are the attributes of professional competency in EMS? Is air medical transport cost-effective?

8. **What are the structural barriers to determining which interventions are effective and efficacious?**
The National EMS Research Agenda cited five barriers to high quality EMS research:
   1) a paucity of highly skilled researchers;
   2) inadequate funding;
   3) failure of EMS professionals to understand the importance of conducting EMS research and translating the findings into clinical practice;
   4) a lack of integrated information systems that provide for meaningful linkage with patient outcome;
   5) logistical problems in obtaining informed consent.

To fill the gaps and advance EMS knowledge, there needs to be substantial work on eliminating these barriers.

9. **What is the prospect for one day knowing if what we do as EMS professionals really makes a difference for our patients?**
Those of you who have literally saved someone's life by your direct and specific actions know when you have done so. The question is: what about all the other stuff we do that is not directly life-saving at the moment – does any of it make a difference? Do we relieve discomfort? Is what we do cost-effective? The good news is that, despite the barriers described in the question above, many necessary steps are taking place. The prehospital studies led by Gausche-Hill and Stiell, respectively looking at pediatric airway management and advanced life support, have shown that controlled clinical trials can be conducted in the prehospital environment. Other groups, such as the EMS Outcomes Project (EMSOP) and the EMS Cost Assessment Project (EMSCAP), are developing the methods and tools to better assess the outcomes from and the costs of prehospital care. One day we'll know how much of a difference we make, but we've got a lot of work to do to get to that day.

Pearls and Pitfalls

1. Avoid the temptation to decide or determine on your own if a prehospital intervention is efficacious or effective.
2. Good research, even in the best of circumstances, is difficult but necessary to demonstrate the effectiveness of prehospital care.
3. Read, read, read. Read the EMS research articles in medical journals such as *Annals of Emergency Medicine*, *Prehospital Emergency Care*, and *Academic Emergency Medicine*.
4. Encourage your system to seek opportunities to participate in clinical research studies and, likewise, participate yourself in the research.
5. Don't stop the routine use of current prehospital interventions because you are unsure if they work. Paramedics and EMTs should rely on their medical directors to provide guidance on what prehospital interventions to employ.
6. Don't do something new in the field that you've seen done in the hospital; instead rely on prehospital research done in the field to guide your practice.

References

1. Brice JH, Garrison HG, Evans AT: Study design and outcomes in out-of-hospital emergency medicine research: a ten-year analysis. Prehosp Emerg Care 2000;4:144-150.
2. Garrison HG, Benson NH, Whitley TW, Bailey BW. Paramedic skills and medications: practice options utilized by local advanced life support medical directors. Prehosp Disaster Med. 1991;6:29-33.
3. Garrison HG, Brice JH. Research and evaluation in out-of-hospital emergency medical services. NC Med J. 2007;68(4):246-8
4. Gausche M, Lewis RJ, Stratton SJ, et al. Effect of out-of-hospital pediatric endotracheal intubation on survival and neurological outcome: a controlled clinical trial. JAMA. 2000;283:783-790.
5. Institute of Medicine. Future of Emergency Care: Emergency Medical Services at the Crossroads. Washington, DC: National Academies Press; 2007.

6. Keim SM, Spaite DW, Maio RF, et al. Establishing the scope and methodological approach to out-of-hospital outcomes and effectiveness research. Acad Emerge Med. 2004;11:1067-1073.
7. Lerner EB, Nichol G, Spaite DW, Garrison HG, Maio RF. A comprehensive framework for determining the cost of an emergency medical services system. Ann Emerg Med. 2007;49:304-313.
8. Rudehill A, Bellander BM, Weitzberg E, Bredbacka S, Backheden M, Gordon E. Outcome of traumatic brain injuries in 1,508 patients: impact of prehospital care. J. Neurotrauma. 2002;19:855-868.
9. Sayre MR, White LJ, Brown LH, McHenry SD, National EMS Research Agenda. Prehosp Emerg Care. 2003;6(3 Suppl): S1-43.
10. Sayre MR, White LJ, Brown LH, McHenry SD, National EMS Research Strategic Plan Writing Team. The National EMS Research Strategic Plan. Prehosp Emerg Care. 2005;9:255-266.
11. Smith E, Jennings P, McDonald S, MacPherson C, O'Brien T, Archer F. The Cochrane Library as a resource for evidence on out-of-hospital health care interventions. Acad Emerg Med. 2007;49:344-350.
12. Spaite DW. Outcome analysis in EMS systems. Ann Emerg Med. 1993;22:1310-1311.
13. Spaite DW, Maio R, Garrison HG, et al. Emergency Medical Services Outcomes Project (EMSOP) II: developing the foundation and conceptual models for out-of-hospital outcomes research. Ann Emergency Med. 2001;37:657-663.
14. Stiell IG, Spaite DW, Field B, et al. Advanced life support for out-of-hospital respiratory distress. N Engl J Med. 2007;356:2156-2164.

Intravenous Access

John Riccio, MD, and Anne Clouatre, MHS, EMT-P

CHAPTER 80

1. **How long has the concept of intravenous therapy existed?**
   Information that dates back to 1628 describes a blood transfusion performed by Dr. Giovanni Francisco Colle, an Italian physician. Twenty-six years later, Dr. Francisco Folli reportedly performed a blood transfusion also. He used animal blood vessels, a silver tube, and a bone cannula.

2. **Does everyone need an intravenous line?**
   No. Intravenous access is not without complications, cost, and pain.

3. **Why should an intravenous line be started?**
   To gain direct access to a patient's circulatory system, which may allow the following to be accomplished:
   - Replacement of fluid
   - Administration of medications
   - Phlebotomy for blood samples for laboratory determinations

4. **What kind of equipment is needed?**
   Typical materials include the following:
   - 70% isopropyl alcohol pads or povidone–iodine pads
   - Small gauze sponges
   - Tourniquet/blood pressure cuff
   - Various sizes and styles of tape or proprietary securing material
   - Various sizes and styles of intravenous over-the-needle catheters
   - Gloves and other body substance isolation gear
   - Intravenous tubing set
   - Intravenous fluid(s)
   - Equipment for obtaining blood samples
   - Sharps container

5. **What are some optimal peripheral sites to use?**
   When starting a peripheral line, the veins in the upper extremities are usually the best choice. There are many options from which to choose. However, the veins in the upper extremities are easily accessible, and placement here is well tolerated by the majority of patients.
   Unless the patient is critically ill, it is best to start the line in the most distal vein. Then, in case the initial puncture does not work, other, more proximal sites are available. Furthermore, leakage problems may result if the clinician initially fails at a proximal puncture and then tries a distal site in the same extremity. Using ultrasound-guided or other blood vessel-locating devices for peripheral IV placement may be of significant assistance in patients with difficult intravenous access.

6. How many choices are there for drips sets?

Typically, there are three:
- a minidrip set that delivers 60 gtts/mL
- a regular or blood pump drip set that delivers 10 gtts/mL
- a regular drip set that delivers 15 gtts/mL

Occasionally, a fourth type of set may be used that delivers 20 drops per milliliter.

7. What does the abbreviation *gtts* stand for and why?

The abbreviation *gtts* stands for drops and *gtt* means drop. The abbreviations come from *guttae* and *gutta,* respectively, and originated in Latin.

8. What steps should be followed to start a peripheral intravenous line?

1. Confirm the need to establish an intravenous line.
2. Choose the appropriate fluid, tubing, and catheter.
3. Connect intravenous fluid and tubing, flush air out of the line.
4. Maintain aseptic technique and observe body substance isolation requirements.
5. Choose appropriate site for puncture and place tourniquet above site.
6. Prepare the site using isopropyl alcohol pads or povidone–iodine pads and let dry.
7. Pull gentle traction on the skin below the puncture site.
8. Puncture site and insert catheter, bevel up, at a 15–30° angle to the skin.
9. Observe for "blood flash" and gently advance the catheter into the vein up to the hub.
10. Briefly occlude the vessel above the catheter, using your fingers.
11. Release the tourniquet or blood pressure cuff.
12. Remove needle and discard in sharps container.
13. Continue to occlude the area above the catheter and then release to draw blood samples as necessary.
14. If no blood samples are needed, then continue to occlude the area above the catheter until you connect the intravenous tubing.
15. Open intravenous tubing to confirm that fluid will infuse.
16. Look for swelling around the site of insertion to rule out infiltration.
17. Tape down the intravenous setup to prevent dislodgment.
18. Adjust the intravenous line to an appropriate flow rate.

9. What are some of the complications of intravenous therapy?

Air embolism
Arterial puncture
Catheter shear
Circulatory overload
Extravasation resulting in tissue damage and sloughing
Hematoma
Infection such as cellulitis

Local infiltration
Pyrogenic reactions
Thrombophlebitis
Venous thrombosis

10. **What kind of findings preclude starting an intravenous line in a given extremity?**
    If the extremity has burns, trauma, thrombosis, cellulitis, phlebitis, sclerosis, or massive edema, an intravenous line should be started elsewhere. If the patient has had a mastectomy or has an indwelling, surgically placed fistula or shunt, the opposite arm should be used to start the line. The vessel that is used to start a line should not empty into the traumatized area; fluids could be lost out of the trauma site.

11. **If the arm veins are inaccessible, is there another peripheral choice?**
    The external jugular vein may be a good alternative. It is easily visualized and is relatively constant in its anatomic position.

12. **Are there any suggestions to keep in mind when starting an external jugular line?**
    Yes. Suggestions include:
    1. Know your anatomic landmarks.
    2. To promote venous distention, use your finger to tamponade the vessel at the base of the neck.
    3. If no cervical spine trauma is suspected, turn the patient's head to the side and try to lower the head (Trendelenburg position).
    4. Once you have successfully placed the catheter, be sure to place pressure just past the tip of the catheter while preparing to attach the intravenous tubing. This will help prevent air from being drawn into the vein and consequently will help to avoid introducing an air embolism.

13. **I've started the intravenous line but it won't run. I'm sure I saw a flash and that I am in the vein. What could be wrong?**
    Any number of things, most of which are easily corrected. The following questions help to troubleshoot the problem:
    - Is the stopcock open?
    - Is the tourniquet/blood pressure cuff off the patient's arm?
    - Is the IV solution hanging up high enough?
    - Is something pinching off the tubing?
    - Is the stretcher wheel sitting on top of the tubing?
    - Is the drip chamber completely full?
    - Has the patient moved and occluded the catheter tip?

14. **What can be done to confirm that the intravenous catheter is in the vein?**
    1. Lower the bag of fluid *below* the level of the IV site; if the catheter is in the vein, some blood will come back into the intravenous tubing. *Or:*
    2. Attach a syringe to the nearest port by the puncture site. Draw back on the syringe and look for blood coming back into the tubing. If blood is visible, the catheter is probably in the vein. *Or:*

3. Attach a syringe to the nearest port to the puncture site and draw back. You should see blood but, in addition, reinject the fluid that you just drew back. Look and palpate carefully around the puncture site. You should *not* see any swelling when you reinject the fluid. If you do, the line is probably not patent.

15. What can be done about swelling around the puncture site?
The fluids have probably infiltrated, which can be confirmed by lowering the IV bag or drawing back with a syringe. If no blood is in the tubing, the line is probably not patent. It should be shut off immediately and the catheter removed. Pressure should be applied to the puncture site and the site dressed appropriately. Document what happened and, if possible, start another line.

16. Can't the infiltrated line be left in, especially if the patient is critically injured and we are low on EMS personnel?
Yes. If you are dealing with a critical patient and do not have time to pull the line, just shut it off. When activities slow down, pull it, apply pressure, and dress the site according to protocol. Document your actions appropriately and report them to the receiving facility.

17. As I punctured the vessel, the back end of the catheter flew off. As I attached the intravenous tubing, I noticed that the blood was bright red. It then began to work its way up the tubing toward the intravenous fluid. What is happening?
It sounds like an inadvertent arterial puncture. You should immediately shut off the line and pull the catheter. Apply direct pressure to the puncture site for at least 5 minutes or until the bleeding is stopped. Document it and report the events appropriately.

18. What should I do if I accidentally give medications or fluids in the interstitial space instead of into the vein where they belong?
Immediately shut off and pull the line. Some fluids and medications cause no problems when they extravasate. Others, however, can be toxic and cause local necrosis of tissue. Notify the receiving physician about this complication in case additional therapy such as an antidote is indicated.

19. What are the best sites in which to start an intravenous line in children?
Good peripheral intravenous sites include the antecubital space of the arms, the top of the hand, and, in infants, the scalp.

20. What if I am unable to start a peripheral intravenous line in a child?
Pediatric lines are often difficult. If it is a critical situation, you may opt to start an intraosseous (IO) line. However, because this procedure is painful, it has been used primarily in patients who are obtunded. If an IO line is not feasible and you only need to give medications, consider intranasal or intramuscular administration. Be aware of which medications can be given by these alternative routes.

21. What materials are needed to start an IO infusion?

Basic Equipment for an Intraosseous Infusion

IO needle or proprietary IO insertion devices/kits

Isopropyl alcohol or povidone-iodine pads

Gauze sponges

Intravenous tubing

Intravenous fluid/medications

10-mL or 20-mL syringe with IV solution inside

Tape

Gloves and other body substance isolation gear

22. What IO sites can be used?
Refer to your local protocols for approved IO insertion sites, which may include:
- The proximal tibia approximately 1–3 cm below the tibial tuberosity
- The distal tibia
- The distal femur
- The proximal humerus
- The sternum

23. What are the steps in starting an IO line?
The technique of IO insertion is device- or needle-specific and requires specialized training prior to use.

24. How do I confirm correct needle placement?
- IV fluid and medication flow freely through the needle.
- There are no signs of infiltration or swelling.
- The needle can stand up by itself.

25. What kinds of fluids/medications can be put through the IO line?
The same fluids and medications that can be given intravenously can be given intraosseously. Note, however, that the efficacy of certain medications with unusual characteristics such as adenosine (very short half-life) is unknown.

26. What are some complications associated with IO infusions?
Bone fracture

Compartment syndrome

Fat embolism

Necrosis of skin

Osteomyelitis

Subperiosteal infusion

Complications are rare, but they tend to be more serious than complications with peripheral IV placements.

27. Doesn't it take a long time for fluids and medications to reach the heart from an IO site?
No. In fact, circulation time from the IO site to the heart is generally less than 20 seconds and may be significantly less based on IO site proximity. Therefore, rapid medication administration and effective volume resuscitation can be accomplished via an IO infusion.

28. Can IO be used in adults?
Yes. A resurgence in adult IO use in the civilian setting has occurred due to its effective use in field military operations. Commercially made devices are available with active EMS civilian deployment.

Prehospital Skills and Interventions

29. **When is central line placement indicated?**
    1. When access for a transvenous pacemaker is needed
    2. When central venous pressure and cardiac monitoring are indicated
    3. When more central drug delivery is needed
    4. When a peripheral IV site is not accessible
30. **What is the best location to start a central line?**
    The subclavian vein, the internal jugular vein, and/or the femoral vein. Each site has its advantages and disadvantages. Most recently, ultrasound-guided central line placement has increased the success rate and decreased the complication rate associated with this procedure.
31. **Why are central lines usually not placed in the field?**
    Complications are more severe and more common than for peripheral IV placement. In addition, the procedure is technically more difficult and requires more training, time, and equipment.

Some Complications of Central Line Placement in the Field

Air embolus
Arterial puncture
Cerebral infarct
Hemothorax
Infection
Intrathoracic catheter fragmentation
Nerve injury
Pneumothorax
Tracheal perforation

32. **True or false? Central lines allow for more rapid fluid delivery than peripheral lines.**
    False. Poiseuille's law states that flow is proportional to the fourth power of the radius of the cannula and inversely related to its length. Therefore, short-length, large-bore intravenous catheters such as peripheral catheters will infuse the greatest amount of fluid in the shortest amount of time.
33. **Can medications and fluids be given through indwelling vascular access lines?**
    Most indwelling lines such as a central venous catheter or a peripherally inserted central catheter can be used safely to give medications and fluids in the emergency setting (based on protocols). When questions arise, it is usually best to ask the patient or caretaker about the line since they will probably be able to provide information concerning its care and capabilities.

Pearls and Pitfalls

1. Not every patient needs an IV; start only as indicated.
2. Unless the patient is critical, start the IV in the distal upper extremity and move proximally if needed.
3. Remember that the external jugular vein is a peripheral option in the patient with difficult access.

Intravenous Access

4. Consider the IO route as an option in the critical child or adult without IV access.
5. Essentially all fluids and medications that can be given IV can also be administered IO.
6. Do not attempt an IO stick in the same bone more than once.
7. Central lines are technically more difficult and have much greater risk of significant complications.
8. Ultrasound guidance for peripheral and central lines aids in increasing success rate for placement and decreasing complication rates.

References

1. Bledsoe BE. Atlas of Paramedic Skills. Englewood Cliffs, NJ, Prentice-Hall, 1987.
2. Bledsoe BE, Porter RS, Shade BR. Paramedic Emergency Care, 2nd ed. Englewood Cliffs, NJ: Prentice-Hall, 1994.
3. Butman AM, Martin SW, Vomacka RW, McSwain NE Jr. Comprehensive Guide to Pre-Hospital Skills: A Skills Manual for EMT-Basic, EMT-Intermediate, EMT-Paramedic. Akron, OH, Emergency Training, 1995.
4. Campbell JE (ed.) Basic Trauma Life Support for Paramedics and Advanced EMS Providers, 3rd ed. Englewood Cliffs, NJ, Prentice-Hall, 1995.
5. Chameides L, Hazinski MF, eds. Pediatric Advanced Life Support. Dallas, TX: American Heart Association, 1994.
6. Cummins RO, ed. Advanced Cardiac Life Support. Dallas, TX, American Heart Association, 1994.
7. Greenwald J. The Paramedic Manual. Englewood Cliffs, NJ: Prentice-Hall, 1988.
8. Heightman AJ. Rebirth of adult IO. JEMS October 30(10):suppl. 4–7, 2005.
9. Roberts JR, Hedges JR. Clinical Procedures in Emergency Medicine, 2nd ed. Philadelphia: W.B. Saunders, 1991.
10. Sanders MJ. Mosby's Paramedic Textbook. St. Louis: Mosby, 1994.
11. Walraven G, Julihn M. Paramedic Review Guide: Case Studies and Self-Assessment Questions. Englewood Cliffs, NJ: Prentice-Hall, 1988.
12. Costantino TG, Parikh AK, Satz WA, Fojtik JP. Ultrasonography-guided peripheral intravenous access versus traditional approaches in patients with difficult intravenous access. Ann Emerg Med 46(5):456-61, 2005.
13. Stein J, George B, River G, et al. Ultrasonographically guided peripheral intravenous cannulation in emergency department patients with difficult intravenous access: A randomized trial. Ann Emerg Med 54:33–40, 2009.
14. Espinet A, Dunning J. Does ultrasound-guided central line insertion reduce complications and time to placement in elective patients undergoing cardiac surgery. Interact Cardiovasc Thorac Surg 3:523–527, 2004.

CHAPTER 81

Prehospital Airway Management

Arthur Hsieh, MA, NREMT-P, and Gregory J. Chapman, BS, RRT, REMT-P

1. **Is airway management essential for good patient care?**
   Absolutely. Airway is the "A" in ABC. It is the first thing that must be assessed and managed for any patient, *critical or not*. It is also the "B" in the ABCs, as breathing is an integral part of airway management. In some patient care situations, the prehospital care providers will spend the entire time and all their energy on addressing an airway problem; in those instances, their time will have been appropriately spent. There is never a fracture, wound, or injury more important than assuring airway patency.

2. **What is the best method of assessing an airway?**
   Look, listen, and feel.
   - Is the face intact? Are teeth broken? Is there facial hair? Is the patient unusually heavy, have a short, wide neck or a recessed mandible? These questions will help you size up the patient's ability to have his/her airway managed if necessary. Affirmative answers to these questions imply a more difficult airway to manage.
   - Is there blood, vomit, or other bodily fluids in the mouth? Turn the patient on his or her side and suction to clear the airway.
   - Is there nasal flaring, intercostal retractions, or accessory muscle use during inhalation? Is chest rise normal or absent? Is the patient tachypneic or hypopneic? There may be restrictions in the airway that require assisted ventilations through basic or advanced means.
     (b) **Listen** to the airway.
         Normal breathing is quiet to the ear. Does it sound like air is moving in and out? Are there any wheezes, gurgling, grunting, stridor, or other abnormal sounds that would indicate difficulty in moving air? Any indication of airway instability requires close monitoring and rapid intervention.
     (c) **Feel** for air exchange in the airway.
         Hold your hand over the patient's mouth and nose to determine respiratory rate and estimate tidal volume. Feel the chest wall to determine stability, crepitus, and symmetry of movement.

3. **What are normal respiratory rates per minute?**

Adults (12 years and older)	12–20
School aged child (6–12 years)	18–30
Preschooler (4–5 years)	22–34
Toddler (1–3 years)	24–40
Infant (1–12 months)	30–60

A better question to ask is how *well* is the patient breathing? Breathing should be effortless. Any findings to the contrary are cause for suspicion and further investigation.

4. **Which patients need supplemental oxygen?**
   Any patient who looks ill and has any reason to be hypoxic. Signs of hypoxia include:
   - Respiratory distress, tachypnea, respiratory effort, noisy respirations, or cyanosis
   - Abnormal vital signs such as hypotension, tachycardia, or, more ominously, bradycardia
   - Altered level of consciousness
   - Cardiac or respiratory arrest

5. **What is the approximate percentage of oxygen in various methods of delivery?**

Inhalation Method	Flow Rate/Min	Oxygen in Inspired Air/%
Room air	0	21
Nasal cannula	2–6	28–40
Face mask	10	50–60
Mask with reservoir	10	90
Bag–mask device	12	40
Bag–mask device with reservoir	10–15	90

6. **Which patients need ventilation?**
   Any patient who has an open airway and inadequate ventilation or no ventilation requires assisted ventilation. This includes patients who are breathing spontaneously but moving inadequate tidal volume.

7. **How should I ventilate a patient?**
   Carefully. Overventilation will cause increased intrathoracic pressure, decreased venous return to the heart, decreased blood pressure, hypocarbia, and gastric distension. Hypoventilation will prolong or exacerbate hypoxia and hypercarbia. Either condition can be fatal. Control ventilation rates to 8–12 breaths per minute. Provide enough pressure to cause the chest to rise *and no more*.

8. **When does an airway need intervention?**
   This is a tough question to answer. Any patient who is not alert, oriented, and breathing comfortably at a normal rate and volume has the potential to need intervention. If the patient can't maintain a clear airway or needs help breathing, the airway needs to be managed.

9. **What is the most common cause of airway obstruction in the unconscious patient?**
   The tongue. As it relaxes, it falls against the posterior pharynx. Position the head and shoulders to allow the head to tilt back. Lift the chin and mandible to move the tongue anteriorly. A modified jaw thrust may be used if a cervical spine injury is suspected. If the patient is spontaneously breathing and spine injury is not a concern, placing the body in a lateral recumbent (recovery) position will help keep the airway clear.

10. **What are other common causes of airway obstruction?**
    Food is the next most common cause. Hot dogs, candy, grapes, or nuts are common obstructive agents in children. Children additionally are at risk because toys, balloons, or small household objects may get lodged in their airways. Steak or other meat obstruction is common in intoxicated or elderly adults with

inadequate chewing ability. Trauma patients further run the risk of teeth, vomit, or blood interfering with the airway.

Less common causes include tissue swelling secondary to tumor, anaphylaxis, infection, or burns.

11. What are ways to remove a foreign body airway obstruction (FBAO)?

Abdominal thrusts, chest thrusts, or a combination of both are effective basic means of dislodging a foreign body from the upper airway. Advanced procedures of FBAO removal include the use of Magill forceps and direct laryngoscopy. For an FBAO located below the glottic opening, an endotracheal (ET) tube cut proximal to the balloon cuff can be attached to suction tubing. Visualize the glottic opening, insert the ET tube through the cords until resistance is felt, and then activate suction. The FBAO may be sucked up into or against the distal end of the ET tube and be withdrawn.

12. What are the first steps in establishing an airway for an unconscious patient?

First use personal protective equipment—gloves, goggles, and mask. Position the patient supine, consider padding the shoulders to lift the torso, and then place more under the head to lift it forward into the sniffing position. Open the airway by using the head tilt/chin lift maneuver if possible, or open the airway by using the jaw thrust maneuver if neck injury is suspected. The key is to lift the jaw, not just tilt the head.

13. When are oropharyngeal or nasopharyngeal airways necessary?

In the unconscious patient who is breathing spontaneously or in the patient who needs bag–mask ventilation. The purpose is to maintain an open airway by keeping the tongue off the posterior pharynx.

14. What are the disadvantages of an oropharyngeal airway (OPA)?

- It cannot be used in a patient with an intact gag reflex.
- If improperly inserted, an OPA can cause airway obstruction.
- It can be easy to dislodge.
- It cannot be inserted through clenched teeth.
- An OPA does not isolate or protect the trachea.

15. What are the advantages and disadvantages of a nasopharyngeal airway (NPA)?

- It is better tolerated in a patient with the gag reflex but still can cause vomiting.
- An NPA is more difficult to dislodge than an oropharyngeal airway.
- It may cause nosebleed and increase the risk of aspiration.
- An NPA should not be used if midface trauma or chance of basilar skull fracture exists.
- An NPA does not isolate or protect the trachea.

16. What are the indications for using a supraglottic airway device?

This is a difficult question to address, as the answer is, "it depends." In general, a patient whose airway is difficult to manage with a basic airway and bag mask, and who is also difficult to intubate with an endotracheal tube, is a candidate for either a first-line or backup/rescue attempt with a supraglottic airway.

17. What are the advantages and disadvantages of supraglottic airways?

Each specific device has its own strengths and weaknesses. Overall:

- Supraglottic airways use a "blind" approach to insertion. With correct head positioning, these airways can be inserted without visualizing the glottic opening.

Prehospital Airway Management

- Compared to an OPA or NPA, these airways use balloons to surround the glottic opening and reduce the possibility of aspiration, although they do not eliminate the risk completely.
- Supraglottic airways cannot be used in a patient with an intact gag reflex.
- The height of the patient (too tall, too short) may limit the use of certain supraglottic airways.

18. What are the indications for endotracheal intubation (ETI)?
The answer is again dependent upon various factors, including operator skill, patient anatomy, and physiological condition. Generally speaking, consider ETI when managing an airway that needs to be controlled and basic maneuvers have proven to be insufficient.

19. What are advantages and disadvantages of ETI?
- ETI provides a patent airway.
- Aspiration is minimized with intubation, as compared to other airway devices.
- Deep tracheal suction may be performed through the endotracheal tube.
- The ventilatory effort of a patient in severe respiratory distress or failure may be better managed with ETI.
- ETI may provide an alternative route for specific medication administration.
- There is an increased risk of overpressurizing the lungs, causing barotrauma.
- There is an increased risk of over-pressurizing the thoracic cavity, reducing preload and causing decreased cardiac output and hypotension.
- There is a risk of overventilating the patient, causing hypocarbia and alkalosis.
- A significant amount of training and experience is needed to maintain proficiency in the skill.
- Prolonged attempts at intubation are often associated with hypoxia and hypercarbia.

20. What size tube should I use?

Age	ET Tube (internal diameter in mm)
Preemie	2.5–3.0
Newborn	3.0–3.5
6 mo	3.5–4.0
1 year	4.0–4.5
2 years	4.5
4 years	5.0
6 years	5.5
8 years	6.0
Adult female	7.0–8.0
Adult male	8.0–8.5

21. Is there any way to remember what size tube to use on a child?
One suggestion is to use a tube the size of the child's little finger; or, for children older than 1 year of age: internal diameter (ID) = 4 + (patient's age in years/4.) In the newly born, the ET tube size may be estimated by dividing the gestational age (in weeks) by 10.

As tube sizes are always approximate, a tube 0.5 mm smaller than predicted size and one 0.5 mm larger should be available.

22. At what age should a cuffed endotracheal tube be used?
Age 6 years is the youngest age to consider using a cuffed tube (size 5.5 mm ID).

23. What are the most commonly used laryngoscope blades?
Curved (MacIntosh) and straight (Miller, Wisconsin, and others).

24. What is the difference in the way the blades are used?
The tip of the curved blade is inserted into the vallecula, under the epiglottis. The tip of the straight blade slides *over* the epiglottis. Both will expose the glottic opening when traction is exerted upward on the handle of the laryngoscope.

25. Sometimes patients start to vomit during the intubation. Is there anything I can do to prevent this?
A technique known as Sellick's maneuver may be helpful. This maneuver involves pressure applied to the cricoid cartilage to occlude the proximal esophagus, minimizing gastric inflation and esophageal regurgitation, thus decreasing the risk of aspiration. Too much pressure, however, can make the intubation attempt more difficult, particularly in children whose tracheas are much less rigid than in adults.

26. When the tube is in the correct position in an adult, what will the depth marking read between the front teeth?
In general, 20–22 cm.

27. How can the tube position be confirmed after intubation?
- Visualize passage of the tube through the vocal cords.
- Listen to the epigastrium first, and then listen to the lungs on both sides.
- Check for expired carbon dioxide with either a colorimetric device or end tidal capnography.
- Visualize chest rise or gastric distension.

28. Which tube placement confirmation technique is best?
None. Use at least two methods of checking tube placement to confirm position.

29. What are the complications of intubation?
The worst complication is an undetected esophageal intubation. Injuries to the airway soft tissues and to the teeth are possible. A tube placed too deeply will usually result in a right mainstem intubation with oxygenation of only the right lung. Overventilation may result in pneumothorax. An endotracheal tube may become obstructed or dislodged.

30. I need to intubate the patient in order to secure the airway, but the patient is still breathing, has an intact gag reflex, or has clenched teeth (trismus). What should I try?
Assuming that basic life support procedures will not maintain a patent airway, attempt a nasal intubation or perform a medication-assisted intubation.

31. What should I know about nasal intubation?
There can be incredible bleeding if a turbinate is torn or dislodged during a nasal intubation attempt. Minimize bleeding by doing the following:

Prehospital Airway Management

- Spray the right nare with neosynephrine spray to constrict the capillary bed.
- Dilate the right nare with a nasal trumpet lubricated with lidocaine jelly.
- Use a tube size one half to one size smaller than one used for an oral intubation attempt.
- Gently insert the tube straight back into the nare, with the bevel facing the septum. DO NOT FORCE the insertion. If needed, slightly turn the tube back and forth as you advance it, to ease past the turbinates.
- If the tube is unable to pass through the right nare, prepare the left side in a similar fashion. Orient the tube so that the bevel faces the septum. When it reaches past the turbinate, twist the tube 180° and proceed with the intubation.

32. How do I know when I have intubated the patient nasally?
Airflow through the tube will increase dramatically as the tube passes through the vocal cords. A Beck airway airflow monitor (BAAM) can help amplify the sounds so they can be heard in a noisy environment.

33. What are the complications of nasal intubation?
There are several. Even done properly, nasal intubation can cause significant epistaxis, which can also increase the risk of aspiration, and trauma to the soft tissues of the nares, nasopharynx, epiglottis, and vocal cords. Sinus infection is also another complication. Using too small diameter of a tube will require higher pressures to ventilate adequately.

34. What about medication-assisted intubation (MAI)?
This certainly is an area of controversy. Many small studies of predominantly air-based prehospital systems have demonstrated the effective use of MAI. However, studies of larger EMS systems using MAI have shown lower and unacceptable success rates of intubation. Recently, studies have reported poorer outcomes in patients intubated in the field. Simultaneously, the efficacy of basic airway management has been demonstrated. What's the "take-away" message then?

- Most airways can be managed with basic procedures.
- There are a few circumstances where ETI may be needed to create a patent airway.
- There are rare circumstances where MAI may be needed to facilitate an ETI on a patient whose airway cannot be maintained by basic procedures.

This specific subset of patients is quite sick and has very unstable airways. Administering a paralytic agent will eliminate any remaining protective reflexes the patient might have left. The success or failure of the airway will be entirely dependent upon you.

35. What should I know about MAI?
If you have committed to managing the patient's airway with MAI, remember to perform the following "seven Ps":

Preparation: Prepare your equipment and medications. Assemble laryngoscopy equipment and medications.

Preoxygenation: Ventilate and oxygenate the patient as best as possible prior to inducing chemical paralysis. Measure oxygen saturation and end tidal carbon dioxide levels constantly.

Pretreatment: Consider the use of LOAD: Lidocaine and Opioids such as fentanyl to blunt an increase of intracranial pressure (ICP), Atropine to reduce the likelihood of bradycardia, especially in pediatric patients, and a Defasiculation agent such as vecuronium to also reduce ICP. Several systems may use a sedating agent such as a benzodiazepine prior to paralyzation.

Paralysis with induction: A short-acting, depolarizing agent such as succinylcholine will create a paralyzed state rapidly and for a relatively short period of time (10 minutes or less). Nondepolarizing agents such as vecuronium, pancuronium, or rocuronium will also paralyze the patient, and without the fasciculating side effects of succinylcholine. However, the effects last much longer, often 30 minutes or more.

Protection and positioning: Suction must be immediately available. Position the head and shoulders to elevate the head so the tragus of the ear is in line with the sternal notch, parallel to the ground.

Placement with proof: Confirm tube placement with a minimum of two methods, as described previously.

36. What should I know about cricothyroidotomy?

Creating an artificial opening in the neck is a highly invasive procedure that can cause severe complications including bleeding, subcutaneous emphysema, and aspiration. However, on the very rare circumstance that securing an airway orally is simply not possible, this may be truly a life-saving procedure. Examples include severe facial trauma, burns to the oropharynx, and severe epiglottitis, all causing complete airway obstruction.

If you use transtracheal jet ventilation to ventilate a needle cricothyroidotomy, recognize that even a short burst of the device will generate a large volume of gas in the lungs. Barotrauma is a distinct possibility.

Pearls and Pitfalls

1. The best airway is the one that works for the patient. You should be familiar with several different techniques in the event you are unable to manage the airway with your first choice. Start with basic airway maneuvers and work your way up to more advanced interventions as needed.
2. Practice makes better. Intubation is a low frequency, high criticality skill that demands training and experience to maintain competency.
3. When in doubt, go back to the beginning. The initial step of your primary assessment is the assessment and management of the patient's airway; however the airway must be continually monitored.
4. There is no such thing as an easy airway, at least until after you are finished securing it.
5. Be aware of the technological imperative which says that if a procedure is taught, it will be performed with a frequency that exceeds its indications. Just because you *can* intubate, it doesn't mean that you *must* intubate; instead, provide the *appropriate* airway management for the situation and the patient.
6. Be careful not to hyperventilate the patient. Inadvertent hyperventilation is a common finding; however, the associated decrease in carbon dioxide levels is not beneficial in head injured patients unless clinical signs of herniation are present. Often, hyperventilation causes increased intrathoracic pressure which decreases venous return to the heart and blood pressure.

References

1. National Association of EMTs. Prehospital Trauma Life Support, 7th ed. St. Louis: Mosby, 2011.
2. Butler K, Clyne B. Management of the difficult airway: Alternative airway techniques and adjuncts. Emerg Med Clin N Am 21;259–289, 2005.

3. Davis DP, Hoyt DB, Ochs M, et al. The effect of paramedic rapid sequence intubation on an outcome in patients with severe trauma brain injury, J Trauma 54:444, 2003.
4. Davis DP, Dunford JV, Poste JC, et al. The impact of hypoxia and hyperventilation on outcome after paramedic rapid sequence intubation of severely head-injured patient. J Trauma 57:1, 2004.
5. Dunford J. Incidence of transient hypoxia and pulse rate reactivity during paramedic rapid sequence intubation. Ann Emerg Med 42(6):721–728, 2003.
6. Garza A, Algren DA, Gratton MC, et al. Populations at risk for intubation nonattempt and failure in the prehospital setting. Prehosp Emerg Care; 9:163–166, 2005.
7. Levitan RM. A Pocket Guide to Intubation. Airway Cam Technologies, Inc., Wayne, PA, 2005.
8. Levitan RM. Patient safety in emergency airway management and rapid sequence intubation: Metaphorical lessons from sky diving. Ann Emerg Med 42:81–87, 2003.
9. O'Connor R, Swor RA. Verification of endotracheal tube placement following intubation. Prehosp Emerg Care 3(3):248–250, 1999.
10. Silvestri S, Ralls GA, Krauss B, et al. The effectiveness of out-of-hospital use of continuous end-tidal carbon dioxide monitoring on the rate of unrecognized misplaced intubation within a regional emergency medical services system. Ann Emerg Med 45(5):497–503, 2005.
11. Spaite D, Criss E. Out-of-hospital rapid sequence intubation: Are we helping or hurting our patients? Ann Emerg Med 42:729–730, 2003.
12. Wang HE, Kupas DF, Greenwood MJ, et al. An algorithmic approach to prehospital airway management. Prehosp Emerg Care; 9:145–155, 2005.

Pharmacologic Agents in Airway Management

Jedd Roe, MD, MBA, FACEP

CHAPTER 82

1. **Why are pharmacologic agents used in airway management?**
   Adjunctive medications assist the provider by creating the optimal intubating environment through sedation and muscle relaxation. This process is called rapid sequence intubation (RSI), and has been commonly used in emergency departments (EDs) for years and more recently been added to the capabilities of certain EMS systems. It is important to note, however, that there is nothing "rapid" about rapid sequence intubation. In fact, this procedure takes some time to accomplish. See question 14 in this chapter.

2. **How does the RSI process work?**
   After preparation and preoxygenation, the patient is given medication, typically a paralytic agent combined with a sedative, and the intubation proceeds. Depending on which drug is chosen or the clinical circumstances, pretreatment with other medications may be necessary.

3. **What else do I need to know before I use a paralytic agent?**
   This sounds obvious, but you must think through if you should paralyze the patient in the first place. The decision rests not just on the clinical need for airway management, but also on your ability to ventilate the patient with basic techniques should you be unable to achieve endotracheal intubation. For instance, if intubation can't be achieved in a patient with massive hematemesis, the patient can't be bagged, as blood will just be forced down into the lungs. In this setting, a surgical approach to airway management is the only option left. Other clinical scenarios that might pose similar difficulties occur in the setting of facial trauma or neck trauma where anatomic and secretion issues may be present.

4. **What paralytic drugs are used and how do they work?**
   These drugs work by blocking the nervous impulses through their acetylcholine (ACh)-like activity at the neuromuscular junction in two different ways:
   Succinylcholine is perhaps the most commonly used paralytic today, and as a mimic of the ACh molecule causes sustained depolarization at the ACh receptor site of the motor end plate. Though ultimately undergoing similar enzymatic breakdown, succinylcholine lasts longer than ACh at the receptor site, causing myocytes to undergo a brief period of tetany prior to the complete relaxation which occurs with depletion of the cell's ready resources.
   Competitive or nondepolarizing muscle blockers, such as *vecuronium* or *rocuronium*, act by preventing ACh access to the receptor sites of the motor end plate, and as the necessary ACh is not present to initiate depolarization, paralysis of the myocytes ensues.

5. **What are the characteristics of these paralytic agents?**
   The pharmacologic criteria of these agents are displayed in Table 82.1.

TABLE 82.1: Pharmacologic Criteria of Paralytic Agents

	Dose	Onset	Duration
Succinylcholine	1.5 mg/kg	45–60 sec	6–10 min
Vecuronium	0.3 mg/kg	2–4 min	Approx 120 min
Rocuronium	1 mg/kg	60–90 sec	Approx 50 min

6. **Which medication should I choose?**
   A useful drug for RSI is one that is fast-acting, consistent in its effect, and short in duration. The reason why succinylcholine has been used for so long and so often is that of the options listed, it is the most predictable in terms of these criteria, as well as being relatively inexpensive. Safety is a concern in certain settings, as hyperkalemia has been seen in denervation syndromes such as amyotrophic lateral sclerosis and in severe burns more than 5 days after the initial trauma. Physiologically, succinylcholine administration can cause increased intracranial and intraocular pressure, and a negative chronotropic effect may be manifested as sinus bradycardia, particularly in pediatric patients. The latter situation is mitigated by the pre-treatment of the patient with atropine (0.01–0.02 mg/kg). Remember to allow 2 minutes for the atropine to take effect.

   Rocuronium is the most advantageous in terms of non-depolarizing muscle blockers, and can be used as a first-line agent or in those situations where succinylcholine is less suitable. Its action is also fairly predictable, but there is the cost of a substantially longer duration of action.

7. **Do I need to add a sedative agent?**
   Absolutely. The paralytics do not affect mentation, sensation, or the ability to feel pain; therefore sedatives must be used in the RSI procedure. Even in patients who are unresponsive the sedative agent may attenuate some of the adverse physiologic effects of airway manipulation and paralytic drugs and at the same time enhance muscular relaxation.

8. **What sedative agents are suitable in the prehospital setting?**
   Ideally, a sedative agent should have all the same characteristics that we look for in our preferred paralytic (e.g., rapid onset, short duration, safe).

   Benzodiazepines have been very useful when sedation is required in emergency settings, and midazolam is the agent that has the most useful profile for RSI.

   Midazolam's pharmacologic profile is seen in Table 82.2. For sedation in ED settings, one often begins with a dose of 2–3 mg in a 70 kg individual and titrate the dose upwards to achieve the desired effect. When performing RSI, we're looking for a deeper level of sedation and rapid onset, so a higher dosing regimen of 0.1–0.2 mg/kg is recommended. Although this dosage is effective, midazolam is a negative inotrope and blood pressure may be lowered substantially. Perhaps because of the greater familiarity with the 2–3 mg dose of midazolam some EMS systems have reported using it with RSI. This practice should be avoided, as not only does it not achieve an effective level of sedation, but it may also not adequately reduce the physiologic response to intubation or achieve optimal relaxation.

   Etomidate is a short-acting barbiturate whose pharmacologic characteristics are also displayed in Table 82.2. Because of these characteristics and etomidate's remarkable ability to lower intracranial pressure without significantly lowering blood pressure or cerebral perfusion pressure, it has become the agent of choice in the majority of emergent RSI settings. Etomidate has been known to cause brief episodes of myoclonus in up to 20–30% of patients, but in RSI many of these episodes are not seen due to the use of a paralytic medication, and usually an optimum intubating environment is achieved.

TABLE 82.2: Characteristics of Midazolam and Etomidate

	Dose	Onset	Duration
Midazolam	0.1–0.2 mg/kg	30 sec	20 min
Etomidate	0.3 mg/kg	<30 sec	5–8 min

9. **Can etomidate be used as a sole agent to facilitate intubation?**
Although one study of 50 patients reported an intubation success rate of 89%, the use of etomidate alone does not create an optimal intubating environment. In the ED's controlled setting, one often has the time to titrate medications to the maximum level of sedation; however, it is not practical in the field, where achieving maximum relaxation must be achieved as quickly as possible.

10. **Are other pretreatment medicines necessary?**
In most cases for the prehospital setting, beyond the use of atropine for pediatric patients receiving succinylcholine, the answer is no.

11. **Is the use of these medications endorsed by our specialty group?**
Yes, with caveats. The National Association of EMS Physicians (NAEMSP) position statement of January 2005 states, "Drug-assisted intubation (DAI) is an advanced airway procedure that should not be considered mandatory, nor is it appropriate, for many prehospital EMS systems. DAI should be utilized only by EMS systems that, in the judgment of the medical director(s), have a specific need for the procedure and possess adequate resources to develop and maintain a prehospital DAI protocol."

12. **This position statement sounds kind of restrictive. Why is that?**
EMS systems began considering the use of RSI mainly to deal with failed intubation attempts that had been attributed to inadequate relaxation, as might be seen in a combative patient with a head injury, for example. Early on, RSI was mostly implemented by air-medical agencies, whose personnel usually had received a higher level of training and whose practice concentrated the experience with this procedure in a small number of providers.
Reported RSI success rates in ground EMS environments range from highs of up to 96% to as low as 85%. Why is there such a large range? The answer may lie in the fact that in the system reporting the higher rate, paramedics intubated 20 operating room patients during their initial training and had 4-12 RSI per year, with at least one of those supervised by an anesthesiologist. This is a fairly intense training regimen. In contrast, the system that reported the lower result conducted one of the few prospective studies on this subject and dealt with 484 paramedics from multiple agencies who received seven one-hour classes on RSI and the use of a combitube as a rescue device.

13. **Are there significant complications of RSI in the field?**
Potentially, yes. In the prospective study mentioned above, 57% of patients demonstrated a drop in oxygen saturation to less than 90%, with a median time duration of hypoxia of 2 minutes and 40 seconds. In addition, 19% of patients experienced bradycardia during these episodes. It is disturbing to note that

paramedics described the RSI as "easy" in 84% of patients that experienced oxygen desaturation. Another study addressed the outcome of severely head-inured patients and showed a mortality of 41% in RSI patients as compared with 22% in a group of matched control patients.

14. **What is the impact of RSI on on-scene time?**
   This has not yet been studied. However, one can infer that the RSI medications will take at least a minute to have their effect, and we know at least 5 minutes of 100% oxygen therapy is necessary to achieve ideal preoxygenation. If 5 minutes is necessary to prepare for intubation (e.g., checking equipment, drawing up medications, etc.), then it would seem that even in the best of circumstances, 10 minutes would be added to the on-scene time. In urban environments where transport times are relatively short, the question must be asked if delaying transport to an environment where definitive care can be provided is in the patient's best interest.

15. **If I do decide to implement a prehospital RSI program, what are the necessary components of that program?**
   As NAEMSP states, the following elements must be present at a minimum:
   - Close medical direction and supervision
   - Extensive training and continuing education on airway procedures, RSI, and rescue methods of airway management
   - Standardized RSI protocols
   - Resources for continuous monitoring, drug storage and delivery, and confirmation of tube placement
   - Programs for continuing quality improvement, skill retention, and plans for remediation

16. **That's a lot to put in place. Do we really need to implement prehospital RSI programs?**
   Prehospital RSI may have a role in settings where long transport times are anticipated, where providers are likely to perform this procedure frequently, and where specialized training and oversight are possible. For many ground EMS systems with large numbers of paramedics, one must question whether or not one will be able to train large numbers of paramedics to the skill level required and if these skills will be maintained, since a paramedic will perform the procedure only rarely. Further prospective research is necessary to measure the effect on patient outcome with prehospital RSI, and until we get more data, the question cannot be answered.

Pearls and Pitfalls

1. When managing an airway with RSI, always be prepared for the worst-case scenario and become skilled in rescue airway management methods.
2. Effective preoxygenation with 100% oxygen will maximize the time you have to safely intubate a patient.
3. RSI creates the optimum intubating environment.
4. Before using a paralytic agent, consider if you will be able to successfully bag a patient if you cannot intubate the patient.
5. Remember to pretreat with atropine if using succinylcholine in pediatric patients.
6. Oxygen desaturation in patients undergoing prehospital RSI occurs more frequently than paramedics may perceive.

7. The training and quality monitoring demands of a prehospital RSI program are substantial.
8. If effectively ventilating a patient with basic techniques and a short transport time is anticipated, ask yourself if the delay in arriving to an ED where definitive care can be provided is worth the time spent to perform RSI.

References

1. Bozeman WP, Young S. Etomidate as a sole agent for endotracheal intubation in the prehospital air medical setting. Air Med J 21:32–36, 2002.
2. Davis BD, Fowler R, Kupas DF, et al. Role of rapid sequence induction for intubation in the prehospital setting: helpful or harmful? Curr Opin Crit Care 8:571–577, 2002.
3. Dunford JV, Davis DP, Ochs M, et al. Incidence of transient hypoxia and pulse rate reactivity during paramedic rapid sequence intubation. Ann Emerg Med 42:721–728, 2003.
4. NAEMSP. Drug-assisted intubation in the prehospital setting position statement. Prehosp Emerg Care 10:260, 2006.
5. Ochs M, Davis D, Hoyt D, et al. Paramedic-performed rapid sequence intubation of patients with severe head injuries. Ann Emerg Med 40:159–167, 2002.
6. Walls RM. The Airway. In Rosen's Emergency Medicine: Concepts and Clinical Practice, 6th ed., Marx JA, ed. Philadelphia: Mosby Elsevier, 2006.
7. Wayne MA, Friedland E. Prehospital use of Succinylcholine: A 20-year review. Prehosp Emerg Care 3:107–109, 1999.

PASG

Robert Suter, DO, and Jeffrey Metzger, MD

1. **What does PASG stand for?**
   Pneumatic antishock garment.
2. **What are some other names for PASG?**
   The most common is MAST which stands for *military antishock trousers*; another is *medical antishock trousers*. Most people use the redundant term *MAST trousers*. Another term is *pneumatic counterpressure device*.
3. **What is the PASG?**
   A medical device that looks like a pair of pants when applied. They are held on the patient with Velcro closures. Air bladders in the legs and abdomen apply circumferential pressure when they are inflated.

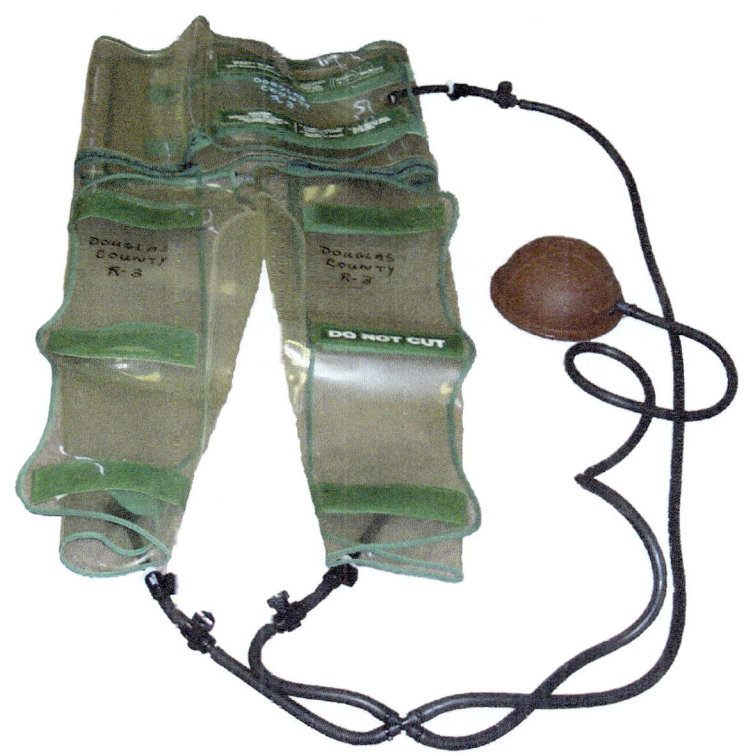

FIGURE 83.1   Pneumatic antishock garment.

4. **Isn't the PASG obsolete?**
   Although most emergency medical services (EMS) systems have discarded their PASGs, there are still some recognized indications for their use.
5. **What is the purpose of the PASG?**
   They were designed to raise blood pressure in patients who are in shock.
6. **What are the effects of the application of the PASG?**
   The PASG has positive effects on blood pressure and cardiac output. These effects occur in patients with hypovolemia caused by hemorrhage or medical hypotension. The mechanism of this effect is still not fully understood. The increases in blood pressure and cardiac output in mild hypovolemia may be a reflex response to the positive pressure exerted on the lower extremities. In more severe hypovolemia, an increase in systemic vascular resistance occurs by compressing the blood vessels in the legs and abdomen.
7. **Why is the PASG controversial?**
   From the 1960s through most of the 1980s, the PASG was in widespread use in prehospital systems based on a number of animal studies and anecdotal reports in humans. A group of researchers then began to question whether the PASG actually helped to keep human trauma patients in shock from dying. In one of these studies, trauma patients in shock died more frequently when the PASG was applied than when it was not used. This study, frequently referred to as the "911 Study," involved victims of penetrating trauma, including many chest injuries, a recognized contraindication to PASG use. Questions were raised as to the validity of the study's conclusions. However, many EMS systems adopted the findings and applied them to all groups of patients. This resulted in many people being completely against use of the PASG in all circumstances.
8. **Does the PASG really increase the blood pressure in shock patients?**
   Yes. A large number of studies have shown that blood pressure increases in patients with shock in whom the PASG has been applied.
9. **How could something that raises blood pressure in shock patients be controversial?**
   More recent research suggests a period of permissive hypotension may be beneficial in patients with uncontrolled bleeding. Patients seem to tolerate a brief period of hypotension followed by control of the bleeding (often in the operating room) followed by resuscitation better than massive resuscitation and restoration of blood pressure followed by control of bleeding. The concept is comparable to the assumption that more water comes out of a faucet under higher pressure. Also, a number of animal studies have shown increased blood loss with PASG use in the setting of uncontrolled hemorrhage. Finally, any benefit gained from the use of the device may be negated by the increased amount of time it takes to apply them.
10. **What is the difference between controlled hemorrhage and uncontrolled hemorrhage?**
    Uncontrolled hemorrhage is any bleeding that continues despite efforts to stop it. Uncontrolled hemorrhage is often due to chest or abdominal injury that it is not easily controlled in the field, though some severe arterial extremity wounds may also be very difficult to control.
11. **It sounds like the PASG was developed about 30 years ago. Who invented them?**
    Actually, antishock garments have existed since 1903. George W. Crile invented a device he called the *pneumatic rubber suit*, noted that it increased blood pressure, and reported his work in an article entitled,

PASG

"The Resuscitation of the Apparently Dead." Their use became more common during the Vietnam War, and it wasn't until then that they became popular in the civilian prehospital environment.

12. **Is there a use for the PASG that everyone agrees is good for the patient?**
    Some trauma practitioners say there is no indication for the PASG, though most will say they have a use in patients with hypotension due to pelvic fractures who have long transport times. This is essentially using the PASG as a compressive air-splint.

13. **In what patients with shock should the PASG be applied?**
    Although system protocols may vary, the literature supports the use of the shock trousers in patients with severe hypotension who have lost blood but who have controlled sources of bleeding or have unstable posterior pelvic fractures.

14. **Are there shock patients who should never have the PASG applied?**
    Yes. Absolute contraindications to the PASG include pulmonary edema, penetrating chest injuries, and diaphragmatic rupture.

15. **Are there other times that the PASG should not be used routinely?**
    Yes. Although the PASG has been widely used by EMS personnel to splint leg injuries and suspected pelvic fractures at accident scenes even when the patient is not in shock, they can cause complications such as compartment syndromes in the legs that make their use for these injuries questionable. Also, if there is an uncontrolled hemorrhage not directly compressed by the PASG, increased hemorrhage may result, and the PASG should not be used. Patients with exposed abdominal contents or who are pregnant are two more conditions in which the PASG may cause more harm than good.

16. **Is it acceptable to use the PASG to splint femur fractures even if the patient is stable?**
    Although some EMS systems allow the PASG to be used as splints, femur fractures are better treated with traction splints. The traction splint provides good stabilization and decreases internal bleeding and pain without putting external pressure on the leg, which can cause compartment syndromes and skin damage. Lower-leg injuries are well stabilized with blanket or pillow splints. To use the PASG as a routine lower-extremity splint, one must make sure to inflate them with only enough air to provide support. Avoid placing too much pressure on the legs. There are also concerns for causing or worsening a compartment syndrome with the PASG.

17. **Why do you need to limit the amount of time that the PASG is left on?**
    The primary concern with prolonged PASG application is related to the pressure they place on the legs and abdomen. There have been a number of cases of compartment syndromes in the legs as well as electrolyte abnormalities similar to crush syndrome with prolonged PASG use. Finally, it may also cause pressure necrosis of the skin.

18. **How do you apply the PASG?**
    There are a number of "right" ways to put on the PASG. The classic way is to lay the garment out flat and open and log roll the patient onto the trousers, fastening all of the Velcro straps and then inflating it one compartment at a time, starting with each leg and ending with the abdomen. To help speed things up using this technique, many emergency medical technicians and paramedics have the PASG laid out on a spine board in their ambulance so that they can place the trauma patient on the back board and the PASG trousers at the same time.

19. Are there quicker ways of applying the PASG?
Yes, in a patient in whom speed is of the essence and who would not appear to be at high risk for a lumbar spinal injury, the trousers may be applied in the same way in which one would dress a small child. With the Velcro straps loosely affixed, one would grab the patient's feet and have an assistant pull the MAST trousers onto the patient just like putting on a pair of pants. One would then inflate the trousers as before.

20. How much should each part of the PASG be inflated?
Inflate each segment, starting with the legs followed by the pelvic section, until you hear the Velcro start to pop. Then recheck vital signs. The pressure in the PASG at this point is about 100 mmHg. Much lower pressure (well below systolic blood pressure) should be used if the PASG is being used to splint a leg in a stable patient.

21. Are any patients with trauma of the abdomen or chest helped by the PASG?
Maybe. The research is inconclusive, but even the 911 study seems to show that the patients with the lowest blood pressures, those with systolic blood pressure of 60 mmHg or below, do improve with the PASG and die less frequently than other patients. This finding was not the official finding of the study and is not universally accepted.

22. Should the PASG be used for cardiac arrests?
No, there has never been any proven benefit.

23. What should I remember about the PASG?
That they definitely improve blood pressure, but improving blood pressure in this way rather than treating the cause of the low blood pressure may not be in the best interest of the patient. If they increase respiratory distress, they should be removed.

Pearls and Pitfalls

1. There is little or no indication for use of the PASG in most urban EMS systems.
2. The PASG may be used as air splints over a fractured femur or pelvis when there are long transport times.
3. Contraindications to the PASG include pulmonary edema, diaphragmatic rupture, and penetrating chest injuries.

References

1. Aprahamian C, Gessert G, Bandyk DF, et al. MAST-associated compartment syndrome (MACS): A review. J Trauma 29:549–555, 1989.
2. Bass RR, Allison EJ Jr, Reines HD, et al. Thigh compartment syndrome without lower extremity trauma following application of pneumatic antishock trousers. Ann Emerg Med 12:382–384, 1983.
3. Batalden DJ, Wichstrom PH, Ruiz E, et al. Value of the G suit in patients with severe pelvic fracture. Controlling hemorrhagic shock. Arch Surg 109:326–328, 1974.
4. Burn N, Lewis DG, Mackenzie A, et al. The G-suit. Its use in emergency surgery for ruptured abdominal aortic aneurysm. Anaesthesia 27:423–428, 1972.
5. Cayten CG, Berendt BM, Byrne DW, et al. A study of pneumatic antishock garments in severely hypotensive trauma patients. J Trauma 34:728–735, 1993.

6. Clarke G, Mardel S. Use of MAST to control massive bleeding from pelvic injuries. Injury 24:628–629, 1993.
7. Crile GW. The resuscitation of the apparently dead and a demonstration of the pneumatic rubber suit as a means of controlling blood pressure. Trans S Surg Gyn Assoc 16:361–370, 1904.
8. Dickinson K, Roberts I. Medical anti-shock trousers (pneumatic anti-shock garments) for circulatory support in patients with trauma. Cochrane Database Syst Rev 1999, 4(CD001856). DOI: 10.1002/14651858.CD001856.
9. Domeier RM, O'Connor RE, Delbridge TR, et al. Use of the pneumatic anti-shock garment (PASG). National Association of EMS Physicians. Prehosp Emerg Care 1:32–35, 1997.
10. Hagman J, Iguchi R, Kinsley J, et al. Diaphragmatic rupture following blunt trauma. Ann Emerg Med 13:49–52, 1984.
11. Mattox KL, Bickell W, Pepe PE, et al. Prospective MAST study in 911 patients. Trauma 29:1104–1112, 1989.
12. McSwain NE: Pneumatic anti-shock garment: State of the art 1988. Ann Emerg Med 17:506–525, 1988.

Needle Decompression

CHAPTER 84

John Riccio, MD, and Anne Clouatre, MHS, EMT-P

1. **Why is it important to understand needle decompression?**
   This simple procedure, executed properly in the field, can save a life.
2. **What is needle decompression?**
   It is the technique of inserting a pointed instrument into a tension-filled chest. This vents the chest, converting a tension pneumothorax into an open pneumothorax, a less lethal entity. Though a relatively simple procedure, needle decompression can be the difference between life and death. Therefore, we must be proficient and knowledgeable about this procedure.
3. **Name the *only* indication for needle decompression.**
   Tension pneumothorax.
4. **What is a tension pneumothorax?**
   A one-way air leak from the lung or chest wall that causes air to enter but not exit the pleural space. Air enters the pleural space during inspiration but becomes trapped with expiration. The continued accumulation of air leads to a significant increase in intrathoracic pressure, which collapses the affected lung, displacing the mediastinum away from the tension pneumothorax, and thereby compressing the mediastinal structures, particularly the vena cava (Figure 84.1).
5. **Why is compression of the vena cava such a big problem?**
   As the vena cava becomes increasingly compressed and narrowed, the amount of blood able to return to the heart becomes diminished. As a result, cardiac output then falls and the patient's blood pressure drops.
6. **When was a tension pneumothorax first identified/recognized?**
   Many centuries ago during the reign of Alexander the Great.
7. **What causes a tension pneumothorax?**
   The most common cause is iatrogenic barotrauma, which means that postintubation patients receiving positive pressure ventilation may develop a tension pneumothorax. Findings of decreased lung compliance as evidenced by increased resistance to bag–valve ventilation and/or patients who are in cardiac arrest who present in pulseless electrical activity should immediately alert the caregiver to the possibility of a tension pneumothorax.
   Other causes of tension pneumothorax include: traumatic chest injuries where a lung leak fails to seal, a sucking chest wound that is improperly occluded (e.g., with a dressing taped on four sides versus three), and a spontaneous pneumothorax from a ruptured bulla that continues to leak. But remember, any form of mechanical ventilation with positive pressure ventilation including bag-valve mask, esophageal/tracheal dual lumen airways, supraglottic airways including but not limited to the laryngeal mask airway, and even continuous positive airway pressure could lead to a tension pneumothorax.

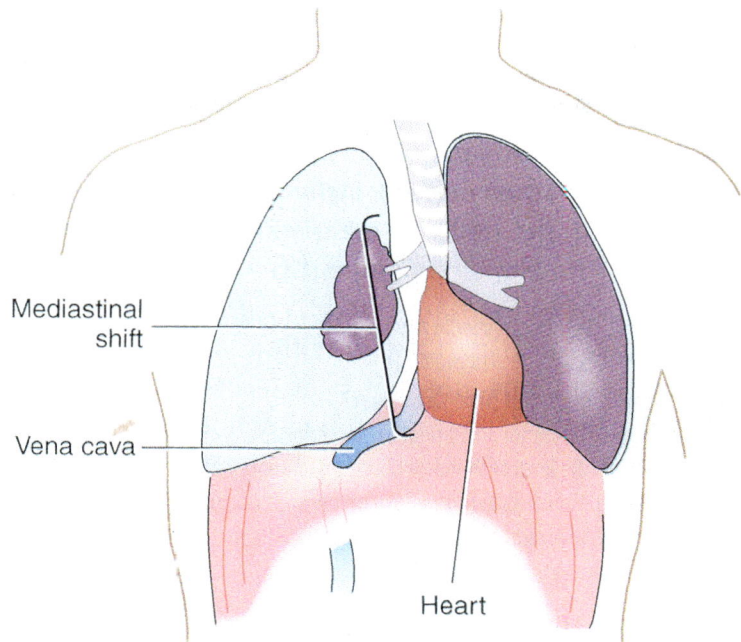

FIGURE 84.1 Tension pneumothorax with mediastinal shift. Reproduced with permission from Salomone JP, Pons PT, eds. PreHospital Trauma Life Support, 7th ed. Elsevier Mosby, 2011.

8. **How is a tension pneumothorax recognizable?**
   A tension pneumothorax is a clinical diagnosis characterized by respiratory distress, hypotension, tachycardia, unilateral absence of breath sounds, neck vein distension, and increasing difficulty in bagging. Late manifestations include subcutaneous emphysema, tracheal deviation, and cyanosis. It rapidly progresses to cardiac arrest, and delayed recognition can be fatal. Therefore, one should be vigilant in looking for a tension pneumothorax.

9. **Define Beck's triad.**
   Hypotension, jugular venous distension, and diminished heart sounds.

10. **Is Beck's triad associated with tension pneumothorax?**
    No. It is associated with cardiac tamponade. A cardiac tamponade has similar symptomatology and initially can be confused with a tension pneumothorax. Both life-threatening conditions share the first two components of hypotension and distended neck veins, but they are differentiated by diminished heart sounds versus diminished breath sounds. A tension pneumothorax has diminished (or absent) breath sounds with hyperresonant percussion on the affected side. These findings are not present with cardiac tamponade. Differentiating between these two life-threatening conditions is critical.

Prehospital Skills and Interventions

11. **People can survive with one lung. Why is a tension pneumothorax life-threatening?**
    People can survive with even less than one full lung. Therefore, something more must be compromising these patients. The displacement of the mediastinum compresses the vena cava, causing a decrease in venous blood return to the heart. The heart does not adequately fill, which leads to diminished cardiac output and, eventually, cardiac arrest.

12. **Is a lot of advanced equipment needed to perform a needle decompression?**
    No. An antiseptic skin preparation solution such as povidine-iodine and a long, large-bore (14-gauge) catheter-over-needle device are the essential pieces of equipment. Follow your airway, breathing, circulation (ABCs), provide supplemental oxygen, and wear appropriate personal protective equipment—universal precautions should always be observed. Commercially manufactured (premade) kits for needle decompression are also available.

13. **Where is the needle inserted into the chest?**
    There are two approaches, anterior and lateral. The anterior approach is at the second intercostal space in the midclavicular line. The level of the second intercostal space can be rapidly identified by palpating the sternum for the angle of Louis, a prominence on the sternum about one-quarter of the way down from the sternal notch. Avoid inserting the needle medial to the midclavicular line, because the internal mammary artery could be lacerated (Figure 84.2).
    The lateral approach is at the fifth intercostal space in the midaxillary line. In men, the nipple is usually over the fifth rib, so it can be used as a quick reference point for the fifth intercostal space. When using the lateral approach, insert the needle during peak inspiration when the diaphragm is at its lowest in the thoracic cavity. If inserted during peak expiration, the needle could puncture the diaphragm, which may rise to the level of the fifth intercostal space during this phase of the respiratory cycle and, at the same time, lacerate the liver. With either approach, the needle is inserted over the top of the rib to avoid the intercostal vessels and nerve which run along the inferior border of each rib.

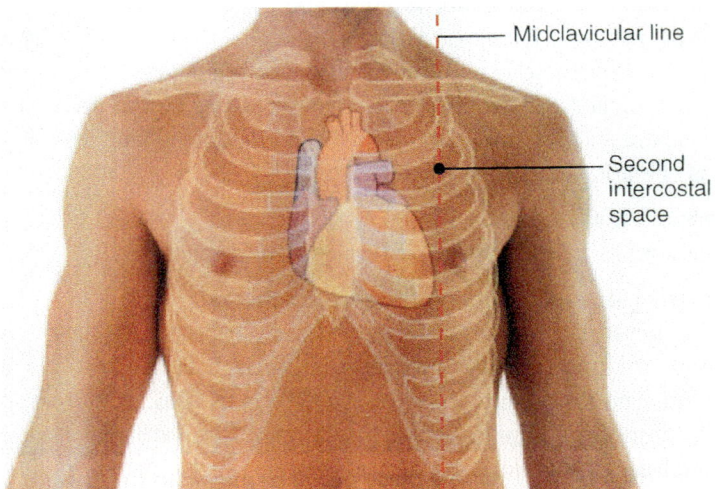

FIGURE 84.2 Needle thoracostomy for prehospital treatment of tension pneumothorax. Reproduced with permission from Salomone JP, Pons PT, eds. PreHospital Trauma Life Support, 7th ed. Elsevier Mosby, 2011.

Needle Decompression

14. What is the procedure for doing a needle decompression?
1. Confirm the diagnosis by physical findings (and obtain base station order if protocols mandate this).
2. Identify needle insertion site.
3. Wear appropriate personal protection equipment.
4. Prepare skin with antiseptic.
5. Insert the catheter-over-needle device over the top of the selected rib.
6. Confirm placement by release of air under pressure.
7. Remove the needle and leave the catheter in place.
8. Secure the catheter and attach a one-way valve, if available.
9. Monitor the patient for any changes in clinical condition.
10. Transport to hospital for chest tube placement.

15. Why might one fail in performing a needle decompression?
Insufficient catheter length or size may lead to procedure failure, as could incorrect landmark identification and needle placement. The catheter must transverse the skin and several muscle layers to reach the parietal pleura. Therefore, a large bore over-the-needle catheter (e.g, 14 gauge) of at least 4-6 cm length should be used. Take into consideration the chest wall thickness of the patient.

16. Can a tension pneumothorax reoccur after needle decompression?
Certainly. If a one-way valve is not used in patients who are breathing spontaneously, air can be sucked back into the pleural space via the catheter, resulting in reaccumulation of intrathoracic pressure. The soft plastic catheter can also become kinked or occluded, preventing the escape of air from the tension pneumothorax. Needle decompression is only a temporizing measure, not definitive care. Therefore, the patient should be reassessed frequently for recurrence of tension pneumothorax following decompression. Repeat needle decompression may be necessary in these cases. In patients who are intubated and being bagged, there is no longer the possibility of air being sucked back into the pleural space and it is acceptable to leave the catheter open or use a one-way valve.

17. Who can perform needle decompression?
A skilled health care provider trained and authorized in needle decompression, which includes physicians, paramedics, flight nurses, and mid level providers with protocol approval.

18. If I believe a patient has a tension pneumothorax but local protocols do not authorize me to perform needle decompression, what can I do?
- Establish an open airway.
- Administer high-flow oxygen.
- Rapidly transport the patient to an appropriate facility.
- Establish intravenous fluid resuscitation en route.
- Provide ventilatory assistance as needed.

19. What are the potential complications of a needle decompression?
- Hemothorax
- Lacerated lung
- Pneumothorax if tension pneumothorax was misdiagnosed

- Intercostal vessel or mammary artery puncture
- Pleural infection or empyema
- Cellulitis
- Hematoma
- Cardiac, liver, splenic or diaphragmatic puncture

20. Are there any absolute contraindications to needle decompression?

No. Tension pneumothorax is a life-threatening condition requiring immediate treatment. In this critical situation, rapid (immediate) identification and action are required to save a life.

Pearls and Pitfalls

1. Not every pneumothorax is a tension pneumothorax; a simple pneumothorax does not require needle decompression in the field.
2. Tension pneumothorax is a clinical diagnosis.
3. Tension pneumothorax is a fatal disease process—act quickly when indicated.
4. The most common cause of a tension pneumothorax is mechanical ventilation (iatrogenic barotrauma).
5. Always insert the needle over the top of the rib to avoid the intercostal nerve and blood vessels underneath.
6. Use a large-gauge over-the-needle catheter of sufficient length to ensure reaching the pleural space.
7. Insert the needle during peak inspiration when the diaphragm is at its lowest point in the chest.
8. Tension pneumothorax can reoccur, so reassess the patient frequently.
9. Needle decompression is only a temporizing measure, not definitive care.

References

1. Salomone JP, Pons PT, eds. PreHospital Trauma Life Support, 7th ed., St Louis: Mosby JEMS/Elsevier, 2011.
2. Roberts JR, Hedges JR: Clinical Procedures in Emergency Medicine, 5th ed. Philadelphia: W.B. Saunders, 2009.
3. Rosen P, ed. Emergency Medicine Concepts and Clinical Practice, 7th ed. St. Louis: Mosby, 2009.
4. Sanders MJ. Mosby's Paramedic Textbook, 3rd ed, revised. St. Louis: Mosby, 2007.
5. Barton ED, Epperson M, Hoyt DB, et al. Prehospital needle aspiration and tube thoracostomy in trauma victims: A six-year experience with aeromedical crews. J Emerg Med 13:155–163, 1995.
6. Baumann MH, Sahn, SA. Tension pneumothorax: diagnostic and therapeutic pitfalls. Crit Care Med 21:177–179, 1993.
7. Britten S, Palmer SH. Chest wall thickness may limit adequate drainage of tension pneumothorax by needle thoracocentesis. J Accid Emerg Med 13:426–427, 1996.
8. Eckstein M, Suyehara D. Needle thoracostomy in the prehospital setting. Prehospital Emergency Care 2:132–135, 1998.
9. Friend KD. Prehospital recognition of tension pneumothorax. Prehosp Emerg Care 4:75–77, 2000.
10. Marinaro J, Kenny C, Smith S, et al. Needle thoracostomy in trauma patients: What catheter length is adequate? Acad Emerg Med 10:495, 2003.

Immobilization and Splinting

Will Chapleau, EMT-P, RN, TNS

CHAPTER 85

1. **What are the basic goals of splinting and immobilization?**
   The goal of splinting is to preserve function and ensure adequate blood flow as well as to reduce the pain associated with musculoskeletal injuries. This is usually accomplished by splinting the affected body part from one joint above to one joint below the site of injury or, in the case of a dislocation or injury to a joint, securing the bone above and the bone below the injured joint. The goals of immobilization of the spine (perhaps better referred to as spinal motion restriction) are to protect the integrity of the spinal column, commonly through the use of cervical collars and spine boards.

2. **What are the most important considerations in deciding when and how to apply splints?**
   When considering splinting a limb, however deformed or injured, you must remember the ABCs of trauma care. Establishment of an adequate airway, insurance of adequate breathing, assessment of circulatory status (including bleeding control and IV access), and protection of the spinal column all take precedence over the evaluation and treatment of injured extremities (except obviously exsanguinating wounds). Even totally ischemic limbs will remain viable for hours, and precedence must be given to intracranial, thoracic, and abdominal injuries.

3. **How well do backboards and cervical collars work to immobilize patients?**
   Frankly, we do not immobilize anything, which is essentially impossible to do. Instead, our actions would better be described as spinal motion restriction. When only cervical collars are compared, it is found that Philadelphia collars permit less movement than either rigid plastic or soft foam collars. When combined with placement of the patient on a long backboard, however, rigid plastic collars provide greater movement restriction than other types of collars. Typically, this results in approximately a 90% reduction in flexion, lateral motion, and rotation, with approximately 50% reduction in extension. Most patients whose head is directly on the backboard have their neck in slight extension. It has been suggested that 1–1.5 inches of padding between the head and backboard will put the neck in a more neutral position (and be more comfortable).
   The opposite occurs with children. Because their heads are relatively large compared to their bodies, placing their heads flat on the board results in flexion of the neck. They benefit from 1–2 inches of padding under their shoulders and upper bodies to bring the neck to a more neutral position.

4. **What is the riskiest part of applying backboards or cervical collars?**
   Of those patients with neurologic deficits after spinal injuries, it is estimated that up to 25% develop the neurologic deficit after medical care has been initiated. Several studies have shown that logrolling patients onto backboards can result in significant movement of unstable thoracolumbar spinal segments, even when performed under ideal conditions by trained personnel. Thus, great care must be taken whenever a patient is being moved in order to restrict motion of the spine. In order for cervical collars to be effective

and not cause complications related to circulation or breathing, they must be properly sized to the patient. Manufacturers provide instruction on how each collar works.

5. **What about the use of towel rolls or sandbags?**
   Blocks of some kind are commonly placed along both sides of the head to provide additional stabilization. Sandbags and IV bags are not recommended. Both have enough mass to exert lateral pressure on the cervical spine if the patient must be rolled to the side (i.e., during vomiting) or if severe lateral G forces are generated while the patient is in the ambulance. Rolled towels and commercial foam products both provide increased stability without significant weight.

6. **What about strapping the patient to the backboard?**
   Strapping the patient to the backboard is commonly used to restrict lateral movement of the spine. Although many different styles of strapping and commercial products for this have been developed, only a few styles of strapping have been shown to reduce lateral motion. The efficiency of straps around the torso (at the armpits) and legs was shown to be greatly improved with the addition of a strap at the superior aspect of the pelvis. Strapping the arms to the chest as well as crossing straps over the chest offers no improvement in reducing lateral motion. Whatever type of strap used, the recommended sequence of applying the straps is first to the trunk, then the legs and finally the head. This is a precaution so that manual stabilization of the head and neck is maintained until the last strap is applied.

7. **Some EMS writers have called for elimination of the use of the backboards, saying that they are harmful. Is that true?**
   No procedure is completely benign. Patients on a rigid board for any length of time may be quite uncomfortable and can develop pressure sores. Patients with curved spines or asymmetrical anatomy will be particularly uncomfortable and at risk for breakdown of compressed tissues. Guidelines are usually published by your EMS system for determining the indication for spinal immobilization. An example of these protocols can be found in the 7th edition of the PHTLS text.

8. **What about vacuum splints?**
   Vacuum splints are widely used in Europe as an alternative to traditional motion restriction with cervical collars and backboards. Vacuum splints are, in effect, thin mattresses filled with small polystyrene balls. They may be easily molded to the body. When air is removed, they form a rigid splint that holds its shape. Vacuum splints with and without cervical collars have been shown to support and stabilize patients as well as backboards with cervical collars and are much more comfortable for the patient.

9. **How well do the Kendrick extrication device and short boards work?**
   Use of the Kendrick extrication device (KED) and strapping the patient to a short board have both been shown to provide immobilization comparable to that of long boards for all planes of movement except lateral motion of the neck. Short-board immobilization can potentially make airway control more difficult because of its chin straps. There are no good controlled trials comparing extrication of the patient directly to a long board versus KED or short-board extrication.

10. **How should you splint pelvic fractures?**
    Some studies have shown that application of the pneumatic antishock garment can effectively compress a fractured pelvis and potentially control bleeding from the fracture. Additionally, studies have shown that tying sheets around the pelvis or using commercially available pelvic binders can close the fractures

(bringing the broken pelvic bones together) and potentially reduce internal hemorrhage; however the benefit of prehospital application of these devices to patients has not yet been established.

11. What about inflatable extremity splints?
Inflatable extremity splints have several disadvantages. Although they are easy to apply, gauging their pressure with fingertip indentation of the splint or resistance to inflation by mouth commonly results in excessive pressure. Only mechanical popoff valves have been shown to reliably control their inflation pressure. In addition, even with healthy volunteers, normal inflation pressures can cause oxygen tension in the limb to drop by two thirds. For patients with increased compartment pressure due to fractures, this can easily result in an ischemic limb when the splint is applied.

12. Besides commercial products, what else can be used to splint extremities?
Blood tubing boxes or newspaper sections make stiff yet light splints for forearm and wrist fractures, whereas pillow or blanket splints work very well for foot and ankle injuries.

13. What extremity injuries require special consideration when splinting?
Several orthopedic injuries cannot be easily reduced in the field or moved to neutral positions on a backboard. Hip fractures are best stabilized with a pillow or blankets between the patient's legs, with a supporting strap around the legs. Posterior hip dislocations (knee versus dashboard) can result in a hip that is flexed and internally rotated and should be supported in place until evaluated. Although uncommon, inferior shoulder dislocations (luxatio erecta) result in the arm being held straight up in the air, and any attempts to bring the arm to the patient's side are very painful.

14. What about open fractures or dislocations?
Most open fractures, particularly those contaminated with foreign material, should be splinted as they lie. This will prevent dragging foreign material back into the wound and increasing the chance of infection. Wounds should be covered with a sterile dressing, with pressure dependent on the degree of hemorrhage.

15. Should you reduce fracture-dislocations with distal ischemia in the field?
Pro. Reduction of fracture-dislocations will often immediately restore blood flow to the affected limb. This allows for transport and evaluation of the patient without the time pressure of having an ischemic limb. In addition, the patient may be much more comfortable after the dislocation has been reduced.
Con. Fracture-dislocations may not be that easily reduced. It is not uncommon for tendons or soft tissue to become trapped in the dislocation, requiring open reduction in the operating room. Because patients can tolerate an ischemic limb for hours, time spent on the scene attempting reductions may be better spent transporting the patient to the hospital for definitive treatment.

16. What should you do with impaled objects?
Whether we are talking splinters of wood or metal, nail gun injuries (fairly common), or pieces of fence or industrial equipment, impaled objects should not be removed. They should be stabilized as best they can, and the patient should be transported to the emergency department for their removal. Objects that may penetrate the eye should be stabilized and both eyes covered to prevent consensual movement of the eyes. The dressing on the eye with the impaled object should not apply pressure to the eye (cups work well) to prevent extrusion of the contents of the globe. The only instance in which you would consider removing an impaled object is in the case of an object impaled into the airway and impairing breathing.

17. What should be done with avulsed or subluxed teeth?

Do not attempt to splint loose teeth or replace avulsed teeth in patients whose mental status is such that they might aspirate them. Aluminum foil, if available, can be folded around subluxed teeth to splint them to stable surrounding teeth, but only with caution. Avulsed teeth should be placed (by the patient) back into the sockets from which they were avulsed. If they cannot be replaced in their sockets, they may be transported in the patient's own saliva, either between cheek and gum or in a cup. In addition, there are commercially available solutions, such as Hank's solution, that can be used to transport an avulsed tooth. Other alternatives are saline or milk which will also serve as a transport medium.

Pearls and Pitfalls

1. Obviously deformed and visually impressive extremity injuries should never distract from the priorities of the airway-breathing-circulation in trauma care.
2. The longer a patient is on a rigid board, the greater the likelihood of developing decubitus ulcers. Expedite the transport of these patients for definitive evaluation and discontinuance of the board.
3. Distal pulses and neurologic function should be checked before and after any extremity manipulation or splinting.
4. Avulsed teeth are ideally managed by replacement into their original socket unless the patient has an altered mental status or other reason for risk of aspiration.
5. Ideal splinting of a fracture involves including the joints above and below the fracture site and for dislocations, splinting the bones above and below the dislocation site.

References

1. Christensen KS, Trautner S, Stockel M, et al. Inflatable splints: Do they cause tissue ischemia? Injury 17:167, 1986.
2. Hamilton RS, Pons PT. The efficacy and comfort of full-body vacuum splints for cervical–spine immobilization. J Emerg Med 14:553, 1996.
3. Mazolewski P, Manix TH. The effectiveness of strapping techniques in spinal immobilization. Ann Emerg Med 23:1290, 1994.
4. McGuire RA, Neville S, Green BA, et al. Spinal instability and the log-rolling maneuver. J Trauma 27:525, 1987.
5. Schriger DL, Larmon B, Gasick T, et al. Spinal immobilization on a flat backboard: Does it result in neutral position of the cervical spine? Ann Emerg Med 20:878, 1991.
6. National Association of Emergency Medical Technicians. Prehospital Trauma Life Support, 7th ed. New York: Elsevier 2011.
7. Chapleau W, Pons PT. Burba A, Page D, eds. The Paramedic. New York: McGraw-Hill 2008.

Prehospital Pain Management

Timothy Howey, BA, NREMT-P

CHAPTER 86

1. **Why is the treatment of pain important in the prehospital setting?**
   Pain is the most common complaint among emergency department patients, with up to 70% of patients reporting pain as part of their chief complaint. Another study showed 20% of all prehospital patients complained of moderate to severe pain. With such a large percentage of patients complaining of pain, prehospital health care workers spend a great deal of time assessing, treating, and monitoring patient pain. A clear understanding of pain pathology and treatment will improve the care of a large number of patients.

2. **What is pain?**
   Pain is what the patient feels or experiences in response to damage or injury.

3. **How do we classify pain, and how can we tell the difference?**
   Pain is generally divided into two categories: acute (nociceptive) and chronic (neuropathic). Acute pain is felt when nerve fibers, called nociceptors, detect harmful stimuli such as tissue damage, inflammation, hypoxia, and obstruction of a hollow organ. Unlike acute pain, chronic pain is not caused by the activation of nerve endings, but by the desensitization, or reduced inhibition, of these nerve pathways. Due to the pathology involved, chronic pain is not always responsive to narcotics. The patient interview and history will help the care provider determine the pathology of the pain.

4. **I've heard it said many times that "nobody ever died from pain." Is this statement true?**
   Pain has many potentially negative side effects, including increased peripheral vascular resistance, increased myocardial oxygen consumption, hypercoagulability, and decreased immune function. In patients sensitive to these changes, such as the elderly, these secondary complications may contribute to morbidity and mortality.

5. **How can we accurately assess pain?**
   Pain should be assessed for both quality and quantity. Assessing the quality of the pain (i.e., sharp, stabbing, dull, aching) will help determine the cause, which may or may not be correctable. The patient is the best judge of pain quantity. Have the patient rate his or her pain on a 0–10 scale, with 0 being no pain, and 10 being "the worst pain imaginable." If a patient is unable to report pain, then the care provider must rely on his or her own perceptions and experience to determine the extent of a patient's pain. Generally, if a patient appears to be in pain, then the patient is in pain and should be treated.

6. **How do we have to change our methods when assessing pain in children?**
   Assessing pain in pediatric patients is often more challenging than assessing pain in adults. In a 2005 study, the reason given 93% of the time for withholding morphine from pediatric patients was the inability to assess pain. In these patients, communication on the child's level is of the utmost importance. Phrases such as "hurts a lot" and "hurts a little" can be helpful with school-age children. FACES is a chart where the child points to the face that most closely correlates to the degree of pain he or she is experiencing

(See Figure 63.2, page 420.) In young toddlers and infants, the parents may help determine the amount of patient pain. Observe infants for facial grimace and squinting. Treat observed pain.

7. **Should we assess and treat pain in patients with an altered mental status?**
   Yes. An altered mental status does not mean the patient is not experiencing pain. During your physical exam, observe the patient for facial grimace upon palpation, withdrawal from stimuli, and verbal signs of pain.

8. **What different methods are available for the treatment of pain?**
   Pain can be controlled by physical, psychological, and pharmacological means. A combination of all three will typically result in the greatest pain relief.

9. **What do you mean by "physical" means of controlling pain?**
   Splinting, positioning, and hot/cold pack application are all physical methods practiced routinely by EMS professionals. Significant levels of pain relief can be achieved through these simple means, and they can be performed by any responder, regardless of level of training.

10. **What is distraction therapy?**
    Distraction therapy is a psychological technique where the patient's attention is drawn away from the pain, decreasing his or her perception of pain. Distraction therapy is very effective but may be limited in patients with one or more injuries requiring the attention of the prehospital provider.

11. **How can you perform distraction therapy in the prehospital setting?**
    The most readily available distraction technique is conversation. Talking with your patient has many benefits, including pain relief and increased trust. Casual conversation also decreases the patient's anxiety levels, allowing you to attempt procedures, such as venous access, that will allow you to further treat the pain through other routes. Also, as care allows, injuries should be removed from patient sight, particularly in children.

12. **What other distraction therapy techniques are available when the transport time is extended, such as transport from a community hospital to a tertiary care facility?**
    Music therapy is effective at distracting a patient from pain. Many ambulances are equipped with rear radio speakers, and tuning the radio to the patient's favorite station can have beneficial effects. With the decreasing costs and size of DVD players, you can also keep a movie selection on hand for longer transport times.

13. **What pharmacological therapies are available?**
    Opiate analgesics and nonsteroidal anti-inflammatory drugs (NSAIDs) are two common classes of drugs used for pain management (Table 86.1). Both have advantages and disadvantages, and a combination of both drugs may provide the most relief for the largest number of patients. Opiate analgesics provide pain relief in most situations, but carry a number of negative side effects, such as respiratory depression. NSAIDs, although perceived to be safer than opiates, also have a list of negative side effects such as gastrointestinal irritation and hemorrhage and renal toxicity that the provider must become familiar with. NSAIDs work particularly well when treating musculoskeletal pain and pain related to inflammation of tissue, such as pericarditis, pleuritis, kidney stones, and biliary colic.

14. **What is the best route for administering pain medications?**
    Intravenous medication administration is the best route. Time of onset is short, results are predictable, and you can easily titrate to effect. If the intravenous route is unavailable, then most medications may

TABLE 86.1: Analgesics Commonly Used in the Prehospital Setting

Generic Name	Trade Name(s)	Classification	Comments
Morphine sulfate	Morphine	Opioid	Standard to which all other opiates are compared. Most commonly used opiate in prehospital care.
Hydromorphone hydrochloride	Dilaudid	Opioid	Used in smaller doses than morphine, with similar side effects.
Fentanyl citrate	Sublimaze	Opioid	Slightly shorter time of onset and time to peak effect than morphine. Large doses may cause muscle rigidity, which may be reversed with neuromuscular blockers.
Meperidine hydrochloride	Demerol	Opioid	Longer half-life and effect than morphine, but metabolism is affected by renal and hepatic disease. Higher CNS toxicity.
Nalbuphine	Nubain	Synthetic opioid	Minimal hemodynamic effects, with a ceiling on respiratory depression. Is an opiate antagonist, and may precipitate withdrawal symptoms in long term opiate users.
Ketorolac tromethamine	Toradol	NSAID	Decreases ability to clot. Not indicated for use in children. Do not use in presence of advanced renal failure.
Nitrous oxide/ oxygen mixture	Nitrous, "laughing gas"	Gas	Self-administered by the patient. Mask should never be secured to patient's head. Ideal for use in children.

be administered subcutaneously. Intramuscular injections should be avoided; the time of onset is comparable to subcutaneous injections, but intramuscular injections are more painful.

15. **What is the difference between an analgesic and a sedative?**
A sedative such as midazolam or etomidate provides relief from anxiety and induces amnesia but has little to no effect on pain. When treating a stable patient, it may be beneficial to administer both an analgesic and a sedative prior to performing a painful procedure, such as reducing a fracture.

16. **What risks are associated with pharmacological pain control?**
All medications have side effects, the extent of which depends on the dose and patient tolerance. Opiates can cause respiratory depression, nausea and vomiting, and hypotension. NSAIDs are associated with gastrointestinal bleeding, kidney failure, and platelet dysfunction, but these side effects are most common in patients receiving NSAIDs over a long period of time and not in the acute setting.

17. **In the case of an accidental overdose, what antidotes are available?**
Naloxone (Narcan™) is effective at antagonizing the effects of opioids. It is important to remember that in most cases the effects of the opiates last much longer than the effect of the naloxone. Therefore, the patient must be observed closely for recurrence of overdose symptoms once the naloxone wears off after approximately 30–45 minutes.

18. **Do any other drugs reduce the undesired effects of opiates?**
Antiemetics, such as promethazine HCl (Phenergan™) and odansetron HCl (Zofran™), are effective at reducing, or prophylactically treating, nausea induced by opiates. If hypotension occurs, a fluid bolus of an isotonic solution may be administered.

19. **What should I do if I think my patient is a drug seeker?**
A previous history of dependence is the best indicator of drug seeking behavior; unfortunately, we do not have the time or resources prehospital for fully exploring or evaluating the patient history, so if in doubt, treat for pain. It is rare for a patient with no other history of dependence to become addicted to pain medication.

20. **Some EMS agencies carry fentanyl, some carry morphine, and some carry both. Which is better?**
Fentanyl is a narcotic analgesic that has a very rapid onset of action; however, it does not last very long. Thus, it is a good choice in EMS systems with short transport times. Morphine, on the other hand, has a slower onset of action but it lasts much longer than Fentanyl. Having both drugs available therefore provides the best of both worlds, one that produces pain relief quickly and one that lasts longer. If both medications are given to a patient, careful observation for respiratory depression is mandatory.

21. **Isn't it true that giving analgesics may mask symptoms and make it more difficult to diagnose the patient at the hospital?**
This has been a traditional viewpoint and commonly taught maxim for decades. As a result, untold numbers of patients have waited in pain in emergency departments until their diagnostic studies were done. Numerous recent studies have now demonstrated that the administration of analgesics does not impair the workup of a patient and, if anything, pain relief makes it easier. Therefore, medication for the relief of pain should be offered and administered to a patient as soon as it is recognized that the patient has pain.

Pitfalls and Pearls

1. Proper assessment of pain levels is essential when treating pain.
2. Most patients are best treated with a combination of physical, psychological, and pharmacological means.
3. Ongoing assessment and treatment is necessary for maintaining adequate pain relief.
4. Symptoms of narcotic overdose treated with naloxone may recur once the naloxone has been metabolized.

References

1. Miner JR, Paris PM, Yealy DM. Procedural sedation and analgesia. In Rosen's Emergency Medicine: Concepts and Clinical Practice, 7th ed., Marx J, Hockberger R, Walls R, eds. Chapter 186. St. Louis Mosby. 2010.
2. Sander MJ., Paramedic Textbook, rev. 3rd ed., St. Louis: Mosby Inc., 2007.
3. Bledsoe BE, Porter RS, Cherry RA, eds. Paramedic Care: Principles and Practice: Trauma Emergencies, 2nd ed. update, p. 328 Upper Saddle River, NJ: Pearson Education, Inc., 2011.
4. Nursing 2007 Drug Handbook, 27th ed., Springhouse, PA: Lippincott Williams & Wilkins, 2007.
5. Aehlert BJ. Comprehensive Pediatric Emergency Care, pp. 390–405 St. Louis: Mosby, Inc., 2005.
6. Dieckmann RA, Brownstein D, Gausche-Hill M. Pediatric Education for Prehospital Professionals, p. 152, Elk Grove Village, IL: American Academy of Pediatrics, 2000.
7. Hennes H, Kim MK, Pirrallo RG. Prehospital pain management: A comparison of providers' perceptions and practices. Prehosp Emerg Care 9(1):32–39, 2005.
8. Dillard JN, Knapp S. Complementary and alternative pain therapy in the emergency department. Emerg Med Clin N Am 23(2):529–549, 2005.
9. McManus JG Jr., Sallee DR Jr. Pain management in the prehospital environment. Emerg Med Clin N Am 2005
10. Markovchick VJ, Pons PT, eds. Emergency Medicine Secrets, 2nd ed., pp. 43–44, 310–314, Philadelphia: Hanley & Belfus, 1999.

Ultrasound in the Field

John Kendall, MD, FACEP

1. **Why is a chapter on ultrasound in a prehospital textbook?**
   The use of ultrasound in the emergency department (ED) has proven to be a rapid and highly effective diagnostic aid that helps expedite triage and guide patient management. Early intervention and appropriate triage are two of the hallmarks of prehospital care, so naturally people have begun to question and research the potential applications for ultrasound in the field. Numerous ED-based studies have demonstrated that relatively minimal training can yield highly accurate results in focused ultrasound exams and the early prehospital data corroborates these findings. In addition, the evolving ultrasound technology has produced small, highly durable machines with excellent image quality that EMS could easily carry in the field. The potential for ultrasound to help guide prehospital diagnosis, triage, and intervention is great and an exciting area of possibility for emergency medical care.

2. **How does ultrasound work?**
   Ultrasound machines emit sound waves at various frequencies, which then reflect off tissue interfaces to generate images. Higher ultrasound frequencies yield greater tissue resolution, but at the cost of reduced penetration, whereas low-frequency studies can penetrate deep tissues but with less resolution. Dense tissues, such as bone or gallstones, appear bright white because most of the ultrasound energy is absorbed or reflected. Solid organs, such as the liver or spleen, show a gray scale of tissue architecture. All of the ultrasound energy passes through fluid or blood, leaving a black, or anechoic (no echo), area on the screen. Ultrasound energy does not propagate through air well, so lung and hollow viscus structures are difficult to visualize. In general, 3.5- to 5-MHz transducers are necessary for sonograms of the heart and abdomen.

3. **What are the potential applications for ultrasound in the prehospital setting?**
   (a) Evaluating trauma patients for hemoperitoneum or hemopericardium (*F*ocused *A*ssessment with *S*onography for *T*rauma [FAST] exam)
   (b) Determining the aortic diameter in patients with suspected abdominal aortic aneurysm (AAA)
   (c) Assessing cardiac activity in patients with cardiac arrest or pulseless electrical activity (PEA)
   (d) Visualizing the pleural line to rule out pneumothorax
   (e) Aiding in procedures such as peripheral or central vascular access

4. **Are there any studies demonstrating the effective use of ultrasound in the prehospital setting?**
   Most of the prehospital ultrasound literature consists of case reports or abstracts. The exceptions are a few studies involving ultrasound use during air transport or studies done in Europe with non-paramedic sonographers. One such study demonstrated a sensitivity, specificity, and accuracy of 93, 99, and 99%, respectively, for a FAST exam done in the prehospital setting. More importantly, in 30% of cases there

was a change in management or therapy resulting from the prehospital FAST and a change in admitting hospital in 22%.

5. **Will performing an ultrasound in the prehospital setting delay transport?**
Not likely. Because emergency ultrasounds are directed studies that focus on one or two easily recognizable findings, one can complete the exams quickly. In most instances, EMS personnel can perform the ultrasound during transport. Two notable exceptions would be using ultrasound in the cardiac arrest patient where it may affect decisions on whether to transport or not, as well as using ultrasound at the scene of a mass casualty incident where it could aid as a triage tool.

6. **How long does it typically take to complete a focused ultrasound exam?**
Although there is a learning curve, most studies show that focused ultrasound exams take 3–5 minutes to complete. Some exams are much easier to perform and can be completed in a matter of seconds. For instance, a quick view of the heart for contractility can be done in conjunction with pulse checks during cardiopulmonary resuscitation. It is likely that the ultimate use of ultrasound in the prehospital setting will be largely dictated by the time it takes to perform specific exams. Those that take too long to complete will not be performed or the technique will be modified to meet the time frame of prehospital care.

7. **What type of training is involved?**
Historically, diagnostic ultrasound training required months of advanced training, the completion of hundreds of ultrasound exams, or a medical residency in the specialty of radiology. Recently, however, numerous specialties have adopted the concept of a limited or focused ultrasound exam. Limited exams are designed to look for one or two specific findings, and their presence or absence are used to diagnose and guide treatment. These are the studies typically performed by emergency physicians. Training for the focused exams involves one or two days of didactic and hands-on education followed by the performance of 25 "practice" or "training" exams for each clinical indication. Emergency physicians have demonstrated excellent results after similar training. To date, there are no specific guidelines for training of prehospital providers to perform focused exams.

8. **What are the primary findings of the FAST exam?**
The FAST exam involves the assessment of the peritoneal and pericardial spaces for abnormal collections of blood. When visualized with ultrasound, most blood appears black or, to use an ultrasound term, anechoic (Figure 87-1). Prior studies have shown that fluid usually collects in the peritoneal cavity in a predictable fashion—specifically, in the dependent portions of the peritoneal cavity. In the supine patient this is either the pelvis or around the liver. In certain instances, fluid can also collect around the spleen as well. The abdominal part of the FAST exam entails three views and is considered to be positive when anechoic fluid around the liver, spleen, or in the pelvis is detected. The FAST exam also evaluates the heart and is a relatively straightforward study. The ultrasound first assesses the presence (or absence) of cardiac activity and once that is established, whether there is fluid in the pericardial space.

9. **Is there a set approach for obtaining FAST exam images?**
Although patients come in different shapes and sizes, there are anatomic clues and standard transducer positions that are used and that are most likely to visualize the dependent recesses where blood often collects. Although the sequence in which the four views are obtained is not important, it is vital that one visualizes all of these regions. There are many different patterns of blood collection, and omitting one view may yield a false negative result.

Prehospital Skills and Interventions

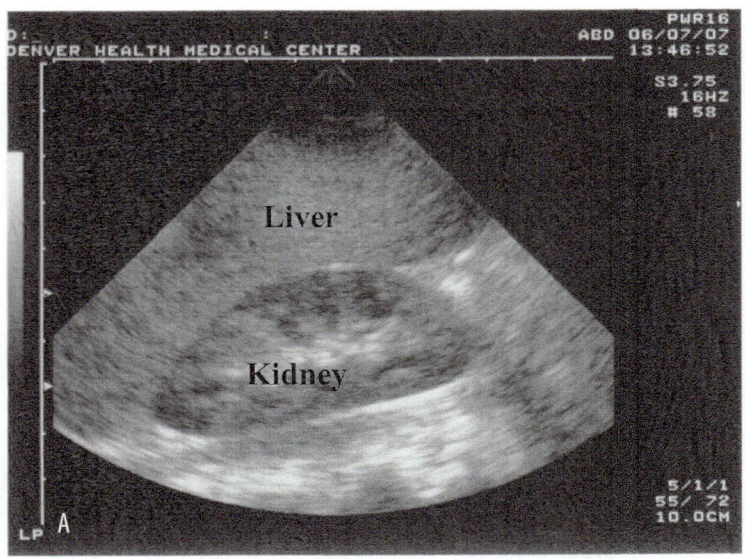

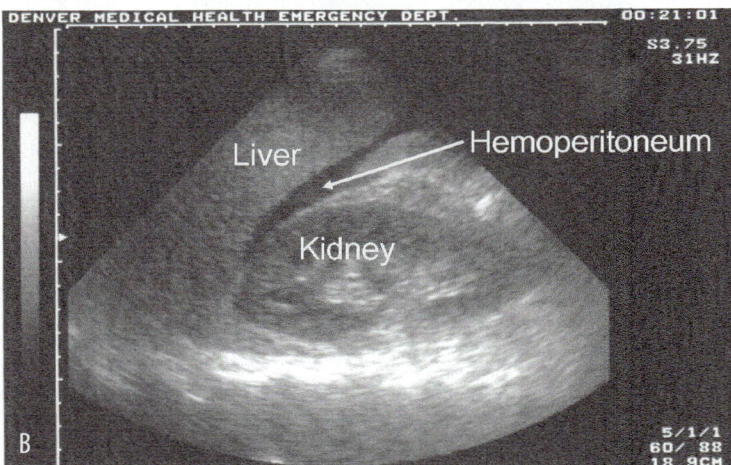

FIGURE 87.1 (a) Ultrasound image demonstrating a normal FAST exam with no fluid between the liver and the kidney. (b) Ultrasound image demonstrating a positive FAST with fluid detected between the liver and kidney.

10. How are findings of the FAST exam used in clinical decision-making?

In the ED setting, findings of the FAST exam are one component in the overall assessment of a trauma patient. The usual approach is the use of positive or negative findings and other clinical parameters, such as vital signs, to determine the appropriate course of action. For instance, a patient with a positive ultrasound and unstable vital signs is a candidate for immediate operative intervention. Although the source of the bleeding is unlikely to be identified by ultrasound, the instability is presumed to be due to the hemoperitoneum.

11. What are the findings of the echocardiography exam?

The focused exam of the heart or echocardiography is directed towards two primary findings: detecting the presence or absence of cardiac activity and, once that is established, determining whether or not there is a pericardial effusion. The recognition of pathology is a fairly straightforward process in cardiac ultrasound. Determining cardiac activity is qualitative, not quantitative, and therefore without much ambiguity. The second finding is the presence of pericardial fluid collections, which appear as anechoic (black) fluid that encircles the heart (Figure 87-2). The difficulty in cardiac ultrasound is not the interpretation of studies, but rather image acquisition. As with any focused study, you are both the one obtaining the images and the one interpreting the findings. Patient habitus, patient cooperation/combativeness, the obscuring of anatomy by nearby anatomy, and the sonographer's understanding of anatomic orientation can all make the heart and pericardial space difficult to image.

12. How can one use these findings in clinical decision-making?

The presence of a pericardial effusion on ultrasound has varying significance, depending on the context in which it is detected. In the setting of trauma, any pericardial effusion should be assumed to be pathologic and either a reflection of cardiac rupture or potentially an aortic tear. These patients need to be transported emergently to the nearest trauma center capable of handling such injuries. Cardiac ultrasound can also be used to detect nontraumatic pericardial effusions which are seen as sequelae of many conditions (i.e., malignancy, uremia [renal failure], pericarditis, rheumatologic disorders). Although many patients may have an incidentally detected nontraumatic pericardial effusion, the presence of fluid around the heart in a patient who is hypotensive, in shock, or in PEA arrest should help direct resuscitation. Cardiac contractility can be assessed in patients presenting in cardiac arrest when there is a question of pulseless electrical activity. In patients with no evidence of cardiac contractility and no reversible cause of PEA, many emergency physicians would terminate resuscitative efforts. It remains to be seen whether similar decision-making can be used with ultrasound in the prehospital setting.

13. Is there equipment made specifically for the prehospital setting?

Technically, the answer to this question is "no." That being said, however, the emergency ultrasound market has changed drastically over the last ten years and many of these developments have allowed for the introduction of ultrasound into the prehospital arena. Probably the most important of these changes is the reduction in size of ultrasound machines. Currently, some machines are the size of a laptop computer and produce extremely high-quality images. In addition, there have been significant improvements in the durability of ultrasound machines. How these changes will affect the prehospital use of ultrasound remains to be seen, but it appears the stage has been set to have machines that can fit within the tight confines of the back of an ambulance or that can be taken to the unpredictable environment of an accident scene.

14. What does a focused ultrasound exam of the abdominal aorta entail?

Evaluation of the abdominal aorta can be useful in elderly patients who present with a pulsatile abdominal mass, nontraumatic abdominal pain or flank pain, hypotension of unknown cause, or unexplained PEA. Aneurysms of the abdominal aortic have a diameter that is greater than 3 cm with patients who are symptomatic, having aneurysms that are typically greater than 5 cm (Figure 87-3). Studies by radiologists and emergency physicians showed a sensitivity and specificity of 100% for the detection of AAA. As well, ultrasound-determined aortic diameters correlated with pathologic specimens 90% of the time.

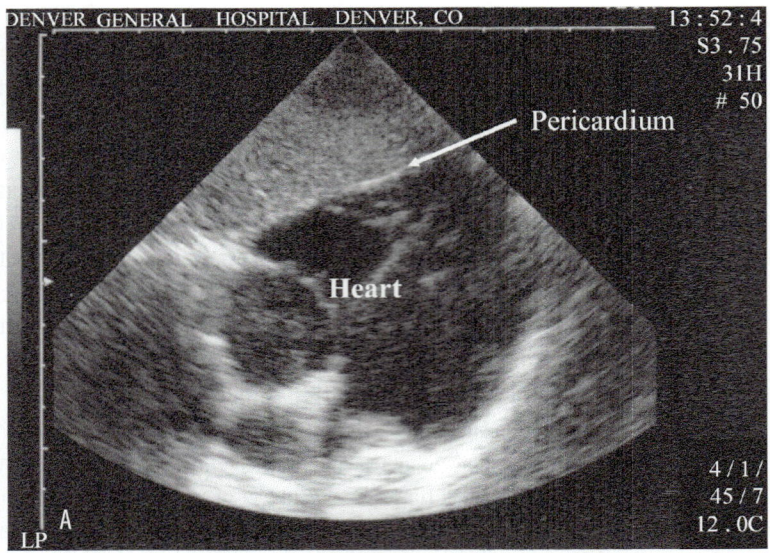
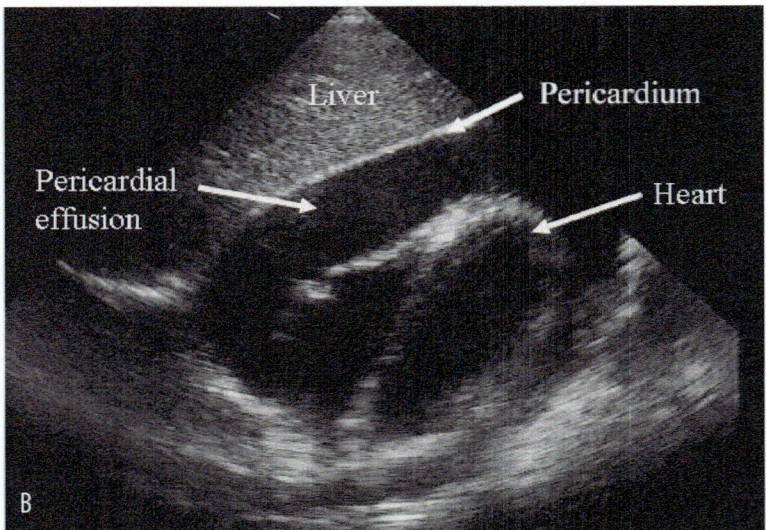

FIGURE 87.2 (a) Ultrasound showing normal exam of the heart and no pericardial fluid. (b) Ultrasound showing the presence of a large pericardial effusion.

15. How can finding an AAA impact prehospital clinical decision-making?

A ruptured AAA is a vascular catastrophe that only a few hospitals are equipped to handle on an emergent basis. Studies have reported mortality rates to be as high as 90% if rupture of an AAA occurs. Interestingly, ED studies have found that patients who had an ultrasound as part of their initial evaluation had a decreased time to diagnosis, operative repair, and mortality. Although no prehospital studies have

Ultrasound in the Field

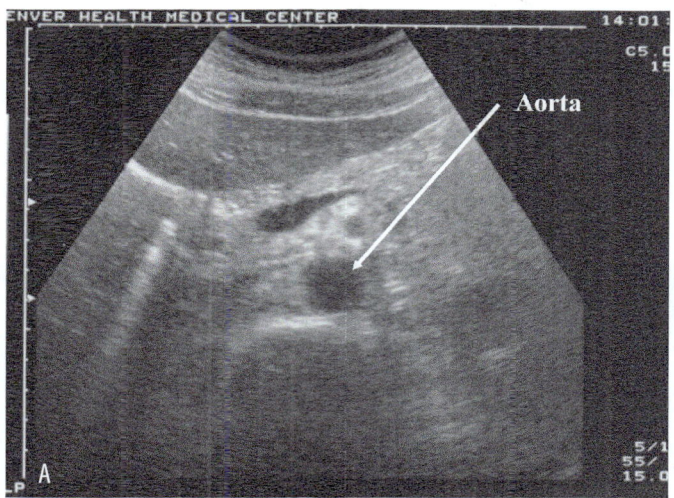

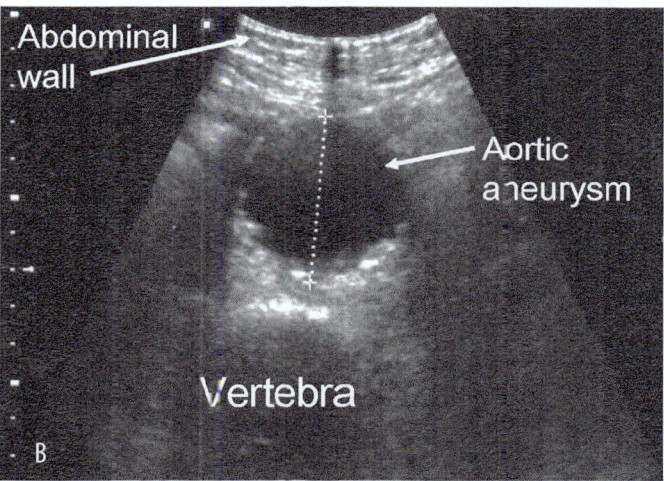

FIGURE 87.3 (a) Ultrasound of the abdomen showing normal aorta. (b) Transverse view of a 4.5-cm AAA.

been performed, it would seem logical that the earlier a suspected ruptured AAA is detected, the greater the chance for a patient's survival. If an AAA is detected, it provides direction for destination to the nearest facility that can perform emergent vascular surgery.

16. **Are there any procedures that ultrasound guidance makes easier, faster, or more successful?**

    Whichever invasive procedure is considered, most likely it can be performed with greater success and a lower complication rate if ultrasound is used to guide it. For instance, one study, which looked at the use of ultrasound in the placement of central lines, demonstrated that the relative risk of failed placement went down by 86% and the relative risk of complications went down by 57%.

Using ultrasound to guide procedures requires that target structures be identified sonographically as well as their surrounding landmarks. If one places the ultrasound transducer over this structure and a needle is inserted in the plane of the ultrasound beam, it can be visualized in real time as it approaches and then enters the target structure, assuring it is correctly placed (Figure 87-4).

In addition to vascular access, other procedures where ultrasound could be useful in the prehospital setting include localization and drainage of pleural or pericardial effusions, confirmation

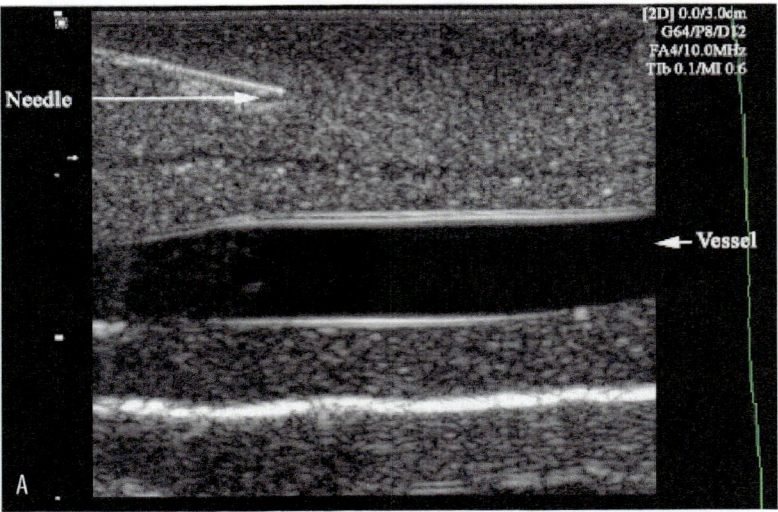

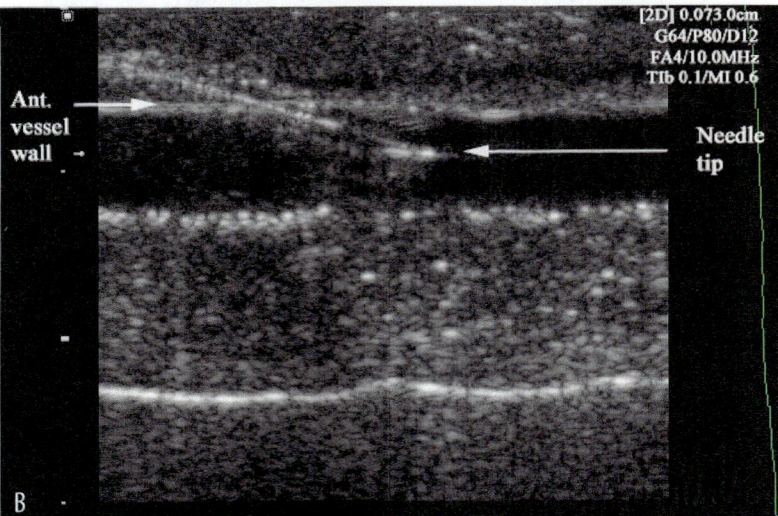

FIGURE 87.4 (a) An image showing the tip and shaft of a needle in the tissue during an ultrasound-guided vascular access. (b) Ultrasound demonstration of successful cannulation of a vessel using real-time guidance.

of endotracheal tube placement, assessing adequacy of compressions during CPR, or confirmation of cardiac pacing.

17. **What other applications may be on the horizon for ultrasound in the prehospital setting?**

    Some possible future areas of ultrasound use in the prehospital setting that have had little or no research as yet include the assessment of patients with undifferentiated hypotension, the early detection of hemoperitoneum in a patient with ectopic pregnancy, the assessment of fetal cardiac activity in the pregnant trauma patient, and evaluating for pneumothorax. Many of these presentations or conditions are currently being studied in the ED environment and may yet make their way to the prehospital setting as well.

Pearls and Pitfalls

1. Emergency ultrasound is a focused exam that can be done quickly in order to answer time-critical diagnostic questions such as whether or not a patient has evidence of intra-abdominal hemorrhage after trauma.
2. The training requirement for focused ultrasound exams is relatively minimal and yields accurate results.
3. Although certain conditions can present with benign peritoneal or pericardial fluid collections, a positive FAST exam in a trauma patient should be assumed to be blood, and the patient should be transported to a trauma center.
4. An abdominal aorta diameter greater than 3 cm is pathologic and considered an aortic aneurysm.
5. If the patient with an ultrasound-documented abdominal aortic aneurysm has hypotension or tachycardia, he or she should be transported emergently to a hospital capable of performing cardiothoracic surgery.

References

1. Walcher F, Weinlich M, Conrad G, et al. Prehospital ultrasound imaging improves management of abdominal trauma. Br J Surg 93:238–242, 2006.
2. Hind D, Calvert N, McWilliams R, et al. Ultrasonic locating devices for central venous cannulation: meta-analysis. BMJ 327:361–367, 2003.

Index

Note: Page references designated as *f* or *t* indicate figures and tables, respectively.

A

Abbreviated Injury Score (AIS-90), 93
Abbreviations, use in documentation, 42, 43*t*
ABCs (airway, breathing, circulation), 542
  of acute coronary syndrome management, 247
  of dysbarism management, 471
  of neck trauma management, 383
  of seizure management, 435–436
  of splinting, 565
  of vomiting management, 297–298
Abdomen
  acute. *see also* Abdominal pain
    definition of, 287
    esophageal rupture-related, 242
  examination of
    in children, 419
    in thoracic trauma patients, 386–387
    unreliable or equivocal, 391
  pain in. *See* Abdominal pain
  traumatic injuries to, 390–393
    pneumatic antishock garment use in, 553
    stab wounds, 388
Abdominal aortic aneurysms
  as abdominal pain cause, 287, 288
  rupture of, 287, 288, 290
Abdominal pain, 287–292
  assessment of, 287, 289
  cardiovascular causes of, 287–288
  in children, 291
  colicky, 289
  in elderly patients, 290–291
  gastrointestinal causes of, 288
  genitourinary causes of, 287, 288–289
  gynecologic-related, in nonpregnant females, 333
  in immunosuppressed patients, 291
  management of, 289–290
  in pregnant patients, 291, 330, 331
Abrasion rings, on entrance wounds, 498
Abruptio placentae, 331, 332
"Accidental Death and Disability, the Neglected Disease of Modern Society," 10

Accreditation
  of EMT-paramedic training, 12
  of medical transport systems, 523
Accrediting agencies, involved with emergency medical services, 75
Acetaminophen, overdose of, 311
Acetazolamide, 328
Acidosis, metabolic
  diabetic ketoacidosis-related, 343, 346–347
  grand mal seizure-related, 281
Acquired immunodeficiency syndrome (AIDS), 117, 118-119. *See also* Human immunodeficiency virus (HIV) infection
Acronyms, 43*t*
Activated charcoal, 310
Acute abdomen. *See also* Abdominal pain
  definition of, 287
  esophageal rupture-related, 242
Acute coronary syndrome (ACS), 228, 245-256. *See also* Myocardial infarction, acute
  assessment of, 247–252, 250*f*, 251*f*, 251*t*
  as chest pain cause, 240
  definition of, 245
  in diabetic patients, 347
  signs and symptoms of, 248
  treatment for, 250*t*, 252–256, 255*f*
Acute mountain sickness (AMS), 326, 327–328
Acute radiation syndrome (ARS), 177–178
Acute respiratory distress syndrome, shock-related, 236
Acyanotic defects, 426–427
Adenosine
  action mechanism of, 220
  contraindication in asthmatic patients, 220
  drug interactions of, 220
  as tachycardia treatment, 219, 220, 220*f*
    failure of, 221
    in supraventricular tachycardia with aberrancy, 222
  use in pregnant patients, 332

583

Index

Adolescents
　delirium in, 259
　drowning-related deaths in, 461
　narcotic overdose in, 426
　vital signs in, 453*f*
Advanced Cardiac Life Support (ACLS), 85–86
　drug dosages in, 231
　efficacy of, 231
　in hypothermic patients, 318
　training course in, 13
Advance directives, 68
Advanced Life Support (ALS) EMS providers, on-line medical direction for, 80
Advanced Life Support (ALS) medical kits, for technical rescues, 511
Aerobic exercise, 103
Aeromedical transport, 515-525. *See also* Helicopter emergency medical services (HEMS); Helicopters
　cost-effectiveness of, 521
　crew members for, 518
　　training of, 518–519
　effect of managed care on, 521
　future of, 524
　versus ground transport, 519–520
　guidelines for, 523
　history of, 7, 515
　integration with ground emergency medical services, 520
　international comparison of, 524
　medical supplies for, 517–518
　models of, 515–516
　patient outcomes in, 522
　physiology of altitude during, 526–528
　program design for, 516
　safety of, 522–523
　selection of aircraft for, 516–517
　start-up and operational costs of, 521
Aggression, in patients, 110-111. *See also* Violent patients
Airborne precautions, 116, 169
Aircraft, pressurized, 527
Air embolism, 183–184, 536
　arterial, 470
　in scuba divers, 37
Air Force, 476
Air Medical Resource Management, 522–523
Air-medical services. *See* Aeromedical transport
Airplane crashes, 146
Airway
　airway, supraglottic devices, 544–545

　cricothyroidostomy, 451–452
　cricothyroidotomy, 548
　injuries to, 382, 383
　pediatric, 417–418
Airway compromise, in spinal cord injury patients, 379
Airway management, 542-549. *See also* Endotracheal intubation; Intubation
　in abdominal trauma patients, 393
　airway assessment in, 199, 542
　in anaphylaxis patients, 337, 338
　in burn patients, 407
　in children, 417–418, 425, 451
　　in respiratory distress, 442–445, 443*f*
　in seizures, 436
　in comatose patients, 264
　in facial burn patients, 404
　in hypothermic patients, 318
　in neck injury patients, 383–384
　pharmacologic agents in, 550–554
　in poisoning patients, 263
　in spinal cord injury patients, 379
　in the tactical environment, 492, 493
　in thoracic trauma patients, 387–388
　in trauma patients, 370–371
　in unconscious patients, 544
Airway obstruction, 386
　common causes of, 543–544
　in infants and children, 417–418, 423, 451, 543
Albuterol, 301, 338, 447–448
Alcoholic patients, thiamine administration in, 348
Alcohols, toxicity of, 310
Alcohol use, adverse effects of, 310
　altered mental status, 260–261, 374
　cancer, 104
　cardiovascular disease, 102, 103
　drowning risk, 461
　emergency calls related to, 108
　gastrointestinal hemorrhage, 294
Alcohol withdrawal, 313
Alexander the Great, 560
Allergies, 335–340
Alpha particles, 174
Altered mental status, 193. *See also* Delirium
　alcohol ingestion-related, 374
　AVPU evaluation system for, 199, 424
　as cerebral perfusion and oxygenation indicator, 193
　in children, 425–426
　definition of, 257
　in diabetic patients, 346, 347

Index

head trauma-related, 373, 374
hyperglycemia-related, 346
implication for hypertension treatment, 274–275
nonketotic hyperosmolar coma-related, 344
pain management in, 570
as violence risk factor, 361
Altitude
　measurement of, 326
　physiology of, 526–528
Altitude illness, 326–329
Amanita muscaria, 314
Amanita phalloides, 314
Ambu bags, 10
Ambulance(s). *See also* Emergency vehicle(s); Emergency vehicle operation
　audible warning devices on, 62
　consistency of care in, 24
　design of, 8
　emergency lights on, 62
　Finley, 5
　"flying," 4, 5
　history of, 3–4, 5–7, 488
　at mass casualty incidents, 154–155, 156
　medicine chests on, 6–7
　parking of, at accident scenes, 112
　physician attendants in, 12
　private services, 73
　response time of, 154
　"undercover," 490f
　volunteer services, 73
Ambulance bypass status, implication for cardiac arrest patients, 37–38
Ambulance companies, quality of, 76
Ambulance drivers, 6
Ambulance personnel, training of, 6, 9
Ambulancias, 4
American Academy of Orthopedic Surgeons, 8
American Association of Poison Control Centers, 309
American Burn Association, 34, 410, 411
American College of Cardiology, 9
American College of Emergency Physicians, 13, 84, 171
American College of Surgeons, 8
　Committee on Trauma, 13, 34
　　Prehospital Care Subcommittee of, 9
American Heart Association
　Guidelines for Cardiopulmonary Resuscitation (CPR) and Emergency Cardiac Care of, 9, 228–230, 229f
　hypertension definition of, 246
American Medical Association, 11, 12, 171

American Nurses Association, 171
American Red Cross, 11
Amiodarone
　dosage in advanced cardiac life support, 231
　ventricular pacemaker-suppressing effect of, 224
　as wide complex tachycardia treatment, 222
Ammonia, 161
Amnesia, lightning strike-related, 481–482
Amphetamines, 313
Amphetamine withdrawal, 314
AMPLE, 199
Amputations
　burn-related, 402
　diabetes-related, 341
　transport destination guidelines for, 36
Anaerobic respiration, 235
Analgesics
　as abdominal pain treatment, 290
　differentiated from sedatives, 572
　masking effect of, 572
　overdose of, 309
Anaphylaxis, 335–340
　bee sting-related, 486
　definition of, 335
　differentiated from allergic reactions, 336
　immune-mediated, 335, 336
　non-immune-mediated, 335, 336
　as shock cause, 235
Aneurysms
　abdominal aortic
　　as abdominal pain cause, 287, 288
　　focused ultrasound examination of, 577, 578–579
　　rupture of, 287, 288, 290
　hypertension-related, 275
　neck injury-related, 383
Angina, 240, 246
　unstable, 240, 246, 247
Angina pectoris, differentiated from acute myocardial infarction, 245
Angioedema, 336
Angiotensin-converting enzyme inhibitors, as angioedema cause, 336
Anthrax, 163
　infection control of, 169
　signs and symptoms of, 165
　transmission of, 114
Anthrax vaccine, 165
Anticholinergic toxidromes, 260, 312t, 313, 314
Anticoagulants, as pesticide components, 313
Antidepressants, overdose of, 310–311

Antiemetics, 299, 572
Antifreeze, toxicity of, 310
Antigens, 335
Antilock braking systems (ABSs), 61
Antiseizure medications, 279, 281
　common, 435t
　noncompliance with, 434
　for pediatric patients, 434, 435t, 436, 437f
Antivenom, for snakebites, 484
Ant stings, 486
Aorta, abdominal
　aneurysms of, 287, 288, 290, 577, 578–579
　focused ultrasound examination of, 577, 578–579, 579f
Aortic dissection, 275
　spontaneous (nontraumatic), 241
Appendicitis, as abdominal pain cause, 288
Arborescent superficial erythema, 481–482, 482f
Army Medical Research Institute of Infectious Diseases, 170–171
Arrington v. Wong, 53–54
Arterial gas embolism, 467, 470, 471
Arteries
　intravenous access-related puncture of, 536, 538
　occlusion of, in extremities, 305–306
Aspiration
　as airway obstruction cause, 543–544
　of foreign objects, 448, 452, 543–544
　vomiting-related, 297–298
　of water, 462
Aspirin
　as acute coronary syndrome treatment, 248, 252–253
　as chest pain treatment, 240
　as gastrointestinal hemorrhage cause, 294
　overdose of, 311
Assessment, prehospital, 198-202. *See also* ABCs (airway, breathing, circulation); *also under specific medical conditions*
　primary, 198–199
　secondary, 199–200, 200f
Assessment, prehospital, 198-202. *See also under specific medical conditions*
　of children, 417–421, 422–423, 426
Association of Air Medical Services, 523
Asterixis, 260, 262
Asthma, 301
　acute attacks of, 447–448
　in children, 447–448
　as contraindication to adenosine, 220

　as pneumothorax cause, 241
　as wheezing cause, 452
Asystole, 210, 223, 223f, 228
Atherosclerosis, 245
Athletes, normal resting pulse in, 223
Ativan. *See* Lorazepam
Atmospheric pressure, 526
Atria, repolarization of, 204
Atrial fibrillation, 209–210, 219, 219f
　with rapid ventricular response, 219
Atrial flutter, 209, 219, 219f, 220f
Atrioventricular (AV) node, 203f, 204
Atrioventricular dissociation, 221f, 222
Atrioventricular heart block, 210
　first degree, 211, 211f
　second degree, 211, 212f, 213f
　　as bradycardia cause, 224, 224f
　third degree, 212, 214f
　　as bradycardia cause, 224, 224f
　　with premature ventricular contractions, 224
Atropine
　as bradycardia treatment, 224
　contraindication as asystole treatment, 223
　dosage in advanced cardiac life support, 231
　as insecticide poisoning treatment, 312–313
　as nerve agent antidote, 159–160, 159f, 160f
Auscultation, abdominal, 391–392
Automatic Vehicle Location systems, 30
Avian influenza virus, 118
AVPU scale, 199, 424

B

Bacillus anthracis. See Anthrax
Backboards, 565–566
Back injuries. *See also* Spinal cord injuries
　avoidance of, 112
Bacteremia, 284
Bag-mask ventilation
　in children, 418, 442, 451–452
　in neck injury patients, 383
　oxygen percentage in, 543
　"squeeze, release, release" technique in, 230, 233, 418
Banks, Sam, 8
Barodentalgia, 467, 470, 471
Barosinusitis, 467, 469, 470
Barotitis, 467, 468–469, 468f
Barotrauma, 242
　in children, 418
　external ear, 467, 469, 470

Index

facial, 467, 469
gastrointestinal, 467, 470, 471
inner ear, 467, 469, 470
middle ear, 467, 468–469, 458f, 470
as pneumothorax cause, 241
Basic Life Support (BLS), 13
Basic Life Support providers, on-line medical direction for, 80
Beck airway airflow monitor (BAAM), 547
Beck's triad, 561
Bedside manner, 46
Bee's stingers, removal of, 486
Bee stings, 335, 486
Behavioral changes, 352
Behavioral emergencies, 350–350
    organic *versus* functional (psychiatric), 350–352
Behavioral factors, in the prehospital environment, 24
Bellevue Hospital, New York City, 5
Benadryl, as hives treatment, 338–339
"Bends," 470
Benner, Ludwig, 503
Benzodiazepines
    adverse effects of, 355
    as chemical restraint, 354–355
    as delirium treatment, 264–265
    as pediatric seizure treatment, 436, 437t
    as sympathomimetic poisoning treatment, 313
    use in rapid sequence intubation, 551
Beta blockers
    as acute coronary syndrome treatment, 254
    overdose of, 311–312
    use in cocaine-using patients, 242
Beta particles, 174
Bethesda Naval Hospital, Casualty Care Research Center of, 488–489
Bezoars, 311
Bias, Ray, 13–14
Bible, references to prehospital care in, 3
Bigelow, Boyd, 7
Binoculars, 504, 505f
"Biocom," 32
Biological terrorism, 67, 163–173
    decontamination in, 167–168, 169
    differentiated from natural epidemics, 163–164, 164
    psychological effects of, 170
    "Ten Commandments of Biological Defense" for, 168–171
    treatment for, 167
Bipolar disorder, 357
Bismuth subsalicylate, 311

Bites
    Gila monster, 485
    snake, 484–485
    spider, 486
Black widow spider bites, 486
Bladder, rupture of, 391
Blast injuries
    common sources of, 180
    mechanistic forces of, 181–182
    nuclear attack-related, 176
    types of, 180–181
Blast lung, 183
Blast overpressure waves, 180, 181, 182–183
Blast winds, 180, 181
Bleeding. *See* Hemorrhage
Blister agents, 158, 161
Blood banks, 488
Blood flow, cerebral, 264
    autoregulation of, 274–275
Blood glucose levels. *See also* Hyperglycemia; Hypoglycemia
    in children, 425
    in diabetic patients, 342, 347
    normal, 341
    unknown, 348
Blood pressure. *See also* Hypertension; Hypotension
    in children, 423
    diastolic, normal, 273
    measurement in supine position, 195
    systolic
        in adolescents, 453t
        age-related differences in, 193–194, 453t
        cerebral blood flow in, 264
        in children, 417, 453t
        in infants, 417, 453t
        normal, 273
Blood pressure measurement
    in acute coronary syndrome patients, 249
    improper sphygmomanometer cuff size in, 196
Blood products, administration of, 237
Blood sugar levels. *See* Blood glucose levels
Blood transfusions, history of, 535
Blood volume, in children, 454
Blunt trauma
    abdominal, 390, 391
    blast-related, 180, 184
    definition of, 368
    to the neck, 382
    spinal, 378

Index

Body armor, concealed, 112
Body composition, 104
Body language, aggressive, 110
Body temperature. *See also* Fever
    in acute coronary syndrome patients, 249
    measurement of, 193, 283
Boerhaave's syndrome, 299
Bone pain, sickle cell disease-related, 306–307
Botulinum toxins/botulism, 163
    protection against, 165
    signs and symptoms of, 166
    treatment for, 167
Bowel
    infarction of, 287
    obstruction of, as abdominal pain cause, 288
    rupture of, 391
Bowel sounds, 391–392
Boyd, John, 499
Boyle, Jon, 13–14
Boyle's law, 465, 466f, 469–470, 526
Bradycardia, 210
    absolute, 223
    atrioventricular block-related, 224, 224f
    butyrophenones-related, 365
    in children, 210, 418, 442
    definition of, 215
    differential diagnosis of, 194–195
    electrocardiogram of, 210–211
    relative, 223
    sinus, 210
        in children, 418
    treatment for, 224, 225
Bradypnea, differential diagnosis of, 195
Brain
    abscess of, as altered mental status cause, 263
    blood flow in, 264
        autoregulation of, 274–275
    herniation of, 373
    in shock, 236
Brainstorming, 94
Brain tumors
    as headache cause, 267
    as seizure cause, 280, 430t
Brake fade, 61
Braking, in emergency vehicle operation, 61–62
Breath, fruity (ketotic) odor of, 261
Breathholding, 461
Breathing. *See also* Airway management; Respiration
    assessment of, 199

    in acute coronary syndrome patients, 249
    "seesaw," 442
    "work of," 440–441, 442
Bronchiolitis, 300, 446
Broselow tape, 442, 443f, 454
Brucellosis, 163, 169
Bruises (contusions), 367
    cardiac, 387
    child abuse-related, 397–398, 457
    pulmonary, 387–388
Bubonic plague, 164
Buddy Care for the Military, 488
Buerger's disease, 306
Buildings
    collapses of, 137f, 508
    fires in, 402
        as multiple casualty incidents, 152, 155–156
        scene safety at, 155
    as protection from lightning, 481
Bulletin of the American College of Surgeons, 8
Bullet-resistant body armor, 112
Bundle-branch blocks, 213–214
    left, 209, 250
    right, 209
Burn centers, 37, 410
    referrals to, 412
Burnout, 124–125
Burn patients, 34
    intravenous access in, 537
    transport destinations for, 37
Burns, 156. *See also* Chemical burns; Electrical burns; Thermal burns in children, 450
    child abuse-related, 398, 406, 407f, 457
    lightning strike-related, 480, 482
    radiation-related, 174–175, 177, 178
Butyrophenones, cardiovascular side effects of, 365

C

CAD. *See* Coronary artery disease
CAD (Computer Aided Dispatch), 30–31, 77
Caesar, 3
Calcium channel blockers
    contraindication as wide complex tachycardia treatment, 221
    overdose of, 311
Callback numbers, 28, 30
Calls, most dangerous, 108
Campbell, John, 13

Index

Cancer
    as abdominal pain cause, 290
    as delirium cause, 258
    as mortality cause, 101
    risk assessment for, 104
    screening tests for, 104, 105t, 107
    smoking-related, 101–102, 104
    warning signs of, 104–105, 105t
Capillary refill time (CRT)
    in children, 418, 423
    in shock patients, 452
Capnography, 303, 441
Carbamate insecticides, 312, 312t
Carbamazepine, interaction with adenosine, 220
Carbon dioxide, end tidal (EtCO$_2$), 303
Carbon monoxide poisoning, 37, 260, 314, 526–527
    in burn patients, 412
    diving-related, 470
Cardiac arrest, 228–233
    chain of survival in, 254–256
    in children, 231, 442, 444
        seizure-related, 436
    information about, 233
    lightning strike-related, 481
    pneumatic antishock garment use in, 553
    in pregnant patients, 232, 332
    survival rate in, 228, 230
        as continuous quality improvement measure, 93
    tension pneumothorax-related, 561
    traumatic *versus* nontraumatic, 232
    treatment for, 222
        mild therapeutic hypothermia, 231–232
    ventilation rate in, 230
Cardiac arrest patients, transport destinations for, 37–38
Cardiac care
    defibrillator use in, 8–9
    training in, 9
Cardiac cycle, 204–205, 205f
Cardiac disease. *See* Cardiovascular disease
Cardiac reserve, age-related differences in, 194
Cardiopulmonary resuscitation (CPR)
    CPR Directives, 68
    before defibrillation, 230
    development of, 9–10
    guidelines for, 228–230, 229f
    in hyperthermic patients, 317
    in lightning strike victims, 481
    termination of, 232
    in ventricular tachycardia patients, 222

Cardiovascular disease. *See also specific types of cardiovascular disease*
    diabetes-related, 341
    as mortality cause, 12, 101
    risk factors for, 101–102, 240
    risk reduction for, 102–103
Cardiovascular endurance, 103
Cardiovascular medications, 248
    overdose of, 311–312
Cardioversion, synchronized, 222
Cardozo, Benjamin, 50–51
Care under fire, 493, 494
Carmona, Richard, 488
Caroline, Nancy, 11
Casualty evacuation care (Casevac), 493, 494, 495f
Catecholamines, 106
Causation, 48
Cell phones, 144
    disruption during disasters, 150
Cellulitis, 307
    implication for intravenous access, 537
Centers for Disease Control and Prevention (CDC), 117, 170–171
Central lines, 540
Central nervous system, effect of hypertension on, 274
Cerebral vascular accidents (CVA). *See* Stroke
Certification, of emergency medical services technicians, 76, 473
Cervical collars, 420, 450, 565–566
Cervical spine
    immobilization of
        with cervical collars, 420, 450, 565–566
        in children, 420
        with Philadelphia collars, 56
        in seizure patients, 281
        in submersion victims, 463–464
        management in anterior neck injury patients, 384
    traumatic injuries to, 262–263
        in children, 418, 450–451
        as respiratory compromise cause, 378
Cesarean sections, 332
Chain of survival, 254–256
    tactical medics' role in, 489–490
Charcot's paralysis, 480
Charity Hospital, New Orleans, Louisiana, 6
Charles' law, 465, 526
CHART format, for medical information organization, 40–41
Chemical agents, of mass destruction, 158–162

589

Index

Chemical burns
  dressings for, 403
  treatment for, 404–405
Chemical restraint, 111, 354–355, 364–365, 364t
Chemical spills, 146
Chemtel, 504
Chemtrec, 504
Chest
  circumferential third-degree burns of, 407
  traumatic injuries to, 386–389
    in children, 452
    evaluation of, 386–387
    pneumatic antishock garments use in, 556, 557, 558
    treatment for, 387–388
Chest compressions, 228–230, 229f, 233
  in water, 464
Chest pain, 239–244
  acute coronary syndrome-related, 247–248
  angina, 240
    unstable, 240, 246, 247
  angina pectoris, differentiated from acute myocardial infarction, 245
  assessment of, 239–240, 247–248
  in children, 243
  in elderly patients, 243
  life-threatening causes of, 239
  pathophysiology of, 239
  pleuritic, 300
  pulmonary embolism-related, 240–241
  treatment for, 240
Chewing tobacco, 102
Chicago Fire Department, 8
Chicken pox, 116
Child abuse, 402, 456–458
  assessment of, 427
  burns as, 398, 406, 407f, 457
  categories of, 397, 456
  cause of, 397
  recognition of, 397–398, 456–457
  reporting of, 398, 456
Child neglect, 397, 398, 456, 457
Child Protective Services (CPS), 456, 457
Children. *See also* Infants; Neonates
  abdominal pain in, 291
  abdominal trauma in, 392
  advanced life support drug doses for, 231
  airway obstruction in, 417–418, 423, 451, 543
  alcohol-related hypoglycemia in, 261
  anaphylaxis treatment in, 339
  anatomy of, 422
  assessment of, 417–421, 422–423
    in children with special health care needs, 426
  backboard use with, 565
  bronchiolitis in, 300
  burns in, 402
    estimation of size of, 405–406
  cardiac arrest in, 231, 436, 442, 444
  cardiac reserve in, 194
  chest pain in, 243
  cigarette smoke exposure in, 102
  critically ill or injured, 425
  deaths of, 130
  delirium in, 259, 263
  diabetic, dextrose administration in, 348
  diarrhea in, 298
  drowning-related deaths in, 461
  endotracheal tube size for, 231, 545–546
  fever in, 259, 284
    as delirium cause, 263
    as seizure cause, 263, 278, 285, 430t, 433–434, 433t, 436
  field approach to, 422–428
  FOOSH injuries in, 304
  gastrointestinal hemorrhage in, 295
  hypothermia in, 316, 319
  intravenous access in, 538
  mortality causes in, 450
  neutral position in, 379, 380
  "nursemaid's elbow" in, 306
  occiput size in, 418, 450
  pain assessment in, 569–570
  poisonings in, 309
  respiratory distress in, 439–449
  seizures in, 429–438
    febrile, 263, 278, 285, 433–434, 433t, 436
  sickle cell crisis in, 307
  stroke in, 271
  trauma in, 450–455
  vital signs in, 193–194, 417, 452–453, 453f
  vomiting in, 298
Children's hospitals, as trauma centers, 36
Chlorine, 161
Cholelithiasis, as abdominal pain cause, 288
Cholesterol, 102, 102t, 103
  as cardiovascular disease risk factor, 240, 246
  high-density lipoprotein (HDL), 246
  low-density lipoprotein (LDL), 102, 102t

Cholinergic toxidromes, 312*t*
Chronic complaints, recurrent, 196
Chronic obstructive pulmonary disease (COPD), 252, 526–527
    as contraindication to morphine, 300
    differentiated from congestive heart failure, 300
Cialis, 248
Cieslak, Ted, 168
Cigarette smoking. *See* Smoking
Cincinnati Prehospital Stroke Scale (CPSS), 269
Circulation assessment, 199
    in children, 418, 422, 423
Civil liberties, violations of, 111
Civil War, 5
Cleveland, Henry, 7
Clinical instability, of cardiac dysrhythmia patients, 218
Clothing
    of chemical burn patients, 404
    protective. *See* Personal protective equipment
    removal of, as hypothermia cause, 319
Coarctation of the aorta, 418
Coast Guard, 476
Cobb, Leonard, 10
Cocaine, 242, 313
Cocaine withdrawal, 313, 314
Codeine, 262
Coelenterate stings, 485
"Coffee grounds," vomiting of, 293, 298
Cold water, submersion in, 463
Cold zones, 405, 504
Colle, Giovanni Francisco, 535
Collicutt, Paul "Skip," 13
Colorado tick fever, 486
Coma
    alcohol use-related, 261
    head injury-related, 263
    nonketotic hyperosmolar, 344, 347*t*
Comatose patients, airway management in, 264
Commission on Accreditation of Allied Health Education Programs (CAAHEP), 76
Commission on Accreditation of Medical Transport Systems (CAMTS), 523
Communicable diseases. *See also* Infectious diseases exposures
    definition of, 114
    signs and symptoms of, 117
    transmission of, 114
Communication(s), 26-33. *See also* Dispatch system; Radio communication
    during biological terrorism events, 170
    during casualty incident responses, 138, 144
    during disaster situations, 150, 151
    disruptions in, 138, 144
    E911, 27
    interoperable systems of, 150
    911, 26
    nonverbal, 361, 361*t*
    Public Safety Answering Point ("peesap"), 27
Community, emergency medical services for, 16–17
Community standard, of care, 47–48
Compartment syndrome, 305
Compazine, 299
Computer Aided Dispatch (CAD), 30–31, 77
Conduction, as heat loss mechanism, 283, 316
Cone shell stings, 485
Confidentiality
    in continuous quality improvement, 95
    patient, 69
Confusion. *See also* Altered mental status
    medical *versus* psychiatric, 257–258
Congestive heart failure, 246, 301
    in children, 426–427
    differentiated from chronic obstructive pulmonary disease (COPD), 300
Consent. *See also* Informed consent
    emergency exception from, 67
    for minors, 51–52
    presumed, 67
Contact precautions, 116
Continuous positive airway pressure (CPAP), 253, 301
Continuous quality improvement (CQI), 90, 91–96
    checksheets in, 94
    components of, 91–92
    differentiated from quality assurance, 90–91
    examples of, 95
    legal issues in, 95–96
    model of, 93
    "six Ds" of, 92
    tools for, 94
Contractures, electrical injury-related, 408
Control charts, 94
Contusions (bruises), 367
    cardiac, 387
    child abuse-related, 397–398, 457
    pulmonary, 387–388
Convection, as heat loss mechanism, 283, 316
Cooling, as heat stroke treatment, 324
Coordination, in incident management, 137, 139

Index

Core temperature afterdrop, 319
Coronary artery disease (CAD)
    as chest pain cause, 239, 240
    definition of, 245
    as mortality cause, 239
    physical examination for, 240
    prevalence of, 245–246
    risk factors for, 246
Cough
    chronic obstructive pulmonary disease-related, 252
    croup-related, 445, 446t
    pneumonia-related, 252
    tuberculosis-related, 117
Counter Narcotics Tactical Operations Medical Support (CONTOMS), 488–489
Coworkers, peer support for, 131–132
CPR Directives, 68
CPSS (Cincinnati Prehospital Stroke Scale), 269
Cricothyroidostomy, 451–452
Cricothyroidotomy, 548
    in the tactical environment, 493, 494
Crile, George W., 9, 556–557
Crimean-Congo hemorrhagic fever, 165, 167
Crimean War, 488
Critical illness, in pregnant patients, 333
Critical incidents, definition of, 122
Critical incident stress, 122–133
    differentiated from everyday stress, 123
Critical incident stress debriefings, 125–126, 128t, 132
    components of, 129
    differentiated from
        critical incident stress defusings, 127, 129
        critical incident stress management, 126
    preeducation about, 127
Critical incident stress defusings, 127, 128t, 129, 130, 132
Critical incident stress management
    definition of, 144
    differentiated from
        critical incident stress debriefings, 126
        therapy, 131
    evaluation of need for, 126–127
    family members' role in, 129–130
    peer support in, 131–132
    preincident education in, 128t, 132
    types of interventions in, 127, 128t
Critical incident stress management teams, 131
Croup, 442, 445–446, 446t
    comparison with epiglottitis, 445t
Crystalloid therapy, in children, 424
"Customers," 23

Cyanide poisoning, 34, 158, 161–162, 314
Cyanogen chloride, 158, 161
Cyanokit, 161
Cystitis, 289
Cysts, ovarian, rupture of, 289

D

Dactylitis, 307
Dalton's law, 465, 526
Danger. *See also* Personal safety and wellness; Scene safety; Violent patients
    in emergency vehicle operation, 62
    red flags of, 110
Dangerous patients. *See also* Violent patients
    psychotic patients as, 352–353
"Deadly dozen," 386
Death
    of children, 130
    preventable, 101–102
    as triage category, 143, 154
"Death in a Ditch" (Farrington), 8
Debriefings, critical incident stress, 125–126, 127, 128t, 129, 132
Decision-making capacity (DMC), 67, 68
Decompression illnesses/sickness, 37, 465–472, 527
Decontamination
    in bioterrorism events, 167–168, 169
    of chemical burn patients, 404–405
    gastrointestinal, 310
    in poison exposures, 264, 310
    in radiologic attacks/disasters, 176, 177, 178
Deep venous thrombosis, 306
Defensive driving courses, 56
Defibrillation
    in children, 231
    in hypothermic patients, 318
    in torsades de pointes patients, 225
    as ventricular fibrillation treatment, 228
    as ventricular tachycardia treatment, 222
Defibrillators
    AC, 8–9
    automated external, 189
    DC, 9
    development of, 9
    training in use of, 29
Dehydration
    diabetic ketoacidosis-related, 261, 343
    fever-related, 285
    hyperglycemia-related, 346
    respiratory syncytial virus (RSV)-related, 446–447

Delayed category, of triage, 143, 149, 154
DELIRIOUS EMT-Ps mnemonic, for delirium etiology, 260
Delirium, 257–266
    causes of, 259–264
    definition of, 257
    diagnosis of, 259
    excited, 363
    hyperactive, 257–258
    hypoactive, 257–258
    postoperative, 258
    prevalence of, 258
    resolution of, 258
    risk for, 258
    treatment for, 264–265
    withdrawal-related, 313
Delusions, 352, 357
Demerol, 262, 571t
Deming, W. Edwards, 91
Denali National Park, 476
Dengue fever, 167
Denver Metropolitan EMS Medical Directors organization, 86
Deployment, fixed *versus* dynamic, 20
Depositions, in malpractice lawsuits, 49–50
Depression, 355
Depth perception, 57, 58
Destinations, in prehospital transport. *See* Transport destinations
Detoxification, of poisoning patients, 263
Dexamethasone, 328
Dextrose, as hypoglycemia treatment, 347–348
Diabetes mellitus, 341–349
    as cardiovascular disease risk factor, 240, 246
    in children, 426
    definition of, 341
    gestational, 342–343
    medical emergencies in, 343–348, 347t
    type II (non-insulin-dependent), 342, 343, 343t
    type 1 (insulin-dependent), 341, 342, 343–344, 343t
Diabetic patients
    assessment of, 261, 345
    bacterial infections in, 285
    management strategies for, 346–348
Diagnosis, in prehospital patient assessment, 201
Diagnostic and Statistical Manual of Mental Disorders (DSM IV-TR), 257
Diaphragm
    penetrating injuries to, 391
    rupture of, as contraindication to pneumatic antishock garments, 557

Diarrhea, 156, 298
    in children, 298
    in geriatric patients, 298
    as mass casualty incident, 156
Diastat™, 281
Diazepam
    as chemical restraint, 364t
    as seizure treatment, 281
    in children, 436, 437t
Dickens, Charles, 148
Diet
    for cancer prevention, 104
    healthful, 106, 107
Differential diagnosis, formulation of, 196
Dignitary protection, 491
Digoxin, overdose of, 312
Dilaudid, 262, 571t
Diltiazem, as tachycardia treatment, 221
Dimick, Alan, 9
Dineen, Joseph, 13–14
Diphenhydramine, as hives treatment, 338–339
Diphenoxylate, 262
Dipyridamole, interaction with adenosine, 220
Disaster(s), 146–151
    definition of, 137, 144, 146
    differentiated from mass casualty incidents, 146
    human-caused, 146
    media relations during, 151
    medical direction during, 87
    natural, 146
    as stress cause, 123, 130
    triage in, 69
    types of, 146
Disaster management teams, 147
Disaster response plans, 147, 153–154
    activation phase of, 147
    command structure of, 148
    implementation phase of, 147, 148
    for mass gatherings, 186–187
    mitigation phase of, 147, 148
    recovery phase of, 147, 148
Dislocations, 306, 567
Dispatchers
    cardiopulmonary resuscitation instructions from, 10
    responsibilities of, 31, 77
    role in medical care, 15
    safety functions provided by, 28
    training of, 77
    transport destination determination by, 31

Index

Dispatch protocols, differentiated from field protocols, 28–29
Dispatch system, 26, 28-29. *See also* Medical directors; Medical direction
    CAD (Computer Aided Dispatch), 30–31, 77
    definition of, 73
    as "heart of the EMS system," 26
    location of, 73
Distraction therapy, 570
Distress, 123
Diver Alert Network, 471, 478
Diverticulitis
    as abdominal pain cause, 288, 290
    as gastrointestinal hemorrhage cause, 294
Diving disorders. *See* Dysbarisms
DNARs (do-not-attempt resuscitation) orders, 68
DNRs (do-not-resuscitate orders), 50
Doan's Pills, 311
Documentation, 39–44
    abbreviation use in, 42, 43*t*
    guidelines for, 39–40
    for malpractice lawsuit prevention, 46, 54
    at mass gatherings, 189
Domestic violence calls, 108. *See also* Intimate partner violence
Do-not-attempt resuscitation (DNAR) orders, 68
Do-not-resuscitate orders (DNRs), 50
Dopamine, as bradycardia treatment, 224
Dressings
    Israeli battle, 496*f*
    use in tactical environment, 495, 496*f*
Droperidol, as chemical restraint, 355, 364*t*, 365
Droplet precautions, 116
Drowning
    in children, 450
    definition of, 461
    "dry," 461–462
    in saltwater *versus* freshwater, 462
Drowning persons, rescue of, 463–464
Drug abuse. *See also* Cocaine
    emergency calls related to, 108
    as violence risk factor, 361
Drug Enforcement Agency (DEA), 488–489
Drug intoxication, as psychosis cause, 352
Drug overdose, 309–315
    in adolescents, 426
    as seizure cause, 281
Drug-seeking behavior, 572
Drug withdrawal syndromes, 352

Duke University Medical Center, Diver Alert Network of, 471, 478
Duodenal ulcers, as abdominal pain cause, 287, 288
Duodote™ autoinjector, 160, 160*f*
DuoNeb, 447–448
Durable powers of attorney, 50, 68
Duty, 67
Dysbarisms, 465–472
    differential diagnoses of, 467–468
    as disorders of ascent, 467, 469–470
    as disorders of depth, 467, 469
    as disorders of descent, 467, 468–469
    recompression therapy for, 470–471
Dyspnea, 300–303
    definition of, 300
    pulmonary embolism-related, 240–241
Dysrhythmias, cardiac, 218-227. *See also* Bradycardia; Tachycardia
    in children, 418
    clinical instability of, 218
    electrical injury-related, 408
    electrocardiogram findings in, 210–215
    hemodynamic instability of, 218
    regularity *versus* irregularity of, 219

E

Ear, anatomy of, 467*f*
"Ear squeeze," 467, 468–469, 468*f*, 470
Earthquakes, 146
Eastern Kentucky University, 12
Eberhardt v. City of Los Angeles, 53
Ebola virus, 163, 164, 165, 167
Echocardiography, 576
Eclampsia, 276, 281
    differentiated from preeclampsia, 331
Edema
    burn-related, 407
    high-altitude cerebral (HACE), 326, 327
    histamine-related, 336
    implication for intravenous access, 537
    pulmonary, 246
        acute, 301
        acute coronary syndrome-related, 254
        as contraindication to pneumatic antishock garments, 557
        high-altitude pulmonary (HAPE), 302, 326, 327
        saltwater aspiration-related, 462
        severe hypertension-related, 274

Index

Education programs. *See also* Training
  involved with emergency medical services, 75
Edwin Smith papyrus, 3
Effectiveness, of prehospital interventions, 531–534
Efficacy, of prehospital interventions, 531–534
Elam, James, 9, 10
Elder abuse, 397, 400
Elderly patients
  abdominal aortic evaluation in, 577
  abdominal pain in, 290–291
  airway obstruction in, 543–544
  chest pain in, 243
  delirium in, 258, 260, 264
  diarrhea in, 298
  gastrointestinal hemorrhage in, 295
  hypothermia in, 316, 319
  vital signs in, 194
  vomiting in, 298
Elder neglect, 400
Electrical burns, 408–409, 409*f*
Electrical flash arc injuries, 409
Electrical stun devices, 265, 365, 498–499
Electrocardiogram (ECG)
  applications of, 203–217
    asystole, 223, 223*f*
    atrial fibrillation, 219*f*
    atrial flutter, 219*f*
    atria repolarization, 204
    atrioventricular heart blocks, 211, 211*f*, 212, 212*f*, 213*f*, 214*f*
    atrioventricular node reentry tachycardia, 218*f*, 220*f*
    bradycardia, 210–211
    dysrhythmias, 210–215, 210*f*, 211*f*, 212*f*, 213*f*, 214*f*, 215*f*, 216*f*
    heart rate calculation, 207–209, 208*f*
    hypothermia, 320*f*
    left bundle-branch blocks, 209
    multifocal atrial tachycardia, 219*f*
    myocardial infarction, 215
    premature atrial contractions (PACs), 209
    premature ventricular contractions (PVCs), 226*f*
    pulseless electrical activity (PEA), 210
    pulseless ventricular tachycardia, 210
    right bundle-branch blocks, 209
    tachycardia, 210, 212–214
    torsades de pointes, 225*f*
    ventricular fibrillation, 210, 210*f*
    Wolff-Parkinson-White syndrome, 218*f*
  axis in, 206, 207*f*
  cardiac cycle in, 204–205, 205*f*
  definition of, 203, 204
  normal, 205
  obtaining of, 205–206
  PR interval in, 205, 205*f*, 211, 212, 214*f*
  PR segment in, 205*f*
  P wave in, 204, 205*f*, 209–210, 211, 212, 214, 214*f*, 221*f*
  QRS complex in, 205, 205*f*, 206, 209–210, 211–212, 214*f*
  QRS interval in, 205
  QRS wave in, 204
  QRS width in, 209
  R wave in, 204
  R' wave in, 204
  ST segment in, 205, 205*f*
  S wave in, 204
  transmission via radio, 32
  T wave in, 205*f*
  12-lead, 205, 216
    for acute coronary syndrome evaluation, 249–250, 250*t*, 251*f*, 251*t*, 252, 254
    for chest pain evaluation, 239
    role in prehospital environment, 243
Electroconvulsive devices (ECDs). *See* Electrical stun devices
Elisha (prophet), 3
Emaciated patients, thiamine administration in, 348
Embolism
  air, 183–184, 536
  arterial, 470
  in scuba divers, 37
  arterial gas, 467, 470, 471
  pulmonary, 240–241, 289, 302, 526–527
"Emergency Care in the Streets," 11
Emergency departments (EDs)
  electrocardiogram (ECG) interpretation in, 203
  as emergency medical system component, 16, 17
  mass casualty incident patient transport to, 157
  mass casualty incident plans of, 157
Emergency exception, from consent, 67
Emergency Medical Dispatch, 28–29. *See also* Dispatch system
Emergency Medical Services Act, 12, 83
Emergency medical services (EMS) providers. *See also* Emergency medical technicians (EMTs)
  lifestyle risks of, 101
  occupational fatality rate of, 101

595

Index

Emergency medical services (EMS) systems
    agencies and organizations involved with, 74–75
    community services of, 16–17
    components of, 15
    definition of, 73
    design and service delivery models of, 16
        comparison of, 18
        definition of, 15
        performance hallmarks for, 21–22
        rationale for, 18–19
        tiered, 19–20
    emergency department component of, 16, 17
    "father" of, 8
    government funding for, 12
    "heart" of, 26
    organization of, 16
    organizations participating in, 73–74
    specialized components of, 16
    standardized performance metrics for, 20–21
    Star of Life emblem of, 11
    status management of, 20
Emergency Medical Technician-Ambulance training programs, 11
Emergency Medical Technician-D (Emergency Medical Technician-Defibrillator), 29
Emergency Medical Technician-Paramedic training programs, 11, 12
Emergency medical technicians (EMTs)
    urban, 473
    wilderness (WEMTs), 473–474
Emergency Medical Treatment and Active Labor Act (EMTALA), 52–54
Emergency Nurses Association, 171
Emergency patients, types of, 12–13
Emergency responses, speed of, 56
"Emergency!" (television program), 11
Emergency vehicle(s)
    audible warning devices on, 62
    emergency lights on, 62
    gridlock of, 155
    ingress and egress routes for, 139–140, 140*f*, 141*f*
    organization of, 139–140, 140*f*, 141*f*
Emergency vehicle operation, 56–63
    braking in, 61–62
    effect of weather conditions on, 60
    most dangerous situations in, 62
    negotiation of skids, 62
    negotiation of turns and curves, 61–62
    at night, 58–59

"onboard computer" use in, 57
    role of vision in, 57–58, 60
    training in, 56–57, 63
    in urban *versus* rural areas, 60
    vehicle handling problems in, 59–60
Emesis. *See* Vomiting
Emotional abuse, of children, 397
Emphysema, 241, 470
EMS Agenda for the Future, 73, 85
EMS Performance Measures Project, 20–21
EMTALA (Emergency Medical Treatment and Active Labor Act), 52–53
Encephalitis
    as altered mental status cause, 263
    as headache cause, 267
    as seizure cause, 280–281, 430*t*
Encephalopathy
    hepatic, 260
    hypertensive, 274
    Wernicke's, 348
Endotracheal intubation
    advantages and disadvantages of, 545
    in children, alternatives to, 442
    in facial burn patients, 404
    in hypothermic patients, 318
    indications for, 545
Endotracheal tubes
    cuffed, 546
    cuff pressure of, 527
    placement of, 546
    size of, 545
        for children, 231, 442, 444, 451, 545–546
E911, 27
Enterococcus, vancomycin-resistant (VRE), 116
Entry wounds, 367–368
    documentation of, 498
Envenomations, 484–487
Environmental Protection Agency (EPA), 405
Epididymitis, as abdominal pain cause, 289
Epiglottitis, 446
    comparison with croup, 445*t*
Epilepsy, 278, 281. *See also* Seizures
    in children, 429
    definition of, 429
    relationship to febrile seizures, 433
Epinephrine
    as anaphylaxis treatment, 337, 338–339
    as asystole treatment, 223
    as bradycardia treatment, 224

Index

as cardiac arrest treatment, 222, 231
contraindication to, 339
dosage in advanced cardiac life support, 231
intramuscular administration of, 338
subcutaneous administration of, 338
Erythema, arborescent superficial, 481–482, 432f
Escharotomy, 407, 408f
Eschars, 407
Esophagus
injuries to, 382, 384
rupture of, 239, 242, 299
Essential List of Supplies for Ambulances, 8
Ethanol, toxicity of, 310
Ethics and ethical dilemmas, in emergency medical services, 67–70
differentiated from the law, 67
in wilderness emergency medical services, 477–478
Ethylene glycol, toxicity of, 310
Etomidate, use in rapid sequence intubation, 551–552, 552t
Eustress, 123
Evaporation, as heat loss mechanism, 283, 315
Everly, George, 126
Exit wounds, 368
documentation of, 498
Expectant category, of triage, 149, 154
Explosions, industrial, 146
Explosives
classes of, 180
as weapons of mass destruction, 180–185
Exposure, of patients, 199
Exsanguination, 391, 493
Extravasation, into interstitial space, 538
Extremities
arterial occlusion of, 305–306
circumferential third-degree burns of, 407, 408f
as intravenous access sites, 535–538
ischemia of, 305–306
pain in, 304–308
pulseless, 305
splinting of, 565–568
Extrication, of patients
from motor vehicles, 155
responsibility for, 473
in urban emergency medical services, 473
in wilderness emergency medical services, 473
Eyes, blast-related injuries to, 183
Eyewear, protective, 115

F

Face, burns to, 404
FACES pain assessment chart, 420f, 424, 569–570
Fainting. See Syncope
Falls
in children, 450
as injury cause, 156
Family
role in stress management, 129–130
withholding of resuscitation requests from, 68
Farrington, J.D. "Deke," 8–9, 11, 12
Farrington era, of emergency medical services, 8–12
FAST (focused assessment with sonography for trauma) examination, 574, 575–576, 576f
Federal agencies. See also specific federal agencies
involved with emergency medical services, 74
Federal Aviation Administration (FAA), 522–523
Federal Emergency Management Agency (FEMA), 476
Femur
fractures of
child abuse-related, 397
splinting of, 557
as intraosseous infusion site, 419, 419f
Fentanyl, 572
Fentanyl citrate, 571t
Ferning, 481–482, 432f
Fetor hepaticus, 260
Fetus, care for, 332
Fever, 283–286
as altered mental status cause, 263
in children, 259
as seizure cause, 263, 278, 285, 430t, 433–434, 433t, 436
definition of, 283
as delirium cause, 259, 263
meningitis-related, 117
methods for lowering of, 285
pulmonary embolism-related, 241
Fibrinolytic therapy, 243–244, 254, 255t, 270
"Fight-or-flight" mechanism, 106, 110
Filoviruses, 167
Fire coral stings, 485
Fire departments. See also Firefighting agencies
as emergency medical services system component, 73
as lead agencies at fire scenes, 155
responsibility for patient extrication, 473
Firefighters
as ambulance attendants, 8
occupational fatality rate of, 101

Index

Firefighting agencies, Incident Command System of, 142
Fires
    in buildings, 402
        as multiple casualty incidents, 152, 155–156
        scene safety at, 155
    wildfires, 142
First aid rooms, 187
"First in, last out" concept, 154–155
Fish, venomous, 485
Fishbone diagrams, 94
"Five Ps," 305
Flail chest, 387–388
    in children, 452
Flashover phenomenon, 480
Floods, 146
Flowcharts, process, 94
Fluid resuscitation
    in abdominal trauma patients, 393
    in burn patients, 411
    in children, 424, 453–454
    in hypothermic patients, 318
    in hypovolemic patients, 371
    as "overresuscitation," 388
    Parkland formula for, 411
    in penetrating chest trauma patients, 387, 388
    in shock patients, 236–237
        pediatric, 453–454
Focused assessment with sonography for trauma (FAST) examination, 574, 575–576, 576*f*
Folli, Francisco, 535
Food, as airway obstruction cause, 543–544
Food allergies, 335
Food Allergy and Anaphylaxis Network, 335
Food and Drug Administration, 8
Food poisoning, 298
FOOSH injuries, 304
Foot, electrical injury of, 409*f*
Foreign bodies, aspiration of, 452
    as airway obstruction cause, 543–544
        removal of, 544
    in children, 448
Fractals, 481–482, 482*f*
Fracture-dislocations, with distal ischemia, 567
Fractures, 367
    electrical injury-related, 408
    of the femur
        child abuse-related, 397
        splinting of, 557
    of the hip, 304
    open, 567
    pelvic, 394–396
        "open-book," 394–395
    splinting of, 566–567
Franciscella tularensis. *See* Tularemia
Free Hospital of New York, 5
Frostbite, 319
Frozen tissues, thawing of, 319
Funeral homes, prehospital transportation provided by, 5, 7
Furosemide (Lasix™), 254, 274
Fusion beats, 214, 215*f*, 222
Futility, of medical treatment, 68

G

Gallstones, 289
Gamma radiation, 174
Gastric ulcers, as abdominal pain cause, 287, 288
Gastritis, as abdominal pain cause, 288
Gastroenteritis, as abdominal pain cause, 288
Gastrointestinal disorders, as abdominal pain cause, 288
Gastrointestinal tract
    blast-related injuries to, 184
    decontamination of, 310
General gas law, 465
General Hospital, Cincinnati, Ohio, 5
Genitouriary system, pelvic frature-related injuries to, 395
Genitourinary disorders, as abdominal pain cause, 287, 288–289
Geriatric patients. *See* Elderly patients
Gila monster bites, 485
Glanders, 163, 169
Glasgow Coma Scale (GCS), 262, 374–375
    pediatric, 424, 454
Glaucoma, as contraindication to ipratropium, 448
Global awareness, 109–110
Gloves, protective, 115
Glucagon, 342, 348
    as anaphylaxis treatment, 339
"Golden hour," 369
Good Samaritan, 3
Good Samaritan laws, 477
Gout, 307
Gowns, surgical, 115
Grand Teton National Park, 475, 476
Gray Hospital, Atlanta, Georgia, 6–7
Greece, ancient, prehospital care in, 3–4
Greenberg, Myles, 92

Index

Gunmen, barricaded, 492
Gunshot wounds, 108, 367–368, 368f
   as multiple casualty incidents, 156
   to the neck, 382
   as pediatric mortality cause, 450
   as spinal cord injury cause, 378

H

HACE (high-altitude cerebral edema), 326, 327
Haldol™, 364t, 365
Hallucinations
   auditory, 352
   definition of, 352
   delirium-related, 257
   olfactory, 352
   tactile, 352
   taste, 352
   visual, 258, 352
   withdrawal-related, 313
Haloperidol
   as chemical restraint, 354, 355, 364t, 365
   as delirium treatment, 264
Hand-foot syndrome, 307
Hand hygiene, 116
HAPE (high altitude pulmonary edema), 302, 326, 327
Hare Traction Splint, 10
Hazardous materials, definition of, 503
Hazardous materials exposure events, 146, 503–507
   control zones for, 405, 504
   scene safety at, 309–310, 503
   as small-scale multiple casualty incidents, 152
Headaches, 267–268
   altitude sickness-related, 326
   cluster, 267
   migraine, 267
Head-tilt-chin lift maneuver, in children, 418
Head trauma, 373–376
   minor, 375–376
   physical examination in, 262–263
   as seizure cause, 430t
Health Insurance Portability and Accountability Act (HIPAA), 52
Health Resource and Service Administration (HRSA), 20–21
Healthy individuals, definition of, 101
Hearing loss
   in helicopter pilots, 527
   lightning strike-related, 481, 482

Heart
   electrical axis of, 206, 207f
   electrical conducting system of, 203–204, 203f
   penetrating injuries to, 391
Heart blocks, 211-212. *See also* Atrioventricular heart block
   complete, 223
Heart disease. *See* Cardiovascular disease
Heart rate
   in adolescents, 453t
   calculation of, 207–209, 208f
   in children, 423, 453t
   in infants, 453t
   temperature-related increase in, 284, 285
Heat cramps, 263, 322
Heat exhaustion, 263, 322
Heat illness, 322–325
Heat loss, mechanisms of, 283, 316
Heat production, mechanisms of, 283
Heat stroke, 263, 322, 323, 324
Heimlich maneuver, 463
Helicopter emergency medical services (HEMS), 515
   history of, 7
   indications for use of, 36
   physiologic risks associated with, 526–527
   versus rotor-wing aircraft use, 517
Helicopters
   crashes of, 101
   use in search and rescue operations, 475–476
Hematemesis, 293, 298
Hematochezia, 293
Hematoma
   epidural, 373–374
   intracerebral, 373–374
   intravenous therapy-related, 536
   subdural, 373–374
   as seizure cause, 280
Hemodynamic instability, of cardiac dysrhythmia patients, 218
Hemoglobin, synthetic oxygen-carrying substitutes for, 237
Hemophilia, 308
Hemophilus influenzae, as epiglottitis cause, 446
Hemorrhage
   abdominal trauma-related, 391
   controlled *versus* uncontrolled, 556
   control of, in tactical emergency medicine, 492–493, 493f, 494
   gastrointestinal, 293–296

599

Hemorrhage *(continued)*
    age differences in, 295
    lower, 293, 294, 295
    treatment for, 295
    upper, 293, 294, 295
    as vomiting cause, 293, 298
    intracranial
        electrical injury-related, 408
        as seizure cause, 261, 280
    neck injury-related, 383, 384
    pelvic fracture-related, 395
    subarachnoid, as seizure cause, 280
    trauma-related, 371
Hemothorax, massive, 386, 387
Henry's law, 465, 469–470, 526
Heparin, 254
Hepatitis, 117, 288
Hepatitis B, 114–115, 118, 119
Hepatitis C, 114–115, 118, 119
Heroin, 262, 313
High-altitude cerebral edema (HACE), 326, 327
High altitude pulmonary edema (HAPE), 302, 326, 327
High-density lipoprotein (HDL) cholesterol, 102, 102*t*, 246
High-voltage injuries, 480
    lightning-related, 479–483
Highway Safety Act, 10
Hip, fractures of, 304
Hippocrates, 3
Histamine, 336
Histograms, 94
History, of Emergency Medical Services (EMS), 3–14
    7000 BCE-1790 (pre-organized EMS era), 3-4
    1790-1865 (Larrey era), 4-5
    1865-1950 (military, mortuaries, and hospitals era), 5-7
    1950-1975 (Farrington era), 8–12
    1970s onward (modern era)), 12–14
Hives, 336, 338–339
Hollow organs, traumatic injury to, 391
Home remedies, for burns, 411
Homicide, in progress, 492
Honeybee stings, 486
Hormones. *See also specific hormones*
    stress-related, 106, 124
Hornet stings, 486
Hospice patients, 69
Hospital divert status, 31
    implication for cardiac arrest patients, 37–38

Hospitalized patients, delirium in, 258
Hospitals. *See also* Transport destinations; Trauma centers; *names of specific hospitals*
    during disasters, 150
    Incident Management Systems of, 142
Hostage situations, 492
Hot zones, 405, 504
HRSA (Health Resource and Service Administration), 20–21
Human immunodeficiency virus infection, 114–115
    as delirium cause, 258
    occupational exposure to, 119–120
    signs and symptoms of, 117
Hurricanes, 146
Hydatidiform mole, 276
Hydrocodone, 262
Hydrogen cyanide (hydrocyanic acid), 158, 161
Hydromorphone, 262
Hydromorphone hydrochloride, 571*t*
Hydroplaning, 60
Hydroxocobalamin, 161, 314
Hymenoptera stings, 486
Hyperbaric oxygen therapy
    for burn patients, 412
    for dysbarism patients, 37, 470–471
Hypercalcemia, as abdominal pain cause, 289
Hypercholesterolemia
    as cardiovascular disease risk factor, 240, 246
    lowering of, 103
Hyperglycemia
    diabetes-related, 261, 342, 343, 344, 347*t*, 348
        differentiated from hypoglycemia, 345–346
    as seizure cause, 430*t*
Hyperkalemia
    electrical burn-related, 408
    as wide complex tachycardia cause, 222
Hypertension, 273–277
    as cardiovascular disease risk factor, 240, 246
    complications of, 275
    definition of, 246, 273
    diagnosis of, 273
    differential diagnosis of, 194
    essential, 273
    most common cause of, 273
    during pregnancy, 260, 275–276, 281, 331
    stage 1, 273
    stage 2, 273
    treatment for, 274–275
Hypertensive emergency, 273–274
Hyperthermia, 283, 285

Hyperventilation/hyperventilation syndrome
  in head injury patients, 375
  management of, 301, 357–358
Hypoglycemia
  alcohol use-related, 261
  in children, 425–426
  as delirium cause, 261
  diabetes-related, 34–345, 261, 343, 347t, 348
    differentiated from hyperglycemia, 345–346
    management of, 347–348
  in pregnant patients, 331
  as seizure cause, 430t, 436
Hypoglycemic agents, oral, 343, 344f
Hypotension
  acute coronary syndrome-related, 254
  as altered mental status cause, 264
  anaphylaxis-related, 337, 338
  beneficial effects of, 556
  differential diagnosis of, 194
  fever-related, 284
  histamine-related, 336
  myocardial ischemia-related, 246
  rattlesnake bite-related, 484
  tension pneumothorax-related, 561
  trauma-related, 370
  traumatic brain injury-related, 376
Hypothalamus, role in body temperature regulation, 283, 284
Hypothermia, 316–321
  accidental, 316
  in burn patients, 319, 403
  diagnosis of, 316–317
  electrocardiogram findings in, 320f
  mild therapeutic, 231–232
  mistaken for death, 317
  submersion incident-related, 463, 464
  treatment for, 317, 318f
Hypoventilation, 543
Hypovolemia. *See also* Shock, hypovolemic
  fluid replacement therapy for, 371
Hypoxia, 260
  oxygen therapy for, 371, 543
  as seizure cause, 430t
  in spinal cord injury patients, 380
  in traumatic brain-injured patients, 376

I

Ice
  contraindication as thermal burn treatment, 402–403
  driving on, 60
  slipping on, 112
Ice water immersion, as heat stroke treatment, 324
Ictus, 278
Identification
  of mass casualty incident patients, 155
  of responder personnel, 138–139, 138f, 139f
IEDs (improvised explosive devices), 180
Immediate category, of triage, 143, 149, 154
Immersion syndrome, 463
Immobilization, 565–568. *See also* Splinting
  basic goal of, 555
  of spinal injury patients, 377–378, 565–566
  children, 450–451
  seizure patients, 281
Immunoglobulin E (IgE), 335, 336
Immunosuppressed patients. *See also* Acquired immunodeficiency syndrome (AIDS); Human Immunodeficiency virus (HIV) infection
  abdominal pain in, 291
Impaled objects, 567
Impedance threshold devices (ITDs), 230
Impetigo, 116
Implied consent, for delirious patients, 265
Implosion-explosion forces, 181, 182
Improvised explosive devices (IEDs), 180
Inapsine™, 364t, 365
Incident, definition of, 137
Incident command
  at mass casualty incidents, 153, 156
  in the tactical environment, 499
Incident Command System (ICS), 141–142
Incident management, 137–145
  coordination in, 137, 139
  critical features of, 137
  identification of personnel in, 138–139, 138f, 139f
  organization in, 137, 139–140, 140f, 141f
Incompetent patients, 68
Incontinence, seizure-related, 260, 261
Indigestion, 240
Infants. *See also* Neonates
  fever in, 284
  field approach to, 422–428
  gastrointestinal hemorrhage in, 295
  hypothermia in, 316
  occiput size in, 418, 450
  vital signs in, 193, 453f

601

Index

Infection, as fever cause, 284, 285
Infectious diseases exposures, 112, 114-121. *See also* Biological terrorism
　airborne precautions for, 116
　as altered mental status cause, 263
　contact precautions for, 116
　droplet precautions for, 116
　at mass casualty incidents scenes, 156
　signs and symptoms of, 117
　transmission of, 114
Inflammatory bowel, as abdominal pain cause, 288
Influenza, airborne precautions for, 116
Influenza viruses, 117, 118
Information, organization of, 40–42
Informed consent, 50–51
　definition of, 67
　for trauma patients, 369
Informed refusal, 51–52
Inhalation injuries, 410
Inhaled poisons, 314
Injuries. *See* Trauma
Insecticide poisoning, 312, 312*t*
Insulin
　definition of, 342
　discovery of, 341
　function of, 342
Insulin pump, 344, 345*f*
Insulin resistance, 342–343
Insulin therapy, 344–345, 345*f*
Intensive care units (ICUs), surgical, compared with burn ICUs, 412
International League Against Epilepsy, 430
International Society of Mountain Medicine, 478
International Society of Travel Medicine, 478
International Trauma Life Support, 13
Interns, as ambulance attendants, 6, 12
Interpersonal violence, 397-401. *See also* Child abuse; Elder abuse; Intimate partner violence
Interstitial space, medication or fluid extravasation into, 538
Interviews, with media personnel, 64, 65–66
Intimate partner violence, 397, 398–400
Intoxicated patients, vomiting in, 298
Intracranial pressure, elevated, head trauma-related, 373, 375
Intramuscular access
　in agitated/violent patients, 355
　contraindication for pain medication administration, 572

Intraosseous (IO) access, 231, 233
　as alternative to intravenous access, 538–539
　in children, 419, 419*f*, 424, 453
　complications of, 539
Intravenous infusion rates, in head-injured patients, 376
Intravenous (IV) access, 535–541
　central lines, 540
　in children, 424, 453, 538
　choice of drip sets for, 536
　complications of, 536–537, 538
　equipment for, 535
　gtts abbreviation for, 536
　indwelling, 540
　intraosseous access as alternative to, 538–539
　optimal peripheral sites for, 535
　for pain medication administration, 570, 572
　peripheral, 535–538
　puncture site swelling associated with, 538
Intubation. *See also* Endotracheal intubation; Nasopharyngeal intubation; Nasotracheal intubation; Orotracheal intubation; Rapid sequence intubation
　in anaphylaxis patients, 338
　in children, 451–452
　complications of, 546
　in intoxicated patients, 298
　medication-assisted, 547–548
　in spinal cord injury patients, 379
　vomiting during, 546
Ionizing radiation
　definition of, 174
　effects of, 177–178
　protection from, 175
Ipratropium, 448
Irrigation, of chemical burn patients, 404–405
Isabella, Queen of Spain, 4
Ischemia
　distal, fracture-dislocation-related, 567
　of the extremities, 305–306
　intestinal, 287
　myocardial, 246, 287
Isolation precautions, 164
Isopropanol alcohol, toxicity of, 310

J

Jacksonian march, 278
Jaundice, liver failure-related, 260, 262
Jaws of Life, 10
Jello™, 294

Index

Jellyfish stings, 485–486
Johnny, of Rescue 51 (television character), 11
Johnson v. University of Chicago Hospitals, 53, 54
Joint Commission on Accreditation of Hospitals, 42, 43*t*
Joint Review Committee for EMT-Paramedic
    Accreditation, 12
Joints
    hemophilia-related disorders of, 308
    warm and red, 307
Journal of the American Medical Association, 5–6
Jugular vein, external, as intravenous access site, 537
JumpSTART triage system, 149

K

Kansas Supreme Court, 51–52
Kendrick extrication device, 450–451, 566
Keraunoparalysis, 480
Ketoacidosis, diabetic, 260, 261, 342, 343–344
    as abdominal pain cause, 289
    signs and symptoms of, 346–347
Ketorolac tromethamine, 571*t*
Kidney, blunt injuries to, 391
Knee pain, 304
Knowledge gaps, in prehospital interventions, 532
Kolman, John, 488
Korean War, 122, 488, 499, 515
    air medical services during, 7
Kussmaul's respirations, 261, 346

L

Labor and delivery, 332-333. *See also* Pregnancy
Lacerations, 367
Laerdal, Åsmund, 10
Langerhans, Paul, 341
LAPSS (Los Angeles Prehospital Stroke Screen), 269, 270
Larrey, Dominique-Jean, 4, 9, 488
Larrey era, of emergency medical services, 4
Laryngoscope blades, 451, 546
Lasix™ (furosemide), 254, 274
Lassa fever, 165, 167
"Laughing gas," 571*t*
Law enforcement. *See also* Police officers
    tactical emergency medicine and, 488–502
Lawsuits. *See also* Malpractice lawsuits
    Emergency Medical Treatment and Active Labor Act-
        related, 52–54
    emergency vehicle operation-related, 56
    Health Insurance Portability and Accountability Act-
        related, 52

Left bundle-branch blocks, 209, 250
Legal isses. *See* Medicolegal issues
Letterman, Jonathan, 5
Levitra, 248
Lewisite, 158, 151
Lice, 116
Lichtenberg's flowers, 481–482, 482*f*
Lidocaine
    dosage in advanced cardiac life support, 231
    ventricular pacemaker-suppressing effect of, 224
Life expectancy, 101
Lifestyle, healthy, 101
Life-sustaining treatments, withholding of, 68
Lifting, safe methods of, 112
Lightning strike injuries, 479–483
Limbs. *See* Extremities
Lincoln Medical Foundation, 13
Lion-tamer theory, 110
Liver failure
    as altered mental status cause, 262
    as jaundice cause, 260, 262
Living wills, 50
Load transfer, 59
Locality rule, 47–48
Lomotil, 262
Lorazepam
    as chemical restraint, 355, 364*t*
    as pediatric seizure treatment, 436, 437*t*
Lorcet, 262
Lortab, 262
Los Angeles County Fire Department, 515, 516
Los Angeles Prehospital Stroke Screen (LAPSS), 269, 270
Los Angeles Sheriff's Emergency Service Detail, 490
Low-density lipoprotein (LDL) cholesterol, 102,
    102*t*, 246
Lund-Browder chart, 405–406
Lung cancer, 101–102
    warning signs of, 104
Lungs
    blast-related injuries to, 183–184
    penetrating injuries to, 391
Lyme disease, 486

M

Maass, Friedrich, 9
MADFOCS mnemonic, for behavioral emergency
    management, 351
Magnesium, dosage in advanced cardiac life
    support, 231

603

Index

Magnesium salicylate, 311
Maguire, B.J., 101
Malpractice lawsuits, 45–55
   depositions in, 49–50
   legal damages recovered from, 49
   proof of causation in, 48–49
   as "records" cases, 46
Managed care, off-line medical direction and, 87
Manic-depression, 357
Marburg virus, 163, 164, 165, 167
Mark I autoinjector, for atropine, 159–160, 159f
Martini's law, 469
Maryland State Police, 495f, 515, 516
Masks, protective, 115–116, 118
Mask squeeze, 467, 469, 470
Mass casualty incidents, 146-151
   definition of, 146
   differentiated from disasters, 146
   "first in, last out" concept of, 154–155
   goal of medical care during, 147
   transport destinations during, 36
   triage in, 69, 142–143, 144
Mass gatherings, 186–190
MASS system, of triage, 149
Mast cells, 335, 336
MAST (military antishock trousers), 237, 555
Material safety data sheets (MSDS), 504
McSwain, Norman, 13
Mean heat index, 323
Measles, airborne precautions for, 116
Mechanical injury, definition of, 367
Mechanism of injury (MOI), 34–35
Medical antishock trousers (MAST), 237, 555
Medical care, refusal of. *See* Refusal, of medical care
Medical control, of mass casualty incidents, 156
Medical direction, of emergency medical services systems, 73–88
   advantages and disadvantages of, 81
   definition of, 15, 83
   during disasters, 87
   need for, 73–74
   off-line (indirect), 86
      components of, 84
      definition of, 83
      differentiated from on-line medical direction, 74
      managed care and, 87
      versus on-scene physician's direction, 87
      patient preferences and, 87
      prospective components of, 85
      retrospective components of, 85
   on-line (OLMD), 79–81, 86
      alternative to, 79
      differentiated from off-line medical direction, 74
      mandated switch to, 86
      priority over off-line medical direction, 87
      system configuration of, 80
      training in, 81
   standing-order protocol system of, 79
Medical directors, 31
   of air medical transport systems, 523–524
   differentiated from physician advisors, 83
   recommended characteristics of, 84
   responsibilities of, 76
   selection of prehospital interventions by, 532
Medical durable powers of attorney, 50, 68
Medic Alert bracelets, 11
Medical Management of Biological Casualties Handbook, 171
Medical threat assessment (MTA), 489
Medical treatment
   futile, 68
   refusal of. *See* Refusal, of medical care
Medications. *See also names of specific medications*
   anaphylactic reactions to, 336
   as body temperature elevation cause, 284
   effect on vital signs, 193, 195
   as gastrointestinal hemorrhage cause, 294
   overdoses of, 309–315
   as vomiting cause, 298
Medicolegal issues, 45-55. *See also* Lawsuits; Malpractice lawsuits
   abused patients, 400
   continuous quality improvement, 95–96
   explosions, 181
   Good Samaritan laws, 477
   restraint of patients, 111
Megahertz, 29
Melena, 293
Meningitis
   as altered mental status cause, 263
   as headache cause, 267
   occupational exposure to, 120
   as seizure cause, 280–281, 430t
   signs and symptoms of, 117
Mental health holds (MHHs), 358
Meperidine, 262
Meperidine hydrochloride, 571t

Methadone, 262
Methanol, toxicity of, 310
Methicillin-resistant *Staphylococcus aureus* (MRSA), 116, 117
Methylprednisolone, 380
Methyl salicylate, 311
Metoclopramide, 299
Michael Reese Hospital, Chicago, 7
Midazolam
    as chemical restraint, 355, 364*t*
    as seizure treatment, 281
        in children, 436, 437*t*
    use in rapid sequence intubation, 551, 552*t*
Migraine headaches, 267
Military antishock trousers (MAST), 237, 555
Military Assistance to Safety and Traffic program, 515
Military special operations units, tactical emergency medicine and, 488–502
Mills, Dawson, 11
Minimal/minor category, of triage, 143, 149, 154
Minors. *See also* Adolescents; Children; Infants; Neonates
    consent to medical treatment for, 51–52
Minowski, Oskar, 341
Miscarriages, 330
Mistakes
    as basis for lawsuits, 45
    documentation of, 40
    media coverage of, 64
Mitchell, Jeffrey, 126
Mobile Computer Terminals (MCTs), 30
Mobile Data Terminals (MDTs), 30
MONA (morphine, oxygen, nitroglycerin, and aspirin) treatment, for acute coronary syndrome, 250*t*, 252–253
Monoamine oxidase inhibitors, as hypertension cause, 273
Morando, Rocco, 11
Morphine, 262
    as abdominal pain treatment, 290
    as acute coronary syndrome treatment, 253–254
    as burn-related pain treatment, 403, 411
    comparison with fentanyl, 572
    contraindication in chronic obstructive pulmonary disease, 300
Morphine, oxygen, nitroglycerin, and aspirin (MONA) treatment, for acute coronary syndrome, 250*t*, 252–253
Morphine sulfate, 571*t*
Mortality, preventable, 101–102

Mortality causes
    leading, 101
    motor vehicle accidents, 450, 490
Mortality rates, occupational, 101
Mosquito-borne diseases, 488
Motor vehicle(s). *See also* Ambulances; Emergency vehicle(s)
    extrication of patients from, 155
    as protection from lightning, 481
Motor vehicle accidents, 60, 101, 146
    emergency medical services' access to, 154
    as mortality cause
        in children, 450
        in police officers, 490
    as multiple casualty incidents, 152, 154, 155
    during pregnancy, 332
    scene safety at, 112, 155
Mountain Rescue Association, 478
Mount Ranier National Park, 476
Mouse poisons, 313
MRSA (methicillin-resistant *Staphylococcus aureus*), 116, 117
Multiple casualty incidents
    definition of, 152
    differentiated from "usual" or "routine" EMS responses, 152
    lightning strike-related, 481
    small-scale, 152–157
        definition of, 152
        errors in management of, 155
        incident and unified command for, 153
        planning for, 153–154
        training for, 152–153
Mumps, airborne precautions for, 116
Muscle endurance exercise, 103
Muscle flexibility exercise, 104
Mushrooms, poisonous, 314
Music therapy, 570
Mutual aid situations, transport destination decisions in, 31
Mycobacterium tuberculosis, 118. *See also* Tuberculosis
Myocardial infarction, acute
    as abdominal pain cause, 289
    as chest pain cause, 240, 247–248
    cocaine use-related, 313
    consequences of, 246
    differentiated from
        angina pectoris, 245
        unstable angina, 240

Myocardial infarction *(continued)*
    electrocardiogram findings in, 216, 249–250, 250*t*, 251*f*, 251*t*, 252
    gastrointestinal hemorrhage-related, 294
    non-ST-segment elevation (NSTEMI), 245, 250, 256
    risk factors for, 246
    signs and symptoms of, 247
    ST-segment elevation (STEMI), 245, 250, 254, 255–256
    thrombolytic therapy for, 244
    in wide complex tachycardia patients, 221
Myocardial ischemia, 246, 287
Myocarditis, as abdominal pain cause, 287
Myoglobinuria, electrical burn-related, 408, 409*f*

N

Nalbuphine, 571*t*
Naloxone (Narcan™), 253–254, 262, 313, 426, 572
Napoleon Bonaparte, 4
Napoleonic Wars, 488
Narcan. *See* Naloxone
Narcotic analgesics. *See also* Opiate analgesics
    as abdominal pain treatment, 290
Nasal intubation, 546–547
Nasopharyngeal intubation, 544
    in children, 436, 444
    use in the tactical environment, 493, 494, 495
Nasotracheal intubation, in children, 451
National Academy of Sciences, National Research Council of, 10
National Association of Emergency Medical Services Physicians (NAEMSP), 20–21, 552
National Association of Emergency Medical Technicians (NAEMT), 8, 13
National Association of Search and Rescue (NASAR), 473, 478
National Association of State Medical Services Directors, 20–21
National Center for Atmospheric Research, 522–523
National Disaster Management System (NDMS), 476
National Emergency Medical Services Education Standards, 14
National Emergency Medical Services Information System, 21
National Emergency Medical Services Research Strategic Plan, 532–533
National Highway Traffic Safety Administration (NHTSA), 11, 20–21, 85
National Incident Management System (NIMS), 85, 141, 504, 508

National Institute of Allergy and Infectious Disease, 335
National Institute of Safety and Health (NIOSH), 405
National organizations, involved with emergency medical services, 74–75
National Outdoor Leadership School (NOLS), 473, 478
National parks, search and rescue operations in, 475–476
National Registry of Emergency Medical Technicians (NREMT), 8, 10–11, 48, 473
National Ski Patrol, 473, 478
National Standard EMT-Ambulance curriculum, 8
National Tactical Officers Association, 488
National Traffic Safety Act of 1966, 10
Natural disasters, types of, 146
Nausea
    abdominal pain-related, 289–290
    middle ear barotrauma-related, 468–469
    radiation exposure-related, 178
Navy SEALS, 493, 500
Near-drowning, 461
Neck. *See also* Cervical spine
    anatomic zones of, 382–383, 382*f*
    traumatic injury to, 382–385, 382*f*
        penetrating injury, 378, 382
        vascular, 382, 383
Needle cricothyroidostomy, 451–452
Needle decompression, 560–564, 561*f*, 562*f*
    during air transport, 527
    in tactical environment, 493, 494
Needle-stick injuries, 119
Needle thoracostomy. *See* Needle decompression
Negligence
    as basis for malpractice lawsuits, 47–50
    per se, 50
Neisseria meningitidis, 120
Neonates
    gastrointestinal hemorrhage in, 295
    naloxone administration in, 426
    shock in, 418
Nephrolithiasis, as abdominal pain cause, 288
Nerve agent exposure, 158–160
    antidotes to, 159–160, 159*f*, 160*f*
    SLUDGE acronym/mnemonic for, 159
Neuroleptic malignant syndrome, 299
Neuroleptics
    adverse effects of, 299, 355
    as chemical restraint, 354–355
Neurologic assessment. *See also* Glasgow Coma Scale
    in children, 424

Neurologic emergencies, acute, 267–272
  headaches, 267–268
  stroke, 268–271
Neurons, in seizures, 429
Neuropathic pain, 569
Neutral position, 379–380, 420
Neutrons, 174
New York Police Department Emergency Service Unit, 490
New York State Department of Health, statement on trauma patient transport, 369–373
Night driving, 58–59
Nightingale, Florence, 488
911 emergency calls, 26
  E (enhanced), 27
"911 Study," 556, 558
Nitrates, 248
Nitrogen narcosis, 467, 469, 470
Nitroglycerin, 253
  sublingual, 240, 274, 301
Nitrous oxide/nitrogen mixture, 571t
Nociceptive pain, 569
Nominals, 94
Nonsteroidal anti-inflammatory drugs (NSAIDs)
  as gastrointestinal hemorrhage cause, 294
  as pain treatment, 570, 572
  side effects of, 294, 572
North American Emergency Response Guidebook, 504
Nubain, 571t
Nuclear bombs, 175
Nuclear disasters/terrorist events, 174–179
  risk perception in, 175
Nuclear power plants, terrorist attacks on, 176
"Nursemaid's elbow," 306
Nurses
  as on-line medical direction providers, 79
  on-scene, during disasters and mass casualty incidents, 149–150
Nursing home patients
  delirium in, 258
  resuscitation of, 68

O

Obesity, health problems associated with, 102, 104
Observe, orient, decide, and act (OODA) loop, 499
Obstetric emergencies. *See* Pregnancy
Occiput size, in children, 418, 450
Occupational exposure
  infection risk associated with, 119–120
  prevention of, 119

Occupational Safety and Health Administration (OSHA), 505, 510
Odansetron hydrochloride, 572
Oil of wintergreen, 311
Olanzapine, 264
Ontario Prehospital Advanced Life Support (OPALS) group, 531–532
OODA (observe, orient, decide, and act) loop, 499
Opiate analgesics, 570, 571t
  as abdominal pain treatment, 290
Opiate withdrawal, 313
Opioid toxidromes/poisoning, 261–262, 312t, 313, 572
Opium, 262
OPQRST mnemonic for chest pain assessment, 199, 247–248
Oral hypoglycemic agents, 343, 344f
Orange Book, 8
Organophosphate insecticides/pesticides, 158, 312, 312t
Organ perfusion, shock-related decrease in, 236
Organs, traumatic injury to, 367
Oropharyngeal airways, 544
Orotracheal intubation
  in children, 444
  in neck injury patients, 383
Osteomyelitis, 307
Otitis media, as seizure cause, 430t
Outcome measures in continuous quality improvement, 92, 93
Outcomes, bad, as basis for lawsuits, 45
Out-of-hospital care providers, levels of, 77
Ovarian cysts, rupture of, 289
Ovarian torsion, as abdominal pain cause, 288
Overdose, 309–315
  in adolescents, 426
  as seizure cause, 281
"Overresuscitation," 388
Oxycodone, 262
Oxygen, supplemental
  in acute coronary syndrome patients, 253
  in asthma patients, 301
  in dyspneic patients, 300, 302
  in hypoxic patients, 511, 543
  indications for, 543
  in pediatric respiratory distress patients, 442
  in pediatric seizure patients, 436
  percentage of oxygen in, 543
  in trauma patients, 371
  use during air transport, 527

Oxygen delivery system, components of, 234
Oxygen saturation
  in children, 425, 441
  measurement of, 196
  in traumatic brain-injured patients, 376
Oxygen saturation monitor, use in trauma patients, 371
Oxygen toxicity, to central nervous system, 467, 469, 470

P

Pacemaker cells, 203–204
Pacemakers
  artificial, 215–216, 216f
  ventricular, suppression of, 224
Pacing, transcutaneous, 225
  contraindication in asystole, 223
Packed red blood cells (PRBCs), 237
Pain. *See also* Abdominal pain; Chest pain
  definition of, 569
  in extremities, 304–308
  limb ischemia-related, 305
  negative side effects of, 569
  referred, 392
Pain assessment
  accuracy of, 569
  in children, 420, 420f, 423–424, 569–570
Pain management, 569–573
  in burn patients, 411
  in extremity injury patients, 306
  pharmacological methods of, 570–572, 571t
  physical methods of, 570
Pain rating scales, pediatric, 420, 420f, 424, 569–570
Pallor, limb ischemia-related, 305
Pancreatitis, as abdominal pain cause, 288
Pantridge, J.F., 8–9
Paper bags, rebreathing into, 301–302
Paralysis
  Charcot's, 480
  limb ischemia-related, 305
Paralytic agents, 550–551, 551t
Paramedic programs, first, location of, 11
Paramedics
  state-licensed, medical direction for, 74
  training programs for, 11, 12, 76
Paresthesias
  compartment syndrome-related, 305
  limb ischemia-related, 305
Pareto charts, 94
Paris Academy of Sciences, 9
Parkinson's disease, antiemetic use in, 299

Parkland formula, for fluid resuscitation, 411
Partial pressure of carbon dioxide CO_2 in arterial blood ($PaCO_2$), 303
Partner violence, 397, 398–400
Pascal's law, 465
PASGs (pneumatic antishock garments), 555–559, 555f
"Path of injury," 304–305
Pathogens, 114
Patient assessment, prehospital. *See* Assessment, prehospital
Patient care, transfer of, 19–20
"Patient dumping," 52–54
Patients, types of, 12–13
Paturas, Jim, 13–14
Pediatric Advanced Medical Cardiac Life Support (PACLS), 85–86
Pediatric Assessment Triangle (PAT), 422–423, 424, 439–441, 440f, 450
  TICLS mnemonic of, 422–423, 439–440
Peer review, 91
"Peesap" (Public Safety Answering Point), 27
Pelvic binders, 395–396
Pelvic examination, in thoracic trauma patients, 386–387
Pelvic fractures, 394–396
  "open-book," 394–395
  splinting of, 566–567
Pelvic inflammatory disease, as abdominal pain cause, 288
Pelvic ring fractures, 394
Penetrating trauma, 367–368
  abdominal, 390, 391, 392
  blast-related, 180, 184
  definition of, 367
  to the neck, 378, 382
  as pediatric mortality cause, 450
Penicillin, 488
Pepper spray, 498
Peptic ulcer disease, 294
Pepto-Bismol™, 311
Percocet, 262
Percodan, 262
Percussion, abdominal, 391–392
Pericardial effusion, 575, 577, 578f
Pericardial tamponade, 232
Pericarditis, as abdominal pain cause, 287
Peritoneal signs, 289, 392
Persantine, interaction with adenosine, 220
Per se negligence, 50

Index

Personality characteristics, of emergency responders, 125
Personal protective equipment, 112
   for biological terrorism agent exposures, 168
   for chemical burn events, 404, 405
   definition of, 115
   for hazardous materials exposure, 505–506
   indications for, 115–116
   for infectious disease prevention, 115
   for law enforcement personnel, 492
   for mass casualty incidents, 156
   for nerve agent incidents, 160
   for radiologic attacks/exposure, 177, 178
   for the tactical environment, 495, 496f
   for technical rescues, 510
Personal safety and wellness, 101–107. *See also* Scene safety
   in behavioral and psychiatric emergencies, 353–354
   in infectious diseases exposures, 114–121
   in wilderness emergency medical services, 477–478
Personnel identification, in incident management, 138–139, 138f, 139f
Pertussis (whooping cough)
   airborne precautions for, 116
   signs and symptoms of, 117
Pesticide poisoning, 312–313, 312t
Pharyngitis, streptococcal, 289
Pharynx, injuries to, 384
Phenergan™, 572
Philadelphia collars, 56
Phlebitis, implication for intravenous access, 537
Phosgene, 158, 161
Phosphodiesterase inhibitors, 248
Physical activity, as body temperature elevation cause, 284
Physical examination
   of delirious patients, 260
   head-to-toe, 200
   vital signs assessment in, 195
Physical findings, documentation of, 42
Physical fitness activities, 103–104
Physical inactivity, as cardiovascular disease risk factor, 102, 246
Physician advisors, 74, 83
Physician orders for life-sustaining treatment (POLST), 68
Physicians
   as ambulance attendants, 12
   as medical dispatch center directors, 32
   as on-line medical direction providers, 79, 81
   on-scene, during disasters and mass casualty incidents, 149–150, 186
   role in incident management, 142, 144
   role in tactical emergency medical services, 490
   transport destination alteration by, 38
Pittsburgh, Pennsylvania Emergency Medical Services system, 92
Placenta previa, 331
Plague, 163
   protection against, 165, 169
   signs and symptoms of, 166
   transmission of, 164
   types of, 166
Plant ingestions, poisonous, 314
Plasma, as shock treatment, 237
Pleural effusions, as abdominal pain cause, 289
Pneumatic antishock garment (PASG), 555–559, 555f
Pneumatic counterpressure device, 555
Pneumatic rubber suit, 556–557
Pneumomediastinum, 242
   diving-related, 470
Pneumonia
   as abdominal pain cause, 289
   aspiration, 297
   as cough cause, 252
   respiratory syncytial virus (RSV)-related, 446
   signs and symptoms of, 302
Pneumothorax, 241–242
   as abdominal pain cause, 289
   diving-related, 467, 470
   misdiagnosis of, 563
   open, 386
      in children, 452
   tension, 242
      air transport-related, 526, 527
      causes of, 560
      in children, 452
      complications of, 563–564
      definition of, 560
      diagnosis of, 387
      as life-threatening condition, 386
      with mediastinal shift, 561f
      needle decompression of, 560–564, 561f, 562f
      recurrent, 563
      in tactical environment, 492, 493, 494, 495
      treatment for, 387, 560–564, 561f, 562f
PoisIndex©, 504
Poison Control Centers, 504

Index

Poisonings, 263, 309–315
   with inhaled poisons, 314
   plant ingestion-related, 314
   toxidromes caused by, 312–313, 312t
   with unknown substances, 314
Police officers
   occupational fatality rate of, 101
   protective role of, 108, 109
   searches of patients by, 111
POLST (physician orders for life-sustaining treatment), 68
Polydipsia, 346, 347t
Polyphagia, 346, 347t
Polyuria, 346, 347t
Pons, Jordan, 429
Postimmersion syndrome, 463
Posttraumatic stress disorder (PTSD), 125
Potassium iodide pills, 178
Pralidoxime, 159–160, 313
PreArrival Instructions, zero response time and, 29
Preeclampsia, 260, 276, 331
   differentiated from eclampsia, 331
Pregnancy, 330–334
   abdominal pain in, 291
   abdominal trauma in, 392
   antiemetic use in, 299
   cardiac arrest in, 232, 332
   chemical restraint use in, 365
   eclampsia in, 276, 281, 331
   ectopic, 330
      as abdominal pain cause, 289
   gestational diabetes in, 342–343
   hypertension in, 275–276, 281
   molar (hydatidiform mole), 276
   physiologic changes in, 331
   preeclampsia in, 260, 276, 331
   seizures in, 281
Prehospital environment, 23–25
   challenges in, 24, 25
   definition of, 23
Prehospital interventions, efficacy and effectiveness of, 531–534
Prehospital Trauma Life Support (PHTLS), 13–14, 500
Prehypertension, 273
Premature atrial contractions (PACc), 209
Premature ventricular contractions (PVCs), 224, 225–226
   butyrophenones-related, 365
   multifocal, 226f
Pressure sores, 566, 568

Presumed consent, 67
Priapism, spinal cord injury-related, 378
Process, 90
Prochlorperazine, 299
Promethazine hydrochloride, 572
Pseudoseizures, 280
Psychiatric emergencies, 350–360
Psychiatric patients
   dangerousness of, 108
   decision-making capacity of, 68
   vital signs in, 258
Psychological abuse, of children, 397, 456
Psychosclerosis, 201
Psychosis, 352
Pubic rami fractures, 394
Public, relationship to emergency medical services systems, 15
Public and media relations, 64–66
   during disasters, 151
Public health, early history of, 3
Public information officers (PIOs), 65, 151
Public Safety Answering Point ("peesap"), 27
Pulmonary embolism, 240–241, 289, 302, 526–527
Pulmonary toxicants, 158, 161
Pulmonary trauma, in children, 452
Pulseless electrical activity (PEA), 210, 228, 577
Pulselessness, 305
Pulseless ventricular tachycardia, 210
Pulse oximetry, 196, 303
   in acute coronary syndrome patients, 249
   in children, 425, 441
Pulse rate
   in acute coronary syndrome patients, 249
   age-related differences in, 193–194
   40-59 bpm, 223
   in children, 417, 418, 423
   in infants, 417, 418
   in supine position, 195
Pupillary constriction, in neck injury patients, 385
Pupillary dilation, 373
Pupillary light response, 262
Purpura, 284

Q

Q fever, 114, 169, 486
QRI (quality review and improvement process), 84
Quality, 89–97
   costs of, 91
   definition of, 89

Index

Quality assurance, 89–90
  definition of, 89
  differentiated from continuous quality improvement, 90–91
Quality control, 92
Quality improvement, 92
Quality planning, 91–92
Quality review and improvement (QRI) process, 84
Quality training programs, 76

R

Radial head, subluxation of, 306
Radiation
  definition of, 174
  dose-related symptoms of, 178
  as heat loss mechanism, 283, 316
Radiation detectors, 178
Radiation injury
  types of, 174–175
Radiation leaks, 146
Radiation sickness, 177–178
Radioactive fallout, 176, 177
Radio communication, 24–25
  as biocom, 32
  duplex systems of, 29, 30
  electrocardiogram transmission via, 32
  frequencies in
    during disasters, 150
    at mass casualty incident scenes, 157
    megahertz, 29, 138
  at mass casualty incident scenes, 157
  simplex systems of, 29–30
  "trunked," 30
Radiologic dispersion devices, 176
Radiologic exposure devices, 176
Radiologic terrorism, 174–179
Rain, driving in, 60
Rales, pulmonary embolism-related, 241
Rampart General Hospital, Rescue 51 of, 11
Rapid sequence intubation (RSI), 370–371
  complications of, 552–553
  pharmacologic agents in, 550–554
"Rapture of the deep," 469
Rat poisons, 313
Rattlesnake bites, 484–485
Recreational drugs, effect on vital signs, 195
Rectal temperature, 283
  differential diagnosis for, 323
  as heat illness indicator, 322, 323

Reed, Walter, 488
Refusal, of medical care, 51–52, 67–68
  by abdominal pain patients, 290
  by behavioral emergency patients, 358
  for children, by parents, 420–421
  by delirious patients, 265
  documentation of, 80
  informed, 51–52
  on-line medical direction and, 80
Reglan, 299
Rehydration, in heat illness, 322
Reissner's membrane, tears of, 469
Remote patient assessment, 494
Renal stones, 289
Reporters, interviews with, 64, 65–66
"Rescue 911" (television program), 11
Research, quality activities as, 95
Resource deployment
  factors in, 21
  fixed *versus* dynamic, 20
  risks of, 29
Respiration
  anaerobic, 235
  as heat loss mechanism, 316
  Kussmaul's, 261, 346
Respirators, N95, 115, 118
Respiratory arrest
  opiate use-related, 261
  as pediatric cardiac arrest cause, 231
Respiratory depression
  antiseizure medication-related, 436
  morphine-related, 253–254
  narcotic analgesics-related, 253–254, 572
Respiratory diseases, smoking-related, 101–102
Respiratory distress
  burn-related, 407
  in children and infants, 418, 419, 423, 439–449
    assessment of, 439–441, 440f
    management of, 442–445, 443f
    signs and symptoms of, 441–442
  in diabetic patients, 346–347
  in neck trauma patients, 384
Respiratory failure, in children, 442
Respiratory rate
  in adolescents, 453t
  age-related differences in, 193–194
  in asthmatics, 301
  in children, 453t, 542
  in pulmonary injury, 452

Respiratory rate *(continued)*
   estimation of, 302
   inaccuracy of, 302
   in infants, 453t, 542
   normal, 542
   temperature-related increase in, 284
   in thoracic trauma patients, 386
Respiratory syncytial virus (RSV), 446–447
   airborne precautions for, 116
Respiratory system/tract
   of adults and children, 439
   burns of, 410
Respondeat superior, 45
Restraint, 111, 354
   chemical, 111, 354–355, 364–365, 364t
   dangers of, 265, 363
   four-point, 111
   inappropriate, 363
   indications for use of, 362–363
   methods of, 364
   as mortality cause, 265, 498
   process of use of, 363
   "soft," 364
   of violent patients, 69
Resusci-Annie, 10
Revised Trauma Score (RTS), 93
Rheumatic disorders, 307–308
Ricin toxin, 163
Rift Valley fever, 165, 167
Right bundle-branch blocks, 209
Right heart failure, 246, 252
Ringers lactated solution, 236, 371, 411
Risk-benefit analysis, 508
Risk perception, 175
Risk reduction, for cardiovascular disease, 102–103
Risperidone, 264
Rocky Mountain spotted fever, 486
Rocuronium, 550, 551, 551t
Rodenticides, 313
Rome, ancient, prehospital care in, 3–4
Roy, of Rescue 51 (television character), 11
Royal Victoria Hospital, Belfast, Northern Ireland, 8–9
Rubbing alcohol, toxicity of, 310
Rucker, Daniel Henry, 5
"Rule of nines," 405–406, 406f
"Rule of 10s," 411
Rural areas
   emergency vehicle operation in, 60
   on-line medical direction in, 86
   trauma centers in, 35, 36

S

Sacco Triage Method, 149
SAD PERSONS scale, 356
Safar, Peter, 9, 10
Safety issues, 24-25, 67. *See also* Personal safety and wellness; Scene safety personal risk management, 67
St. Anthony Hospital, Denver, Colorado, 7, 515
Salassi, Gene, 13–14
Saline, intravenous, 236, 371
Salmonella, 163
SALT system, of triage, 149
Saltwater, aspiration of, 462
SAM Pelvic Sling, 395
SAMPLE history, 247, 248–249
Sandbags, as stabilizing devices, 56
Sarin, 158, 159
SARS (severe acute respiratory syndrome), 116, 117
Saturday Evening Post, 9
Scabies, 116
Scalding burns, 402
   as child abuse, 406, 407f
Scene safety, 108–113
   in behavioral and psychiatric emergencies, 353–354
   at building fires, 155
   with delirious patients, 264
   following explosions, 181
   in hazardous materials exposure events, 309–310, 503
   at mass casualty incidents, 155
   at motor vehicle crash sites, 155
   at technical rescue sites, 508, 509f
   in unknown exposures events, 309–310
Scherlis, Leonard, 9
Schizophrenia, 352, 357
Schizophrenic diseases, differentiated from delirium, 257–258
SCIWORA (spinal cord injury without radiologic abnormality), 380
Sclerosis, implication for intravenous access, 537
Scoop stretchers, 396
Scorpion stings, 485
Scromboid fish poisoning, 336–337
Scuba divers, dysbarism in, 466–467
Scuba-diving accidents, 37
Sea anemone stings, 485
Search and rescue (SAR), 475–477
   "extended," 476
   responsibility for, 475–476
Search and rescue (SAR) organizations, 478

Index

Searches, of patients, 111
Seatbelt sign, in children, 454
Sedatives
    differentiated from analgesics, 572
    use in rapid sequence intubation, 551–552, 552t
Seizures, 278–282
    antidepressants-related, 311
    assessment for, 434–435
    atonic, 431t, 433
    causes of, 280–281, 311, 430t
    in children, 429–438
        as fever cause, 263, 278, 285, 430t, 433–434, 433t, 436
        prevalence of, 429–430
    classification of, 430, 431t
    complex partial, 431–432, 431t
    cryptogenic, 279
    definition of, 278
    differential diagnosis of, 279, 280
    eclamptic, 331
    febrile, 263, 285, 433–434
        classification of, 433t
        definition of, 278
        treatment for, 436
    generalized tonic-clonic (grand mal), 278, 280, 431t, 432
    metabolic causes of, 279
    myoclonic, 431t, 432
    new onset, 281
    partial, 430
    pathophysiology of, 429
    petit mal (absence), 278, 431t, 432
    postictal period of, 261
    during pregnancy, 281, 331
    psychogenic, 280
    relationship to epilepsy, 278, 281
    SAMPLE history of, 434–435
    serum electrolytes in, 281
    signs and symptoms of, 430–433, 431t
    simple partial or focal, 278, 430–431, 431t, 432
    tonic, 431t, 432
    traumatic, 281
    treatment for, 279, 281, 435–437, 437f
    withdrawal-related, 313
Seizure threshold, 279
Self-neglect, 400
Sensory deprivation, in delirious patients, 265
Sepsis, 284–285
"7 Ds of Stroke Care," 269
Severe acute respiratory syndrome (SARS), 116, 117

Sexual abuse, of children, 397, 456
Sexual assault victims, 333
Sexually-transmitted diseases, 114
Shaken baby syndrome, 398
Shearing forces, 181–182
Shift work, 104–105, 105t
Shigella, 163
Shipping papers, for hazardous materials, 504
Shock, 234–238
    as altered mental status cause, 264
    anaphylactic, 235
    cardiogenic, 234, 237, 240, 246, 249
    in children, 452–453
        blood pressure in, 423
        compensated, 423
        hypovolemic, 453–454
    diabetic, 237
    hemorrhagic, 234, 236
        hematochezia associated with, 293
    hypovolemic, 234
        in children, 453–454
        fluid resuscitation for, 453–454
        pneumatic antishock garment use in, 555–559
    in neonates, 418
    neurogenic, 234, 237
        differentiated from spinal shock, 379
    organs affected by, 236
    oxygen saturation monitor use in, 371
    in pregnant patients, 392
    septic, 234
    spinal, 379
    stages of, 235
    treatment for, 236–237
Shootings. *See also* Gunshot wounds as multiple casualty incidents, 156
Sick-call bags, 497
Sickle cell crisis, 307
Sickle cell disease
    as bone pain cause, 306–307
    as chest pain cause, 242
    as extremity pain cause, 306–307
"Silent chest," 442
Simple triage and rapid transport (START) system, 143, 149
Sinoatrial (SA) node, 203f, 204
Sinus squeeze, 467, 469, 470
Situational (global) awareness, 109–110
Skids, during driving, 62
Skin
    of hypotensive patients, 194
    in shock, 236

Index

Skin cancer, 104
Skin temperature, in children, 423
Skull, bullets lodged in, 368f
Sleep/sleep patterns, 105–106, 106t
SLUDGE mnemonic, for cholinergic toxidromes, 312t
Smallpox, 163
    airborne precautions for, 169
    signs and symptoms of, 165–166
    transmission-based precautions for, 116
    transmission of, 164
Smallpox vaccine, 165
Smith-Cummins-Sherman Visual Development System, 58
Smoke inhalation, 155–156
Smoking, 101–102
    as cancer cause, 104
    as cardiovascular disease cause, 240, 246
Smoking cessation, 102, 103
Snake bites, 484–485
Sniffing position, 423
Snow, driving on, 60
Snuff, 102
SOAP(IER) format, for medical information organization, 41–42
Society for the Recovery of Drowned Persons, 9
Soman, 158
Spaite, Dan, 531–532
Spalling forces, 181, 182
Spanish-American War, 488
Specialty care centers, 34–37
Spider bites, 486
Spinal cord injuries, 377–381
    airway management in, 379
    electrical injury-related, 408
    immobilization in, 377–378, 565–566
        in children, 450–451
        in seizure patients, 281
    neck injury-associated, 385
    penetrating injuries, 391
    secondary, 380
    signs and symptoms of, 378
    spinal motion restriction (SMR) of, 377–378
Spinal cord injury without radiologic abnormality (SCIWORA), 380
Spinal motion restriction (SMR), 377–378
Spine board, rigid, 378
Spleen
    blunt injuries to, 391
    stab wounds to, 388

Splinting, 305, 565–568
    basic goal of, 565
    inflatable extremity, 567
    pain control effects of, 570
    of pelvic fractures, 395–396
    in the tactical environment, 494
    vacuum splints, 566
Spokespersons, for the media, 64
"Squeeze, release, release" technique, in mechanical ventilation, 230, 233, 418
Stabbings and stab wounds, 108, 367
    abdominal, 388
    as multiple casualty incidents, 156
    to the neck, 382
    spinal cord injury associated with, 378
    thoracic, 388
Standard of care, 47–48
    community-defined, 67
    definition of, 86
    duty to provide, 67
    medical director's responsibility for, 86
    violation of, 47
Standard precautions
    for bioterrorism agent exposures, 164
    for infectious diseases exposures, 115–116
Standing orders, 77, 79, 150
Staphylococcus aureus, methicillin-resistant, 116, 117
Star of Life emblem, 11
START (simple triage and rapid transport) system, 143, 149
Statistical charts, 94
Status epilepticus, 260, 279, 285, 433, 436, 437
Statute of limitations, for medical negligence cases, 47
Steam burns, 410
Steroids, as spinal cord injury treatment, 380
Stethoscopes, for pediatric respiratory assessment, 441
Stingray stings, 485
Stings
    coelenterate, 485
    cone shell, 485
    Hymenoptera, 486
    jellyfish, 485–486
    scorpion, 485
    venomous fish, 485
Stomach, penetrating injuries to, 391
Stool
    blood in, 293, 298
    color of, 293, 294

Stout, Jack, 20
Strategic National (Pharmaceutical) Stockpile, 167
Street drugs, 313
Stress, 102, 105. *See also* Critical incident stress
 as burnout cause, 124–125
 as cardiovascular disease cause, 246
 physiology of, 124
 positive aspects of, 123
 tolerance for, 122
Stress management, 105–106, 132
Stridor, 441–442
Stroke, 268–271
 as altered mental status cause, 264
 aortic dissection-related, 241
 as body temperature elevation cause, 284
 in children, 271
 cocaine use-related, 313
 as contraindication to glucose administration, 348
 definition of, 268
 determination of type of, 269
 diabetes-related, 341
 as headache cause, 267, 268
 hemorrhagic, 264, 268, 269, 274
 hypertension-related, 274
 ischemic, 264, 274
 neck injury-related, 385
 occlusive, 268, 269
 prehospital management of, 270–271
 as seizure cause, 280
 "7 Ds of Stroke Care," 269
"Stroke chain of survival," 271
Stun devices, electrical, 265, 365, 498–499
Styner, James, 13
Sublimaze, 571*t*
Submersion incidents, 461–464
Substance abuse, as delirium cause, 258
Succinylcholine, 408, 550, 551, 551*t*, 552
Sudden cardiac death, 239
 in custody, 498–499
 "dry" drowning-related, 461
 immersion syndrome-related, 463
 taser-related, 365
Suicide/suicidal patients, 309, 355–356, 357
Sulfa drugs, 488
Sulfuric acid burns, 404–405
Sulfur mustard, 158, 161
Supraglottic airway devices, 544–545
SWAT (Special Weapons and Tactics) teams, 488, 490, 491, 492, 495, 496*f*

Symbols, use in documentation, 43*t*
Sympathomimetic toxidrome, 312*t*, 313
Syncope
 pulmonary embolism-related, 241
 vasovagal, differentiated from seizures, 280
System status management, 20

T

Tabun, 158
Tachycardia, 210
 atrial multifocal, 219*f*
 atrioventricular node reentry, 218*f*
 in children, 418, 423
 differential diagnosis of, 194
 management of, 212–213
 narrow complex
  definition of, 218
  irregular, 219
  regular, 213, 218
  stable, 219
 pulmonary embolism-related, 241
 supraventricular, 219
  with aberrancy, 221–222
  in children, 418
  paroxysmal, 332
 tension pneumothorax-related, 561
 ventricular
  as cardiac arrest cause, 222
  differentiated from supraventricular rhythms, 214–215, 221–222
  monomorphic, 225
  pulseless, 210
  with visible P waves, 221*f*
  wide complex, 213–214, 221, 222
Tachypnea
 differential diagnosis of, 195
 pediatric respiratory distress-related, 441
 shock-related, 452
Tactical emergency medical support (TEMS), 488–502
 decision making in, 499–500
 definition of, 488
 development of, 488–489
 forensic topics in, 497
 future of, 500–501
 medical equipment packs for, 495–497, 496*f*
 patients in, 491
 phases of care in, 493–494
 types of mission in, 491–492

Index

Tactical field care, 493, 494
Tamponade, cardiac
  Beck's triad of, 561
  as life-threatening condition, 386
  treatment for, 387
Tarantulas, 486
Target organ damage (TOD), hypertension-associated, 273–274
Tasers, 265, 365, 498–499
Technical rescues, 508–512, 510f
Teeth, avulsed or subluxed, 568
Tegretol, interaction with adenosine, 220
Telemetry, 32
Telephone systems, disruption during disasters, 150
"Ten Commandments of Biological Defense," 168–171
Terminally ill patients
  hospice patients, 69
  withholding of life-sustaining treatment from, 68
Terrorism, 108, 146
  biological, 163–173, 168–171
  chemical, 158–162
  exposure, 180–185
  nuclear/radiological, 174–179
  as small-scale multiple casualty incidents, 152
Tertiary care centers, radiation exposure treatment at, 178
Testicular torsion, as abdominal pain cause, 289
Tetany, 408
Thermal burns, 402–413
  classification of, 410
  dressings for, 403
  estimation of size of, 405–406, 406f
  evaluation of, 405–407, 406f
  first-degree, 402
  fourth-degree, 402, 403f
  home remedies for, 411
  pain management of, 411
  second-degree, 402
  third-degree, 402
    circumferential, of limbs or chest, 407, 408f
  treatment of, 410, 411
  zone of coagulation in, 402
  zone of hyperemia in, 402–403
  zone of stasis in, 403
Thermoregulation, 283
Thiamine, 348
Thoracic trauma. *See* Chest, traumatic injuries to
Thoracotomy, "slash," 388
Threshold braking, 61

Thrombolytic therapy, 243–244, 254, 255t, 270
Thrombosis
  deep venous, 306
  implication for intravenous access, 537
Tibia, as intraosseous infusion site, 419, 419f
Tick bites, 486
Tick paralysis, 486
TICLS mnemonic, of Pediatric Assessment Triangle (PAT), 422–423, 439–440
Tobacco products. *See also* Smoking
  smokeless, 102
Tobacco smoke, passive exposure to, 101–102
Tobacco use. *See also* Smoking
  as cardiovascular disease risk factor, 240, 246
Tongue
  as airway obstruction cause, 439, 543
  seizure-related biting of, 260, 261
Toothache, as barodentalgia, 467, 470, 471
Toradol, 571t
Tornadoes, 146
Torsades de pointes, 222, 225, 225f
Total body surface area (TBSA), of burns, 405–406, 410, 411
Total cholesterol, 102, 103t
Tourniquets, 492, 493f, 494, 495
Towels, as stabilizing devices, 56
Toxidromes, 312–313, 312t
Traffic law violations, by emergency vehicles, 57
Train crashes, 146
Training
  of aeromedical transport crew members, 518–519
  of ambulance personnel, 6, 9
  of dispatchers, 77
  of emergency medical services technicians
    development of, 8–9
    in emergency vehicle operation, 56–57, 63
    in multiple casualty incident management, 152–153
    in on-line medical direction, 81
    in pediatric care, 427
    standardized curriculum for, 85
    in ultrasound, 575
    in wilderness emergency medical technology, 473–474, 478
  of paramedics, 11, 12, 76, 77
  of tactical medics, 500
Transfers, of patients, Emergency Medical Treatment and Active Labor Act (EMTALA) regulations regarding, 52–54

Index

Transient ischemic attacks (TIAs), 268
Transmission-based precautions, for infectious diseases prevention, 116–117
Transport. *See also* Transport destinations
　of abdominal pain patients, 290
　of abdominal trauma patients, 392
　of children, parental refusal of, 420–421
　coordination of, 140
　effect of triage on, 149
　of hyperthermic patients, 317
　policies for, 77
　of pregnant patients, 331
　of seizure patients, 281
　of shock patients, 237
　of trauma patients, 150, 368–370
　ultrasound performance prior to, 575
Transportation, fatality rate associated with, 101
Transportation officers, 150–151
Transport destinations
　for amputation patients, 36
　for cardiac arrest patients, 37–38
　choice of, 34
　determination of, 31
　during disasters, 150–151
　for emergent medical patients, 37
　for mass casualty incident patients, 36, 157
　physicians' alteration of, 38
　for trauma patients, 368–370
Trauma. *See also* Fractures
　abdominal, 390–393
　blunt trauma
　　abdominal, 390, 391
　　blast-related, 180, 184
　　definition of, 368
　　to the neck, 382
　　spinal, 378
　as cardiac arrest cause, 232
　in children, 450–455
　　child abuse-related, 397–398, 456–457
　definition of, 367
　elder abuse-related, 400
　to extremities, 304–308
　at fire scenes, 156
　general principles of, 367–372
　head trauma, 373–376
　　minor, 375–376
　　physical examination in, 262–263
　　as seizure cause, 430*t*
　identification and classification of, 93

　on-scene interventions in, 370–371
　partner violence-related, 399–400
　"path of injury" of, 304–305
　pelvic, 394–395
　penetrating trauma, 367–368
　　blast-related, 180, 184
　　definition of, 367
　　to the neck 378, 382
　　as pediatric mortality cause, 450
　as pneumothorax cause, 241
　radiologic attack/disaster-related, 176–177
　seizure-related, 433–434, 435
　serious, indicators of, 34–35
　spinal cord injuries, 377–381
　thoracic, 386–389
　triage of, 142–143
Trauma centers
　emergent transport to, 34–35
　Level I, 35, 368–369
　Level II, 35, 368–369
　Level III, 35, 369
　Level IV, 35
　patient transport to, 150
　pediatric, 36
　with pediatric commitment, 36
　radiation exposure treatment at, 178
Trauma patients, 12, 13
　airway obstruction in, 544
　intravenous access in, 537
　mortality causes in, 13
　prehospital assessment of, 200
　specialty care for, 34
Trauma Score-Injury Severity Score (TRISS), 93
Treat and release strategies, 187–188
Treatment protocols, 77, 84–85
　conflict with, 87–88
　during disasters, 150
　national medical guidelines for, 85–86
　standard of care of, 86
Treitz, Wenzel, 293
Tremors
　delirium-related, 260
　liver disease-related, 262
Trench rescues, 511
Trends charts, 94
Triage
　of burn patients, 405
　categories of, 142–143, 149, 154
　definition of, 148, 154

617

Index

Triage (continued)
  in disasters, 69
  factors affecting, 370
  guidelines for, 370
  importance of, 149
  in incident management, 140
  in mass casualty incidents, 69, 142–143, 144
  systems of, 149, 154
    JumpSTART system, 149
    MASS system, 149
    Sacco Triage Method, 149
    SALT system, 149
    simple triage and rapid transport (START) system, 143, 149
Triage tags, 149
Tricyclic antidepressants
  overdose of, 310–311
  as wide complex tachycardia cause, 222
Triglycerides, 102, 103t
Tripoding, 423
Tuberculosis, 114–115
  airborne precautions for, 116
  drug-resistant, 118
  signs and symptoms of, 117
  transmission of, 118
Tularemia, 114, 163, 486
  protection against, 165
  signs and symptoms of, 166–167
Tumors, as body temperature elevation cause, 284
"Tunnel vision," 109
Tylenol #3, 262
Tylox, 262
Tympanic membrane
  rupture of, 183, 468–469, 481, 482
  temperature of, 283
Tyramine, as hypertension cause, 273

U

Ulcers
  decubitus, 566, 568
  duodenal, 287, 288
  gastric, 287, 288
  peptic, 294
Ultrasound, in the prehospital environment, 574–581
  effectiveness of, 574–575
  training in, 575
Unified incident command, at mass casualty incidents, 153, 156

U.S. Air Force, 476
U.S. Army Medical Research Institute of Infectious Diseases, 170–171
U.S. Coast Guard, 476
U.S. Department of Health, Education, and Welfare, 12
U.S. Department of Health and Human Services, National Disaster Management System (NDMS) of, 476
U.S. Department of Transportation, 10, 11, 473
  KKK 1822 standards of, 8
U.S. Food and Drug Administration, 8
U.S. Navy SEALS, 493, 500
Unit hour utilization, 20
Universal precautions, in nuclear attacks/exposure, 177
Universal respiratory etiquette, 117
University of Toronto, 341
Unpredictability, in the prehospital environment, 23, 24, 25
Urban areas
  emergency vehicle operation in, 60
  trauma centers in, 36
Urban emergency medical technicians, 473
Uremia, as altered mental status cause, 262
Urticaria, acute (hives), 336, 338–339

V

Vaginal bleeding, in pregnant patients, 330
Valium. See Diazepam
Values, of emergency medical services providers, 69
Vancomycin-resistant Enterococcus (VRE), 116
Variola major. See Smallpox
Vasopressin, 223, 231
Vecuronium, 550, 551, 551t
Veins, occlusion of, 306
Venezuelan equine encephalitis, 169
VENTIDC mnemonic, for central nervous system oxygen toxicity, 469
Ventilation, 543
Ventricular dysrhythmias. See also Tachycardia, ventricular
  butyrophenones-related, 365
Ventricular fibrillation, 210, 210f, 228, 246
  in hypothermic patients, 318
  survival rate in, 230
  treatment for, 228–230, 229f
Verapamil, 221
Verapamil, as tachycardia treatment, 221
Verbal control, of violent patients, 111
Verbal de-escalation, of violence, 363, 364

Index

Versed. *See* Midazolam
Vesicants, 158
Vests, labeled, 138–139, 139f
Viagra, 248
Vicodin, 262
Victims
    categories of, 122–123
    primary, 122
    secondary, 122
    tertiary, 123
Videotaping, of interviews with the media, 66
Vietnam War, 7, 488, 492–493, 494, 515, 557
Violence. *See also* Gunshot wounds; Stabbings and stab wounds; Tactical emergency medical services; Violent patients
    as multiple casualty incident cause, 156
    prediction of, 353
    risk factors for, 361
    signs of impending, 362
Violent behavior, warning signs of, 110–111
Violent patients
    management of, 361–366
    physical restraint of, 69
    psychotic, 352–353
    restraint of, 111
Viral hemorrhagic fever (VHF), 163
    contact precautions for, 169
    protection against, 165
    signs and symptoms of, 167
    South American, 167
    transmission of, 114, 164
Vision
    components of, 57
    focal, 57–58
    implication for emergency vehicle operation, 57–58, 60
    improvement of, 58
    peripheral, 57, 58
Visual acuity, 57
Visual analogue pain scores, 424, 569–570
Vital signs, 193–197
    in acute coronary syndrome patients, 249
    in asthmatics, 301
    in children, 417, 452–453, 453f
    definition of, 193
    in delirious patients, 260
    factors affecting, 193–194
    in febrile patients, 284
    "fifth," 196, 289
    orthostatic, 195
    as patient assessment component, 200
    in psychiatric patients, 258
    in vomiting patients, 297
Volcanic eruptions, 146
Vomacka, Rick, 13–14
Vomiting, 297–299
    altitude sickness-related, 326
    blast injury-related, 184
    of blood (hematemesis), 293, 298
    in children, 298, 436
    of "coffee grounds," 293, 298
    complications of, 297
    in elderly patients, 298
    during intubation, 546
    as mass casualty incident, 156
    middle ear barotrauma-related, 468–469
    in pediatric seizure patients, 436
    radiation exposure-related, 178
von Mering, Joseph, 341
VRE (vancomycin-resistant *Enterococcus*), 116
VX, 158, 159

W

"Walking wounded," 143, 154
Warfarin, 313
Warm zones, 405, 504
Warning process, for emergency vehicles, 62
Warrants, high-risk 491–492
Wasp stings, 486
Water emergencies, 461–464
    drowning
        in children, 450
        definition of, 461
        "dry," 461–462
        in saltwater *versus* freshwater, 462
    drowning persons, rescue of, 463–464
    dysbarisms, 465–472
Water rescues, 511
Weapons
    less lethal, 498
    searches for, 111
Weapons of mass destruction (WMDs), 500–501
    biological, 163–173
    chemical, 158–162
    explosives, 180–185
    radiologic/nuclear, 174–179
Weight estimation
    in infants, 193

Index

Weight estimation of
   in children, 454
Weight transfer, 59
Wellness, personal. *See* Personal safety and wellness
Wheezing
   anaphylaxis-related, 338
   asthma-related, 447
   in children, 442, 452
   differentiated from stridor, 442
   diffuse, 300
Whooping cough (pertussis)
   airborne precautions for, 116
   signs and symptoms of, 117
Wilderness emergency medical services, 473–478
Wilderness Emergency Medical Services Institute (WEMSI), 473, 478
Wilderness emergency medical technicians (WEMTs), 473–474, 478
Wilderness Medical Society, 473, 478
Wilderness medicine, definition of, 473
Wilderness Medicine Institute, National Outdoor Leadership School of, 478
Wilderness rescue, preparation for, 475
Wilderness rescue teams, standards for, 474
Wildfires, 142
Williams, Greer, 9

Windshield washer fluid, toxicity of, 310
Winter storms, 146
WISER database, 504
Withdrawal, 313–314, 352
   in neonates, 426
Withdrawal syndromes, 352
Wolff-Parkinson-White syndrome, 218, 218*f*
Women, intimate partner violence toward, 398–400
Wong-Baker FACES scale, 420*f*, 424, 569–570
World War I, 7
World War II, 515

X
X-rays, chest, 300

Y
Yellow fever, 488
Yosemite National Park, 475, 476

Z
Zero response time, 29
Zofran™, 572
Zone of coagulation, 402
Zone of hyperemia, 402–403
Zone of stasis, 403
Zoonoses, 114